# चरक संहिता सूत्रस्थान

## ENGLISH TRANSLATION

डा. जनार्धन वि हेब्बार

Made with ❤ on the Notion Press Platform
www.notionpress.com

|| Jai Guruji ||

I, Dr. Janardhana V. Hebbar, dedicate this book at the holy feet of Sri Guruji – Swami Vivekananda and my spiritual Guru, Dr. A. Chandrashekhara Udupa MBBS, FAGE, Managing Director, Divine Park Trust (R), Saligrama, Udupi. (www.divinepark.org)

*He guides, He energizes, He shows the path,*
*He holds my hand and makes me walk!*

# क्रम-सूची

# भूमिका

This book covers the 30 chapters of Sutrasthana of Charaka Samhita.

Charaka Samhita is a popular Ayurvedic treatise. As the name indicates, it is a compilation of Ayurveda lessons comprising various aspects including basic concepts (Sutra sthana), diagnosis of diseases (Nidana sthana), treatment concepts (Chikitsa sthana) etc. and is written by Charaka. (Charaka Samhita means 'treatise written by Charaka').

Acharya Charaka redacted the treatise 'Agnivesha Tantra' which has become popular in the name of 'Charaka Samhita'. This means the text 'Agnivesha Tantra' written by Agnivesha was re-modulated by Charaka, which later came to be called 'Charaka Samhita'.

Charaka Samhita is the first and foremost authentic treatise of Ayurveda and is one of the 'greatest trio' (Brihat-Trayee).

Master Charaka was so keen to help people with Ayurveda that he used to roam from one place to the other continuously. Hence he got the name Charaka.

Charati iti Charakaha – One who moves continuously.

## Charaka Samhita

Charaka Samhita, a part of Brihat Trayi or greater trio of Ayurveda occupies a significant place in the history of world's medical science.

Atreya Punarvasu has many intelligent students. Punarvasu was the most respected, learned Guru (teacher) and preacher of Ayurveda. Among the clan of his elite students Agnivesha was the best.

According to the directions and teachings of his teacher Punarvasu Atreya, Agnivesha recorded, documented and composed his work on Ayurveda.

It was called Agnivesha Tantra. It was subsequently redacted by Charaka which in due course of time got popular in the name 'Charaka Samhita'. This Charaka Samhita was further redacted by Dridhabala.

In Charaka Samhita, we can find that justice has been done in covering all the aspects and 8 branches of Ayurveda. But the emphasis has been given in covering the concepts of Kaya Chikitsa (General medicine) in detail. That is why, Charaka Samhita is considered to be the best reference and authentic text of Kaya Chikitsa.

More than 40 commentaries are written on Charaka Samhita. It is translated into all the Indian languages. It is also translated into many foreign languages including Persian, Simhali, Nepali, Arabic etc.

## Sections and Chapters of Charaka Samhita:

Charaka Samhita has been dealt with in 8 sections and 120 chapters.

Sutrasthana – Basic Principles – 30 chapters, 1952 Verses.

Nidana Sthana – Pathology – 8 chapters, 247 verses

Vimana Sthana – Specific determination – 8 chapters, 354 verses

Shareera Sthana – Anatomy – 8 chapters , 382 verses

Indriya Sthana – Sensory organ based prognosis – 12 chapters, 378 verses

Chikitsa Sthana – Therapeutics – 30 chapters, 4904 verses

Kalpasthana – Pharmaceutics and toxicology – 12 chapters – 378 verses

Siddhi Sthana – Success in treatment – 12 chapters – 700 verses

Total – 9295 verses (Sutras)

## Sutra sthana

Deals with fundamental principles of Ayurveda covered in 30 chapters
Sutra Sthana is subdivided into Sapta Chatushkas (7 quadrates), having 4 chapters each.

**They are:**
Bheshaja Chatushka – quadrate on drugs
Swasta Chatushka – quadrate on regimen for the maintenance of health
Nirdesha Chatushka – quadrate on various instructions
Kalpana Chatushka – quadrate on description of therapeutic procedures
Roga Chatushka – quadrate on description of diseases
Yojana Chatushka – quadrate on administration of various therapies
Annapana Chatushka – quadrate on description of diet and drinks
Sangraha adhyaya – 2 chapters at the end of Sutra Sthana are known by the name Sangraha Adhyaya, the concluding chapters

**Vimana Sthana**
Deals with the principles governing the bodily factors that cause diseases – drugs and medicaments covered in 8 chapters
a. In the Rasa Vimana chapter, sweet, sour etc. tastes, qualities, functions, effect on Dosha, oils, ghee, honey etc., their effect on health and asta vidha vishesha Ayatana are explained.

b. In Trividha Kuksheeya Vimana, GI tract, quantity of food to be taken, what happens if the food is taken excessively or in low quantities, Visuchika, Alasaka etc. digestive tract disorders are mentioned.

c. In Janapadodhvamsaneeya chapter – communicable disorders, endemic diseases, reasons, preventive measures are mentioned.

d. In Trividha Roga VIshesha Vijnaneeya chapter, Pratyaksha – direct observation, Anumana, Aptaopadesha – means of knowledge, etc. are explained.

e. In Sroto Vimana chapter, all the body channels, causes, symptoms and treatment of vitiation of body channels are mentioned.

f. In Roganeeka Vimana – types of diseases – mental, physical, types of Agni, Prakriti – body types etc. are mentioned.

g. In Vyadhita Rupeeya Vimana – Guru, Laghu etc. patient features, Krumi causes and treatment are mentioned.

h. In the Roga Bhishag Jiteeya chapter, causes for diseases, sambhasha – discussion, 10 types of patient examination etc. are explained.

**Nidana Sthana**
Deals with aetiology, pathogenesis and diagnosis of diseases covered in 8 chapters.
For each disease, causative factors, prodromal symptoms, signs and symptoms, pathogenesis, prognosis are explained in detail.
Jwara, Rakthapitha, Gulma, Prameha, Kushta etc. diseases are explained in detail.

**Shareera Sthana**
Deals with embryology, anatomy and physiology covered in 8 chapters. This section gives detailed description

about Human Anatomy and its application in treatment, panchamahabhutha (Basic 5 elements of earth), conception, embryology, signs of pregnancy, monthwise fetal development, manas prakruti (constitution of mind), determination of prakruti in the fetus, procedure of labour, diseases of children, bala samskara (Agewise ceremony), child nutrition and treatment of child disease.

### Indriya Sthana

Deals with prognostic signs and symptoms covered in 12 chapters

In this section signs and symptoms of bad prognosis, inauspicious symptoms pertaining to skin complexion, voice, odour, taste, touch, sight, sound, mind, tongue, nose, fire, hygiene, behavioural activities, memory, tolerance capacity of patient, strength, structure of body, dryness, unctuousness, heaviness, digestion of food etc.

Importance of inauspicious symptoms in the origin of disease, pain, advice, shadow, dreams, to see inauspicious signs on the road, auspicious and inauspicious signs related to sense organs and its perceived senses, curable and incurable signs of disease and patients life span are mentioned.

### Chikitsa Sthana

Deals with treatment of various diseases covered in 30 chapters

This section explains in detail under Rasayana chapters – Rasayana medicines, intake procedure of rasayana, types of rasayana, rasayana properties of hareethaki and amalaki, procedure of its preparation, intake and its doses. It also deals with acharya rasayana.

Vachikarana chapters deal with – causes, types and treatment of infertility, use of vajikaran medicines, its method of preparation and intake.

Causes, signs and symptoms, types and treatment of various diseases beginning from jwara, rakthapitha, gulma, prameha, doshagatha diseases, mental disorders, alcoholism,poisoning etc. are mentioned here.

### Kalpa Sthana

Deals with formulations for vamana (emesis), virechana (purgation) etc. covered in 12 chapters.

This section deals with various medicinal formulations of madanaphala, jeemuthaka, dhamargava, krethavedhana, trivruth, aaragvadha, bilva, sapthala, danthi, dravathi etc., its origin, collection, types and properties are also mentioned here.

### Siddhi Sthana

Deals with principles governing the administration of elimination therapies covered in 12 chapters

This section explains in detail – procedure of administration of elimination therapies( panchakarma), its indication and contraindications, complications developed due to improper administration of elimination therapy and its treatment. It also explains signs and symptoms produced due to excess, improper and proper administration of elimination therapy.

The three stages of Panchakarma – preliminary therapy (purvakarma), main therapy (pradhanakarma), post therapy procedures (paschathkarma) are explained in an order.

Persons indicated and contraindicated for elimination therapy and purificatory procedure for contraindicated persons are also explained here.

### Salient features of Charaka Samhita –

The titles of some chapters are based on the first word occurring in the chapter and others are based on the subject matter discussed in that particular chapter

4 types of Sutras are found in Charaka Samhita such as:
Guru Sutra – statements made by the teacher
Shishya Sutra – statements / enquiries made by the disciple
Pratisamskarta Sutra – Statement of the redactor
Ekiya Sutra – statements made by individual scholars

Subject matter of each chapter is described as Uddeshya (brief statement and intention of chapter) followed by Nirdesha (detailed expansion of the above statement) and Lakshana (definition)
The colophons give the information of the author's name, name of redactor, title of the section and chapter and also the serial number of the chapter
The explanation of topics like Swabhavoparama vada highlights the influence of Buddhism on Charaka Samhita

Scientific explanation of the Ayurvedic fundamental principles like Tridoshas, Pancha Mahabhutas and Rasa Panchakas etc. can be seen
Importance of Roga and Rogi Pareeksha (examination of disease and the diseased) has been emphasised
At the end of each chapter, the complete contents of the chapter are enlisted

**Commentaries**
More than 40 Sanskrit Commentaries were written on Charaka Samhita. Out of them the following are available partly or in full form.

Charakanyasa – By Bhattara Harishchandra in 4th century AD
Charaka Panjika – By Swami Kumara after 4th century AD
Nirantarapada Vyakhya – By Jejjata in 6th century AD
Ayurveda Deepika – By Chakrapani in 11th century AD
Tatwa Chandrika – By Shivadas Sen in 15th century AD
Jalpakalpataru – By Gangadhar Sen in 19th century AD
Charakopaskara – By Yogendranath Sen in 20th century AD
Charaka Pradipika – By Jyotishchandra Saraswati in 20th century AD

**Charaka, the highly valued**
Since 4th century A.D. onwards great scholars of Ayurveda, authors, scientists, commentators etc. gave utmost respect to the sage 'Charaka'.
Famous commentators like Bhattara Harischandra, Swami Kumara, Yogendranatha Sen etc., paid their tributes to Acharya Charaka by naming their works as Charakanyasa, Charaka Panjika and Charakopaskara respectively. There are as many as 43 Sanskrit commentaries on this work.
In the beginning of 8th century AD Charaka Samhita was translated into Arabic language.
According to the Colophon, Agnivesha, on the advice of his preceptor Punarvasu Atreya, composed this work which was subsequently redacted by Charaka and Dridhabala

**Charaka's Club** – It is a medical organisation which was established in New York in November 1898. It was founded by a group of 4 doctors named Charles. L. Dana, Joseph Colliers, Fredrick Peterson and Barnad Sachs. This club discussed a wide array of subjects involving fields like medical, medical history, literature, poetry etc.
- Dr Raghuram YS BAMS MD (Ayu)

# पावती (स्वीकृति)

Special thanks to Dr Raghuram YS for painstakingly editing the entire book.
Special thanks to my family members who have been supporting me unconditionally throughout this journey of Easy Ayurveda. Thank you for tolerating all the pains.
Smt. Padmakshamma (mother), Karthyayini (wife and staff), Smt. Vanamala (mother-in-law).
Daughters – Sadhvi & Chinmayi

Sister Sharada, brother-in-law Mr ShashiKumar, Tushar, Ms Sharada.
All my staff who make Easy Ayurveda possible, everyday.
Dr Sudarshan CH, Dr Shilpa Ramdas, Dr Renita D'Souza,
Mr Sachidananda Bhat, Smt. Nayana, Mr Nikhil and Smt. Sumangala.
My mentors - Dr MB Gururaja, Dr MS Krishnamurthy and Dr Prashanth BK

आमुख

**Many Academic Firsts from Charaka Samhita**
Charaka Sutra Sthana Chapter 1
First ever medical conference – The meeting of the sages in the Himalayas could be the first ever conference held for a medical purpose, ever known to mankind.
First representative for a medical cause – Sage Bharadwaja could well be the first ever representative selected to gather knowledge related to a medical cause from a higher authority.

First ever celestial medical guide who taught an earthly being – Lord Indra would well be the first ever celestial medical guide after having taught Ayurveda to an earthly being, sage Bharadwaja.
First ever instance of inter-terrain knowledge transfer in medical science – Sage Bharadwaja bringing the knowledge of Ayurveda from heaven to the earth could have marked the first event of inter-terrain knowledge transfer in medical science wherein Ayurveda came down from the celestial world to the mortal world for the benefit of mankind.

First lessons of Ayurveda on Earth – Sage Bharadwaja teaching Ayurveda to his students and other sages were probably the first lessons of Ayurveda on earth.
First ever medical dictation – Sage Atreya's teachings to his disciples including Agnivesha could be the first ever instance of dictation of notes related to a medical science, though not with that intention. Agnivesha and other students documenting the teachings gave the purpose and shape to Atreya's dictation.

First documentation of Ayurveda in a written form – Agnivesha, student of master Atreya could have been the first ever student on Earth to record and document the medical knowledge (of Ayurveda) in a written form.

First six books of an Ayurvedic library and first medical books to be written in author's name – Below mentioned are the first six books of an Ayurvedic library, any medical science in fact. These are also the first medical treatises which were written and published in the author's name. This reflected the trust the teachers had on their students and the liberty and loyalty given to the students to publish their works in their name. This also reflected the goodness, selflessness and humbleness of the Ayurvedic teachers.

Agnivesha Tantra (which became Charaka Samhita in future) – by master Agnivesha
Bhela Samhita – by master Bhela / Bheda
Jatukarna Samhita – by master Jatukarna
Parashara Samhita – by master Parashara
Harita Samhita – by master Harita
Ksharapani Samhita – by master Ksharapani

First ever submission of completed medical works and first ever approval of the same – Agnivesha and his five friends submitting the completed works of Ayurveda documented and edited by them to their master Atreya Punarvasu and other teachers was probably the first evidence of completed medical works being submitted to their teacher. The acknowledgment of master Atreya and other sages could have been the first ever approval of medical works.

First ever convocation and graduation – The appraisal given to Agnivesha and his friends by master Atreya, the great sages, Gods and divine sages was the first ever celebration of completed works in medical science, the first evidence of convocation and graduation.

First ever 'standardised and approved medical reference books' – In Charaka Samhita it is given that the Gods and sages, including master Atreya gave approval to the treatises written by their students Agnivesha and others. This marks the declaration of the first standard and approved 'medical reference books' which are authenticated references even till today and would be even in future.

First ever redactions of an already published medical book – Charaka Samhita was the first redaction of a standard reference book which had already been published in Ayurveda. Master Charaka takes the credit for re editing and redacting Agnivesha Tantra and shaping it into Charaka Samhita. Master Dridhabala takes the credit of re-redaction and for adding the lost chapters of Charaka Samhita in later years.

First ever 'point of reference' and due credits given to the main author / authors in a medical treatise – Charaka Samhita would be the first treatise in which the point of reference and due credits are given to the main author at the end of each chapter, apart from the treatise bearing the name of the author. At the end of each chapter of Charaka Samhita we can find the phrase 'Thus ends the chapter originally written by the main author Agnivesha and redacted by master Charaka'.

 - Dr Raghuram YS BAMS MD(Ayu)

# 1

# Sutrasthana Chapter 1 Deergham Jeevityeeyam

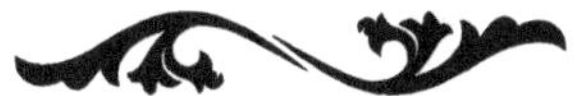

अथातो दीर्घञ्जीवितीयमध्यायं व्याख्यास्यामः||१||

इति ह स्माह भगवानात्रेयः||२||

We shall now expound the Chapter on "The Quest for Longevity." Thus said Lord Atreya [ 1-2]

दीर्घं जीवितमन्विच्छन्भरद्वाज उपागमत्|

इन्द्रमुग्रतपा बुद्ध्वा शरण्यममरेश्वरम्||३||

ब्रह्मणा हि यथाप्रोक्तमायुर्वेदं प्रजापतिः|

जग्राह निखिलेनादावश्विनौ तु पुनस्ततः||४||

अश्विभ्यां भगवाञ्छक्रः प्रतिपेदे ह केवलम्|

ऋषिप्रोक्तो भरद्वाजस्तस्माच्छक्रमुपागमत्||५||

**Origin of Ayurveda:**

Lord Brahma recollected the knowledge of Ayurveda and passed it on to Daksha Prajapati. From him, the sacred knowledge of Ayurveda was passed on to Ashwini Kumaras (Ashwini twins who are considered as doctors for Devatas (divine souls). From them, Lord Indra learnt Ayurveda.

Saint Bharadwaja, being desirous of long life, having known about Indra, approached Indra and learnt about Ayurveda. [3-5]

**Chain and sequence of transfer of Ayurveda Knowledge from Lord Brahma to Sage Bharadwaja**

Lord Brahma (recollects the knowledge of Ayurveda) passes the knowledge of Ayurveda to

↓

Daksha Prajapati

↓

Ashwini twins (divine physicians, doctors for Gods and Goddesses)

↓

Lord Indra

↓

Sage Bharadwaja

↓

To his disciples

**Purpose of sages desiring longevity**

विघ्नभूता यदा रोगाः प्रादुर्भूताः शरीरिणाम्|

तपोपवासाध्ययनब्रह्मचर्यव्रतायुषाम् ||६||
तदा भूतेष्वनुक्रोशं पुरस्कृत्य महर्षयः|
समेताः पुण्यकर्माणः पार्श्वे हिमवतः शुभे ||७||
अङ्गिरा जमदग्निश्च वसिष्ठः कश्यपो भृगुः|
आत्रेयो गौतमः साङ्ख्यः पुलस्त्यो नारदोऽसितः||८||
अगस्त्यो वामदेवश्च मार्कण्डेयाश्वलायनौ|
पारिक्षिर्भिक्षुरात्रेयो भरद्वाजः कपिञ्ज(ष्ठ)लः||९||
विश्वामित्राश्मरथ्यौ च भार्गवश्च्यवनोऽभिजित्|
गार्ग्यः शाण्डिल्यकौण्डिल्यौ(न्यौ)वार्क्षिर्देवलगालवौ||१०||
साङ्कृत्यो बैजवापिश्च कुशिको बादरायणः|
बडिशः शरलोमा च काप्यकात्यायनावुभौ||११||
काङ्कायनः कैकशेयो धौम्यो मारीचकाश्यपौ|
शर्कराक्षो हिरण्याक्षो लोकाक्षः पैङ्गिरेव च||१२||
शौनकः शाकुनेयश्च मैत्रेयो मैमतायनिः|
वैखानसा वालखिल्यास्तथा चान्ये महर्षयः||१३||
ब्रह्मज्ञानस्य निधयो द(य)मस्य नियमस्य च|
तपसस्तेजसा दीप्ता हूयमाना इवाग्नयः||१४||

## Purpose of sages desiring longevity

In ancient times, sages were desirous of having long life so that

- they can perform religious practices, Brahmacharya, sacred studies, Upavasa (fasting), Yama and Niyama (rules of auspicious living), Homa etc spiritual activities
- they (sages also wanted to) can help the people to get their diseases relieved

The above said purposes also became the agenda for the sages to have a meeting in the Himalayas. Meeting of the sages in Himalayas to address the key points of their agenda and the names of those sages. All the Sages sat together for a meeting in the Himalayas. Those sages included Angeerasa, Jamadagni, Vasistha, Kashyapa, Bhrugu, Atreya, Gautama, Sankhya, Pulastya, Naarada, Asita, Agastya, Vamadeva, Markandeya, Ashvalayana, Parikshi, Bhiksu, Atreya, Bharadvaja, Kapinjala, Vishvamitra, Ashmarathya, Bhargava, Chyavana (after whom Chyavanprash is named), Abhijit, Gargya (one of the rare lady Sages), Shandilya, Kaundilya, Varkshi, Devala, Galava, Sankrutya, Baijavapi, Kushika, Badarayana, Badisha, Saraloman, Kapya, Katyayana, Kankayana (after whom Kankayana vati tablet is named), Kaikasheya, Dhaumya, Maricha, Kashyapa, Sharkaraksha, Hiranyaksha, Lokaksha, Paingi, Shaunaka Shakuneya, Maitreyi (another rare lady sage), Maimatayani, Vaikhanasas and Valakhilyas. [ 6 – 14]

## Ayurveda - Chaturvidha Purushartha

धर्मार्थकाम मोक्षाणामारोग्यं मूलमुत्तमम्||१५||
रोगास्तस्यापहर्तारः श्रेयसो जीवितस्य च|
प्रादुर्भूतो मनुष्याणामन्तरायो महानयम्||१६||
कः स्यातेषां शमोपाय इत्युक्त्वा ध्यानमास्थिताः|
अथ ते शरणं शक्रं ददृशुर्ध्यानचक्षुषा||१७||
स वक्ष्यति शमोपायं यथावदमरप्रभुः|१८|

During the conference, the sages learnt that it is only the knowledge and practice of Ayurveda that can save the lives of people and help them in gaining longevity in life.
Good health stands at the very root of
Dharma – righteousness, virtuous acts,

Artha – acquirement of wealth and prosperity,
Kama – fulfilling desires
Moksha – Renunciation

Diseases are destroyers of health, well being and life. They are the greatest obstacles towards the smooth progress of human life and life activities.
Sage Bharadwaja assigned to approach Lord Indra to procure the knowledge of Ayurveda.

So, what could be the remedy for these diseases? – Keeping this question in their mind and this important point in view, the sages entered into meditation. The sages through their divine and spiritual vision saw that (realised that) Lord Indra could be their saviour. They also were assured that Lord Indra, the Lord of Gods would explain to them the proper and comprehensive ways of counteracting the diseases troubling mankind. All the sages took a collective and unanimous decision and decided to send Sage Bharadwaja to Lord Indra to learn Ayurveda from Him. Accordingly, Sage Bharadwaja went to Indra's abode. There he saw Lord Indra, the destroyer of Bala, sitting amidst the gods and sages and was glittering like fire. [15-17]

**Sage Bharadwaja's Plea to Lord Indira**

कः सहस्राक्षभवनं गच्छेत् प्रष्टुं शचीपतिम्||१८||
अहमर्थे नियुज्येयमत्रेति प्रथमं वचः|
भरद्वाजोऽब्रवीतस्मादृषिभिः स नियोजितः||१९||
स शक्रभवनं गत्वा सुरर्षिगणमध्यगम् |
ददर्श बलहन्तारं दीप्यमानमिवानलम्||२०||
सोऽभिगम्य जयाशीर्भिरभिनन्द्य सुरेश्वरम्|
प्रोवाच विनयाद्धीमानृषीणां वाक्यमुत्तमम्||२१||
व्याधयो हि समुत्पन्नाः सर्वप्राणिभयङ्कराः|
तद्ब्रूहि मे शमोपायं यथावदमरप्रभो||२२||
तस्मै प्रोवाच भगवानायुर्वेदं शतक्रतुः|
पदैरल्पैरमितं बुद्ध्वा विपुलां परमर्षये||२३||

Bharadwaja pleaded and humbly submitted his request to Lord Indra and said – "Oh Lord! The diseases are terrifying all living beings and have manifested themselves. Kindly advise proper remedial measures for these diseases." Then, Lord Indra, considering Sage Bharadwaja's depth of wisdom, expounded Ayurveda i.e., the science of life to the sage in brief. [18 – 23]

Bharadwaja learnt Ayurveda and preached the noble science to this world. Sage Punarnava Atreya learnt Ayurveda from Sage Bharadwaja. Later Agnivesha etc sages learnt Ayurveda from Sage Atreya. Sage Agnivesha later wrote Agnivesha Tantra (which later became popular as Charaka Samhita treatise). Agnivesha Tantra was later refined and redacted by Master Charaka and Master Drudabala.

**Trisutra**

हेतुलिङ्गौषधज्ञानं स्वस्थातुरपरायणम्|
त्रिसूत्रं शाश्वतं पुण्यं बुबुधे यं पितामहः||२४||

**Three Principles of Ayurveda:**
Lord Indra expounded the immortal and sacred science of life (Ayurveda) consisting of three principles viz.,
Hetu – causative factors of disease
Linga – symptomatology
Aushadha Jnana – knowledge of therapeutics, treatments and medicines. [24]

Hetu, Linga and Aushadha are known as **Trisutra** – the three formulas of treating disease.

सोऽनन्तपारं त्रिस्कन्धमायुर्वेदं महामतिः।
यथावदचिरात् सर्वं बुबुधे तन्मना मुनिः॥२५॥
तेनायुरमितं लेभे भरद्वाजः सुखान्वितम्।
ऋषिभ्योऽनधिकं तच्च शशंसानवशेषयन्॥२६॥

Bharadwaja – the sage of great wisdom and devotion, enjoyed an infinitely long and happy life, and passed on his sacred knowledge of Ayurveda to other sages. [25 – 26]

ऋषयश्च भरद्वाजाज्जगृहुस्तं प्रजाहितम्।
दीर्घमायुश्चिकीर्षन्तो वेदं वर्धनमायुषः॥२७॥
महर्षयस्ते दृदृशुर्यथावज्ज्ञानचक्षुषा।
सामान्यं च विशेषं च गुणान् द्रव्याणि कर्म च॥२८॥
समवायं च तज्ज्ञात्वा तन्त्रोक्तं विधिमास्थिताः।
लेभिरे परमं शर्म जीवितं चाप्यनित्वरम्॥२९॥

### Six Padarthas (Shat Padartha)

These sages with their divine intuitive powers visualised the 6 padarthas i.e. materials:
Samanya (common),
Vishesha (specialty),
Guna (qualities),
Dravya (substance),
Karma (action),
Samavaya (inseparable).

These are the various categories of padarthas as enumerated in the Nyaya system of philosophy. After having known all this, the sages acted on the prescriptions as available in science and attained the highest levels of well-being and an inexhaustibly long life. [27 – 29]

### Sage Atreya Punarvasu and his disciples

अथ मैत्रीपरः पुण्यमायुर्वेदं पुनर्वसुः।
शिष्येभ्यो दत्तवान् षड्भ्यः सर्वभूतानुकम्पया॥३०॥
अग्निवेशश्च भेलश्च जतूकर्णः पराशरः।
हारीतः क्षारपाणिश्च जगृहुस्तन्मुनेर्वचः॥३१॥

Then Atreya Punarvasu, who by nature is friendly to all and also having compassion for all, taught Ayurveda to his six disciples – Agnivesha, Bhela, Jatukarna, Parashara, Harita and Ksharapani. [30 – 31]

### Presentation of works by Bhela etc.

बुद्धिविशेषस्तत्रासीन्नोपदेशान्तरं मुनेः।
तन्त्रस्य कर्ता प्रथममग्निवेशो यतोऽभवत्॥३२॥
अथ भेलादयश्चक्रुः स्वं स्वं तन्त्रं कृतानि च।
श्रावयामासुरात्रेयं सर्षिसङ्घं सुमेधसः॥३३॥
श्रुत्वा सूत्रणमर्थानामृषयः पुण्यकर्मणाम्।
यथावत्सूत्रितमिति प्रहृष्टास्तेऽनुमेनिरे॥३४॥
सर्व एवास्तुवंस्तांश्च सर्वभूतहितैषिणः।

साधु भूतेष्वनुक्रोश इत्युच्चैरब्रुवन् समम्॥३५॥
तं पुण्यं शुश्रुवुः शब्दं दिवि देवर्षयः स्थिताः।
सामराः परमर्षीणां श्रुत्वा मुमुदिरे परम्॥३६॥
अहो साध्विति निर्घोषो लोकांस्त्रीनन्ववा(ना)दयत्।
नभसि स्निग्धगम्भीरो हर्षादभूतैरुदीरितः॥३७॥
शिवो वायुर्ववौ सर्वा भाभिरुन्मीलिता दिशः।
निपेतुः सजलाश्चैव दिव्याः कुसुमवृष्टयः॥३८॥
अथाग्निवेशप्रमुखान् विविशुर्ज्ञानदेवताः।
बुद्धिः सिद्धिः स्मृतिर्मेधा धृतिः कीर्तिः क्षमा दया॥३९॥
तानि चानुमतान्येषां तन्त्राणि परमर्षिभिः।
भ(भा)वाय भूतसङ्घानां प्रतिष्ठां भुवि लेभिरे॥४०॥

**Presentation of works by Bhela etc. to their masters led by Atreya** - Then the wise ones like Bhela and others expounded their respective works and presented them to master Atreya who was accompanied by a group of sages. Having heard the exposition of the science by the holy ones i.e. disciples of Atreya, the sages were extremely delighted to find that the exposition was well done and they welcomed it. Admiring these disciples of Atreya Punarvasu who were desirous of doing good to all the creatures, all the sages exclaimed at a time in a loud voice "This sympathy by all of you towards living beings is simply brilliant!"

The divine sages accompanied by the Gods residing in heaven heard these sacred words of great sages and were extremely delighted to hear this. "Oh! Excellent," this deep and melodious sound produced in heaven by the delighted gods resounded in all the three worlds. The auspicious wind blew and all directions were illuminated by divine light. Divine showers of flowers and water dropped down and then the gods of wisdom viz. Intellect, Accomplishment, Memory, Understanding, Patience, Fame, Forbearance, and Pity entered Agnivesha and other disciples. These works of the disciples of Atreya accepted by the great sages were established on this earth for the good of all creatures. [32-40]

हिताहितं सुखं दुःखमायुस्तस्य हिताहितम्।
मानं च तच्च यत्रोक्तमायुर्वेदः स उच्यते॥४१॥

**Definition of Ayurveda:**

Ayurveda is the science of life which explains about good and bad things applicable for -

Hitayu – advantageous life

Ahita Ayu – disadvantageous life

Sukhayu – happy state of health and mind

Ahitayu – unhappy state of health and mind. It also explains what is good and bad for life and measurement of life [41]

शरीरेन्द्रियसत्वात्मसंयोगो धारि जीवितम्।
नित्यगश्चानुबन्धश्च पर्यायैरायुरुच्यते॥४२॥

**Definition of Ayu (life)** – The term 'Ayus' stands for the combination of the

Shareera – body,

Indriya – sense organs,

Satva – mind and

Atma – soul.

This means that when the body is intact with sense organs, mind and soul, then one has life, otherwise not.

Synonyms of ayu are

Dhari – the one that prevents the body from decay,

Jeevita – that which keeps one alive,

Nityaga – that which keeps the soul, mind and sense intact with the body all the time, without discontinuation

Anubandha – that which transmigrates from one body to another (after death). [42]

तस्यायुषः पुण्यतमो वेदो वेदविदां मतः|
वक्ष्यते यन्मनुष्याणां लोकयोरुभयोर्हितम्‌ ||४३||

Ayurveda is beneficial to mankind in terms of both the worlds i.e. this life and the life beyond. Such Ayurveda, which is the most sacred and also honoured by those proficient in the Vedas will now be expounded. [43]

**Samanya Vishesha Siddhanta - Theory of common and difference:**

सर्वदा सर्वभावानां सामान्यं वृद्धिकारणम्‌|
ह्रासहेतुर्विशेषश्च, प्रवृत्तिरुभयस्य तु||४४||
सामान्यमेकत्वकरं, विशेषस्तु पृथक्त्वकृत्‌|
तुल्यार्थता हि सामान्यं, विशेषस्तु विपर्ययः||४५||

Common features and characteristics lead to increase / growth. For example, Kapha dosha has oiliness and if we take oily food, Kapha dosha increases in the body.

Difference or specialties in characteristics lead to division and degeneration or depletion. [44 - 45]
For example: Dryness is opposite to Kapha Dosha. If we eat foods having dryness, it decreases the Kapha Dosha.

**Tridanda**

सत्त्वमात्मा शरीरं च त्रयमेतत्त्रिदण्डवत्‌|
लोकस्तिष्ठति संयोगात्तत्र सर्व प्रतिष्ठितम्‌||४६||
स पुमांश्चेतनं तच्च तच्चाधिकरणं स्मृतम्‌|
वेदस्यास्य, तदर्थं हि वेदोऽयं सम्प्रकाशितः||४७||

**Tridanda** – Satva (Mind), Atma (soul) and Shareera (body) – these three are Tripods of life. The world is sustained by their combination. They constitute the basis for everything. [46-47]

**Dravya – Basic matter:**

खादीन्यात्मा मनः कालो दिशश्च द्रव्यसङ्ग्रहः|
सेन्द्रियं चेतनं द्रव्यं, निरिन्द्रियमचेतनम्‌||४८||

**Five basic elements –**
Prithvi – earth
Ap – water,
Tejas – fire,
Vayu – air and
Akasha – ether
These five basic elements along with Atma (soul), Mana (mind), Kala (time) and Disha (direction) form nine kinds of basic matter.

**The substances are of two categories:**
1. Sa Indriya (Sendriya) – having sense organs and soul – living substances
2. Nirindryia Dravya – which do not have sense organs and soul – non living substances [48]

**Guna – qualities:**

सार्था गुर्वादयो बुद्धिः प्रयत्नान्ताः परादयः|
गुणाः प्रोक्ताः ...|४९|

The qualities are – 5 Sartha Gunas + 20 Guru adi gunas + Buddhi + 6 Prayatnanta Guna + 8 Paradi Gunas are the total qualities.

**5 Sartha Gunas - Objects of sense organs:**
Shabda (sound- perceived by ears),
Sparsha (touch - perceived by skin),
Roopa (shape - perceived by eyes),
Rasa (taste - perceived by tongue),
Gandha (smell - perceived by nose)

**20 Guru adi gunas:**
Guru (heavy) X laghu (light in weight)
Manda (slow) X tiksna (quick, fast)
Hima (cold) X ushna (hot)
Snigdha (unctuous) X ruksa (dry)
Slaksna (smooth) X khara (rough)
Sandra (solid) X drava (liquid)
Mrdu (soft) X kathina (hard)
Sthira (stable) X cala (moving, unstable)
Suksma (minute, small) X sthula (big, gross)
Vishada (non slimy, clear) X picchila (slimy)

**Buddhi – knowledge / intellect** which includes
Smriti (recollection),
Chetana (living),
Dhriti (intelligence, retaining power),
Ahamkara (ego).

**Prayatnanta Gunas (qualities ending with prayatna) - 6 Qualities of Atma (soul):**
Iccha – desire
Dvesha – hatred
Sukha – comfort, happiness
Dukha – grief
Buddhi – intellect
Prayatna – effort.

**Paradai gunas**
Para – great,
Apara – not great,
Yukti – planning,
Samkhya – number,
Samyoga – combination,
Vibhaga – division,
Pruthaktva – individuality,
Parimana – quantity,
Samskara – processing,
Abhyasa – habituation,
All these together constitute qualities. [49]

**Definition of Karma – action:**
...प्रयत्नादि कर्म चेष्टितमुच्यते||४९||
The act done with effort is called action. [49]

**Definition of Samavaya – inseparable relationship:**
समवायोऽपृथग्भावो भूम्यादीनां गुणैर्मतः|
स नित्यो यत्र हि द्रव्यं न तत्रानियतो गुणः||५०||
Samavaya is an inseparable relationship. Such a relationship exists between
Prithvi and Gandha (earth and smell),
Ap and rasa (water and taste)
Tejas and Rupa (fire and shape / form)
Vayu and Sparsha (air and touch)
Akasha and Shabda (ether and sound)
This relationship is eternal because where there is matter, its distinctive quality is always there. [50]

**Definition of Dravya (matter):**
यत्राश्रिताः कर्मगुणाः कारणं समवायि यत्|
तद्द्रव्यं ...
...समवायी तु निश्चेष्टः कारणं गुणः||५१||
The one having qualities (Guna) and action (Karma) in an inseparable relation is called as matter (Dravya). For example, ghee (matter) has oiliness (quality) and decreases Vata (action).

**Definition of qualities (Guna):**
That which has inseparable relationship with matter but does not have its own action, is called as Guna. For example, the oiliness (quality) in ghee (matter) lives inseparably. But oil itself does not have any action. The action of 'decreasing vata' is done by the ghee (matter). [51]

**Definition of Karma (action):**
संयोगे च विभागे च कारणं द्रव्यमाश्रितम्|
कर्तव्यस्य क्रिया कर्म कर्म नान्यदपेक्षते||५२||.
इत्युक्तं कारणं...|५३|
कार्यं धातुसाम्यमिहोच्यते|
धातुसाम्यक्रिया चोक्ता तन्त्रस्यास्य प्रयोजनम्||५३||
That which lives (resides within) inseparably with matter (Dravya) and brings about / causes combination and separation is called karma. Karma makes the matter to act without depending on anything else. [52-53]

**Karya – aim of work (in Ayurveda)**
कालबुद्धीन्द्रियार्थानां योगो मिथ्या न चाति च|
द्वयाश्रयाणां व्याधीनां त्रिविधो हेतुसङ्ग्रहः||५४||
The aim of the work in Ayurveda is to bring balance to all the factors in the body (Dhatu Samya). Restoring this balance is the purpose of Ayurveda.

**Cause for disease:**
The cause of the diseases relating to both (mind and body) are

- Atiyoga – excessive utilisation or indulgence, Heena Yoga - less utilisation or indulgence or Mithya Yoga – wrong utilisation or indulgence of the below mentioned –

- Kala – time (like prolonged summer, short summer or heat of summer in other seasons),
- Artha – objects of sense organs (smell, touch etc) (like excessive smelling, not at all seeing, or seeing in dark areas, seeing of sharp objects etc
- Buddhi – mental faculties – like excess thinking, less thinking or wrong thinking and doing etc [54]

## Two places where disease occurs:

शरीरं सत्त्वसञ्ज्ञं च व्याधीनामाश्रयो मतः।

तथा सुखानां, योगस्तु सुखानां कारणं समः॥५५॥

The body and mind constitute the substrata of diseases and happiness. Balanced utilisation of time, mental faculties and object of sense organs is the cause of happiness. [55]

## Definition of Atman (Soul / God):

निर्विकारः परस्त्वात्मा सत्त्वभूतगुणेन्द्रियैः।

चैतन्ये कारणं नित्यो द्रष्टा पश्यति हि क्रियाः॥५६॥

Nirvikara – The soul is essentially devoid of all deformities.

He is the cause of consciousness through the mind and the specific qualities of basic elements (touch, shape, smell, taste and sound). He is eternal. He is an observer – he observes all activities. [56]

## Physical and mental Doshas:

वायुः पित्तं कफश्चोक्तः शारीरो दोषसङ्ग्रहः।

मानसः पुनरुद्दिष्टो रजश्च तम एव च॥५७॥

Pathogenic factors in the body are Vayu (Vata), Pitta and Kapha

Mental Doshas are Rajas and Tamas. [57]

## Three types of treatments:

प्रशाम्यत्यौषधैः पूर्वो दैवयुक्तिव्यपाश्रयैः।

मानसो ज्ञानविज्ञानधैर्यस्मृतिसमाधिभिः॥५८॥

Three types of treatments for these two types of Doshas –

The physical Doshas – Vata, Pitta and Kapha are balanced by

a. Daiva Vyapashraya Chikitsa – religious rites / divine therapies and

b. Yukti Vyapashraya Chikitsa – done by a physician with proper planning.

c. Sattvavajaya Chikitsa – Psychotherapy - The psychological Doshas – Rajas and Tamas are balanced by spiritual and scriptural knowledge, patience, memory and meditation. These treatments help to win over the weakness of mind. Hence, they are called Satva Avajaya Chikitsa. [58]

## Qualities of Vata Dosha:

रूक्षः शीतो लघुः सूक्ष्मश्चलोऽथ विशदः खरः।

विपरीतगुणैर्द्रव्यैर्मारुतः सम्प्रशाम्यति॥५९॥

सस्नेहमुष्णं तीक्ष्णं च द्रवमम्लं सरं कटु।

विपरीतगुणैः पित्तं द्रव्यैराशु प्रशाम्यति॥६०॥

गुरुशीतमृदुस्निग्धमधुरस्थिरपिच्छिलाः।

श्लेष्मणः प्रशमं यान्ति विपरीतगुणैर्गुणाः॥६१॥

**Qualities of Vata Dosha** - Rooksha (rough), Sheeta (cool), Laghu (light), Sookshma (subtle, minute), Chala – mobile, Vishada – clarity, non-slimy and Khara (coarse) are the qualities of Vata. It is balanced by the medicines having opposite qualities to the mentioned qualities of vata.

**Qualities of Pitta Dosha** – Sneha (unctuous), Ushna (hot), Teekshna (sharp, piercing), Drava (liquid), Amla (sour), Sara (fluidity) and Katu (pungent) are the qualities of pitta. It is balanced by the medicines having opposite qualities to the mentioned qualities of pitta.

**Qualities of Kapha are** – Guru (heavy), Sheeta (cool), Mrudu (soft), Snigdha (unctuous, oily) Madhura (sweet), Sthira (immobile) and Picchila (slimy) are the qualities of kapha. It is balanced by the medicines having opposite qualities to the mentioned qualities of kapha. [59-61]

विपरीतगुणैर्देशमात्राकालोपपादितैः|
भेषजैर्विनिवर्तन्ते विकाराः साध्यसम्मताः||६२||
साधनं न त्वसाध्यानां व्याधीनामुपदिश्यते|६३|
**Principle of Tridosha Balance** – The curable diseases are cured by medicines possessing opposite qualities, when administered with due regard to the place, dose and time. No medicine is to be prescribed for incurable diseases. [62-63]

भूयश्चातो यथाद्रव्यं गुणकर्माणि वक्ष्यते||६३||
And so Agnivesha will explain in detail the qualities and actions of drugs. [63]

**Tastes:**
रसनार्थो रसस्तस्य द्रव्यमापः क्षितिस्तथा|
निर्वृत्तौ च विशेषे च प्रत्ययाः खादयस्त्रयः||६४||
स्वादुरम्लोऽथ लवणः कटुकस्तिक्त एव च|
कषायश्चेति षट्कोऽयं रसानां सङ्ग्रहः स्मृतः||६५||
Ap (water) and Prithvi (earth) constitute the substratum for the manifestation of taste (Rasa). Taste is the object of the tongue (Rasanendriya). Akasha (ether), Vayu (air) and Tejas are responsible for the manifestation of different types of taste.
Sweet (Madhura),
Sour (Amla),
Salt (Lavana),
Katu (pungent),
Tikta (bitter) and
Kashaya (astringent) are the six types of Tastes. [65]

स्वाद्वम्ललवणा वायुं, कषायस्वादुतिक्तकाः|
जयन्ति पित्तं, श्लेष्माणं कषायकटुतिक्तकाः||६६||
(कट्वम्ललवणाः पित्तं, स्वाद्वम्ललवणाः कफम्|
कटुतिक्तकषायाश्च कोपयन्ति समीरणम्||१||)|
Medicines and foods having sweet, sour and saline taste balance Vata;
Those having astringent, sweet and bitter (taste) balance Pitta and
those having astringent, pungent and bitter tastes balance Kapha. [66]

**Three types of medicines:**
किञ्चिद्दोषप्रशमनं किञ्चिद्धातुप्रदूषणम्|
स्वस्थवृत्तौ मतं किञ्चित्त्रिविधं द्रव्यमुच्यते||६७||
**Dosha prashamana** – those which balance the increased Doshas
**Dhatu pradushana** – those which imbalance / contaminate the normal Doshas / tissues (and make them abnormal)
**Swasthavrutta** – those which help in maintaining the health in its normal state (balancing health) [67]

**Another three types of substances (Dravya):**

तत् पुनस्त्रिविधं प्रोक्तं जङ्गमौद्भिदपार्थिवम् |
मधूनि गोरसाः पित्तं वसा मज्जाऽसृगामिषम्||६८||
विण्मूत्रचर्मरेतोऽस्थिस्नायुशृङ्गनखाः खुराः|
जङ्गमेभ्यः प्रयुज्यन्ते केशा लोमानि रोचना||६९||
सुवर्णं समलाः पञ्च लोहाः ससिकताः सुधा|
मनःशिलाले मणयो लवणं गैरिकाञ्जने||७०||
भौममौषधमुद्दिष्टमौद्भिदं तु चतुर्विधम्|
वनस्पतिस्तथा वीरुद्वानस्पत्यस्तथौषधिः||७१||
फलैर्वनस्पतिः पुष्पैर्वानस्पत्यः फलैरपि|
ओषध्यः फलपाकान्ताः प्रतानैर्वीरुधः स्मृताः||७२||
मूलत्वक्सारनिर्यासनाल(ड)स्वरसपल्लवाः|
क्षाराः क्षीरं फलं पुष्पं भस्म तैलानि कण्टकाः||७३||
पत्राणि शुङ्गाः कन्दाश्च प्ररोहाश्चौद्भिदो गणः|७४|

**Another three types of substances (Dravya) are as below described:**

**Jangama** - those of animal origin. Example – Different types of honey, dairy products, bile, fats of muscle tissue, marrow, blood, flesh, faeces, urine, skin, semen, bone, ligament, horn, nail, hoof, hair, Loman (hair of the body excluding those of the head and face), Gorochana (purified Ox bile) – these are some of the drugs of animal origin used in medicine.

**Audbhida** - those of vegetables origin

**Parthiva** - metals including minerals which are obtained from underneath the ground. Gold, five Lohas (copper, silver, tin, lead and iron) along with their by-products (different types of bitumen), calcites along with silica, red arsenic, yellow arsenic, gems, salt, red chalk, collyrium – these are in brief the metals and minerals used in medicine.

**Audbhida (plant source) are further divided into four types –**

Vanaspati – which bear fruits without flowers

Vanaspatya – which bear flowers and fruits

Virudha – which spread on ground, with branches

Oshadhi – are those which die out when their fruits mature

The root, bark, sara (aqueous extract), secretions, fibre, juice, tender leaves, alkali preparations, latex, fruits, flowers, ashes, oil, thorns, matured leaves, adventitious roots, rhizomes, sprouts – all these belong to the group of drugs of vegetable origin. [68-73]

मूलिन्यः षोडशैकोना फलिन्यो विंशतिः स्मृताः||७४||
महास्नेहाश्च चत्वारः पञ्चैव लवणानि च|
अष्टौ मूत्राणि सङ्ख्यातान्यष्टावेव पयांसि च||७५||
शोधनार्थाश्च षड् वृक्षाः पुनर्वसुनिदर्शिताः|
य एतान् वेत्ति संयोक्तुं विकारेषु स वेदवित्||७६||

As indicated by Atreya Punarvasu,

those having therapeutically useful roots are sixteen,

those having therapeutically useful fruits are nineteen,

important fats are four,

salts are five,

varieties of urine are eight,

milk is also eight.

Plants used for elimination therapy are six.

It is only those who know how to apply these to various diseases really know the science. [74-76]

## 16 Moolikas

हस्तिदन्ती हैमवती श्यामा त्रिवृद्धोगुडा|
सप्तला श्वेतनामा च प्रत्यक्श्रेणी गवाक्ष्यपि||७७||
ज्योतिष्मती च बिम्बी च शणपुष्पी विषाणिका|
अजगन्धा द्रवन्ती च क्षीरिणी चात्र षोडशी||७८||
शणपुष्पी च बिम्बी च च्छर्दने हैमवत्यपि|
श्वेता ज्योतिष्मती चैव योज्या शीर्षविरेचने||७९||
एकादशावशिष्टा याः प्रयोज्यास्ता विरेचने|
इत्युक्ता नामकर्मभ्यां मूलिन्यः...|८०|

**Sixteen herbs** having therapeutically **useful roots** are

Hastidanti (Croton oblongifolius Roxb.)

Haimavati (Vacha – Acorus calamus Linn.),

Shyama – Shyama Trivrit (Operculina turpethum R.B. – black variety),

Trivrt (Operculina turpethum R.B. – white variety),

Adhoguda (Euphorbia nivulia),

Saptala (Acacia concinna D.C.),

Svethanama (Clitoria ternatea Linn. – variety alba),

Pratyaksreni (Baliospermum montanum Muell. – Danti),

Gavakshi (Citrullus colocynthis Schrad.)

Jyotishmati (Celastrus paniculatus Willd),

Bimbi (Coccinia indica W. and A.),

Shanapuspi (Crotalaria verrucosa Linn.)

Vishanika (Helicteres isora Linn.),

Ajagandha (Gynandropsis gynandra Linn.),

Dravanti (Jatropha glandulifera Roxb.),

Ksheerini (Mimusops hexandra Roxb.).

Out of them, Shanapushpi (Crotalaria verrucosa Linn.), Bimbi (Coccinia indica W. and A.) and Haimavati (Acorus calamus Linn.) are used for emesis (vomiting treatment).

Shveta (Clitoria ternatea Linn.) and Jyotismati (Celastrus paniculatus Willd.) are used for the elimination (of Doshas) from the head and the remaining eleven are for purgation (Virechana).

Thus, the names and actions of plants having therapeutically most useful roots are described here. [77-80]

## Phala Vrukshas

...फलिनीः शृणु||८०||
शङ्खिन्यथ विडङ्गानि त्रपुषं मदनानि च|
धामार्गवमथेक्ष्वाकु जीमूतं कृतवेधनम्|
आनूपं स्थलजं चैव क्लीतकं द्विविधं स्मृतम्||८१||
प्रकीर्या चोदकीर्या च प्रत्यक्पुष्पा तथाऽभया|
अन्तःकोटरपुष्पी च हस्तिपर्ण्याश्च शारदम्||८२||
कम्पिल्लकारग्वधयोः फलं यत् कुटजस्य च|
धामार्गवमथेक्ष्वाकु जीमूतं कृतवेधनम्||८३||
मदनं कुटजं चैव त्रपुषं हस्तिपर्णिनी|

एतानि वमने चैव योज्यान्यास्थापनेषु च||८४||
नस्तः प्रच्छर्दने चैव प्रत्यक्पुष्पा विधीयते|
दश यान्यवशिष्टानि तान्युक्तानि विरेचने||८५||
नामकर्मभिरुक्तानि फलान्येकोनविंशतिः|८६|

The plants having therapeutically **most useful fruits** are:
Shankhini (Canscora decussata Roem. et. Sch.)
Vidanga (Embelia ribes Burm.),
Trapusha (Cucumis sativus Linn.),
Varieties of Madana (Randia dumetorum Lam.),
Dhamargava (Luffa cylindrica Linn. M. Roem.),
Ikshvaku (Lagenaria siceraria Standl.),
Jimuta (Luffa echinata Roxb.),
Kirtavedhana (Luffa acutangula Roxb.)

Two types of Klitaka (Glycyrrhiza glabra Linn.) – the one which grows in marshy land and the other which grows in dry land:
Prakirya (Caesalpinia crista Linn.),
Udakirya (Pongamia pinnata Merr.),
Pratyakpuspa (Achyranthes aspera Linn.),
Abhaya (Terminalia chebula Linn.)
Antahkotarapuspi (Argyreia speciosa),
Autumnal fruit of hastiparnini (Leea macrophylla), fruit of Kampillaka (Mallotus philippinensis Muell. – Arg.)
Aragvadha (Cassia fistula Linn.) and also of Kutaja (Holarrhena antidysenterica Wall.).

Dhamargava (Luffa cylindrica Linn. M. Roem.), Ikshvaku (Lagenaria siceraria Standl.), Jimuta (Luffa echinata Roxb.), Kritavedhana (Luffa acutangula Roxb.), Madana (Randia dumetorum Lam.), Kutaja (Holarrhena antidysenterica Wall.), Trapusa (Cucumis sativus Linn.), Hastiparnini (?) – all these are used in emesis (vamana) and also in Asthapana (a type of medicated enema).

Pratyakpuspa (Achyranthes aspera Linn.) is employed for elimination of Doshas by inhalation. Remaining ten are used for purgation treatment. Thus, the names and actions of nineteen plants having therapeutically most useful fruits have been described. [80-86]

**4 types of fat substances:**
सर्पिस्तैलं वसा मज्जा स्नेहो दिष्टश्चतुर्विधः ||८६||
पानाभ्यञ्जनबस्त्यर्थं नस्यार्थं चैव योगतः|
स्नेहना जीवना वर्ण्या बलोपचयवर्धनाः||८७||
स्नेहा ह्येते च विहिता वातपित्तकफापहाः|८८|
**Four varieties of fats** are ghee, oil, muscle-fat and marrow. They are prescribed for internal use, massage, enema and inhalation. All these varieties of fats add to the unctuousness, invigoration, luster, strength, corpulence (of the body) and alleviate Vata, Pitta and Kapha. [86-88]

सौवर्चलं सैन्धवं च विडमौद्भिदमेव च||८८||
सामुद्रेण सहैतानि पञ्च स्युर्लवणानि च|
स्निग्धान्युष्णानि तीक्ष्णानि दीपनीयतमानि च||८९||
आलेपनार्थं युज्यन्ते स्नेहस्वेदविधौ तथा|
अधोभागोर्ध्वभागेषु निरूहेष्वनुवासने||९०||

अभ्यञ्जने भोजनार्थे शिरसश्च विरेचने।
शस्त्रकर्मणि वर्त्यर्थमञ्जनोत्सादनेषु च॥९१॥
अजीर्णानाहयोर्वाते गुल्मे शूले तथोदरे।
उक्तानि लवणा(नि)...॥९२॥

**Five varieties of salt** are Sauvarchala (sochal salt), Saindhava (rock salt), Vit (Ammonium chloride), Audbhida (salt from the earth), and Samudra (sea salt).

They are all unctuous, hot, sharp and most exceedingly appetising. They are also used for anointment, causing unctuousness, fomentation, purgation, emesis, Niruha, Anuvasana (types of enema – basti treatment), massage, intake, elimination (of Doshas) from the head, surgical measures, suppositories, collyrium, unction, and also for the correction of indigestion, constipation, treatment of diseases due to Vata, Gulma (abdominal tumour), Shoola (colic pain) and Udara (abdominal diseases including ascites). This is about salts. [88-92]

**Types of urine**

... न्यूर्ध्वं मूत्राण्यष्टौ निबोध मे॥९२॥
मुख्यानि यानि दिष्टानि सर्वाण्यात्रेयशासने।
अविमूत्रमजामूत्रं गोमूत्रं माहिषं च यत्॥९३॥
हस्तिमूत्रमथोष्ट्रस्य हयस्य च खरस्य च।
उष्णं तीक्ष्णमथोऽरूक्षं कटुकं लवणान्वितम्॥९४॥
मूत्रमुत्सादने युक्तं युक्तमालेपनेषु च।
युक्तमास्थापने मूत्रं युक्तं चापि विरेचने॥९५॥
स्वेदेष्वपि च तद्युक्तमानाहेष्वगदेषु च।
उदरेष्वथ चार्शःसु गुल्मिकुष्ठिकिलासिषु॥९६॥
तद्युक्तमुपनाहेषु परिषेके तथैव च।
दीपनीयं विषघ्नं च क्रिमिघ्नं चोपदिश्यते॥९७॥
पाण्डुरोगोपसृष्टानामुत्तमं शर्म चोच्यते।
श्लेष्माणं शमयेत् पीतं मारुतं चानुलोमयेत्॥९८॥
कर्षेत् पित्तमधोभागमित्यस्मिन् गुणसङ्ग्रहः।
सामान्येन मयोक्तस्तु पृथक्त्वेन प्रवक्ष्यते॥९९॥
अविमूत्रं सतिक्तं स्यात् स्निग्धं पित्ताविरोधि च।
आजं कषायमधुरं पथ्यं दोषान्निहन्ति च॥१००॥
गव्यं समधुरं किञ्चिद्दोषघ्नं क्रिमिकुष्ठनुत्।
कण्डूं च शमयेत् पीतं सम्यग्दोषोदरे हितम्॥१०१॥
अर्शःशोफोदरघ्नं तु सक्षारं माहिषं सरम्।
हास्तिकं लवणं मूत्रं हितं तु क्रिमिकुष्ठिनाम्॥१०२॥
प्रशस्तं बद्धविण्मूत्रविषश्लेष्मामयार्शसाम्।
सतिक्तं श्वासकासघ्नमर्शोघ्नं चौष्ट्रमुच्यते॥१०३॥
वाजिनां तिक्तकटुकं कुष्ठव्रणविषापहम्।
खरमूत्रमपस्मारोन्मादग्रहविनाशनम्॥१०४॥
इतीहोक्तानि मूत्राणि यथासामर्थ्ययोगतः॥१०५॥

**Mutra – Types of urine -**

The most useful varieties of urine as explained by Atreya, are eight, viz., urine of sheep, goat, cow, buffalo, elephant, camel, horse and ass.

**General qualities of urine** - They are hot, sharp, unctuous, pungent and salty. They are used for unction, anointment,

Asthapana, purgation, fomentation, treatment of constipation, alleviation of diseases in general, to treat diseases like Udara (diseases of abdomen including ascites), Arsha (piles), Gulma (abdominal tumour), Kushta (skin diseases), Kilasa (a type of leucoderma), and for preparing poultices.

They are prescribed as appetisers, antitoxins and bactericides. They are also known as best remedies for those affected by Panduroga (anaemia). When taken it also alleviates Kapha and Vata and also brings down aggravated Pitta. These are the general properties (of urine), the specific ones are as follows:

**Urine of sheep** is bitter, unctuous, and not opposed to Pitta.

**Urine of goat** - is astringent, sweet, wholesome and balances all the three Doshas.

**Cow Urine** is slightly sweet; it also alleviates Doshas; it is bactericidal; it cures Kustha (skin diseases). If taken in, it alleviates itching. It is equally useful for the Doshas and Udara (abdominal diseases including ascites).

**Buffalo urine** is alkaline, laxative; it cures piles, Shopha (Oedema) and Udara (abdominal diseases including ascites).

**Elephant urine** is saline; it is useful against bacterial infection and Kustha (skin diseases); it is specifically useful in cases of constipation, Dysuria, toxic conditions, diseases due to Kapha and piles.

**Camel urine** is bitter; it alleviates Shwasa (dyspnoea, asthma), Kasa (bronchitis, cough) and piles.

**Horse urine** is bitter and pungent; it cures Kustha (skin diseases), Vrana (ulcers) and toxic conditions.

**Donkey urine** cures epilepsy, insanity and Grahadosha (demoniac seizures).

Thus different varieties of urine have been described keeping in view their potentiality and applicability. [92-105]

**Milk Types, Qualities:**

अतः क्षीराणि वक्ष्यन्ते कर्म चैषां गुणाश्च ये||१०५||

अविक्षीरमजाक्षीरं गोक्षीरं माहिषं च यत्|

उष्ट्रीणामथ नागीनां वडवायाः स्त्रियास्तथा||१०६||

प्रायशो मधुरं स्निग्धं शीतं स्तन्यं पयो मतम्|

प्रीणनं बृंहणं वृष्यं मेध्यं बल्यं मनस्करम्||१०७||

जीवनीयं श्रमहरं श्वासकासनिबर्हणम्|

हन्ति शोणितपित्तं च सन्धानं विहतस्य च||१०८||

सर्वप्राणभृतां सात्म्यं शमनं शोधनं तथा|

तृष्णाघ्नं दीपनीयं च श्रेष्ठं क्षीणक्षतेषु च||१०९||

पाण्डुरोगेऽम्लपित्ते च शोषे गुल्मे तथोदरे|

अतीसारे ज्वरे दाहे श्वयथौ च विशेषतः ||११०||

योनिशुक्रप्रदोषेषु मूत्रेष्वप्रचुरेषु च|

पुरीषे ग्रथिते पथ्यं वातपित्तविकारिणाम्||१११||

नस्यालेपावगाहेषु वमनास्थापनेषु च|

विरेचने स्नेहने च पयः सर्वत्र युज्यते||११२||

यथाक्रमं क्षीरगुणानेकैकस्य पृथक् पृथक्|

अन्नपानादिकेऽध्याये भूयो वक्ष्याम्यशेषतः||११३||

**Milk – types and properties:** The best types of milk which can be used are those of sheep, she-goat, cow, she-buffalo, she-camel, she-elephant, mare and woman.

**General qualities of milk** - Milk is generally sweet, unctuous (oily), coolant, lactogenic, refreshing, nourishing, aphrodisiac, good for intellect, provides strength, useful for mental faculties, invigorating, dispels fatigue, relieves dyspnoea and bronchitis. It cures Raktapitta (bleeding from different parts of the body) and helps healing of the wound. It is wholesome for all living beings. It also alleviates and eliminates the morbid / imbalanced doshas. It quenches thirst and is an appetizer.

It is extremely useful in Kshataksina (phthisis), Pandu (anaemia), Amlapitta (hyperacidity), Shosha (consumption), Gulma (abdominal tumour), Udara (abdominal diseases including ascites), Atisara (diarrhoea), Jwara (fever), Daha (burning sensation) and especially in Shvavathu (edema). It is also useful in diseases of female genital tract, semen (male reproductive fluid), depleted sperm count and hard stool. It is a wholesome diet for those suffering from Vata and Pitta imbalance disorders.

Milk is always used for inhalation, anointment, bathing, emesis, Asthapana (a type of medicated enema), purgation and unctous. We will explain in greater details the properties of milk separately one by one in the chapter Annapanadi (Sutrasthana, 27th chapter). [105-113]

**Three special herbs:**
अथापरे त्रयो वृक्षाः पृथग्ये फलमूलिभिः|
स्नुह्यर्कश्मन्तकास्तेषामिदं कर्म पृथक् पृथक्||११४||
वमनेऽश्मन्तकं विद्यात् स्नुहीक्षीरं विरेचने|
क्षीरमर्कस्य विज्ञेयं वमने सविरेचने||११५||
Apart from the plants having most useful fruits and roots, there are three others viz.,
Snuhi (Euphorbia neriifolia Linn.),
Arka (Calotropis procera R. Br.) and
Ashmantaka (Bauhinia malabarica) whose actions are indicated separately (as follows).
Ashmantaka (Bauhinia malabarica) is useful for emesis, latex of Snuhi (Euphorbia neriifolia Linn.), for purgation; and that of Arka (Calotropis gigantea Linn.) for both emesis and purgation. [114-115]

इमांस्त्रीनपरान् वृक्षानाहुर्येषां हितास्त्वचः|
पूतीकः कृष्णगन्धा च तिल्वकश्च तथा तरुः||११६||
विरेचने प्रयोक्तव्यः पूतीकस्तिल्वकस्तथा|
कृष्णगन्धा परीसर्पे शोथेष्वर्शःसु चोच्यते||११७||
दद्रुविद्रधिगण्डेषु कुष्ठेष्वप्यलजीषु च|
षड्वृक्षाञ्छोधनानेतानपि विद्यादिवचक्षणः||११८||
इत्युक्ताः फलमूलिन्यः स्नेहाश्च लवणानि च|
मूत्रं क्षीराणि वृक्षाश्च षड् ये दिष्टपयस्त्वचः||११९||
There are **three other trees** whose barks are useful viz.,
Putika (Caesalpinia crista Linn.), Krishnagandha (Drumstick – Moringa oleifera Lam.) and Tilvaka (Symplocos racemosa Roxb.).
Putika (Caesalpinia crista Linn.) and Tilvaka (Symplocos racemosa Roxb.) are to be used for purgation.
Krishnagandha (Moringa oleifera Lam.) is used in Parisarpa (erysipelas), different types of Shotha (oedema), piles, ringworm, abscess, goitre and Alaji.
The wise should know all these six plants which are useful in elimination therapy.
Thus, the plants with most useful fruits and roots, varieties of fat, salt, urine and milk and also the plants having most useful latex and bark have been enumerated. [116-119]

**Goatherds, shepherds, cowherds**
ओषधीर्नामरूपाभ्यां जानते ह्यजपा वने|
अविपाश्चैव गोपाश्च ये चान्ये वनवासिनः||१२०||
न नामज्ञानमात्रेण रूपज्ञानेन वा पुनः|
ओषधीनां परां प्राप्तिं कश्चिद्वेदितुमर्हति||१२१||

योगवित्त्वप्यरूपज्ञस्तासां तत्त्वविदुच्यते|
किं पुनर्यो विजानीयादोषधीः सर्वथा भिषक्||१२२||
योगमासां तु यो विद्याद्देशकालोपपादितम्|
पुरुषं पुरुषं वीक्ष्य स ज्ञेयो भिषगुत्तमः||१२३||

The goatherds, shepherds, cowherds and other forest dwellers know the drugs by name and form. No one can know the principles governing correct application of drugs simply by knowing their names and forms. A physician, even ignorant of their forms can be said to be a knower of the essence [of this science] if he is acquainted with the principles of the correct application of drugs, let alone the one who knows drugs in their entirety. One who knows the principles of their correct application in consonance with the place, time and individual variation, should be regarded as the best physician. [120-123]

**Wisdom of right usage of medicine:**
यथा विषं यथा शस्त्रं यथाऽग्निरशनिर्यथा|
तथौषधमविज्ञातं विज्ञातममृतं यथा||१२४||
औषधं ह्यनभिज्ञातं नामरूपगुणैस्त्रिभिः|
विज्ञातं चापि दुर्युक्तमनर्थायोपपद्यते||१२५||

A drug not known is similar to poison, weapon, fire and thunderbolt while the drug which is well known is equivalent to the nectar. A drug known in respect of its name, form and properties or even if known, improperly administered, leads to bad consequences. [124-125]

योगादपि विषं तीक्ष्णमुत्तमं भेषजं भवेत्|
भेषजं चापि दुर्युक्तं तीक्ष्णं सम्पद्यते विषम्||१२६||
तस्मान्न भिषजा युक्तं युक्तिबाह्येन भेषजम्|
धीमता किञ्चिदादेयं जीवितारोग्यकाङ्क्षिणा||१२७||
कुर्यान्निपतितो मूर्ध्नि सशेषं वासवाशनिः|
सशेषमातुरं कुर्यान्नत्वज्ञमतमौषधम्||१२८||
दुःखिताय शयानाय श्रद्दधानाय रोगिणे|
यो भेषजमविज्ञाय प्राज्ञमानी प्रयच्छति||१२९||
त्यक्तधर्मस्य पापस्य मृत्युभूतस्य दुर्मतेः|
नरो नरकपाती स्यात्तस्य सम्भाषणादपि||१३०||
वरमाशीविषविषं क्वथितं ताम्रमेव वा|
पीतमत्यग्निसन्तप्ता भक्षिता वाऽप्ययोगुडाः||१३१||
नतु श्रुतवतां वेशं बिभ्रता शरणागतात्|
गृहीतमन्नं पानं वा वित्तं वा रोगपीडितात्||१३२||
भिषग्बुभूषुर्मतिमानतः स्वगुणसम्पदि|
परं प्रयत्नमातिष्ठेत् प्राणदः स्याद्यथा नृणाम्||१३३||

Even an acute poison can become an excellent drug if it is properly administered. On the other hand even a drug, if not properly administered, becomes an acute poison.

So a wise patient desirous of longevity and health should not accept any medicine prescribed by a physician ignorant of the principles governing its application.

Sometimes, one might escape death even when a thunderbolt of Indra has fallen on his head, but one can never survive if he takes medicine prescribed by a physician ignorant of the principles governing its application.

If the one pretending to be a wise physician, without knowing the principles governing its applicability, prescribes a medicine for a patient, distressed, lying on bed and having faith (in the former's prescription), he, the mischievous one is a sinner, devoid of virtuous acts and a messenger of death. Even talking to him would lead a man to hell.

One can take the poison of a serpent, melted copper; one can take iron-pills heated with fire, but the one (physician) wearing the garment of wise ones should not accept food, drink or wealth from a patient seeking his shelter. Thus, the wise one who aspires to be a physician should make special efforts to maintain his good qualities so that he can be the life-giver to human beings. [126-133]

तदेव युक्तं भैषज्यं यदारोग्याय कल्पते|
स चैव भिषजां श्रेष्ठो रोगेभ्यो यः प्रमोचयेत्||१३४||

Only that, which can bring about a cure, is the correct medicine. It is only he who can relieve his patients of their ailments is the best physician. [134]

सम्यक्प्रयोगं सर्वेषां सिद्धिराख्याति कर्मणाम्|
सिद्धिराख्याति सर्वैश्च गुणैर्युक्तं भिषक्तमम्||१३५||
Accomplishment of all objects i.e., actual prevention and cure of diseases implies the proper application of medicine. Success also implies the presence of the best physician endowed with all good qualities. [135]

**Summing up the contents: -**
तत्र श्लोकाः:-
आयुर्वेदागमो हेतुरागमस्य प्रवर्तनम्|
सूत्रणस्याभ्यनुज्ञानमायुर्वेदस्य निर्णयः||१३६||
सम्पूर्णं कारणं कार्यमायुर्वेदप्रयोजनम्|
हेतवश्चैव दोषाश्च भेषजं सङ्ग्रहेण च||१३७||
रसाः सप्रत्ययद्रव्यास्त्रिविधो द्रव्यसङ्ग्रहः|
मूलिन्यश्च फलिन्यश्च स्नेहाश्च लवणानि च||१३८||
मूत्रं क्षीराणि वृक्षाश्च षड् ये क्षीरत्वगाश्रयाः|
कर्माणि चैषां सर्वेषां योगायोगगुणागुणाः||१३९||
वैद्यापवादो यत्रस्थाः सर्वे च भिषजां गुणाः|
सर्वमेतत् समाख्यातं पूर्वाध्याये महर्षिणा||१४०||
Thus, the transmission of Ayurveda, object of transmission, spread, approval of the codification in a seminar, definition of Ayurveda, entire cause (means), object of Ayurveda, aetiology of diseases, enumeration of Doshas, collection of most useful medicines, enumeration of Rasas (tastes) along with their corresponding material objects, threefold classification of material objects, drugs, with most useful roots and fruits, important fats, varieties of useful salt, urine, and milk, those six plants whose latex and bark are most useful, actions of all these (drugs), their applicability and otherwise, good as well as bad qualities of theirs, abuse of physicians, the good qualities of physicians – all these have been explained by the sage in the first chapter. [136-140]

इत्यग्निवेशकृते तन्त्रे चरकप्रतिसंस्कृते सूत्रस्थाने दीर्घञ्जीवितीयो नाम प्रथमोऽध्यायः||१||
Thus, ends the first chapter on "Deergham Jeevityeeyam Adhyayam - The Quest for Longevity" chapter of the Sutra section of Agnivesa's work as redacted by Charaka.

# 2

# Sutrasthana Chapter 2 Apamarga Tanduleeyam

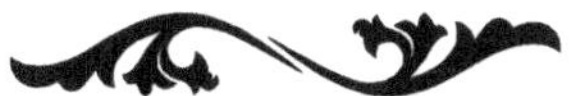

अथातोऽपामार्गतण्डुलीयमध्यायं व्याख्यास्यामः||१||

इति ह स्माह भगवानात्रेयः||२||

Apamarga is an herb called Prickly Chaff Flower (Achyranthes aspera Linn.). Tandula means its de-husked seeds. This chapter is named as Apamargatanduleeya Adhyaya because it starts with the explanation of dehusked seeds of Apamarga.

We shall now expound the chapter on the Dehusked Seeds of Apamarga. Thus said Lord Atreya. [ 1-2].

**Herbs used For Nasya treatment:**

अपामार्गस्य बीजानि पिप्पलीर्मरिचानि च|

विडङ्गान्यथ शिग्रूणि सर्षपांस्तुम्बुरूणि च||३||

अजाजीं चाजगन्धां च पीलून्येलां हरेणुकाम्|

पृथ्वीकां सुरसां श्वेतां कुठेरकफणिज्झकौ||४||

शिरीषबीजं लशुनं हरिद्रे लवणद्वयम्|

ज्योतिष्मतीं नागरं च दद्याच्छीर्षविरेचने||५||

गौरवे शिरसः शूले पीनसेऽर्धावभेदके|

क्रिमिव्याधावपस्मारे घ्राणनाशे प्रमोहके||६||

**Herbs used For Nasya treatment** - to treat diseases pertaining to head, ear, nose and throat –
In order to eliminate Doshas from the head in the event of heaviness of head, headache, rhinitis, hemicrania (single side headache / migraine), infectious diseases of the head, epilepsy, insomnia and fainting, one should prescribe
Apamarga - seeds of Apamarga (Achyranthes aspera Linn.),
Pippali - Piper longum Linn.,
Maricha – Long pepper / Piper nigrum Linn.,
Vidanga – False Black Pepper / Embelia ribes Burm. F.,
Shigru – Moringa / Moringa oleifera Lam.,
Sarshapa – Mustard / Brassica nigra Kotch
Tumburu - Zanthoxylun alatum. Roxb.,
Ajaji - Cuminum cyminum Linn.
Ajagandha - Gynandropsis gynandra Briquet,
Pilu - Salvadora persica Linn.,
Ela – Cardamom / Elettaria cardamomum Maton,
Harenuka - Pisum sativum Linn.,

Prithvika - Nigella sativa Linn.,
Surasa – Holy Basil / Ocimum sanctum Linn.,
Shveta Aparajita - Clitoria ternatea Linn. White variety,
Kutheraka - Ocimum basilicum Linn.,
Phanijjaka (?),
Seeds of Sirisa - Albizia lebbeck Benth,
Lashuna – Garlic / Allium sativum Linn.,
Haridra – Turmeric / Curcuma longa Linn.,
Daruharidra - Berberis aristata Dc.,
Saindhava - Rock salt,
Sauvarcala - Sonchal salt,
Jyotishmati - Celastrus paniculatus Willd.
Nagara – Ginger – Zingiber officinale Rose [3-6]

## Herbs used for Vamana – Emesis therapy:

मदनं मधुकं निम्बं जीमूतं कृतवेधनम्‌ ।
पिप्पलीकुटजेक्ष्वाकूण्येलां धामार्गवाणि च ॥७॥
उपस्थिते श्लेष्मपित्ते व्याधावामाशयाश्रये ।
वमनार्थं प्रयुञ्जीत भिषग्देहमदूषयन्‌ ॥८॥

## Herbs used for Vamana treatment:

**In the event of gastro-intestinal diseases** caused by vitiated Kapha and Pitta, Vamana (emesis) therapy is advised. For this purpose, the physician should prescribe the below mentioned herbs to avoid injury to the body and to conduct the emesis therapy safely.
Madana (Randia dumetorum Lam.),
Madhuka (Glycyrrhiza glabra Linn.),
Nimba (Azadirachta indica A. Juss.),
Jimuta (Luffa echinata Roxb.),
Kirtavedhana (Luffa acutangula Roxb.),
Pippali (Piper longum Linn.),
Kutaja (Holarrhena antidysenterica Wall.)
Ikshvaku (Lagenaria siceraria Standl.),
Ela – cardamom (Elettaria cardamomum Maton.),
Dhamargava (Luffa cylindrica M. Roem.) [7-8]

## Herbs for Virechana (purgation) Treatment :

त्रिवृतां त्रिफलां दन्तीं नीलिनीं सप्तलां वचाम्‌ ।
कम्पिल्लकं गवाक्षीं च क्षीरिणीमुदकीर्यकाम्‌ ॥९॥
पीलून्यारग्वधं द्राक्षां द्रवन्तीं निचुलानि च ।
पक्वाशयगते दोषे विरेकार्थं प्रयोजयेत्‌ ॥१०॥

## Herbs for Virechana (purgation) Treatment :

In the event of the vitiated Doshas in the intestines, the physician should prescribe the below mentioned herbs for purgation therapy –
Trivrit (Operculina turpethum R.B),
Haritaki (Terminalia chebula Linn.),
Amalaki (Emblica officinalis Gaertn.),

Bibhitaka (Terminalia bellirica Roxb.),
Danti (Baliospermum montanum Muell – Arg),
Neelini (Indigofera tinctoria Linn.),
Saptala (Acacia concinna Dc.),
Vacha (Acorus calamus Linn.),
Kampillaka (Mallotus philippinensis muell – Arg.),
Gavakshi (Citrullus colocynthis Schrad.),
Ksheerini (Mimusops hexandra Roxb.),
Udakeeryaka (Pongamia pinnata Merr.),
Peelu (Salvadora persica Linn.)
Aragvadha (Cassia fistula Linn.),
Draksha – raisins (Vitis vinifera Linn.)
Dravanti (Jatropha glandulifera Roxb.),
Nichula (Barringtonia acutangula Gaertn.). [9-10]

**Herbs used for Asthapana type of Basti:**
पाटलां चाग्निमन्थं च बिल्वं श्योनाकमेव च|
काश्मर्यं शालपर्णीं च पृश्निपर्णीं निदिग्धिकाम्||११||
बलां श्वदंष्ट्रां बृहतीमेरण्डं सपुनर्नवम्|
यवान् कुलत्थान् कोलानि गुडूचीं मदनानि च||१२||
पलाशं कतृणं चैव स्नेहांश्च लवणानि च|
उदावर्ते विबन्धेषु युञ्ज्यादास्थापनेषु च||१३||
अत एवौषधगणात् सङ्कल्प्यमनुवासनम्|
मारुतघ्नमिति प्रोक्तः सङ्ग्रहः पाञ्चकर्मिकः||१४||

**Herbs used for Asthapana type of Basti (enema therapy with Kashayam):**
For Asthapana (a variety of enema) in the event of Udavarta (bloating), Vibandha (constipation), one should prescribe
Patala (Stereospermum suaveolens DC.),
Agnimantha (Clerodendrum phlomidis Linn. F.),
Bilva – Bael tree (Aegle marmelos (L.) Correa),
Shyonaka (Oroxylum indicum Vent.),
Kashmarya (Gmelina arborea Linn.),
Shalaparni (Desmodium gangeticum DC.),
Prishniparni (Uraria picta Desv.),
Nidigdhika (Solanum xanthocarpum Schrad.),
Bala (Sida cordifolia Linn.),
Svadamstra (Tribulus terrestris Linn.),
Brihati (Solanum indicum Linn.),
Eranda (Ricinus communis Linn.).
Punarnava (Boerhavia diffusa Linn.),
Yava – Barley (Hordeum vulgare Linn.),
Kulattha – Horse gram (Dolichos biflorus Linn.),
Kola (Ziziphus jujuba Lam.),
Guduchi (Tinospora cordifolia Miers.),
Madana – emetic nut (Randia dumetorum Lam.),
Palasha (Butea monosperma Kuntze),

Kattruna (Cymbopogon schoenanthus Spreng.),
fats and salts.

These very drugs are also to be prescribed for Anuvasana (fat enema) for the cure of imbalanced Vata. Thus, the five elimination therapies (Panchakarma) are mentioned here in brief. [11-14]

तान्युपस्थितदोषाणां स्नेहस्वेदोपपादनैः|
पञ्चकर्माणि कुर्वीत मात्राकालौ विचारयन्||१५||

In Panchakarma, first, Snehana (oleation treatment) and Swedana (sweating treatment) are done. Due to this, the doshas are brought out (from the tissues into the gut – stomach and intestine). From here, these morbid doshas are eliminated by Panchakarma treatment. While performing Panchakarma treatment, due regard to the dose and time should be given. [15]

### Efficacy of treatment :

मात्राकालाश्रया युक्तिः, सिद्धिर्युक्तौ प्रतिष्ठिता|
तिष्ठत्युपरि युक्तिज्ञो द्रव्यज्ञानवतां सदा||१६||

Efficacy of treatment depends upon the dose of medicine and duration and time of administration (of medicine). Success of treatment depends upon efficient handling of dose and time of medicine. A physician, proficient in these two principles is always superior to those who are acquainted only with the medicine knowledge (ingredients and indication) [16].

अत ऊर्ध्वं प्रवक्ष्यामि यवागूर्विविधौषधाः|
विविधानां विकाराणां तत्साध्यानां निवृत्तये||१७||

Hereafter, I will explain different varieties of gruels prepared with different medicines to eradicate various diseases. [17]

### Different types of Gruels – Yavagu :

पिप्पलीपिप्पलीमूलचव्यचित्रकनागरैः|
यवागूर्दीपनीया स्याच्छूलघ्नी चोपसाधिता||१८||
दधित्थबिल्वचाङ्गेरीतक्रदाडिमसाधिता|
पाचनी ग्राहिणी, पेया सवाते पाञ्चमूलिकी||१९||
शालपर्णीबलाबिल्वैः पृश्निपर्ण्या च साधिता|
दाडिमाम्ला हिता पेया पित्तश्लेष्मातिसारिणाम्||२०||
पयस्यर्धोदके च्छागे ह्रीवेरोत्पलनागरैः|
पेया रक्तातिसारघ्नी पृश्निपर्ण्या च साधिता||२१||
दद्यात् सातिविषां पेयां सामे साम्लां सनागराम्|
श्वदंष्ट्राकण्टकारीभ्यां मूत्रकृच्छ्रे सफाणिताम्||२२||
विडङ्गपिप्पलीमूलशिग्रुभिर्मरिचेन च|
तक्रसिद्धा यवागूः स्यात् क्रिमिघ्नी ससुवर्चिका||२३||
मृद्वीकासारिवालाजपिप्पलीमधुनागरैः|
पिपासाघ्नी, विषघ्नी च सोमराजीविपाचिता||२४||
सिद्धा वराहनिर्यूहे यवागूर्बृंहणी मता|
गवेधुकानां भृष्टानां कर्शनीया समाक्षिका||२५||
सर्पिष्मती बहुतिला स्नेहनी लवणान्विता|
कुशाम्लकनिर्यूहे श्यामाकानां विरूक्षणी||२६||

दशमूलीशृता कासहिक्काश्वासकफापहा|
यमके मदिरासिद्धा पक्वाशयरुजापहा||२७||
शाकैर्मांसैस्तिलैर्माषैः सिद्धा वर्चो निरस्यति|
जम्ब्वाम्रास्थिदधित्थाम्लबिल्वैः साङ्ग्राहिकी मता||२८||
क्षारचित्रकहिङ्ग्वम्लवेतसैर्भेदिनी मता|
अभयापिप्पलीमूलविश्वैर्वातानुलोमनी ||२९||
तक्रसिद्धा यवागूः स्याद्धृतव्यापत्तिनाशिनी|
तैलव्यापदि शस्ता स्यात्क्रपिण्याकसाधिता||३०||
गव्यमांसरसैः साम्ला विषमज्वरनाशिनी|
कण्ठ्या यवानां यमके पिप्पल्यामलकैः शृता||३१||
ताम्रचूडरसे सिद्धा रेतोमार्गरुजापहा|
समाषविदला वृष्या घृतक्षीरोपसाधिता||३२||
उपोदिकादधिभ्यां तु सिद्धा मदविनाशिनी|
क्षुधं हन्यादपामार्गक्षीरगोधारसैः शृता||३३||

**Different types of Gruels – Yavagu :**

**Panchakola Yavagu –** The gruel prepared with Panchkola – Pippali fruit (Piper longum Linn.), root of Pippali, Chavya (Piper chaba Hunter), Chitraka (Plumbago zeylanica Linn.) and Nagara – ginger (Zingiber officinale Rosc.) stimulates digestion, and cures abdominal colic pain. (1)

Gruel prepared with Dadhittha (Feronia limonia Swingle), Bilva (Aegle marmelos Corr.), Changeri (Oxalis corniculata Linn.), Buttermilk and Dadima – Pomegranate (Punica granatum Linn.) is carminative (improves digestion) and absorbs moisture (grahini) (2)

**Vatahara – Laghu Panchamoola Yavagu -** Gruel of Shalaparni (Desmodium gangeticum DC.), Prishniparni (Uraria picta Desv.), Brihati (Solanum indicum Linn.), Kantakari (Solanum xanthocarpum Schrad and Wendle) and Gokshura – (Tribulus terrestris Linn.) is useful for Vata type of diarrhea. (3)

**Yavagu for Atisara -** Gruel prepared with Shalaparni (Desmodium gangeticum DC.), Bala (Sida cordifolia Linn.), Bilva (Bael – Aegle marmelos Corr.), Prishniparni (Uraria picta Desv.) and soured with Dadima – Pomegranate (Punica granatum Linn.) is useful in Atisara (diarrhoea / dysentery) of Pitta and Kapha origin. (4)

**Yavagu for Ratka Atisara -** Gruel of Hribera (Pavonia odorata Willd.), Utpala (Nymphaea alba Linn.), Nagara – Ginger (Zingiber officinale Rosc.) Prishniparni (Uraria picta Desv.) prepared with semi-diluted goat's milk cures dysentery with bleeding. (5)

One should prescribe the gruel prepared with Ativisha (Aconitum heterophyllum Wall.) and Nagara – Ginger (Zingiber officinale Rosc.), and soured with pomegranate for diarrhea in its Ama stage – early stage of diarrhea, with indigestion. (6)

**Yavagu for Dysuria –** Gruel of Shvadamstra (Tribulus terrestris Linn.) Kantakari (Solanum xanthocarpum) along with Phanita (a preparation of sugarcane) should be prescribed in difficulty in urination – Dysuria. (7)

**Yavagu for intestinal worms -** Gruel of Vidanga (Embelia ribes Burm.), root of Pippali (Piper longum Linn.), Shigru (Moringa oleifera Lam.), Maricha (Piper nigrum Linn.) prepared with buttermilk and salted with Suvarchala lavana (black salt) cures infections (8).

**Yavagu for excessive thirst** - Gruel prepared with Mrduveeka (Raisins – Vitis vinifera Linn.), Sariva (Hemidesmus indicus R. B.), fried paddy, Pippali (Piper longum Linn.), honey and Nagara (Zingiber officinale Rosc.), cures excessive thirst. (9)

Gruel of Somaraji (Psoralea corylifolia Linn.) is anti-poisonous. (10)

**Nourishing Yavagu** - Gruel prepared with pork extract is nourishing. (11)

**Yavagu to lose weight** - Gruel prepared with fried Gavedhuka (Triticum aestivum Linn.) along with honey is emaciating. (12)

Gruel prepared with Tila (Sesame seeds – Sesamum indicum Linn.), and added with ghee and salt causes unctuousness, oleating. (13)

Gruel of Shyamaka (Panicum italicum Linn.) prepared with the extract of Kusha (Desmostachya bipinnata Staff.) and Amalaki causes roughness. (14)

**Dashamoola Yavagu** – Gruel prepared with Bilva (Aegle marmelos Corr.), Shyonaka (Oroxylum indicum Vent.), Gambhari (Gmelina arborea Linn.) Patala (Stereospermum suaveolens DC.), Ganikarika (Clerodendrum phlomidis Linn. f.), Shalaparni (Desmodium gangeticum DC.), Prishniparni (Uraria picta Desv.), Brihati (Solanum indicum Linn.), Kantakari (Solanum xanthocarpum Schrad and Wendle), and Gokshura (Tribulus terrestris Linn.) cures coughing, hiccough, dyspnoea and diseases due to Kapha. (15)

The gruel prepared of ghee and oil with Madira wine alleviates pain in intestines (16)

Gruel of vegetables, meat, Tila (Sesame) and Masha (Black gram – Phaseolus mungo Linn.) evacuates the bowel. (17)

Gruel of Jambu (Syzygium cumini Skeels), seeds of Amra (Mango – Mangifera indica Linn.), sour Dadhittha (Feronia limonia Swingle), Bilva (Aegle marmelos Corr.), is astringent. (18)

**Bhedani Yavagu** – Gruel of Yavakshara (alkali preparation from Hordeum vulgare Linn.), Chitraka (Plumbago zeylanica Linn.), Hingu (Asafoetida) and Amlavetasa (Rheum emodi Wall.) causes purgation. (19)

**Vata Anulomana Yavagu** – Gruel prepared with Abhaya (Terminalia chebula Linn.) root of Pippali (Piper longum Linn.) and Vishva (Zingiber officinale Rosc.) helps elimination of flatus. (20)

The gruel prepared with buttermilk eradicates untoward effects caused by (incorrect intake of) ghee. (21)

The gruel prepared with buttermilk and oil cake would alleviate such defects as caused by the incorrect intake of oil. (22)

The gruel prepared with beef extract and soured with Dadima (Punica granatum Linn.) cures irregular fever. (23)

The gruel prepared of Yava (Hordeum vulgare Linn.) with ghee and oil, and boiled with Pippali (Piper longum Linn.) and Amalaka (Emblica officinalis Gaertn.) is useful for the throat. (24)

Gruel of chicken extract alleviates diseases pertaining to the seminal passage. (25)

Gruel of split Masha (Black gram – Phaseolus mungo Linn.) prepared with ghee and milk is aphrodisiac. (26)

Gruel prepared with Upodika (Basella rubra Linn.) and curd cures narcosis. (27)

**Yavagu to suppress hunger** – Gruel of Apamarga (Achyranthes aspera Linn.) boiled with milk and extract of Iguana flesh kills hunger. (28) [18-33]

**Summary**
तत्र श्लोकः-
अष्टाविंशतिरित्येता यवाग्वः परिकीर्तिताः|
पञ्चकर्माणि चाश्रित्य प्रोक्तो भैषज्यसङ्ग्रहः||३४||
Thus, all the twenty-eight varieties of gruel have been described and the drugs in connection with the five elimination therapies have been enumerated in brief. [34]

पूर्वं मूलफलज्ञानहेतोरुक्तं यदौषधम्|
पञ्चकर्माश्रयज्ञानहेतोस्तत् कीर्तितं पुनः||३५||
The drugs, which were described in the previous chapter just for the sake of knowledge as to their most useful roots and fruits, the same have again been described here to indicate their usefulness in the five elimination therapies. [35]

**Characteristics of a good physician -**
स्मृतिमान् हेतुयुक्तिज्ञो जितात्मा प्रतिपत्तिमान्|
भिषगौषधसंयोगैश्चिकित्सां कर्तुमर्हति||३६||
Only the physician who has been endowed with the below mentioned qualities shall be considered as a good physician :
Smrutiman – has a good memory
Hetu yuktijna – knows appropriate cause behind disease
Jitatma – who has mastered excellent control over his sense organs and mind
Pratipattiman – who has presence of mind
is entitled to practice medicine through the combination of various herbs. [36]
इत्यग्निवेशकृते तन्त्रे चरकप्रतिसंस्कृते श्लोकस्थानेऽपामार्गतण्डुलीयो नाम द्वितीयोऽध्यायः||२||
Thus, ends the second chapter of Shloka Sthana of treatise written by Acharya Agnivesha and redacted by Acharya Charaka.

# 3

# Sutrasthana  Chapter 3
# Aragvadheeyam

अथात आरग्वधीयमध्यायं व्याख्यास्यामः||१|| इति ह स्माह भगवानात्रेयः||२||

The third chapter of Charaka Samhita is called Aragvadheeya Adhyaya. It deals with 32 formulae to prepare creams and powder mixes used externally for various skin diseases.

We shall now expound the Chapter on "Aragvadha (Cassia fistula Linn.)." Thus, said Lord Atreya. [1–2]

**Skin creams for external application in a variety of skin diseases:**

आरग्वधः सैडगजः करञ्जो वासा गुडूची मदनं हरिद्रे|

श्र्याह्वः सुराह्वः खदिरो धवश्च निम्बो विडङ्गं करवीरकत्वक्||३||

ग्रन्थिश्च भौर्जो लशुनः शिरीषः सलोमशो गुग्गुलुकृष्णगन्धे|

फणिज्झको वत्सकसप्तपर्णौ पीलूनि कुष्ठं सुमनःप्रवालाः||४||

वचा हरेणुस्त्रिवृता निकुम्भो भल्लातकं गैरिकमञ्जनं च|

मनःशिलाले गृहधूम एला काशीसलोध्राजुर्नमुस्तसर्जाः||५||

इत्यर्धरूपैर्विहिताः षडेते गोपित्तपीताः पुनरेव पिष्टाः|

सिद्धाः परं सर्षपतैलयुक्ताश्चूर्णप्रदेहा भिषजा प्रयोज्याः||६||

कुष्ठानि कृच्छ्राणि नवं किलासं सुरेशलुप्तं किटिभं सदद्रु|

भगन्दरार्शांस्यपचीं सपामां हन्युः प्रयुक्तास्त्वचिरान्नराणाम्||७||

**Skin creams for external application in variety of skin diseases :**

The below six formulae which are in the form of powder shall be used by the physician for external application. Before usage, they are impregnated (triturated with liquids) with Go Pitta – purified ox bile. After this they are ground again and mixed up with mustard oil (Sarshapa taila). Their application immediately cures obstinate skin diseases including Kushta – leprosy, leucoderma of recent origin, alopecia, Kitibha – keloids, Dadru – ringworm, Bhagandhara – fistula–in–ano, Arsha – piles, Apachi – cervical adenitis and Pama – eruptions. The paste combinations are :

(1) Aragvadha (Cassia fistula Linn.), Edagaja (Cassia tora Linn.), Karanja (Pongamia pinnata Merr.), Vasa (Adhatoda vasica Nees.), Guduchi (Tinospora cordifolia Miers.), Madanaphala (Randia dumetorum Lam.), Haridra (Curcuma longa Linn.), and Daruharidra (Berberis aristata DC.);

(2) Sryahva (The lotus), Surahva (Cedrus deodara), Khadira (Acacia catechu Willd.), Dhava (Anogeissus latifolia Wall.), Nimba (Neem – Azadirachta indica A. Juss.), Vidanga (False black pepper – Embelia ribes Burm. F.), and the bark of Karaviraka (Nerium indicum Mill.);

(3) Node of Bhurja (Betula utilis D. don.), Lashuna (Garlic – Allium sativum Linn.), Shireesha (Albizia lebbeck Benth.), Lomasha (Ferri sulphas), Guggulu (Commiphora mukul Engl.), and Krishnagandha (Drumstick – Moringa oleifera Lam.);

(4) Phanijjhaka (a variety of Parnasa), Vatsaka (Kutaja – Holarrhena antidysenterica Wall.), Saptaparna (Alstonia scholaris R. Br.), varieties of Pilu (Salvadora persica Linn.), Kushta (Saussurea lappa C. B. Clarke.) and tender leaves of Sumanas (Jasminum officinale Linn. Var grandiflorum Bailey);

(5) Vacha (Acorus calamus Linn.), Harenu (Pisum sativum Linn.), Trivrit (Operculina turpethum R. B.), Nikumbha (Baliospermum montanum Muell–Ang.), Bhallataka (Semecarpus anacardium Linn f.), Gairika – Ferrum haematite and Anjana – Antimoni isulphidum;

(6) Manashila – Arsenic disulphide, Ala – Arsenic trisulphide, Grihadhooma – kitchen soot, Ela (Elettaria cardamomum Maton), Kaseesa – Ferrous sulphate, Lodhra (Symplocos racemosa Roxb.), Arjuna (Terminalia arjuna W & A.), Musta (Cyperus rotundus Linn.) and Sarja (Vateria indica Linn.) [3–7]

**Powder massage (Udvartana) for skin diseases – Kushtadi Lepa**
कुष्ठं हरिद्रे सुरसं पटोलं निम्बाश्वगन्धे सुरदारु शिग्रू|
ससर्षपं तुम्बुरुधान्यवन्यं चण्डां च चूर्णानि समानि कुर्यात्||८||
तैस्तक्रपिष्टैः प्रथमं शरीरं तैलाक्तमुद्वर्तयितुं यतेत|
तेनास्यकण्डूः पिडकाः सकोठाः कुष्ठानि शोफाश्च शमं व्रजन्ति||९||

**Powder massage (Udvartana) for skin diseases – Kushtadi Lepa**
Powder of the below mentioned herbs shall be used for administering udvarthana – powder massage in skin diseases –

- Kushta (Saussurea lappa C. B. Clarke),
- Haridra (turmeric – Curcuma longa Linn.),
- Daruharidra (Tree turmeric – Berberis aristata DC.),
- Surasa (Black variety of Holy Basil),
- Patola (Trichosanthes cucumerina Linn.),
- Nimba – Neem (Azadirachta indica),
- Ashvagandha (Withania somnifera Dunal),
- Suradaru (Cedrus deodara),
- Shigru (Drumstick – Moringa oleifera Lam.),
- Sarshapa (Mustard – Brassica nigra Koch.),
- Tumburu (Zanthoxylum alatum. Roxb.),
- Dhanya (Coriandrum sativum Linn.),
- Vanya (Cyperus tenuiflorus), and
- Chanda

These herbs are taken in equal quantities. Powders of these herbs are mixed together. The resultant mixture of powders of the mentioned herbs is ground with buttermilk and made into paste. Abhyanga with sesame oil is done on the patient. After that, the above paste is smeared over the body with gentle massage (Udvartana) given in upward direction (from below upwards on whichever part of the body it is done i.e. opposite to the direction of body hair).

This is useful in Kandu – pruritus, Pidaka – pimples, eruptions, Kota – urticaria, Kushta – obstinate skin diseases and

Shotha (inflammation)[8–9]

## Powder for dusting in skin diseases – Kushtadi Churna

कुष्ठामृतासङ्गकटङ्कटेरीकासीसकम्पिल्लकमुस्तलोध्राः।
सौगन्धिकं सर्जरसो विडङ्गं मनःशिलाले करवीरकत्वक्||१०||
तैलाक्तगात्रस्य कृतानि चूर्णान्येतानि दद्यादवचूर्णनार्थम्।
दद्रूः सकण्डूः किटिभानि पामा विचर्चिका चैव तथैति शान्तिम्||११||

## Powder for dusting in skin diseases – Kushtadi Churna

Powder of the below mentioned herbs is used for dusting in skin disorders :

- Kushta (Saussurea lappa),
- Amrutasanga – Cuprum sulphas,
- Katankateri (Tree turmeric – Berberis aristata DC.),
- Kasisa – Ferrous sulphate ,
- Kampillaka (Mallotus philippinensis Muell–Arg.),
- Musta (Cyperus rotundus Linn.),
- Lodhra (Symplocos racemosa), Sulphur,
- Sarjarasa (extract of Vateria indica Linn.),
- Vidanga (Embelia ribes Burm.f.),
- Manashila – realgar,
- Ala (Haratala) – orpiment,
- bark of Karavira (Nerium indicum Mill.).

The above mentioned herbs are taken in equal quantities.
The powders of these herbs are pounded and mixed together to prepare a homogenous mixture. The body of the patient suffering from skin disorders is smeared with sesame oil. Then the body is dusted with the powder prepared as mentioned above. This process of dusting is called Avachurnana.
It relieves Kitibha – ringworm, Kandu – pruritus, Pama – keloids, Vicharchika – Eczema. [10–11]

## Paste for skin disease – Manashiladi Pralepa

मनःशिलाले मरिचानि तैलमार्कं पयः कुष्ठहरः प्रदेहः।
तुत्थं विडङ्गं मरिचानि कुष्ठं लोध्रं च तद्वत् समनःशिलं स्यात्||१२||

## Paste for skin disease – Manashiladi Pralepa

The paste prepared with the below mentioned drugs constitutes a good ointment for curing chronic skin diseases –

- Manashila – Realgar,
- Ala – Orpiment,
- varieties of Maricha (Black pepper – Piper nigrum Linn.),
- Sesame Oil, and
- the latex of Arka (Calotropis gigantea Linn.)

## Ointment for skin disease – Tutthadi Lepa

The mixture of the below mentioned drugs constitute an ointment for the cure of chronic skin diseases :

- Tuttha – Copper Sulphate,
- Vidanga (Embelia ribes Burm. F.)
- varieties of Maricha (Piper nigrum Linn.),
- Kushta (Saussurea lappa),
- Lodhra (Symplocos racemosa) along with
- Manashila – Realgar [12]


**Skin Ointments :**
रसाञ्जनं सप्रपुन्नाडबीजं युक्तं कपित्थस्य रसेन लेपः|
करञ्जबीजैडगजं सकुष्ठं गोमूत्रपिष्टं च परः प्रदेहः||१३||

**Skin ointment :**
**Rasanjanadi Lepa** – Rasanjana (concentrated aqueous extract from Berberis aristata DC.) along with the seeds of Prapunnata (Cassia tora Linn.) mixed with juice of Kapittha (Feronia limonia) constitutes a skin ointment.

**Karanjadi Lepa** – Seeds of Karanja (Pongamia pinnata), Edagaja (Cassia tora) along with Kushta (Saussurea lappa), pounded with cow's urine constitute an ointment par excellence for skin diseases. [13]

उभे हरिद्रे कुटजस्य बीजं करञ्जबीजं सुमनःप्रवालान्|
त्वचं समध्यां हयमारकस्य लेपं तिलक्षारयुतं विदध्यात्||१४||

**Haridradi Lepa** – Combination of the below mentioned drugs is also used as an ointment for skin diseases –

- both types of Haridra (Haridra – turmeric and Daru Haridra – Tree turmeric),
- seeds of Kutaja – Connessi (Holarrhena antidysenterica Wall.) and
- Karanja (Pongamia pinnata),
- tender leaves of Sumanas (Jasminum officinale),
- bark along with the pith of Hayamaraka (Nerium indicum) mixed with
- the ash of Tila – Sesame (Sesamum indicum) [14]


मनःशिला त्वक् कुटजात् सकुष्ठात् सलोमशः सैडगजः करञ्जः|
ग्रन्थिश्च भौर्जः करवीरमूलं चूर्णानि साध्यानि तुषोदकेन||१५||
पलाशनिर्दाहरसेन चापि कर्षोद्धृतान्याढकसम्मितेन|
दर्वीप्रलेपं प्रवदन्ति लेपमेतं परं कुष्ठनिसूदनाय||१६||

**Manashiladi Lepa** – 1 karsha (12 grams) of the powders of each of the above said herbs should be taken –

- Manashila – Realgar,
- Bark of Kutaja – Connessi (Holarrhena antidysenterica Wall.) along with that of Kushta (Saussurea lappa),
- Lomasha – Ferri–sulphas, Edagaja (Cassia tora Linn.),
- Karanja (Pongamia pinnata),
- node of Bhurja (Betula utilis D. Don.), and
- root of Karavira (Nerium indicum Mill.)

All the above said powders should be boiled on mild heat mixed in 1 adhaka each of (3.072 kg) of tushodaka and juice extracted by burning Palasa (Butea monosperma Lam.). When the contents gain semi solid consistency the vessel shall be removed from the fire. This preparation is called darvi pralepa. This paste is said to be the most useful in eradicating chronic skin diseases when applied over them. [15–16]

## Chaturanguladi / Aragwadhadi Lepa

पर्णानि पिष्ट्वा चतुरङ्गुलस्य तक्रेण पर्णान्यथ काकमाच्याः|
तैलाक्तगात्रस्य नरस्य कुष्ठान्युद्वर्तयेदश्वहनच्छदैश्च||१७||

Equal quantities of the leaves of Chaturangula (Cassia fistula), Kakamachi (Solanum nigrum Linn.) and Ashvahana (Nerium indicum Mill.) should be taken. These should be collectively ground with buttermilk and applied as an ingredient on the parts of the body affected by skin diseases. This paste shall be applied only after applying the oil to the body. This paste destroys the skin disorders. [17]

## Vata balancing creams and ointments :

आनूपमत्स्यामिषवेसवारैरुष्णैः प्रदेहः पवनापहः स्यात्|
स्नेहैश्चतुर्भिर्दशमूलमिश्रैर्गन्धौषधैश्चानिलहः प्रदेहः||१९||
तक्रेण युक्तं यवचूर्णमुष्णं सक्षारमर्तिं जठरे निहन्यात्|
कुष्ठं शताह्वां सवचां यवानां चूर्णं सतैलाम्लमुशन्ति वाते||२०||

## Koladi Lepa / KolaKulathadi Churna :

Powder should be prepared using the below mentioned herbs :

- Kola (Ziziphus jujuba Lam.),
- Kulattha – Horse gram (Dolichos biflorus Linn.),
- Suradaru – Devadaru – (Cedrus deodara),
- Rasna (Vanda roxburghii / Pluchea lanceolata),
- Masha – Black gram (Phaseolus radiatus L.),
- Atasi (Linum usitatissimum Linn.)
- Taila phala – mustard, castor seeds, sesame etc. oil yielding seeds
- Kushta – Saussurea lappa
- Vacha – Acorus calamus
- Shatahva – Indian Dill – Anethum sowa
- Yava – Barley – Hordeum vulgare.

The powder prepared with the above said herbs shall be soured by mixing it in kanji (sour and fermented liquid) or vinegar. This paste should be applied warmly. It constitutes a good ointment for those suffering from Vata / vata disorders. [18]

## Other vata mitigating ointments / anointments

The Veshavara prepared with the meat of marshy animals and birds and equal quantity of meat of fish should be applied warm as an ointment / anointment for those suffering from disorders caused due to aggravated vata. This would alleviate pain and reduce pain associated with vata disorders. [19]

The ointment made of the aromatic drugs mixed up with the Dashamula and four types of fat (ghee, oil, fat and marrow) is also useful for the cure of vitiated Vata and vata disorders. [19]

## Udarashula Nashaka Lepa

Powder of Yava – Barley (Hordeum vulgare) and yava kshara (alkali of barley plant / barley) shall be mixed and ground in buttermilk. The contents are made warm and applied over the abdomen. This paste / anointment eradicates abdominal pain. [20]

## Vatahara / Vata Vyadhihara Lepa

Kushta (Saussurea lappa), Shatahva (Foeniculum vulgare Mill.), Vacha (Acorus calamus Linn.), and powder of Yava – Barley (Hordeum vulgare) should be ground in made sour by grinding them in kanji (sour and fermented liquid / vinegar). This paste should be mixed with sesame oil, made warm and applied on the body / parts of the body of the patient afflicted by aggravated vata. This is a good remedy for vata disorders. [20]

## Creams for gout (Vatarakta)

उभे शताह्वे मधुकं मधूकं बलां प्रियालं च कशेरुकं च।
घृतं विदारीं च सितोपलां च कुर्यात् प्रदेहं पवने सरक्ते॥२१॥

Paste prepared with both types of Shatahva (Foeniculum vulgare Mill.), Madhuka (Glycyrrhiza glabra Linn.), Madhuka (Madhuca indica I. F. Gmel.), Bala (Sida cordifolia Linn.), Priyala (Buchanania lanzan), Kasheruka (Scirpus grossus), ghee, Vidari (Ipomoea paniculata / Pueraria tuberosa) and Sugar forms an useful anointment / ointment in cases of vatarakta (gout). [21]

## Vataraktaja Vedanahara Lepa

रास्ना गुडूची मधुकं बले द्वे सजीवकं सर्षभकं पयश्च।
घृतं च सिद्धं मधुशेषयुक्तं रक्तानिलार्तिं प्रणुदेत् प्रदेहः॥२२॥

Equal quantity of the powders of the below mentioned herbs shall be taken –

- Rasna (Vanda roxburghii / Pluchea lanceolata),
- Guduchi (Tinospora cordifolia Willd.),
- Madhuka (Glycyrrhiza glabra Linn.),
- two types of Bala (Sida cordifolia) along with
- Jivaka – (Malaxis acuminata / Microstylis wallichii) / Root tuber of Pueraria tuberosa (Official substitute)
- Rishabhaka – (Malaxis muscifera) / Root tuber of Pueraria tuberosa (Official substitute)

Powders of all these herbs shall be mixed with 4 times ghee and 16 times cow's milk and boiled / processed. When the milk evaporates and only ghee is left over, wax is added and mixed thoroughly. When applied, this paste / anointment would help in eradicating the pain arising from / associated with vatarakta (gout). [22]

## Godhumadi Lepa / Vataraktahara Lepa

वाते सरक्ते सघृतं प्रदेहो गोधूमचूर्णं छगलीपयश्च।२३।

In Vatarakta (gout), the ointment made of ghee, the powder of Godhuma – wheat and goat's milk are prescribed. [23]

नतोत्पलं चन्दनकुष्ठयुक्तं शिरोरुजायां सघृतं प्रदेहः॥२३॥
प्रपौण्डरीकं सुरदारु कुष्ठं यष्ट्याह्वमेला कमलोत्पले च।
शिरोरुजायां सघृतः प्रदेहो लोहैरकापद्मकचोरकैश्च॥२४॥

## Creams for headache :

Nata (Valeriana wallichii), Utpala (Nymphaea alba), Chandana (Sandalwood – Santalum album) and Kushta

(Saussurea lappa) – these drugs mixed up with ghee constitute an unguentum useful for headache.

The paste of the below mentioned drugs mixed with ghee and applied on head forms another unguentum for those having headache –

- Prapanundarika (Nymphaea lotus Linn. red variety),
- Suradaru (Cedrus deodara),
- Kushta (Saussurea lappa),
- Yashtyahra (Glycyrrhiza glabra Linn.),
- Ela (Elettaria cardamomum Maton),
- Kamala (Nelumbo nucifera Gaertn.),
- Utpala (Nymphaea alba),
- Loha (Aquilaria agallocha Roxb.),
- Eraka (Typha angustifolia Linn.),
- Padmaka (Prunus cerasoides D. Don.),
- Choraka (Angelica glauca) [24]


## Cream for chest pain

रास्ना हरिद्रे नलदं शताह्वे द्वे देवदारूणि सितोपला च।
जीवन्तिमूलं सघृतं सतैलमालेपनं पार्श्वरुजासु कोष्णम्||२५||

The paste of the below mentioned drugs mixed well with ghee and oil, slightly warmed up and applied, makes a good ointment for chest / flank (sides of the chest) pain. The drugs used herein are

- Rasna (Pluchea lanceolata Oliver & Hiern),
- Haridra (turmeric – Curcuma longa),
- Daruharidra (Berberis aristata DC.),
- Nalada (Nardostachys jatamansi DC.),
- two varieties of Shatahva (Foeniculum vulgare Mill. and Foeniculum capillaecum),
- two varieties of Devadaru (Cedrus deodara Loud.),
- Sugar,
- root of Jivanti (Leptadenia reticulata) [25]


## Creams for burning sensation

शैवाल पद्मोत्पल वेत्रतुङ्ग प्रपौण्डरीकाण्यमृणाल लोध्रम्।
प्रियङ्गुकालेयक चन्दनानि निर्वापणः स्यात् सघृतः प्रदेहः||२६||

## Creams for burning sensation

The below mentioned herbs are ground together to prepare their paste. This paste shall be mixed with ghee and applied in the form of ointment to relieve burning sensation. The drugs used herein are –

- Shaivala (Vallisneria spiralis),
- Padma – Lotus (Nelumbo nucifera),
- Utpala (Nymphaea alba),
- Vetra (Salix caprea),
- Tunga (Calophyllum inophyllum),
- Prapaundarika (Nymphaea lotus) – red variety),

- Amrunala (Vetiveria zizanioides Nash),
- Lodhra (Symplocos racemosa),
- Priyangu (Callicara macrophylla),
- Kaleyaka (Santalum flavum),
- Chandana (Sandalwood – Santalum album), [26]


सितालतावेतसपद्मकानि यष्ट्याह्वमैन्द्री नलिनानि दूर्वा|
यवासमूलं कुशकाशयोश्च निर्वापणः स्याज्जलमेरका च||२७||
The ointment prepared with the below mentioned herbs relieves burning sensation

- Sugar,
- Lata (Rubia cordifolia Linn.),
- Vetasa (Salix caprea Linn.),
- Padmaka (Prunus cerasoides D. Don.),
- Yashtyahva (Glycyrrhiza glabra Linn.),
- Aindri (Citrullus colocynthis Lehrad.),
- Nalina (Nelumbo nucifera Gaertn.)
- Durva (Cynodon dactylon),
- root of Yavasa (Alhagi pseudalhagi),
- Kusha (Desmostachya bipinnata),
- Kasa (Saccharum spontaneum Linn.),
- Jala (Pavonia odorata Willd.), and
- Eraka (Typha angustifolia Linn.) [27]


## Cream for toxic conditions

शैलेयमेलागुरुणी सकुष्ठे चण्डा नतं त्वक् सुरदारु रास्ना|
शीतं निहन्यादचिरात् प्रदेहो विषं शिरीषस्तु ससिन्धुवारः||२८||
शिरीषलामज्जकहेमलोधैस्त्वग्दोषसंस्वेदहरः प्रघर्षः|
पत्राम्बुलोध्राभयचन्दनानि शरीरदौर्गन्ध्यहरः प्रदेहः||२९||

## Cream for cold sensation

The ointment prepared with the paste of the below mentioned herbs instantaneously relieves cold sensation –

- Shaileya (Parmelia perlata),
- Ela (Elettaria cardamomum Maton),
- Aguru (Aquilaria agallocha Roxb.),
- Kushta (Saussurea lappa), Chanda,
- Nata (Valeriana wallichii),
- Tvak (Cinnamomum zeylanicum Blume.),
- Suradaru (Cedrus deodara),
- Rasna (Vanda roxburghii / Pluchea lanceolata)


## Cream for toxic conditions

Cream or anointment prepared with Shirisha (Albizia lebbeck Benth.) along with Sindhuvara (Vitex negundo) alleviates toxic conditions. [28]

## Cream to relieve excess sweating
The paste of the below mentioned herbs when applied as ointment or their powder rubbed over the skin / afflicted part of the body, alleviates skin diseases and reduces sweating. The herbs used herein are –

- Shirisha (Albizia lebbeck Benth),
- Lamajjaka (Cymbopogon jwarancusa Schult.),
- Hema (Mesua ferrea) and
- Lodhra (Symplocos racemosa)

## Cream for body odour
The ointment prepared from the below mentioned herbs removes bad smell from the body
Patra – Cinnamomum tamala,
Ambu – Pavonia odorata,
Lodhra – Symplocos racemosa,
Abhaya – Terminalia chebula,
Chandana – Sandalwood – Santalum album

तत्र श्लोकः–
इहात्रिजः सिद्धतमानुवाच द्वात्रिंशतं सिद्धमहर्षिपूज्यः|
चूर्णप्रदेहान् विविधामयघ्नानारग्वधीये जगतो हितार्थम्||३०||
Thus, for the sake of the well–being of all, Lord Atreya respected by the Siddhas and Maharishis (great sages) expounded in the chapter on Aragvadheeya – 32 types of most efficacious powders and pradehas useful in different diseases.

इत्यग्निवेशकृते तन्त्रे चरकप्रतिसंस्कृते श्लोकस्थाने आरग्वधीयो नाम तृतीयोऽध्यायः||३||
Here ends the third chapter of the Sutrasthana of Agnivesha's work as redacted by Charaka.

# 4

# Sutrasthana Chapter 4 Shad Virechana Shatashriteeyam

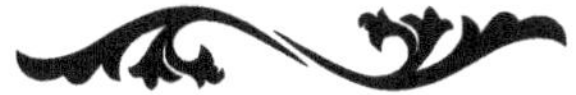

The 4th Chapter of Charak Samhita deals with 50 different groups of 10 herbs each with common action. It also deals with five basic Ayurvedic dosage forms like Swarasa (juice extract), Kalka (paste), Kashaya (decoction) etc.

अथातः षड्विरेचनशताश्रितीयमध्यायं व्याख्यास्यामः||१||

इति ह स्माह भगवानात्रेयः||२||

इह खलु षड् विरेचनशतानि भवन्ति, षड् विरेचनाश्रयाः, पञ्च कषाययोनयः, पञ्चविधं कषायकल्पनं, पञ्चाशन्महाकषायाः, पञ्च कषायशतानि, इति सङ्ग्रहः||३||

There are 600 purgatives:

- Six different parts of the plant useful for purgation (Virechana Ashraya) (Virechana means purgation treatment, it is one among Panchakarma treatments).
- Five varieties of drugs for the preparation of decoction (Kashaya).
- Five basic dosage forms.
- Fifty important decoctions.
- And five hundred decoctions. This is, in brief, the subject matter of this chapter. [3]

षड् विरेचनशतानि, इति यदुक्तं तदिह सङ्ग्रहेणोदाहृत्य विस्तरेण कल्पोपनिषदि व्याख्यास्यामः; (तत्र) त्रयस्त्रिंशद्योगशतं प्रणीतं फलेषु, एकोनचत्वारिंशज्जीमूतेषु योगाः, पञ्चचत्वारिंशदिक्ष्वाकुषु, धामार्गवः षष्टिधा भवति योगयुक्तः, कुटजस्त्वष्टादशधा योगमेति, कृतवेधनं षष्टिधा भवति योगयुक्तं, श्यामात्रिवृद्योगशतं प्रणीतं दशापरे चात्र भवन्ति योगाः, चतुरङ्गुलो द्वादशधा योगमेति, लोध्रं विधौ षोडशयोगयुक्तं, महावृक्षो भवति विंशतियोगयुक्तः, एकोनचत्वारिंशत् सप्तलाशङ्खिन्योर्योगाः, अष्टचत्वारिंशद्दन्तीद्रवन्त्योः, इति षड्विरेचनशतानि||४||

## 600 Virechana formulations

The number of purgation formulations and the herb from which they are prepared are enlisted below:

Madana Phala (Randia dumetorum Lam.) - 133

Jimuta (Luffa echinata Roxb.) - 39

Ikhsvaku (Lagenaria siceraria Standl.)- 45

Dhamargava (Luffa cylindrica M. Roem.)- 60

Kutaja – Connessi (Holarrhena antidysenterica Wall.) - 18

Kritavedhana (Luffa acutangula Roxb.) - 60

Black variety of Trivrit (Operculina turpethum R. B.) - 110

Chaturangula (Cassia fistula Linn.) - 12

Lodhra (Symplocos racemosa) - 16
Mahavruksha (Euphorbia neriifolia Linn.) - 20
Saptala (Acacia concinna DC.) and Shankini (Canscora decussate) - 39
Danti (Baliospermum montanum Muell-Arg.) and Dravanti (Jatropha glandulifera Roxb.) - 48
These are the six hundred varieties of purgatives including emetics. [4]

षड् विरेचनाश्रया इति क्षीरमूलत्वक्पत्रपुष्पफलानीति||५||
पञ्च कषाययोनय इति मधुरकषायोऽम्लकषायः कटुकषायस्तिक्तकषायः कषायकषायश्चेति तन्त्रे सञ्ज्ञा||६||

The six different parts of the plant useful for purgation are latex, root, bark, leaves, flowers and fruits. [5]. Five varieties of decoctions as found in the work are sweet, sour, pungent, bitter and astringent. [6].

**Five types of basic formulations – Pancha Vidha Kashaya Kalpana**
पञ्चविधं कषायकल्पनमिति तद्यथा- स्वरसः, कल्कः, शृतः, शीतः, फाण्टः, कषाय इति|
Five basic dosage forms of Ayurveda are –
Swarasa – juice extract
Kalka – paste
Shruta – Kashaya - astringent – water decoction
Sheeta – cold infusion
Fanta – Hot infusion.

**Definition of Swarasa – juice extract:**
यन्त्रनिष्पीडिताद्रव्यादसः स्वरस उच्यते |
Juice extracted from a drug pressed by a machine is known as Svarasa;

**Definition of Kalka – paste**
यः पिण्डो रसपिष्टानां स कल्कः परिकीर्तितः ||
When a fresh herb is converted into paste form, with the juice intact, in a spherical shape, it is called as Kalka.

**Definition of Kashaya**
वह्नौ तु क्वथितं द्रव्यं शृतमाहुश्चिकित्सकाः |
**Shruta** - Kashayam or herbal decoction of herb – Medicine prepared by boiling a drug on fire is called Shruta (Kashaya)

**Definition of Sheeta – Cold infusion**
द्रव्यादापोत्थितात्तोये प्रतप्ते निशि संस्थितात् ||
कषायो योऽभिनिर्याति स शीतः समुदाहृतः |
**Sheeta** - cold infusion – cold infusion prepared by putting the coarsely ground drug in boiled water and preserved over night is known as Sheeta;

**Definition of Fanta – Hot infusion:**
क्षिप्त्वोष्णतोये मृदितं तत् फाण्टं परिकीर्तितम् ||
When a medicine is prepared by putting the drug in boiled water and then squeezed, the resultant filtrate is known as Phanta or hot infusion.

तेषां यथापूर्वं बलाधिक्यम्; अतः कषायकल्पना व्याध्यातुरबलापेक्षिणी; न त्वेवं खलु सर्वाणि सर्वत्रोपयोगीनि भवन्ति||७||
Among these five, Phanta is most light to digest and has least strength and Swarasa is hardest to digest and is the

strongest. These preparations should be prescribed with due regard to the strength of the patient and seriousness of the disease. All these preparations are not equally useful in all cases. [7]

**Panchashat Mahakashaya – 50 main decoctions / group of herbs**

'पञ्चाशन्महाकषाया' इति यदुक्तं तदनुव्याख्यास्यामः; तद्यथा- जीवनीयो बृंहणीयो लेखनीयो भेदनीयः सन्धानीयो दीपनीय इति षट्कः कषायवर्गः; बल्यो वर्ण्यः कण्ठ्यो हृद्य इति चतुष्कः कषायवर्गः; तृप्तिघ्नोऽर्शोघ्नः कुष्ठघ्नः कण्डूघ्नः क्रिमिघ्नो विषघ्न इति षट्कः कषायवर्गः; स्तन्यजननः स्तन्यशोधनः शुक्रजननः शुक्रशोधन इति चतुष्कः कषायवर्गः; स्नेहोपगः स्वेदोपगो वमनोपगो विरेचनोपग आस्थापनोपगोऽनुवासनोपगः शिरोविरेचनोपग इति सप्तकः कषायवर्गः; छर्दिनिग्रहणस्तृष्णानिग्रहणो हिक्कानिग्रहण इति त्रिकः कषायवर्गः; पुरीषसङ्ग्रहणीयः पुरीषविरजनीयो मूत्रसङ्ग्रहणीयो मूत्रविरजनीयो मूत्रविरेचनीय इति पञ्चकः कषायवर्गः; कासहरः श्वासहरः शोथहरो ज्वरहरः श्रमहर इति पञ्चकः कषायवर्गः; दाहप्रशमनः शीतप्रशमन उदर्दप्रशमनोऽङ्गमर्दप्रशमनः शूलप्रशमन इति पञ्चकः कषायवर्गः; शोणितस्थापनो वेदनास्थापनः सञ्ज्ञास्थापनः प्रजास्थापनो वयःस्थापन इति पञ्चकः कषायवर्गः; इति पञ्चाशन्महाकषाया महतां च कषायाणां लक्षणोदाहरणार्थं व्याख्याता भवन्ति| तेषामेकैकस्मिन् महाकषाये दश दशावयविकान् कषायाननुव्याख्यास्यामः; तान्येव पञ्च कषायशतानि भवन्ति||८||

Now we shall expound the 50 important varieties of de-coctives mentioned before.

**First six are –**
Jeevaneeya – Elivening, Invigorating
Bruhmaneeya – Nourishing, increasing weight
Lekhaneeya – Scraping, decreasing weight
Bhedaneeya – Cathertics, piercing deep
Sandhaneeya – wound healing and bone healing
Deepaneeya – improving digestion strength

**Next four are –**
Balya – improving strength
Varnya – improving skin complexion
Kanthya – improving quality of voice
Hrudya – improving heart strength

**Next six are –**
Truptighna – relieving pseudo-satiation
Arshoghna – curing piles
Kushtaghna – relieving skin diseases
Kandughna – relieving itching sensation
Krimighna – relieving worm infestation
Vishaghna – anti toxic

**Next four are –**
Stanyajanana – improving breast milk
Stanyashodhana – cleansing and detoxifying breast milk
Shukrajanana -improving quality of semen and ovum
Shukrashodhana – cleansing and detoxifying semen and ovum

**Next seven are –**
Snehopaga – adjuvants of Snehana (oleation treatment)
Svedopaga -adjuvants of Swedana (sweating treatment)

Vamanopaga – adjuvant to Vamana (vomiting therapy)
Virechanopaga – adjuvant to Virechana (purgation therapy)
Asthapanopaga – adjuvant to Kashaya Basti – decoction enema
Anuvasanopaga -adjuvant to Snehabasti – oil enema
ShiroVirechanopaga – adjuvants useful in Nasya treatment

**Next three are –**
Chardi Nigrahana – relieving vomiting
Trushna Nigrahana – relieving thirst
Hikka Nigrahana – relieving hiccups

**Next five are –**
Purisha Sangrahaneeya – bowel binders, which helps to improve the bulk of stools
Purisha Virajaneeya – which helps to bring back proper colour of stools
Mutra Sangrahaneeya – which helps to restore normal quantity of urine
Mutra Virajaneeya -which helps to restore proper colour of urine
Mutra Virechaneeya – which helps to cleanse urine (and bladder)

**Next 5 are –**
Kasahara – relieving cough, cold
Shwasahara – relieving asthma, difficulty in breathing
Shothahara – relieving inflammation
Jwarahara – relieving fever
Shramahara – relieving tiredness

**Next 5 are –**
Daha Prashamana – relieving burning sensation
Sheeta Prashamana – relieving cold sensation
Udarda Prashamana – relieving allergic skin rashes
Angamarda Prashamana – relieving body pain
Shula Prashamana -relieving abdominal colic pain

**Next 5 are –**
Shonitasthapana – stopping bleeding, restoring proper quantity of blood
Vedanasthapana – relieving pain
Sanjnasthapana – restoring consciousness
Prajasthapana – procreative, useful in begetting child
Vayaha Sthapana -rejuvenating, anti aging.

**1. Jeevaneeya Gana – Enlivening, anti aging group of herbs**
तद्यथा- जीवकर्षभकौ मेदा महामेदा काकोली क्षीरकाकोली मुद्गपर्णीमाषपर्ण्यौ जीवन्ती
मधुकमिति दशमानि जीवनीयानि भवन्ति (१),

**1. Jeevaneeya Gana – Enlivening, anti ageing group of herbs**
Jeevaka – (Malaxis acuminata / Microstylis wallichii) / Root tuber of Pueraria tuberosa (Official substitute)
Rishabhaka – (Malaxis muscifera) / Root tuber of Pueraria tuberosa (Official substitute)
Meda – Polygonatum cirrhifolium
Mahameda – Polygonatum verticillatum

Kakoli – Roscoea purpurea / Root of Withania somnifera (Official substitute)
Kshira Kakoli – (Lilium polyphyllum) / Root of Withania somnifera (Official substitute)
Mudgaparni – Phaseolus trilobus,
Mashaparni – Teramnus labialis,
Jivanti – Leptadenia reticulata and
Madhuka– Licorice – Glycyrrhiza glabra

## 2. Bruhmaneeya Gana – Nourishing, increasing weight

क्षीरिणी राजक्षवकाश्वगन्धा काकोली क्षीरकाकोली वाट्यायनी भद्रौदनी भारद्वाजी
पयस्यर्ष्यगन्धा इति दशेमानि बृंहणीयानि भवन्ति (२)

## 2. Bruhmaneeya Gana – Nourishing, increasing weight

Ksheerini – Mimusops hexandra Roxb.
Rajakshavaka – Euphorbia microphylla,
**Ashwagandha** – Winter Cherry / Indian ginseng (root) – Withania somnifera,
Kakoli – Fritillaria roylei / Roscoea purpurea
Ksheerakakoli – Roscoea purpurea / Lilium polyphyllum,
Vatyayani – Country mallow (root) – Sida cordifolia,
Bhadraudani (Sida cordifolia Linn.),
Bharadvaji – Thespesia lampas,
Payasya – Ipomoea paniculata and
Rushyagandha (Withania coagulans)

## 3. Lekhaneeya Gana – Scraping, decreasing weight

मुस्त कुष्ठ हरिद्रा दारुहरिद्रा वचातिविषा कटुरोहिणी चित्रक चिरबिल्व हैमवत्य इति दशेमानि लेखनीयानि भवन्ति (३)

## 3. Lekhaneeya Gana – Scraping, decreasing weight

Musta (Cyperus rotundus Linn.),
Kushta – Saussurea lappa,
Haridra (turmeric – Curcuma longa),
Daru Haridra – Tree Turmeric (stem) – Berberis aristata,
Vacha (Acorus calamus Linn.),
Ativisa (Aconitum heterophyllum Wall.),
Katurohini – Picrorhiza kurroa,
Chitraka – Leadword – Plumbago zeylanica,
Chirabilva – Holoptelea integrifolia and
Haimavati – Iris versicolor

## 4. Bhedaneeya Kashaya – Cathertics, Piercing deep

सुवहाकार्ोरुबुकाग्निमुखी चित्रा चित्रक चिरबिल्व शङ्खिनी शकुलादनी स्वर्णक्षीरिण्य इति दशेमानि भेदनीयानि भवन्ति (४)

### 4. Bhedaneeya Kashaya – Cathartics, Piercing deep

Suvaha (Operculina turpethum R.B.),
Arka – Calotropis gigantea,
Urubuka – Castor – Ricinus communis
Agnimukhi – Gloriosa superba,
Chitra – Baliospermum montanum,
Chitraka – Leadwort – Plumbago zeylanica,

Chirabilva – Holoptelea integrifolia,
Shankini – Canscora decussata,
Shakuladani – Picrorhiza kurroa and
Svarnaksheerini – Argemone mexicana Linn

## 5. Sandhaneeya – wound healing and bone healing
मधुक मधुपर्णी पृश्निपर्ण्यम्बष्ठकी समङ्गा मोचरस धातकी लोध्र प्रियङ्गु कट्फलानीति दशेमानि सन्धानीयानि भवन्ति (५)

## 5. Sandhaneeya – wound healing and bone healing
Madhuka – Licorice (Glycyrrhiza glabra Linn.),
Madhuparni – Indian tinospora (stem) – Tinospora cordifolia,
Prishnaparni – Uraria picta,
Ambasthaki (Cissampelos pareira Linn.),
Samanga – Rubia cordifolia,
Mocharasa (Salmania malabarica Schott & Endl.),
Dhataki – Woodfordia fruticosa,
Lodhra (Symplocos racemosa),
Priyangu (Callicarpa macrophylla) and
Katphala – Myrica nagi

## 6. Deepaneeya – improving digestion strength
पिप्पली पिप्पलीमूल चव्य चित्रक शृङ्गवेराम्लवेतस मरिचाजमोदा भल्लातकास्थि हिङ्गुनिर्यासा इति दशेमानि दीपनीयानि भवन्ति (६)
इति षट्कः कषायवर्गः||९||

## 6. Deepaneeya – improving digestion strength
Pippali – Long pepper fruit – Piper longum,
Pippalimoola – Long pepper root – Piper longum,
Chavya (Piper chaba Hunter.),
Chitraka – Leadwort – Plumbago zeylanica,
Shringavera – Ginger – Zingiber officinale,
Amlavetasa – Garcinia pedunculata Roxb. / Rheum emodi Wall.,
Maricha – Black pepper fruit – Piper nigrum,
Ajamoda – Celery fruit – Trachyspermum roxburghianum,
stone of Bhallataka (Semecarpus anacardium Linn.) and
Hingu Niryasa – Asa foetida

## 7. Balya Gana – improving strength
ऐन्द्र्यृषभ्यतिरसर्ष्यप्रोक्ता पयस्याश्वगन्धा स्थिरा रोहिणी बलातिबला इति दशेमानि बल्यानि भवन्ति (७)

## 7. Balya Gana – improving strength
Aindri (Citrullus colocynthis Schrad.),
Rishabhi – Rishabhaka – Manilkara hexandra
Atirasa – Asparagus root – Asparagus racemosus,
Rishyaprokta – Teramnus labialis,
Payasya – Ipomoeapaniculata,
Ashwagandha – Winter Cherry / Indian ginseng (root) – Withania somnifera,
Sthira – Desmodium gangeticum,
Katukarohini – Picrorhiza kurroa,

Bala – Country mallow (root) – Sida cordifolia,
Atibala – Abutilon indicum

## 8. Varnya Gana – improving skin complexion
चन्दन तुङ्ग पद्मकोशीर मधुक मञ्जिष्ठा सारिवा पयस्या सितालता इति दशेमानि वर्ण्यानि भवन्ति (८)

## 8. Varnya Gana – improving skin complexion
Chandana (Santalum album Linn.),
Tunga (Calophyllum inophyllum),
Padmaka – Prunus cerasoides,
Ushira – Vetiver – Vetiveria zizanioides,
Madhuka– Licorice – Glycyrrhiza glabra,
Manjistha (Rubia cordifolia Linn.),
Sariva – Indian Sarsaparilla – Hemidesmus indicus,
Payasya – Ipomoeapaniculata,
Sita – white variety of Cynodon dactylon and
Lata (black variety of Cynodon dactylon Pers.)

## 9. Kanthya Gana – improving quality of voice
सारिवेक्षुमूल मधुक पिप्पली द्राक्षा विदारी कैटर्य हंसपादी बृहती कण्टकारिका इति दशेमानि कण्ठ्यानि भवन्ति (९)

## 9. Kanthya Gana – improving quality of voice
Sariva – Indian Sarsaparilla – Hemidesmus indicus,
Iksumula – Sugarcane root – Saccharum officinarum,
Madhuka– Licorice – Glycyrrhiza glabra,
Pippali – Long pepper fruit – Piper longum,
Darksha – Raisin – Vitis vinifera,
Vidari (Ipomoea paniculata / Pueraria tuberosa),
Kaitarya – Myrica nagi,
Hamsapadi – Adiantum lunulatum,
Brihati – Solanum indicum
Kantakarika – Solanum xanthocarpum – these ten drugs are useful for the throat.

## 10. Hrudya – improving heart strength
आम्राम्रातक लिकुच करमर्द वृक्षाम्लाम्लवेतस कुवल बदर दाडिम मातुलुङ्गानीति दशेमानि हृद्यानि भवन्ति (१०), इति चतुष्कः
कषायवर्गः||१०||

## 10. Hrudya – improving heart strength
Amra – mango – Mangifera indica,
Amrataka – Spondias pinnata,
Lakucha – Artocarpus lakoocha,
Karamarda – Carissa carandas,
Urksamla (Tamarindus indica Linn.),
Amlavetasa – Garcinia pedunculata Roxb. / Rheum emodi Wall.,
Kuvala – Zizyphus sativa,
Badara – Zizyphus jujuba,
Dadima – Pomegranate – Punica granatum,
Matulunga – Lemon variety – Citrus decumana / Citrus limon

## 11. Truptighna Gana- relieving pseudo-satiation

नागर चव्य चित्रक विडङ्ग मूर्वा गुडूची वचा मुस्त पिप्पली पटोलानीति दशेमानि तृप्तिघ्नानि भवन्ति (११)

## 11. Truptighna Gana- relieving pseudo-satiation

Nagara – Ginger (Zingiber officinale Rosc.),

Chavya (Piper chaba Hunter.),

Chitraka – Leadwort – Plumbago zeylanica,

Vidanga (Embelia ribes Burm f.),

Murva (Marsdenia tenacissima (Roxb.) / Clematis triloba Heyne ex Roth.),

Guduci (Tinospora cordifolia Miers.),

Vacha (Acorus calamus Linn.),

Musta (Cyperus rotundus),

Pippali – Long pepper fruit,

Patola – Pointed gourd (Trichosanthes cucumerina Linn.)

## 12. Arshoghna Gana- curing piles

कुटज बिल्व चित्रक नागरातिविषाभया धन्वयासक दारुहरिद्रा वचा चव्यानीति दशेमान्यर्शोघ्नानि भवन्ति (१२)

## 12. Arshoghna Gana- curing piles

Kutaja – Connessi (Holarrhena antidysenterica Wall.),

Bilva (Aegle marmelos Corr.),

Chitraka – Leadwort – Plumbago zeylanica,

Nagara (Zingiber officinale Rosc.),

Ativisa (Aconitum heterophyllum Wall.),

Abhaya (Terminalia chebula),

Dhanvayasaka (Fagonia cretica Linn.),

Daru Haridra – Tree Turmeric (stem) – Berberis aristata,

Vacha (Acorus calamus Linn.),

Chavya (Piper chaba Hunter.)

## 13. Kushtaghna Gana – relieving skin diseases

खदिराभयामलक हरिद्रारुष्कर सप्तपर्णारग्वध करवीर विडङ्ग जातीप्रवाला इति दशेमानि कुष्ठघ्नानि भवन्ति (१३)

## 13. Kushtaghna Gana – relieving skin diseases

Khadira (Acacia catechu Willd.),

Abhaya (Terminalia chebula),

Amalaka (Emblica officinalis Gaertn.),

Haridra (turmeric – Curcuma longa),

Arushkara (Semecarpus anacardium Linn. f.),

Saptaparna (Alstonia scholaris R, Br.),

Aragvadha (Cassia fistula),

Karavira (Nerium indicum Mill.),

Vidanga (Embelia ribes Brum. f.)

Jatipravala (tender shoots of Jasminum officinale Linn. var. grandiflorum Bailey.)

## 14. Kandughna Gana – relieving itching sensation

चन्दन नलद कृतमाल नक्तमाल निम्ब कुटज सर्षप मधुक दारुहरिद्रा मुस्तानीति दशेमानि कण्डूघ्नानि भवन्ति (१४)

## 14. Kandughna Gana – relieving itching sensation
Chandana – Sandalwood (Santalum album),
Nalada (Nardostachys jatamansi DC.),
Krtamala (Cassia fistula Linn.),
Naktamala – Karanja (Pongamia pinnata Merr.),
Nimba – Neem (Azadirachta indica),
Kutaja – Connessi (Holarrhena antidysenterica Wall.),
Sarshapa – Mustard – (Brassica nigra Koch.),
Madhuka– Licorice – Glycyrrhiza glabra,
Daru Haridra – Tree Turmeric (stem) – Berberis aristata
Musta (Cyperus rotundus)

## 15. Krimighna Gana – relieving worm infestation
अक्षीव मरिच गण्डीर केबुक विडङ्गनिर्गुण्डी किणिही श्वदंष्ट्रा वृषपर्णिकाखुपर्णिका इति दशेमानि क्रिमिघ्नानि भवन्ति (१५)

## 15. Krimighna Gana – relieving worm infestation
Aksheeva (Moringa oleifera Lam.),
Maricha – Black pepper fruit (Piper nigrum),
Gandira (Euphorbia antiquorum Linn.),
Kebuka (Costus speciosus)
Vidanga – False Black Pepper (Embelia ribes Burm. f.),
Nirgundi (Vitex negundo),
Kinihi (Achyranthes aspera Linn.),
Shwadamstra (Tribulus terrestris Linn.),
Vrsaparnika (a variety of Ipomoea reniformis Chois),
Akhuparnika (Ipomoea reniformis Chois)

## 16. Vishaghna Gana – anti toxic
हरिद्रा मञ्जिष्ठा सुवहा सूक्ष्मैला पालिन्दी चन्दन कतक शिरीष सिन्धुवार श्लेष्मातका इति दशेमानि विषघ्नानि भवन्ति (१६), इति षट्कः कषायवर्गः॥११॥
### 16. Vishaghna Gana – anti toxic
Haridra (turmeric – Curcuma longa),
Manjistha (Rubia cordifolia Linn.),
Suvaha– (Operculina turpethum),
Sukshma Ela – Cardamom (Elettaria cardamomum Maton.),
Palindi – (Ichnocarpus frutescens (Linn.) R.Br. / Operculina turpethum),
Chandana – Sandalwood (Santalum album),
Kathaka (Strychnos potatorum Linn. f.),
Shirisha (Albizia lebbeck Benth.),
Sindhuvara (Vitex negundo) and
Shleshmataka (Cordia dichotoma Forst. f.)

## 17. Stanyajanana – improving breast milk
वीरण शालिषष्टिकेक्षुवालिका दर्भ कुश काश गुन्द्रेत्कट कतृणमूलानीति दशेमानि स्तन्यजननानि भवन्ति (१७)

## 17. Stanyajanana – improving breast milk
Virana (Vetiveria zizanioides Nash.),

Shali – Rice (Oryza sativa Linn.),
Shastika (a variety of rice – Oryza sativa Linn.),
Ikhsuvalika (Asteracantha longifolia Nees),
Darbha (Desmostachya bipinnata Staff.),
Kusha (Desmostachya bipinnata),
Kasha (Saccharum spontaneum Linn.),
Gundra (Saccharum sara),
Itkata – Sesbania bispinosa and
Katruna (Cymbopogon schoenanthus Spreng.)

## 18. Stanyashodhana – cleansing and detoxifying breast milk

पाठा महौषध सुरदारु मुस्त मूर्वा गुडूची वत्सकफल किराततिक्तक कटुरोहिणी सारिवा इति दशेमानि स्तन्यशोधनानि भवन्ति (१८)

## 18. Stanyashodhana – cleansing and detoxifying breast milk

Patha (Cissampelos pareira Linn.),
Mahausadha – Ginger (Zingiber officinale Rosc.),
Suradaru (Cedrus deodara),
Musta (Cyperus rotundus),
Murva (Clematis triloba Heyne ex Roth.),
Guduchi (Tinospora cordifolia Miers.),
fruit of Vatsaka – Kutaja (Holarrhena antidysenterica Wall.),
Kiratatikta (Swertia chirata Buch-Ham.),
Katurohini – Picrorhiza kurroa and
Sariva – Indian Sarsaparilla – Hemidesmus indicus

## 19. Shukrajanana -improving quality of semen and ovum

जीवकर्षभक काकोली क्षीरकाकोली मुद्गपर्णी माषपर्णी मेदा वृद्धरुहा जटिला कुलिङ्गा इति दशेमानि शुक्रजननानि भवन्ति (१९)

## 19. Shukrajanana -improving quality of semen and ovum

Jeevaka – Malaxis acuminata
Rishabhaka – Manilkara hexandra
Kakoli – Fritillaria roylei
Kshira Kakoli – Roscoea purpurea / Lilium polyphyllum
Mudgaparni (Phaseolus trilobus Ait.),
Mashaparni – Teramnus labialis,
Meda – Polygonatum cirrhifolium,
Vriddharuha (Asparagus racemosusWilld.),
Jatila (Nardostachys jatamansi D C.),
Kulinga – Rhus acuminata

## 20. Shukrashodhana – cleansing and detoxifying semen and ovum

कुष्ठैलवालुक कट्फल समुद्रफेन कदम्बनिर्यासेक्षु काण्डेक्षिविक्षुरक वसुकोशीराणीति दशेमानि शुक्रशोधनानि भवन्ति (२०), इति चतुष्कः कषायवर्गः ||१२||

## 20. Shukrashodhana – cleansing and detoxifying semen and ovum

Kustha (Saussurea lappa C. B. Clarke.),
Elavaluka (Prunus cerasus Linn.),
Katphala – Myrica nagi,

Samudraphena (Internal-cell of Sepia officinalis.),
Gum of Kadamba (Anthocephalus indicus A. Rich.),
Ikshu – Sugarcane (Saccharum officinarum Linn.),
Kandeksu (Saccharum spontaneum Linn.),
Ikhsuraka (Asteracantha longifolia Nees.),
Vasuka (Indigofera enneaphylla Linn.),
Ushira – Vetiver – Vetiveria zizanioides

## 21. Snehopaga – adjuvants of Snehana (oleation treatment)

मृद्वीका मधुक मधुपर्णी मेदा विदारी काकोली क्षीरकाकोली जीवक जीवन्ती शालपर्ण्य इति दशेमानि स्नेहोपगानि भवन्ति (२१)

## 21. Snehopaga – adjuvants of Snehana (oleation treatment)

Mrudvika (Vitis vinifera Linn.),
Madhuka– Licorice – Glycyrrhiza glabra,
Madhuparni – Indian tinospora (stem) – Tinospora cordifolia,
Meda – Polygonatum cirrhifolium,
Vidari (Ipomoea paniculata / Pueraria tuberosa),
Kakoli – Fritillaria roylei,
Ksheerakakoli – Lilium polyphyllum,
Jivaka – Malaxis acuminata,
Jivanti – Leptadenia reticulata and
Shalaparni (Desmodium gangeticum D C.)

## 22. Svedopaga -adjuvants of Swedana (sweating treatment)

शोभाञ्जनकैरण्डार्क वृश्चीर पुनर्नवा यव तिल कुलत्थ माष बदराणीति दशेमानि स्वेदोपगानि भवन्ति (२२)

## 22. Svedopaga -adjuvants of Swedana (sweating treatment)

Shobhanjanaka Moringa seed (Moringa oleifera Lam.),
Erandaka – Castor (Ricinus communis Linn.),
Arka – Calotropis gigantea,
Vrischira (white variety of Boerhaavia diffusa Linn.),
Punarnava (red variety of Boerhaavia diffusa Linn.),
Yava – Barley (Hordeum vulgare),
Tila – Sesame (Sesamum indicum),
Kulattha (Dolichos biflorus Linn.),
Masha (Phaseolus mungo L.),
Badara – Zizyphus jujuba

## 23. Vamanopaga – adjuvant to Vamana (vomiting therapy)

मधु मधुक कोविदार कर्बुदार नीप विदुल बिम्बी शणपुष्पी सदापुष्पा प्रत्यक्पुष्पा इति दशेमानि वमनोपगानि भवन्ति (२३)

### 23. Vamanopaga – adjuvant to Vamana (vomiting therapy)

Madhu (honey),
Madhuka– Licorice – Glycyrrhiza glabra,
Kovidara (red variety of Bauhinia variegata Linn.),
Karbudara (white variety of Bauhinia variegata Linn.),
Neepa (Anthocephalus indicus A. Rich.),
Vidula (Barringtonia acutangula Gaertn.),

Bimbi (Coccinia indica W. & A.),
Shanapushpi (Crotalaria verrucosa Linn.),
Sadapushpa (Calotropis gigantea R. Br. Ait.),
Pratyakpushpa (Achyranthes aspera Linn.)

## 24. Virechanopaga – adjuvant to Virechana (purgation therapy)

द्राक्षा काश्मर्य परूषकाभयामलक बिभीतक कुवल बदर कर्कन्धु पीलूनीति दशमानि विरेचनोपगानि भवन्ति (२४)

## 24. Virechanopaga – adjuvant to Virechana (purgation therapy)

Draksha – Raisin – Vitis vinifera,
Kashmarya (Gmelina arborea Linn.),
Parushaka (Grewia asiatica Linn.),
Abhaya – Haritaki – Terminalia chebula,
Amalaka (Emblica officinalis Gaertn.),
Bibhitaka (Terminalia belerica Roxb.),
Kuvala – Zizyphus sativa,
Badara – Zizyphus jujuba,
Karkandhu (Zizyphus nummularia W. & A.),
Pilu (Salvadora persica Linn.)

## 25. Asthapanopaga – adjuvant to Kashaya Basti – decoction enema

त्रिवृद्बिल्व पिप्पली कुष्ठ सर्षप वचा वत्सकफल शतपुष्पा मधुक मदनफलानीति दशेमान्यास्थापनोपगानि भवन्ति (२५)

## 25. Asthapanopaga – adjuvant to Kashaya Basti – decoction enema

Trivrt (Operculina turpethum R. B.),
Bilva (Aegle marmelos Corr.),
Pippali – Long pepper fruit – Piper longum,
Kushta – Saussurea lappa,
Sarshapa (Brassica nigra Koch.),
Vacha (Acorus calamus Linn.),
Fruit of Vatsala (Holarrhena antidysenterica Wall.),
Shatapushpa (Foeniculum vulgare Mill.),
Madhuka– Licorice – Glycyrrhiza glabra,
fruits of Madanaphala (Randia dumetorum Lam.)

## 26. Anuvasanopaga -adjuvant to Snehabasti – oil enema

रास्ना सुरदारु बिल्व मदन शतपुष्पा वृश्चीर पुनर्नवा श्वदंष्ट्राग्निमन्थ श्योनाका इति दशमान्यनुवासनोपगानि भवन्ति (२६)

## 26. Anuvasanopaga -adjuvant to Snehabasti – oil enema

Rasna (Pluchea lanceolata Oliver & Hiern.),
Suradaru (Cedrus deodara),
Bilva (Aegle marmelos Corr.),
Madana (Randia dumetorum Lam.),
Shatapushpa (Foeniculum vulgare Mill.),
Vruscheera (white variety of Boerhaavia diffusa Linn.),
Punarnava (red variety of Boerhaavia diffusa Linn.),
Shvadamstra (Tribulus terrestris Linn.),
Agnimantha (Clerodendrum phlomidis Linn. f.),

Shyonaka (Oroxylum indicum Vent.)

## 27. Shiro Virechanopaga – Group of herbs useful in Nasya treatment (nasal drops)

ज्योतिष्मती क्षवक मरिच पिप्पली विडङ्ग शिग्रु सर्षपापामार्गतण्डुल श्वेतामहाश्वेता इति दशेमानि शिरोविरेचनोपगानि भवन्ति (२७), इति सप्तकः कषायवर्गः॥१३॥

## 27. Shiro Virechanopaga – Group of herbs useful in Nasya treatment (nasal drops)

Jyotishmati (Celastrus paniculatus Willd.),
Kshavaka (Centipeda minima A. Br. Et. Aschers.),
Maricha – Black pepper fruit – Piper nigrum,
Pippali – Long pepper fruit – Piper longum,
Vidanga – False Black Pepper (Embelia ribes Burm. f.),
Shigru – Moringa leaves (Moringa oleifera Lam.),
Sarshapa (Brassica nigra Koch.),
Seed of Apamarga (Achyranthes aspera Linn.),
Shveta (white variety of Clitoria ternatea Linn.),
Mahashveta (a variety of Clitoria ternatea Linn.).

## 28. Chardi Nigrahana – antiemetic – relieving vomiting

जम्ब्वाम्रपल्लव मातुलुङ्गाम्ल बदर दाडिम यव यष्टिकोशीर मृल्लाजा इति दशेमानि छर्दिनिग्रहणानि भवन्ति (२८)

## 28. Chardi Nigrahana – antiemetic – relieving vomiting

Jambu – Jamun (Syzygium cumini Skeels.),
Tender leaves of Amra – mango – Mangifera indica,
Matulunga – Lemon variety – Citrus decumana / Citrus limon,
Badara – Zizyphus jujuba of sour variety,
Dadima – Pomegranate – Punica granatum,
Yava – Barley (Hordeum vulgare),
Yashtika (Glycyrrhiza glabra Linn.),
Ushira – Vetiver – Vetiveria zizanioides,
Mrit (earth),
Laja (fried paddy).

## 29. Trushna Nigrahana – relieving thirst

नागर धन्वयवासक मुस्त पर्पटक चन्दन किराततिक्तक गुडूची ह्रीवेर धान्यक पटोलानीति दशेमानि तृष्णानिग्रहणानि भवन्ति (२९)

## 29. Trushna Nigrahana – relieving thirst

Nagara – Ginger (Zingiber officinale Rosc.),
Dhanvayasaka (Fagonia cretica Linn.),
Musta (Cyperus rotundus),
Parpataka (Fumaria parviflora Lam.),
Chandana – Sandalwood – Santalum album,
Kiratatikta (Swertia chirata Buch. – Ham.),
Guduchi (Tinospora cordifolia Miers.),
Hrivera (Pavonia odorata Willd.),
Dhanyaka (Coriandrum sativum Linn.),
Patola (Trichosanthes cucumerina Linn.)

### 30. Hikka Nigrahana Gana – herbs relieving hiccups
शटी पुष्करमूल बदरबीज कण्टकारिका बृहती वृक्षरुहाभया पिप्पली दुरालभाकुलीर शृङ्ग्य इति दशेमानि हिक्कानिग्रहणानि भवन्ति (३०),
इति त्रिकः कषायवर्गः ||१४||

### 30. Hikka Nigrahana Gana – herbs relieving hiccups
Shati (Hedychium spicatum Ham. ex Smith.),
Pushkaramula (Inula racemosa Hook. f.),
Stone of Badara – Zizyphus jujuba,
Kantakarika – Solanum xanthocarpum,
Brihati – Solanum indicum,
Vruksharuha (Dendrophthoe falcata Linn. f.),
Abhaya – Terminalia chebula,
Pippali – Long pepper fruit – Piper longum,
Duralabha (Fagonia cretica Linn.),
Kulirashrungi (Rhus succedanea Linn.)

### 31. Pureesha Sangrahaneeya – bowel binders, which helps to improve the bulk of stools
प्रियङ्ग्वनन्तामास्थि कट्वङ्ग लोध्र मोचरस समङ्गा धातकीपुष्प पद्मा पद्मकेशराणीति दशेमानि पुरीषसङ्ग्रहणीयानि भवन्ति (३१)

### 31. Pureesha Sangrahaneeya – bowel binders, which helps to improve the bulk of stools
Priyangu (Callicarpa macrophylla),
Ananta (Hemidesmus indicus R. B.),
Seed of Amra – Mango seed – Mangifera indica,
Katvanga (Oroxylum indicum Vent.),
Lodhra (Symplocos racemosa),
Mocharasa (Salmalia malabarica Schott & Endl.),
Samanga – Rubia cordifolia,
flower of Dhataki – Woodfordia fruticosa,
Padma – Lotus (Nelumbo nucifera),
Filaments of Padma – Lotus (Nelumbo nucifera)

### 32. Pureesha Virajaneeya – which helps to bring back proper colour of stools
जम्बु शल्लकीत्वक्कच्छुरा मधूक शाल्मली श्रीवेष्टक भृष्टमृत्पयस्योत्पल तिलकणा इति दशेमानि पुरीषविरजनीयानि भवन्ति (३२)

### 32. Pureesha Virajaneeya – which helps to bring back proper colour of stools
Jambu (Syzygium cumini Skeels.),
Bark of Shallaki (Boswellia serrata Roxb.),
Kacchura – Curcuma zedoaria,
Madhuka– Licorice – Glycyrrhiza glabra,
Shalmali (Salmalia malabarica Schott & Endl.),
Shriveshtaka (extract of Pinus roxburghii Sargent.),
fired earth (mud) – purified red ochre
Payasya – Ipomoeapaniculata,
Utpala (Nymphaea alba),
grains of Tila – Sesame seeds (Sesamum indicum)

### 33. Mutra Sangrahaneeya – which helps to restore normal quantity of urine – anti-diuretics

जम्ब्वाम्र प्लक्ष वट कपीतनोडुम्बराश्वत्थ भल्लातकाश्मन्तक सोमवल्का इति दशेमानि मूत्रसङ्ग्रहणीयानि भवन्ति (३३)

### 33. Mutra Sangrahaneeya – which helps to restore normal quantity of urine – anti-diuretics

Jambu (Syzygium cumini Skeels),
Amra – mango – Mangifera indica,
Plaksha (Ficus lacor Buch-Ham.),
Vata (Ficus benghalensis Linn.),
Kapeetana (Albizia lebbeck Benth.),
Udumbara (Ficus racemosa Linn.)
Ashvattha (Ficus religiosa Linn.),
Bhallataka (Semecarpus anacardium Linn.),
Ashmantaka (Bauhinia racemosa Lam.),
Somavalka (Acacia catechu Willd.).

### 34. Mutra Virajaneeya -which helps to restore proper colour of urine

पद्मोत्पल नलिन कुमुद सौगन्धिक पुण्डरीक शतपत्र मधुक प्रियङ्गु धातकीपुष्पाणीति दशेमानि मूत्रविरजनीयानि भवन्ति (३४)

### 34. Mutra Virajaneeya -which helps to restore proper colour of urine

Padma – Lotus (Nelumbo nucifera),
Utpala (Nymphaea alba),
Nalina (a variety of Nelumbo nucifera Gaertn.),
Kumuda (Nymphaea alba Linn.),
Saugandhika (?),
Pundarika (red variety of Nymphaea lotus Linn.),
Shatapatra (a variety of Nelumbo nucifera Gaertn.),
Madhuka– Licorice – Glycyrrhiza glabra,
Priyangu (Callicarpa macrophylla),
flowers of Dhataki (Woodfordia fruticosa Kurz.)

### 35. Mutra Virechaneeya – which helps to cleanse urine (and bladder)

वृक्षादनी श्वदंष्ट्रा वसुक वशिर पाषाणभेद दर्भ कुश काश गुन्द्रेत्कटमूलानीति दशेमानि मूत्रविरेचनीयानि भवन्ति (३५),
इति पञ्चकः कषायवर्गः||१५||

### 35. Mutra Virechaneeya – which helps to cleanse urine (and bladder)

Vrukshadani (Dendrophthoe falcata Linn. f.),
Shvadamstra (Tribulus terrestris Linn.),
Vasuka (Indigofera enneaphylla Linn.),
Vasira (Gynandropsis gynandra Briquet),
Pashanabheda (Bergenia ligulata Engl.),
Darbha (a variety of Desmostachya bipinnata Staff.),
Kusha (Desmostachya bipinnata)
Kasa (Saccharum spontaneum Linn.),
Gundra (Saccharum sara),
root of Itkata – Sesbania bispinosa.

### 36. Kasahara – relieving cough, cold

द्राक्षाभयामलक पिप्पली दुरालभा शृङ्गी कण्टकारिका वृश्चीर पुनर्नवा तामलक्य इति दशेमानि कासहराणि भवन्ति (३६)

## 36. Kasahara – relieving cough, cold

Darksha – Raisin – Vitis vinifera,

Abhaya – Terminalia chebula,

Amalaka (Emblica officinalis Gaertn.),

Pippali – Long pepper fruit – Piper longum,

Duralabha (Fagonia cretica Linn.),

Shrungi (Rhus succedanea Linn.),

Kantakarika – Solanum xanthocarpum,

Vrushchira (white variety of Boerhaavia diffusa Linn.),

Punarnava (red variety of Boerhaavia diffusa Linn.,

Tamalaki (Phyllanthus niruri Linn.)

## 37. Shwasahara – relieving asthma, difficulty in breathing

शटी पुष्करमूलाम्लवेतसैला हिङ्ग्वगुरु सुरसा तामलकी जीवन्ती चण्डा इति दशेमानि श्वासहराणि भवन्ति (३७)

## 37. Shwasahara – relieving asthma, difficulty in breathing

Shati (Hedychium spicatum Ham. ex Smith.),

Puskaramula (Inula racemosa Hook. f.),

Amlavetasa – Garcinia pedunculata Roxb. / Rheum emodi Wall.,

Ela (Elettaria cardamomum Maton),

Hingu – Asa foetida,

Aguru (Aquilaria agallocha Roxb.),

Surasa – Holy Basil (Ocimum sanctum Linn.),

Tamalaki (Phyllanthus niruri Linn.),

Jivanti – Leptadenia reticulata,

Chanda.

## 38. Shothahara – relieving inflammation

पाटलाग्निमन्थ श्योनाक बिल्व काश्मर्य कण्टकारिका बृहती शालपर्णी पृश्निपर्णी गोक्षुरका इति दशेमानि श्वयथुहराणि भवन्ति (३८)

## 38. Shothahara – relieving inflammation

Patala (Stereospermum suaveolens DC.),

Agnimantha (Clerodendrum phlomidis Linn. f.),

Shyonaka (Oroxylum indicum Vent.),

Bilva (Aegle marmelos Corr.),

Kashmarya (Gmelina arborea Linn.).,

Kantakarika – Solanum xanthocarpum,

Brihati – Solanum indicum,

Shalaparni (Desmodium gangeticum DC.),

Prishnaparni – Uraria picta,

Goksuraka (Tribulus terrestris Linn.)

## 39. Jwarahara – relieving fever

सारिवा शर्करा पाठा मञ्जिष्ठा द्राक्षा पीलु परूषकाभयामलक बिभीतकानीति दशेमानि ज्वरहराणि भवन्ति (३९)

## 39. Jwarahara – relieving fever

Sariva – Indian Sarsaparilla – Hemidesmus indicus,

Sharkara – sugar,
Patha (Cissampelos pareira Linn.),
Manjistha (Rubia cordifolia Linn.),
Draksha – Raisin – Vitis vinifera,
Pilu (Salvadora persica Linn.),
Parushaka (Grewia asiatica Linn.),
Abhaya – Terminalia chebula,
Amalaka (Emblica officinalis Gaertn.),
Vibhitaka (Terminalia belerica Roxb.).

## 40. Shramahara – relieving tiredness

द्राक्षा खर्जूर प्रियाल बदर दाडिम फल्गु परूषकेक्षु यवषष्टिका इति दशेमानि श्रमहराणि भवन्ति (४०), इति पञ्चकः कषायवर्गः॥१६॥

## 40. Shramahara – relieving tiredness

Darksha – Raisin – Vitis vinifera,
Kharjura – Dates – (Phoenix sylvestris Roxb.),
Priyala (Buchanania lanzan),
Badara – Zizyphus jujuba,
Dadima – Pomegranate – Punica granatum,
Phalgu (Ficus hispida Linn. f.),
Parushaka (Grewia asiatica Linn.),
Ikshu – Sugarcane (Saccharum officinarum Linn.),
Yava – Barley (Hordeum vulgare) and
Shashtika (a variety of rice – Oryza sativa Linn.).

## 41. Daha Prashamana – relieving burning sensation

लाजा चन्दन काश्मर्यफल मधूक शर्करा नीलोत्पलोशीर सारिवा गुडूची ह्रीबेराणीति दशेमानि दाहप्रशमनानि भवन्ति (४१)

## 41. Daha Prashamana – relieving burning sensation

Laja (fried paddy),
Chandana – Sandalwood – Santalum album,
fruit of Kashmarya (Gmelina arborea Linn.),
Madhuka– Licorice – Glycyrrhiza glabra,
Sharkara – Sugar,
Nilotpala (Nymphaea stellata Willd.),
Usheera – Vetiver – Vetiveria zizanioides,
Sariva – Indian Sarsaparilla – Hemidesmus indicus,
Guduchi (Tinospora cordifolia Miers.),
Hribera (Pavonia odorata Willd.)

## 42. Sheeta Prashamana – relieving cold sensation

तगरागुरु धान्यक शृङ्गवेर भूतीक वचा कण्टकार्यग्निमन्थ श्योनाक पिप्पल्य इति दशेमानि शीतप्रशमनानि भवन्ति (४२)

## 42. Sheeta Prashamana – relieving cold sensation

Tagara (Valeriana wallichii DC.),
Aguru (Aquilaria agallocha Roxb.),
Dhanyaka (Coriandrum sativum Linn.),
Shringavera – Ginger – Zingiber officinale,

Bhutika (Trachyspermum ammi Sprague.),
Vacha (Acorus calamus Linn.),
Kantakari – Solanum xanthocarpum,
Agnimantha (Clerodendrum phlomidis Linn. f.),
Shyonaka (Oroxylum indicum Vent.),
Pippali – Long pepper fruit – Piper longum

## 43. Udarda Prashamana – relieving allergic skin rashes

तिन्दुक प्रियाल बदर खदिर कदर सप्तपर्णाश्वकर्णार्जुनासनारिमेदा इति दशेमान्युदर्द प्रशमनानि भवन्ति (४३)

## 43. Udarda Prashamana – relieving allergic skin rashes

Tinduka ( Diospyros peregrina Gurke.),
Priyala (Buchanania lanzan),
Badara – Zizyphus jujuba,
Khadira (Acacia catechu),
Kadara (a variety of Acacia catechu Willd.)
Saptaparna (Alstonia scholaris R. Br.),
Ashvakarna (Dipterocarpus alatus Roxb.),
Arjuna (Terminalia arjuna),
Asana (Terminalia tomentosa W. & A.) and
Arimeda (a variety of Acacia catechu Willd.)

## 44. Angamarda Prashamana – relieving body pain

विदारीगन्धा पृश्निपर्णी बृहती कण्टकारिकैरण्ड काकोली चन्दनोशीरैला मधुकानीति दशेमान्यङ्गमर्द प्रशमनानि भवन्ति (४४)

## 44. Angamarda Prashamana – relieving body pain

Vidarigandha (Desmodium gangeticum DC.),
Prushniparni (Uraria picta Desv.),
Brihati – Solanum indicum,
Kantakarika – Solanum xanthocarpum,
Eranda (Ricinus communis Linn.),
Kakoli – Fritillaria roylei,
Chandana – Sandalwood – Santalum album,
Ushira – Vetiver – Vetiveria zizanioides,
Ela (Elettaria cardamomum Maton),
Madhuka– Licorice – Glycyrrhiza glabra.

## 45. Shula Prashamana -relieving abdominal colic pain

पिप्पली पिप्पलीमूल चव्य चित्रक शृङ्गवेर मरिचाजमोदाजगन्धाजाजी गण्डीराणीति दशमानि शूलप्रशमनानि भवन्ति (४५), इति पञ्चकः
कषायवर्गः||१७||

## 45. Shula Prashamana -relieving abdominal colic pain

Pippali – Long pepper fruit – Piper longum,
root of pippali,
Chavya (Piper chaba Hunter),
Chitraka – Leadwort – Plumbago zeylanica,
Shringavera – Ginger – Zingiber officinale,
Maricha – Black pepper fruit – Piper nigrum,

Ajamoda – Ajowan (fruit) – Trachyspermum roxburghianum,
Ajagandha (Gynandropsis gynandra Briquet.),
Ajaji (Cuminum cyminum Linn.),
Gandira (Euphorbia antiquorum Linn.)

## 46. Shonitasthapana – stopping bleeding, restoring proper quantity of blood

मधु मधुक रुधिर मोचरस मृत्कपाल लोध्र गैरिक प्रियङ्गु शर्करा लाजा इति दशेमानि शोणितस्थापनानि भवन्ति (४६)

## 46. Shonitasthapana – stopping bleeding, restoring proper quantity of blood

Honey,
Madhuka– Licorice – Glycyrrhiza glabra,
Rudhika (Crocus sativus Linn.),
Mocharasa (resin of Salmalia malabarica Schott & Endl.),
Earthen pot pieces,
Lodhra (Symplocos racemosa),
Gairika (Ferrum haematite),
Priyangu (Callicarpa macrophylla),
Sugar,
Fried paddy

## 47. Vedanasthapana – relieving pain

शाल कट्फल कदम्ब पद्मक तुम्ब मोचरस शिरीष वञ्जुलैलवालुकाशोका इति दशेमानि वेदनास्थापनानि भवन्ति (४७)

## 47. Vedanasthapana – relieving pain

Shala (Shorea robusta Gaertn. f.),
Katphala – Myrica nagi,
Kadamba (Anthocephalus indicus A. Rich.),
Padmaka – Prunus cerasoides,
Tumba (Zanthoxylum alatum Roxb.),
Mocharasa (resin of Salmalia malabarica Schott and Endl.),
Shirisha (Albizia lebbeck Benth.),
Vanjula (Salix caprea Linn.),
Elavaluka (Prunus cerasus Linn.),
Ashoka (Saraca indica Linn.).

## 48. Sanjnasthapana – restoring consciousness

हिङ्गु कैटर्यारिमेदा वचा चोरक वयस्था गोलोमी जटिला पलङ्कषाशोक रोहिण्य इति दशेमानि सञ्ज्ञास्थापनानि भवन्ति (४८)

## 48. Sanjnasthapana – restoring consciousness

Hingu – Asa foetida,
Kaitarya – Myrica nagi,
Arimeda (a variety of Acacia catechu Willd.),
Vacha (Acorus calamus Linn.),
Choraka (Angelica glauca),
Vayastha – Brahmi (Bacopa monnieri Pennell.),
Golomi (a variety of Acorus calamus Linn.),
Jatila (Nardostachys jatamansi DC.),
Palankasha (Commiphora mukul Engl.) and

Ashokarohini (Picrorhiza kurroa Royle ex Benth.)

## 49. Prajasthapana – procreative, useful in begetting child

ऐन्द्री ब्राह्मी शतवीर्या सहस्रवीर्या ऽमोघा ऽव्यथा शिवा ऽरिष्टा वाट्यपुष्पी विष्वक्सेन कान्ता इति दशेमानि प्रजास्थापनानि भवन्ति (४९)

## 49. Prajasthapana – procreative, useful in begetting child

Aindri – Colocynth – Citrullus colocynthis,

Brahmi (Bacopa monnieri Pennel.),

Shatavirya (Cynodon dactylon Pers.),

Sahasravirya (a variety of Cynodon dactylon Pers.),

Amogha (Emblica officinalis Gaertn.),

Avyatha (Tinospora cordifolia Miers.),

Shiva (Terminalia chebula Linn.),

Arishta (Picrorhiza kurroa Royle ex Benth.),

Vatyapuspi (Sida rhombifolia Linn.),

Visvaksenakanta (Callicarpa macrophylla Vahl.)

## 50. Vayaha Sthapana -rejuvenating, anti aging.

अमृता ऽभया धात्री मुक्ताश्वेता जीवन्त्यतिरसा मण्डूकपर्णी स्थिरा पुनर्नवा इति दशेमानि
वयःस्थापनानि भवन्ति, इति पञ्चकः कषायवर्गः||१८||
इति पञ्चकषायशतान्यभिसमस्य पञ्चाशन्महाकषाया महतां च कषायाणां लक्षणोदाहरणार्थं व्याख्याता भवन्ति||१९||

## 50. Vayaha Sthapana -rejuvenating, anti ageing.

Amruta (Tinospora cordifolia Miers.),

Abhaya – Terminalia chebula,

Dhatri (Emblica officinalis Gaertn.),

Mukta (pearl),

Shveta (white variety of Clitoria ternatea Linn.),

Jivanti – Leptadenia reticulata,

Atirasa – Asparagus root – Asparagus racemosus,

Mandukaparni (Centella asiatica Urban),

Sthira – Desmodium gangeticum and

Punarnava (Boerhaavia diffusa Linn.)

Thus 500 herbs, grouped in 10 each, based on therapeutic action have been classified. [19].

## Brief explanation of a wide concept:

नहि विस्तरस्य प्रमाणमस्ति, न चाप्यतिसङ्क्षेपोऽल्पबुद्धीनां सामर्थ्यायोपकल्पते, तस्मादनतिसङ्क्षेपेणानतिविस्तरेण चोपदिष्टाः|
एतावन्तो ह्यलमल्पबुद्धीनां व्यवहाराय, बुद्धिमतां च स्वालक्षण्यानुमानयुक्तिकुशलानामनुक्तार्थज्ञानायेति||२०||

The grouping of medicines, as done above and explanation of benefits of each group etc. can be done very elaborately. But as per the context, the grouping has been explained, in neither-too-short nor-too-elaborate manner, so as to make both fool and intelligent understand the concepts in an easier way. An intelligent scholar would understand the hidden concepts with his intelligence, observation, assumptions and his experience. [20]

## Agnivesha's question:

एवंवादिनं भगवन्तमात्रेयमग्निवेश उवाच- नैतानि भगवन्! पञ्च कषायशतानि पूर्यन्ते, तानि तानि ह्येवाङ्गान्युपप्लवन्ते तेषु तेषु
महाकषायेष्विति||२१||

While Lord Atreya was explaining (about these drugs), Agnivesa inquired," Respected Sir! To say that there are five hundred de-coctives does not seem to be correct because the same drug is repeated in a number of groups of de-coctives?" [21]

**Reply by Lord Atreya:**
तमुवाच भगवानात्रेयः- नैतदेवं बुद्धिमता द्रष्टव्यमग्निवेश|
एकोऽपि ह्यनेकां सञ्ज्ञां लभते कार्यान्तराणि कुर्वन्, तद्यथा- पुरुषो बहूनां कर्मणां करणे समर्थो भवति, स यद्यत् कर्म करोति तस्य तस्य कर्मणः कर्तृ-करण-कार्यसम्प्रयुक्तं तत्तद्गौणं नामविशेषं प्राप्नोति, तद्वदौषधद्रव्यमपि द्रष्टव्यम्|
यदि चैकमेव किञ्चिद्द्रव्यमासादयामस्तथागुणयुक्तं यत् सर्वकर्मणां करणे समर्थ स्यात्, कस्ततोऽन्यदिच्छेदुपधारयितुमुपदेष्टुं वा शिष्येभ्य इति||२२||
Lord Atreya - "A wise man like yourself should not view things like that. Even one and the same person performing different acts, is called by different names. For example, a person who is capable of performing many acts gets different designations according to the act performed, nature of acts and the means adopted. Similar is the case with drugs as well. So if we could find one single drug possessing many curative properties to such an extent that it will be effective in curing all diseases, then who would care to enumerate or advise the use of any other drug to his disciples?" [22]

**Summing up content:**
तत्र श्लोकाः-
यतो यावन्ति यैर्द्रव्यैर्विरेचनशतानि षट्|
उक्तानि सङ्ग्रहेणेह तथैवैषां षडाश्रयाः||२३||
रसा लवणवर्ज्याश्च कषाय इति सञ्ज्ञिताः|
तस्मात् पञ्चविधा योनिः कषायाणामुदाहृता||२४||
तथा कल्पनमप्येषामुक्तं पञ्चविधं पुनः|
महतां च कषायाणां पञ्चाशत् परिकीर्तिता||२५||
पञ्च चापि कषायाणां शतान्युक्तानि भागशः|
लक्षणार्थ, प्रमाणं हि विस्तरस्य न विद्यते||२६||
न चालमतिसङ्क्षेपः सामर्थ्यायोपकल्पते|
अल्पबुद्धेरयं तस्मान्नातिसङ्क्षेपविस्तरः||२७||
मन्दानां व्यवहाराय, बुधानां बुद्धिवृद्धये|
पञ्चाशत्को ह्ययं वर्गः कषायाणामुदाहृतः||२८||
तेषां कर्मसु बाह्येषु योगमाभ्यन्तरेषु च|
संयोगं च प्रयोगं च यो वेद स भिषग्वरः||२९||

**Summing up the contents: -**
All the six hundred purgatives along with their ingredients, various preparations of each one of them have been explained here in brief; and so, their six sources have been explained.Drugs of all tastes except salt can be made into water decoction (Kashayam). Thus, there are five-fold sources of de-coctives. Again five-fold pharmaceutical preparations of all the de-coctives and fifty important groups of decoctive have been enumerated.

These 50 important groups of decoctives are further divided into ten each thereby constituting 500 decoctives – such grouping is for the convenience of description; There is no limit to the detailed description of these decoctions. Again, too much of brevity will not be conducive to the understanding of disciples of lower intelligence; so the description of decoction presented in this chapter is neither too brief nor too elaborate. With a view to guiding the disciples of lower intelligence and also to stimulate the imaginative power of the wise, these fifty groups of decoctives have been explained. The one who is acquainted with the internal use as well as external application and prescription by combination of all these drugs, alone is the real physician. [23-29]

इत्यग्निवेशकृते तन्त्रे चरकप्रतिसंस्कृते श्लोकस्थाने षड्विरेचनशताश्रितीयो नाम चतुर्थोऽध्यायः||४||
इति भेषजचतुष्कः||१||
Here ends the fourth chapter on "The Six Hundred Purgatives".

# 5

# Sutrasthana Chapter 5
# Matrashiteeyam

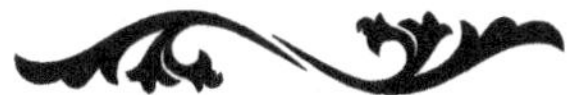

अथातो मात्राशितीयमध्यायं व्याख्यास्यामः||१||

इतिह स्माह भगवानात्रेयः||२||

The fifth chapter of Charak Samhita Sutrasthana deals with Ayurvedic dietetics. What is the right quantity of food in relation to the strength of digestion? Personal hygiene, herbal smoking, nasal drops, oral hygiene, gargling, head massage, foot massage, etc.

The objective of Ayurveda – the science of medicine is two-fold,
1. Treatment of patients suffering from diseases and
2. Maintenance of positive health.
In the first four chapters, and in the next four chapters, various ways of maintenance of normal health are described.

Of all the factors for the maintenance of positive health, food taken in proper quantity occupies the most important position. So the first topic of this chapter deals with the quantity of foods to be consumed.

मात्राशी स्यात्|

आहारमात्रा पुनरग्निबलापेक्षिणी||३||

One should eat in proper quantity. The quantity of food to be taken depends upon the strength of digestion. (3)

**Quantity of food and digestion:**

यावद्ध्यस्याशनमशितमनुपहत्य प्रकृतिं यथाकालं जरां गच्छति तावदस्य मात्राप्रमाणं वेदितव्यं भवति||४||

- Proper quantity of food' shall be defined as that amount / quantity of food which
- gets digested and metabolised in proper time and also so
- without disturbing the equilibrium or balance of doshas and tissues (without harming the constitution) (4)

**Laghu (easy to digest) and Guru (heavy to digest) types of foods :**

तत्र शालिषष्टिकमुद्गलावकपिञ्जलैणशशशरभशम्बरादीन्याहारद्रव्याणि प्रकृतिलघून्यपि मात्रापेक्षीणि भवन्ति|

तथा पिष्टेक्षुक्षीरविकृतितिलमाषानूपौदकपिशितादीन्याहारद्रव्याणि प्रकृतिगुरूण्यपि मात्रामेवापेक्षन्ते||५||

न चैवमुक्ते द्रव्ये गुरुलाघवमकारणं मन्येत, लघूनि हि द्रव्याणि वाय्वग्निगुणबहुलानि भवन्ति; पृथ्वीसोमगुणबहुलानीतराणि, तस्मात् स्वगुणादपि लघून्यग्निसन्धुक्षणस्वभावान्यल्पदोषाणि चोच्यन्तेऽपि सौहित्योपयुक्तानि, गुरूणि पुनरग्निसन्धुक्षणस्वभावान्यसामान्यात्, अतश्चातिमात्रं दोषवन्ति सौहित्योपयुक्तान्यन्यत्र व्यायामाग्निबलात्; सैषा

भवत्यग्निबलापेक्षिणी मात्रा||६||

**Laghu (easy to digest) and Guru (heavy to digest) types of foods :**
The food items like the below mentioned are light in nature (laghu) and are also easy to digest –

- Shali (rice),
- Shashtika (a variety of rice that matures in 60 days) ,
- Mudga (green gram – Vigna radiata),
- Common Quail,
- Grey Partridge,
- Antelope,
- Rabbit,
- Wapiti,
- Indian sambar etc.

Easiness in digestion should be understood according to the quantity of the food.
A light to digest (laghu) food can also become hard to digest (guru) if consumed in very high quantities.

Similarly preparations of flour, sugarcane and milk, tila (Sesame), Masha (Black gram) and meats of marshy and aquatic animals even though heavy in digestion by nature are also required to be taken in proper quantity.

But it should not be concluded that the description of heaviness or lightness does not carry any importance. Because, the light food articles are predominant in the qualities of Vayu and Agni (air and fire) and heavy ones in Prithvi and Ap (earth and water) Mahabhutas. Therefore, according to their qualities, the light articles of food, being stimulants of appetite and by nature are considered to be less harmful even if taken in excess.

On the other hand, heavy articles of food suppress appetite. They are harmful if taken in excess unless there is a strong power of digestion and metabolism achieved by physical exercise.

Thus the quantity of food depends upon the power of digestion. (5-6).

By nature, light food is said to be conducive to good health. Heavy food on the other hand is considered to be detrimental. But for both the types of food, if quantity is to be taken into account, lightness and heaviness of food do not seem to have any implication. Thus, it is true that the quantity rather than heaviness / lightness of food is important in the present context.

**Quantity of food to be taken in relation with stomach volume / capacity of the stomach :**
न च नापेक्षते द्रव्यं; द्रव्यापेक्षया च त्रिभागसौहित्यमर्धसौहित्यं वा गुरूणामुपदिश्यते, लघूनामपि च नातिसौहित्यमग्नेर्युक्त्यर्थम्||७||
We have learnt that the right quantity of food depends on the quality of food. If the food is heavy, only one third or half of the stomach capacity is to be filled up. Even in the case of light food articles excessive intake is not conducive to the maintenance of the power of digestion and metabolism. (7)

**The importance of food taken in proper quantity:**
मात्रावदध्यशनमशितमनुपहत्य प्रकृतिं बलवर्णसुखायुषा योजयत्युपयोक्तारमवश्यमिति||८||

**The importance of food taken in proper quantity:**
Taken in appropriate quantity, food certainty helps the individual in bringing about strength, complexion, happiness

and longevity without distributing the equilibrium of Dhatus (body tissues) and Doshas of the body. (8)

**After meals, avoid heavy food articles:**

भवन्ति चात्र-

गुरु पिष्टमयं तस्मात्तण्डुलान् पृथुकानपि।
न जातु भुक्तवान् खादेन्मात्रां खादेद्बुभुक्षितः||९||

**After meals, avoid heavy food articles:**
Thus, it is said – After having taken food, one should never take such heavy articles like pastries, rice and Pruthuka (boiled and Flattened rice). Even when hunger, one should take these articles only in proper quantity (9)

**Contra Indicated foods:**

वल्लूरं शुष्कशाकानि शालूकानि बिसानि च।
नाभ्यसेद्गौरवान्मांसं कृशं नैवोपयोजयेत्||१०||
कूर्चिकांश्च किलाटांश्च शौकरं गव्यमाहिषे।
मत्स्यान् दधि च माषांश्च यवकांश्च न शीलयेत्||११||

**Contraindicated foods:**
One should not regularly take heavy food items such as Vallura (dried meat), dry vegetables, Lotus Rhizomes and Lotus stalk. One should never take meat from a diseased animal. One should not regularly take Kurchika (Boiled Buttermilk), Kilata (A sweet milk product), pork, beef, Buffalo meat, fish, curd, Masha (Black gram) and Yavaka (a variety of Barley). (10-11)

**Pathya foods – Indicated foods:**

षष्टिकाञ्छालिमुद्गांश्च सैन्धवामलके यवान्।
आन्तरीक्षं पयः सर्पिर्जाङ्गलं मधु चाभ्यसेत्||१२||

**Pathya foods – Indicated foods:**
One should regularly take shashtika (a kind of rice harvested in sixty days), Shali (rice), Mudga (green gram – Vigna radiata), Rock salt, Amalaki (Amla – Emblica officinalis Gaertn.), Rain water, ghee, Meat of animals dwelling in arid climate and honey (12)

तच्च नित्यं प्रयुञ्जीत स्वास्थ्यं येनानुवर्तते।
अजातानां विकाराणामनुत्पत्तिकरं च यत्||१३||
One should regularly take such articles which are conducive to the maintenance of good health and are capable of preventing the attacks. Over-dosage or usage for a longer period than prescribed may cause diseases. (13)

**Personal hygiene:**
अत ऊर्ध्वं शरीरस्य कार्यमक्ष्यञ्जनादिकम्।
स्वस्थवृत्तिमभिप्रेत्य गुणतः सम्प्रवक्ष्यते||१४||
Hereafter collyrium (Kajal) etc. daily activities of personal hygiene are explained for the maintenance of good health. (14)

**Anjana – Collyrium – Kajal**
सौवीरमञ्जनं नित्यं हितमक्ष्णोः प्रयोजयेत्।
पञ्चरात्रेऽष्टरात्रे वा स्रावणार्थं रसाञ्जनम्||१५||
One should regularly apply the collyrium made of antimony because it is useful for the eyes.

Rasanjana – Aqueous extract of Berberis aristata (a preparation of Berberis aristata DC.) is to be applied once in every 5-8 nights for lacrimation of the eyes.

चक्षुस्तेजोमयं तस्य विशेषाच्छ्लेष्मतो भयम्|
ततः श्लेष्महरं कर्म हितं दृष्टेः प्रसादनम्||१६||
दिवा तन्न प्रयोक्तव्यं नेत्रयोस्तीक्ष्णमञ्जनम्|
विरेकदुर्बला दृष्टिरादित्यं प्राप्य सीदति||१७||
तस्मात् स्राव्यं निशायां तु ध्रुवमञ्जनमिष्यते|१८|

Of all the Mahabhutas, Tejas (Fire, in the form of light) dominates in the composition of eyes. Therefore they are susceptible to be afflicted by kapha. Applying anjana regularly protects the eyes from the effect of kapha. Therefore, the therapy (collyrium etc.) which alleviates Kapha is good for keeping the vision clear.

A strong collyrium must not be applied to the eyes during the day time (strong collyrium would drain the eyes). This is because the eyes weakened by drainage (caused by collyrium) will be adversely affected at the sight of the Sun. Thus, the collyrium meant for draining should be applied only during night. (15- 17)

**Simile to explain benefits of Anjana :**
यथा हि कनकादीनां मलिनां विविधात्मनाम्||१८||
धौतानां निर्मला शुद्धिस्तैलचेलकचादिभिः|
एवं नेत्रेषु मर्त्यानामञ्जनाश्च्योतनादिभिः||१९||
दृष्टिर्निराकुला भाति निर्मले नभसीन्दुवत्|२०|

As different types of tarnished gold ornaments are spotlessly cleared by means of oil, cloth and hair brush, so also by the use of Anjana (collyrium) and eye drops, the eyes become spotlessly bright like the moon in a clear sky. (18-19)

**Dhumapana – Herbal Smoking:**
हरेणुकां प्रियङ्गुं च पृथ्वीकां केशरं नखम्||२०||
ह्रीवेरं चन्दनं पत्रं त्वगेलोशीरपद्मकम्|
ध्यामकं मधुकं मांसी गुग्गुल्वगुरुशर्करम्||२१||
न्यग्रोधोदुम्बराश्वत्थप्लक्षलोध्रत्वचः शुभाः|
वन्यं सर्जरसं मुस्तं शैलेयं कमलोत्पले||२२||
श्रीवेष्टकं शल्लकीं च शुकबर्हमथापि च|
पिष्ट्वा लिम्पेच्छरेषीकां तां वर्तिं यवसन्निभाम्||२३||
अङ्गुष्ठसम्मितां कुर्यादष्टाङ्गुलसमां भिषक्|
शुष्कां निगर्भां तां वर्तिं धूमनेत्रार्पितां नरः||२४||
स्नेहाक्तामग्निसम्प्लुष्टां पिबेत् प्रायोगिकीं सुखाम्|२५|

**Dhumapana – Herbal Smoking:**
The below mentioned herbs shall be used in preparing the wick to be used in medicated / herbal smoking –

- Harenua (Pisum sativum Linn),
- Priyangu – Callicarpa macrophylla Vahl.
- Prithvika (Nigella sativa Linn),
- Keshara (Mesua ferrea Linn),
- Nakha – Capparis sepiaria,
- Hrivera (Pavonia odorata Willd),

- Chandana (Sandalwood),
- Patra (Cinnamomum tamala Nees and Eberum ),
- Twak (Cinnamomum zeylanicum)
- Ela – Cardamom – Elettaria cardamomum
- Usheera – Vetiver,
- Padmaka – Wild Himalayan Cherry – Prunus cerasoides
- Dhyamaka (Cymbopogon schoenanthus Spring),
- Madhuka – Licorice – Glycyrrhiza glabra
- Mamsi – Nardostachys jatamansi
- Guggulu (Commiphoramukul Engl.),
- Aguru (Aquilaria agallocha Roxb. ),
- Sharkara (Sugar),
- bark of Nyagrodha (Ficus benghalensis Linn),
- Udumbara (Ficus racemosa Linn),
- Ashvattha (Ficus religiosa Linn),
- Plaksha (Ficus lacor Buch- Ham), and
- Lodhra (Symplocos racemosa)
- Vanya (Cyperus tenuiflorus),
- Sarjarasa (Resin of Vateria indica Linn).
- Musta (Cyperus rotundus)
- Shaileya (Parmelia perlata),
- Kamala (Nelumbo nucifera Gaertn),
- Utpala (Nymphaea alba),
- Shrivestaka (resinous extract from Pinus roxburghii Sargent ),
- Shallaki (Boswellia serrata Roxb.),
- Sukararha

The above mentioned drugs should be ground into paste. The paste should be applied on a reed so as to make a cigar. The cigar shall be of the shape of a barley grain. It should have the thickness of the thumb at its center. Its length should be of eight fingers.

It should then be dried up and the reed be taken out of it. With the help of a pipe, one should regularly smoke that cigar after smearing it with some unctuous substance like ghee and applying fire to it. This is altogether harmless. (20-24)

**Unctuous (Oily) herbal smoking: Vasadi Snaihika Dhumavarti**

वसाघृतमधूच्छिष्टैर्युक्तियुक्तैर्वरौषधैः||२५||

वर्तिं मधुरकैः कृत्वा स्नैहिकीं धूममाचरेत्|२६|

**Unctuous (Oily) herbal smoking:**

One should smoke unctuous cigars made of useful drugs of sweet taste along with fat of muscle, ghee and bee wax according to the prescribed method. (25)

**Herbal smoking for elimination of Doshas: - Svetadi Shirovairechanika Dhuma**

श्वेता ज्योतिष्मती चैव हरितालं मनःशिला||२६||

गन्धाश्चागुरुपत्राद्या धूमं मूर्धविरेचने |२७|

**Herbal smoking for elimination of Doshas:**

For the elimination of Doshas from the head, smoking of cigars made of the below mentioned drugs shall be used –

- Shveta (white variety of Clitoria ternatea Linn),
- Jyotishmati (Celastrus paniculatus Wild).
- Orpiment,
- realgar
- other fragrant articles like Agaru (Aquilaria agallocha Roxb), Patra – Cinnamomum tamala Nees and Eberum. etc. (26)

## Health benefits of herbal smoking:

गौरवं शिरसः शूलं पीनसार्धावभेदकौ||२७||
कर्णाक्षिशूलं कासश्च हिक्काश्वासौ गलग्रहः|
दन्तदौर्बल्यमास्रावः श्रोत्रघ्राणाक्षिदोषजः||२८||
पूतिघ्राणास्यगन्धश्च दन्तशूलमरोचकः|
हनुमन्याग्रहः कण्डूः क्रिमयः पाण्डुता मुखे||२९||
श्लेष्मप्रसेको वैस्वर्यं गलशुण्ड्युपजिह्विका|
खालित्यं पिञ्जरत्वं च केशानां पतनं तथा||३०||
क्षवथुश्चातितन्द्रा च बुद्धेर्मोहोऽतिनिद्रता|
धूमपानात् प्रशाम्यन्ति बलं भवति चाधिकम्||३१||
शिरोरुहकपालानामिन्द्रियाणां स्वरस्य च|
न च वातकफात्मानो बलिनोऽप्यूर्ध्वजत्रुजाः||३२||
धूमवक्त्रकपानस्य व्याधयः स्युः शिरोगताः|३३|

## Health benefits of herbal smoking:

Smoking cures heaviness of head, headache, Rhinitis, Migraine, Earache, Pain in eye, Cough, hiccup, Dyspnea, Obstruction in throat, weakness of teeth, Discharge from the morbid ear, nose and eye, purulent smell from nose and mouth toothache, Anorexia, Lock jaw, Torticollis, Pruritus, Infective condition, Paleness of face, excessive salivation, impaired voice, Tonsillitis, uvulitis, Alopecia, greying of hair, falling of hair, sneezing, excessive drowsiness, loss of consciousness, and excess sleep. It also strengthens hair, skull bones, sense organs and voice. The diseases pertaining to head and neck arising out of Vata and Kapha do not affect the person who is used to smoking (27- 32).

## Schedule for smoking:

प्रयोगपाने तस्याष्टौ कालाः सम्परिकीर्तिताः||३३||
वातश्लेष्मसमुत्क्लेशः कालेष्वेषु हि लक्ष्यते|
स्नात्वा भुक्त्वा समुल्लिख्य क्षुत्वा दन्तान्निघृष्य च|
नावनाञ्जननिद्रान्ते चात्मवान् धूमपो भवेत्|
तथा वातकफात्मानो न भवन्त्यूर्ध्वजत्रुजाः||३५||

## Schedule for smoking:

Eight timings are prescribed for habitual smoking because Vata, Pitta and Kapha get vitiated during these times. These timings are –

- after bathing,
- after eating,

- after tongue scraping,
- after sneezing,
- after brushing the teeth,
- after Nasya – nasal instillation of medicines,
- after application of collyrium and
- after sleep


Herbal smoking at these timings prevents diseases of head and neck resulting from the vitiation of Kapha and vata. Smoking is to be done thrice- three puffs each time. (33-35)

## Time for Dhumapana:

रोगास्तस्य तु पेयाः स्युरापानास्त्रिस्त्रयस्त्रयः|३६|
परं दिवकालपायी स्यादहनः कालेषु बुद्धिमान्||३६||
प्रयोगे, स्नैहिके त्वेकं, वैरेच्यं त्रिचतुः पिबेत्|
हृत्कण्ठेन्द्रियसंशुद्धिर्लघुत्वं शिरसः शमः||३७||
यथेरितानां दोषाणां सम्यक्पीतस्य लक्षणम्|३८|

## Time for Dhumapana:

During the prescribed times, a wise person should smoke twice for habitual variety of smoking (Prayogika), once for unctuous variety (Snaihika) and three to four times for the elimination variety (Vairechanika) of smoking (36)

Clarity of mind, throat and sense organs, lightness of head and elimination of the above mentioned Doshas are features of correct / properly administered smoking. (37)

If untimely done or overdone, smoking causes such troubles as deafness, blindness, dumbness, bleeding from different parts of the body and giddiness. (38)

## Treatment of complications:

बाधिर्यमान्ध्यमूकत्वं रक्तपित्तं शिरोभ्रमम्||३८||
अकाले चातिपीतश्च धूमः कुर्यादुपद्रवान्|
तत्रेष्टं सर्पिषः पानं नावनाञ्जनतर्पणम्||३९||
स्नैहिकं धूमजे दोषे वायुः पित्तानुगो यदि|
शीतं तु रक्तपित्ते स्याच्छ्लेष्मपित्ते विरूक्षणम्||४०||

## Treatment of complications:

If such troubles due to untimely and over smoking arise, intake of ghee, administration of nasal drops, collyrium and demulcent drinks are prescribed. These should be prepared with unctuous drugs in the event of vitiation of Vayu associated with Pitta, with cooling drugs in case of Raktapitta, and with arid drugs in Kapha and Pitta imbalance. (39-40)

## Contraindications for herbal smoking :

परं त्वतः प्रवक्ष्यामि धूमो येषां विगर्हितः|
न विरिक्तः पिबेद्धूमं न कृते बस्तिकर्मणि||४१||
न रक्ती न विषेणार्तो न शोचन्न च गर्भिणी|
न श्रमे न मदे नामे न पित्ते न प्रजागरे||४२||
न मूर्च्छाभ्रमतृष्णासु न क्षीणे नापि च क्षते|

न मद्यदुग्धे पीत्वा च न स्नेहं न च माक्षिकम्||४३||
धूमं न भुक्त्वा दध्ना च न रूक्षः क्रुद्ध एव च|
न तालुशोषे तिमिरे शिरस्यभिहिते न च||४४||
न शङ्खके न रोहिण्यां न मेहे न मदात्यये|
एषु धूममकालेषु मोहात् पिबति यो नरः||४५||
रोगास्तस्य प्रवर्धन्ते दारुणा धूमविभ्रमात्|४६|

## Contraindications for herbal smoking :

A person after taking emesis or purgative or enema (Vamana, virechana or Basti), or a person having bleeding through different orifices of the body, or one afflicted with toxins or a grief- stricken person should not smoke. A pregnant woman should also refrain from smoking; similarly one should not smoke when he is fatigued or intoxicated. Smoking is also prohibited in the event of vitiation of digestion and metabolism, vitiation of Pitta, fainting, giddiness, excess thirst and phthisis.

One should not smoke after having taken liquor or milk or fatty substances or honey or curd; nor should one smoke when there is roughness in his body or he is enraged. Smoking is also prohibited in the event of the dryness of palate, fainting, injury to the head, Shankhaka (a type of headache in the temporal region marked by excessive pain and swelling usually killing a patient in three days), diabetes and narcosis. One who, out of ignorance, smokes in contravention of these situations, subjects himself to various serious diseases. These diseases become severe due to the adverse effect of improper smoking. (41-45)

## Routes of smoking:

धूमयोग्यः पिबेद्दोषे शिरोघ्राणाक्षिसंश्रये||४६||
घ्राणेनास्येन कण्ठस्थे मुखेन घ्राणपो वमेत्|
आस्येन धूमकवलान् पिबन् घ्राणेन नोद्वमेत्||४७||
प्रतिलोमं गतो ह्याशु धूमो हिंस्यादिध चक्षुषी|४८|

## Routes of smoking:

One for whom smoking is prescribed should smoke through the nose in diseases of head, nose and eyes.
One should exhale through the mouth. But if one smokes through the mouth, he should not exhale through the nose because the smoke moving in the reverse direction instantaneously affects the eyes. (46-48)

## Method of herbal smoking –Dhumanetra – smoking tube

ऋज्वङ्गचक्षुस्तच्चेताः सूपविष्टस्त्रिपर्ययम्||४८||
पिबेच्छिद्रं पिधायैकं नासया धूममात्मवान्|४९|

While keeping the body erect and eyes looking to the front, with concentration of mind and having self-control, one should sit at ease. In this position one should smoke three times, thrice during each time, through one nostril while closing the other one. (48)

## Measurement of Dhuma Nadi

चतुर्विंशतिकं नेत्रं स्वाङ्गुलीभिर्विरेचने||४९||
द्वात्रिंशदङ्गुलं स्नेहे प्रयोगेऽध्यर्धमिष्यते|
ऋजु त्रिकोषाफलितं कोलास्थ्यग्रप्रमाणितम्||५०||
बस्तिनेत्रसमद्रव्यं धूमनेत्रं प्रशस्यते|५१|

For the elimination type of smoking (Virechana Dhumapana), the length of the pipe should be 24 finger breadth;

For unctuous smoking (Snaihika), the length of the pipe should be of 32 finger breadth;
For habitual smoking (Prayogika), the length of the pipe should be of 36 finger breadth (finger breadth is to be measured with one's own finger). (49)

## Qualities of best smoking pipe -

ऋजु त्रिकोषाफलितं कोलास्थ्यग्रप्रमाणितम्||५०||
बस्तिनेत्रसमद्रव्यं धूमनेत्रं प्रशस्यते|५१|

The best pipe is the one which is

- Ruju - straight,
- Trikosha Phalita - having three knots,
- whose mouth is of the size of the stone of a Kola fruit (Zizyphus jujuba Lam)
- which is made of the same material as that of the enema pipe [50]


दूरादिवनिर्गतः पर्वच्छिन्नो नाडीतनूकृतः||५१||

The smoke used according to the prescribed dose and time does not affect the sense organs as it is not inhaled directly. It is interrupted by knots and is attenuated by its flow through the passage of the pipe. [51]

## Signs of good herbal smoking:

यदा चोरश्च कण्ठश्च शिरश्च लघुतां व्रजेत्||५२||
कफश्च तनुतां प्राप्तः सुपीतं धूममादिशेत्|

Signs like lightness of the chest, throat, head and liquification of Kapha are the features of correct smoking. [52]

## Ayoga – Signs of insufficient smoking :

अविशुद्धः स्वरो यस्य कण्ठश्च सकफो भवेत्||५३||
स्तिमितो मस्तकश्चैवमपीतं धूममादिशेत्|

## Ayoga – Signs of insufficient smoking :

Impairment of voice, presence of Kapha (phlegm) in the throat and heaviness of head are the features of insufficient smoking. [53]

## Atiyoga – If one smokes in excess:

तालु मूर्धा च कण्ठश्च शुष्यते परितप्यते||५४||
तृष्यते मुह्यते जन्तू रक्तं च स्रवतेऽधिकम्|
शिरश्च भ्रमतेऽत्यर्थं मूर्च्छा चास्योपजायते||५५||
इन्द्रियाण्युपतप्यन्ते धूमेऽत्यर्थं निषेविते|५६|

**Atiyoga** – If one smokes in excess, his palate, head and throat get dried up and burns a lot. One feels thirsty and he becomes unconscious; there may be excessive bleeding, dizziness. fainting and hotness in sense organs. [54-55]

## Anu taila - Ideal nasya taila:

वर्षे वर्षेऽणुतैलं च कालेषु त्रिषु ना चरेत्||५६||

**Nasya Nasal drops** – One should use "**Anu taila**" every year during the three seasons, viz the rainy season, the autumn and the spring, when the sky is free from clouds. [56]

## Benefits of nasal drops :

प्रावृट्शरद्वसन्तेषु गतमेघे नभस्तले|
नस्यकर्म यथाकालं यो यथोक्तं निषेवते||५७||
न तस्य चक्षुर्न घ्राणं न श्रोत्रमुपहन्यते|
न स्युः श्वेता न कपिलाः केशाः श्मश्रूणि वा पुनः||५८||
न च केशाः प्रमुच्यन्ते वर्धन्ते च विशेषतः|
मन्यास्तम्भः शिरःशूलमर्दितं हनुसङ्ग्रहः||५९||
पीनसार्धावभेदौ च शिरःकम्पश्च शाम्यति|
सिराः शिरःकपालानां सन्धयः स्नायुकण्डराः||६०||
नावनप्रीणिताश्चास्य लभन्तेऽभ्यधिकं बलम्|
मुखं प्रसन्नोपचितं स्वरः स्निग्धः स्थिरो महान्||६१||
सर्वेन्द्रियाणां वैमल्यं बलं भवति चाधिकम्|
न चास्य रोगाः सहसा प्रभवन्त्यूर्ध्वजत्रुजाः||६२||
जीर्यतश्चोत्तमाङ्गेषु जरा न लभते बलम्|६३|

The eyes, nose and ears of those who practice nasal therapy at proper time according to the prescribed method would not be affected by any kind of morbidity. His hairs and head would never become white or grey. He would never experience hair fall. The hairs would rather grow luxuriously. Diseases like torticollis, headache, facial paralysis, locked jaw, rhinitis, migraine and tremors of the head are cured thereby.

Being nourished by inhalation, his veins, joints, ligaments and tendons of head and neck gain greater strength. His face becomes cheerful and plumpy; and his voice becomes sweet, stabilized and stertorous.

All the sense organs become clear and there is considerable strength. Diseases relating to the head and neck do not attack such a person. Even though he might be growing old, old age does not affect his head (in the form of grey hair etc). [57 - 63]

## Preparation of Anu taila:

चन्दनागुरुणी पत्रं दार्वीत्वङ्मधुकं बलाम्||६३||
प्रपौण्डरीकं सूक्ष्मैलां विडङ्गं बिल्वमुत्पलम्|
ह्रीबेरमभयं वन्यं त्वङ्मुस्तं सारिवां स्थिराम्||६४||
जीवन्तीं पृश्निपर्णीं च सुरदारु शतावरीम्|
हरेणुं बृहतीं व्याघ्रीं सुरभीं पद्मकेशरम्||६५||
विपाचयेच्छतगुणे माहेन्द्रे विमलेऽम्भसि|
तैलाद्दशगुणं शेषं कषायमवतारयेत्||६६||
तेन तैलं कषायेण दशकृत्वो विपाचयेत्|
अथास्य दशमे पाके समांशं छागलं पयः||६७||
दद्यादेषोऽणुतैलस्य नावनीयस्य संविधिः|
अस्य मात्रां प्रयुञ्जीत तैलस्यार्धपलोन्मिताम्||६८||

## Preparation of Anu taila:

Chandana (Sandalwood – Santalum album),
Aguru (Aquilaria agallocha Roxb),
Patra (Cinnamomum tamala Nees and Eberum.),
Bark of Darvi (Berberis aristata Linn),
Prapaundarika (Nymphaea lotus Linn),
Sookshma - Ela – cardamom
Vidanga (Embelia ribes Brum. F),
Bilva (Aegle marmelos Corr),

Utpala (Nymphaea alba),

Hrivera (Pavonia odorata willd),

Abhaya – Terminalia chebula

Usheera – (Vetiveria zizanioides Nash),

Vanya (Cyperus tenuiflorus),

Tvak (Cinnamomum zeylanicum Blume f),

Musta (Cyperus rotundus),

Sariva – Indian Sarsaparilla – Hemidesmus indicus,

Sthira – Desmodium gangeticum,

Jivanti – Leptadenia reticulata and A,

Prishnaparni – Uraria picta,

Suradaru (Cedrus deodara),

Shatavari (Asparagus racemosus Willd),

Harenu (Pisum sativum Linn),

Brihati – Solanum indicum ,

Vyaghri (Solanum xanthocarpum Schrader and wendl),

Surabhi (Pluchea lanceolata Oliver and Hiern),

Padmakesara (Filaments of Nelumbo nucifera Gaertn)

These drugs should be boiled with hundred times of pure rainwater (of the oil in quantity), till it is reduced to ten times of the oil (in quantity). The oil should be boiled in that decoction for ten times. At the final (that is the tenth) stage of boiling, an equal quantity of goat's milk should be added to it. This is the prescribed method for preparing Anu Taila which is useful for inhalation. The prescribed dosage of oil is half Pala or 24 ml (this is the quantity to be used in twenty-four hours).

**Nasal drops administration :**

स्निग्धस्विन्नोतमाङ्गस्य पिचुना नावनैस्त्रिभिः।
त्र्यहात्र्यहाच्च सप्ताहमेतत् कर्म समाचरेत्||६९||
निवातोष्णसमाचारी हिताशी नियतेन्द्रियः।
तैलमेतत्त्रिदोषघ्नमिन्द्रियाणां बलप्रदम्||७०||
प्रयुञ्जानो यथाकालं यथोक्तानश्नुते गुणान्||७१|

**Nasal drops administration :**

After a head massage with oil and sweating therapy, Anu Taila is to be administered into the nostril with the help of a cotton swab on alternate days- thrice daily- for seven days. This oil is useful for alleviating all the Tridosha and gives strength to the sense organs. The benefit of this oil as envisaged above can be derived if it is used in proper time. The patient using it should reside in a place which is neither too airy nor too warm, he should take wholesome food and have self-control. [63-70]

**Teeth brushing:**

आपोथिताग्रं द्वौ कालौ कषायकटुतिक्तकम्||७१||
भक्षयेद्दन्तपवनं दन्तमांसान्यबाधयन्।
निहन्ति गन्धं वैरस्यं जिह्वादन्तास्यजं मलम्||७२||

**Teeth brushing:**

One should use the tooth-cleaning stick whose top portion is crushed. The stick should be astringent, pungent or bitter in taste. This should be done in such a way that the gums are not affected. This removes the foul smell and tastelessness. It removes the dirt of the tongue, teeth and mouth. It improves taste. This cleans the teeth instantaneously. [71-72]

**Plants for dental brush:**

निष्कृष्य रुचिमाधत्ते सद्यो दन्तविशोधनम्|
करञ्जकरवीरार्कमालतीककुभासनाः||७३||

**Plants for dental brush:** The branches or twigs for brushing the teeth (to be used as toothbrush) should be chosen from one of the below mentioned plants –

- Karanja (Pongamia pinnata Merr),
- Karavira (Nerium indicum Mill),
- Arka – (Calotropis gigantea R.Br.exAit),
- Malati (Aganosma dichotoma K. Schum),
- Kakubha (Terminalia arjuna W.&A),
- Asana (Terminalia tomentosa W.&A)

These and other trees having identical properties are recommended as toothbrush. [73]

**Tongue scraping:**

शस्यन्ते दन्तपवने ये चाप्येवंविधा द्रुमाः|
सुवर्णरूप्यताम्राणि त्रपुरीतिमयानि च||७४||
जिह्वानिर्लेखनानि स्युरतीक्ष्णान्यनृजूनि च|
जिह्वामूलगतं यच्च मलमुच्छ्वासरोधि च||७५||

**Tongue scraping:**

Tongue scrapers, which should not be sharp edged and are curved, are to be made of metals like gold, silver, cropper, tin and brass. [74]
The dirt deposited at the root of the tongue, obstructs expiration and gives rise to foul smell; so the tongue should be scraped regularly.[75]

**Betel leaf chewing :**

दौर्गन्ध्यं भजते तेन तस्माज्जिह्वां विनिर्लिखेत् |
धार्याण्यास्येन वैशद्यरुचिसौगन्ध्यमिच्छता||७६||
जातीकटुकपूगानां लवङ्गस्य फलानि च|
कक्कोलस्य फलं पत्रं ताम्बूलस्य शुभं तथा|
तथा कर्पूरनिर्यासः सूक्ष्मैलायाः फलानि च||७७||

**Betel leaf chewing:**

One desirous of clarity, taste and good smell of mouth should chew the fruits of Jati (Myristica fragrans Houtt), Lavanga (clove) Kauka (Hibiscus abelmoschus Linn), Puga (Areca catechu Linn), Kakkola (Piper cubeba Linn), Sukshma Ela (Cardamom), flower stalk of Tambula (Piper betle Linn).and the extract of Karpura (Cinnamomum camphora). [76-77]

**Gargling :**

हन्वोर्बलं स्वरबलं वदनोपचयः परः|
स्यात् परं च रसज्ञानमन्ने च रुचिरुत्तमा||७८||
न चास्य कण्ठशोषः स्यान्नौष्ठयोः स्फुटनादभयम्|
न च दन्ताः क्षयं यान्ति दृढमूला भवन्ति च||७९||

न शूल्यन्ते न चाम्लेन हृष्यन्ते भक्षयन्ति च|
परानपि खरान् भक्ष्यांस्तैलगण्डूषधारणात्||८०||

**Gargling:**

Sesame oil gargling is beneficial for the strength of jaws, depth of voice, flabbiness of face, excellent gustatory sensation and good taste for food.

Benefits of gargling :

- One will never get dryness of throat,
- The lips will never get cracked
- The teeth will never develop caries
- The teeth would remain deep rooted
- Toothache will not occur
- Teeth will not tingle after taking sour foods
- The teeth will become so strong that they would chew even the hardest and toughest eatables / foods easily [78-80]


**Head massage:**

न खालित्यं न पालित्यं न केशाः प्रपतन्ति च||८१||
बलं शिरःकपालानां विशेषेणाभिवर्धते|
दृढमूलाश्च दीर्घाश्च कृष्णाः केशा भवन्ति च||८२||
इन्द्रियाणि प्रसीदन्ति सुत्वग्भवति चाननम् |
निद्रालाभः सुखं च स्यान्मूर्ध्नि तैलनिषेवणात्||८३||
न कर्णरोगा वातोत्था न मन्याहनुसङ्ग्रहः|
नोच्चैः श्रुतिर्न बाधिर्यं स्यान्नित्यं कर्णतर्पणात्||८४||

**Head massage :**

Benefits of head massage - One who applies sesame oil on his head regularly would have the below mentioned benefits –

- he does not suffer from headache, baldness, greying of hair, or hair fall
- the strength of his head and forehead is specially enhanced;
- his hair becomes black, long and deep-rooted;
- his sense organs work properly;
- the skin of his face becomes brightened;
- he enjoys sound sleep and happiness [81-83]

Ear diseases due to vitiated Vata, torticollis, lock jaw, hardness of hearing and deafness are prevented if oil is regularly dropped into the ears. [84]

**Benefits of massage – Simile:**

स्नेहाभ्यङ्गाद्यथा कुम्भश्चर्म स्नेहविमर्दनात्|
भवत्युपाङ्गादक्षश्च दृढः क्लेशसहो यथा||८५||
तथा शरीरमभ्यङ्गाद्दृढं सुत्वक् च जायते|
प्रशान्तमारुताबाधं क्लेशव्यायामसंसहम्||८६||
स्पर्शनेऽभ्यधिको वायुः स्पर्शनं च त्वगाश्रितम्|

त्वच्यश्च परमभ्यङ्गस्तस्मात्तं शीलयेन्नरः||८७||

**Benefits of massage – Simile:**

As a picture, dry skin, and an axis (of a cart) become strong and resistant by the application of oil, the human body too becomes strong and smooth-skinned by the effect of oil massage. It is not susceptible to the diseases due to Vata. It becomes resistant to exhaustion and exertions. [85-86]

Vata dominates in the tactile sensory organ, and this sensory organ is lodged in the skin. The massage is exceedingly beneficial to the skin; so one should practice it (oil massage) regularly. [87]

**Advantages of regular massage :**

न चाभिघाताभिहतं गात्रमभ्यङ्गसेविनः|
विकारं भजतेऽत्यर्थं बलकर्मणि वा क्वचित्||८८||
सुस्पर्शोपचिताङ्गश्च बलवान् प्रियदर्शनः|
भवत्यभ्यङ्गनित्यत्वान्नरोऽल्पजर एव च||८९||

**Advantages of regular massage:**

In those who practices oil massage regularly, the body, even if subjected to injuries or strenuous work, is not much injured; His physique is smooth, flabby, strong and charming. By regular oil massage, the onslaught of ageing is slackened. [88-89]

**Foot massage :**

खरत्वं स्तब्धता रौक्ष्यं श्रमः सुप्तिश्च पादयोः|
सद्य एवोपशाम्यन्ति पादाभ्यङ्गनिषेवणात्||९०||
जायते सौकुमार्यं च बलं स्थैर्यं च पादयोः|
दृष्टिः प्रसादं लभते मारुतश्चोपशाम्यति||९१||
न च स्याद्गृध्रसीवातः पादयोः स्फुटनं न च|
न सिरास्नायुसङ्कोचः पादाभ्यङ्गेन पादयोः||९२||

**Foot massage :**

By massaging oil in the feet, roughness, immobility, dryness, tiredness and numbness are instantaneously cured; Tenderness, strength and steadiness of feet are improved.

The eyesight becomes clear and Vata (Vitiated) is relieved.

Prevention from sciatica, cracking of feet, constriction of vessels and ligaments of feet is ensured by foot massage with oil. [90-92]

**Parimarjana – applying cream / paste over the body :**

दौर्गन्ध्यं गौरवं तन्द्रां कण्डूं मलमरोचकम्|
स्वेदबीभत्सतां हन्ति शरीरपरिमार्जनम्||९३||

**Parimarjana – applying cream / paste over the body:**

Applying herbal creams over the body eliminates bad smell, cures heaviness, drowsiness, itching and removes undesirable dirt and unpleasantness due to sweating.[93]

**Effects of bathing:**

पवित्रं वृष्यमायुष्यं श्रमस्वेदमलापहम्|
शरीरबलसन्धानं स्नानमोजस्करं परम्||९४||

**Effects of bathing:**

Bathing is purifying, improves sexual strength, stimulant and life-giving; removes fatigue, sweating and dirt, it brings about strength in body and is an aid par excellence for the enhancement of Ojas. [94]

**Role of clean dress in life:**
काम्यं यशस्यमायुष्यमलक्ष्मीघ्नं प्रहर्षणम्|
श्रीमत् पारिषदं शस्तं निर्मलाम्बरधारणम्||९५||

**Role of clean dress in life:**
Wearing clean apparel adds to the bodily charm, reputation, longevity and prevents inauspiciousness. It brings about pleasure, grace, competence to participate in conferences and good looks. [95]

**Use of fragrance:**
वृष्यं सौगन्ध्यमायुष्यं काम्यं पुष्टिबलप्रदम्|
सौमनस्यमलक्ष्मीघ्नं गन्धमाल्यनिषेवणम्||९६||

**Use of fragrance:**
Use of scents and garlands stimulates libido, produces good smell in the body, enhances longevity and charm; it gives corpulence and strength to the body; it is pleasing to the mind and it prevents inauspicious.[96]

**Use of ornaments:**
धन्यं मङ्गल्यमायुष्यं श्रीमद्व्यसनसूदनम्|
हर्षणं काम्यमोजस्यं रत्नाभरणधारणम्||९७||
Wearing of gems and ornaments adds to the prosperity, auspiciousness, longevity, grace, prevents dangers from snakes, evil spirits etc. it is pleasant and charming. It is also conducive to Ojas [97]

**Cleaning of orifices:**
मेध्यं पवित्रमायुष्यमलक्ष्मीकलिनाशनम्|
पादयोर्मलमार्गाणां शौचाधानमभीक्ष्णशः||९८||

**Cleaning of orifices:**
If one frequently cleans the feet and excretory orifices (with water, earth, etc), it promotes intelligence, brings about purity cleanliness and longevity; it also eliminates inauspicious and the bad effects of Kali (i.e., age of vice MW) [98]

**Care for hair and nails:**
पौष्टिकं वृष्यमायुष्यं शुचि रूपविराजनम्|
केशश्मश्रुनखादीनां कल्पनं सम्प्रसाधनम्||९९||

**Care for hair and nails:**
The dressing and cutting of hair, beard (including moustaches) and nails, etc. adds to the corpulence, libido, longevity, cleanliness and beauty.[99]

**Use of foot wears:**
चक्षुष्यं स्पर्शनहितं पादयोर्व्यसनापहम्|
बल्यं पराक्रमसुखं वृष्यं पादत्रधारणम्||१००||

**Use of foot wears:**
Use of foot wears is conducive to eyesight and skin (of feet); it protects the feet from reptiles, etc. it gives strength

and facilitates the display of physical force and is also a stimulant of libido. [100]

**Use of hand stick:**

ईतेः प्रशमनं बल्यं गुप्त्यावरणशङ्करम्‌।
घर्मानिलरजोम्बुघ्नं छत्रधारणमुच्यते॥१०१॥
स्खलतः सम्प्रतिष्ठानं शत्रूणां च निषूदनम्‌।
अवष्टम्भनमायुष्यं भयघ्नं दण्डधारणम्‌॥१०२॥

**Use of hand stick:**

The use of walking stick prevents slipping, and averts the enemy; it gives strength and longevity; it averts fear (from the attacks of reptiles etc) [102]

**Simile on personal vigilance:**

नगरी नगरस्येव रथस्येव रथी यथा।
स्वशरीरस्य मेधावी कृत्येष्ववहितो भवेत्‌॥१०३॥

A wise person should be vigilant about his duties towards his own body like an officer- in-charge of a city and a charioteer towards the city and the chariot respectively.[103]

भवति चात्र-
वृत्त्युपायान्निषेवेत ये स्युर्धर्माविरोधिनः।
शममध्ययनं चैव सुखमेवं समश्नुते॥१०४॥

Thus, it is said: One should adopt only such a means of livelihood which does not clash with virtuous paths. One should follow the path of peace and engage himself in studies. This is how one can attain happiness. [104]

**To sum up:**

तत्र श्लोकाः-
मात्रा द्रव्याणि मात्रां च संश्रित्य गुरुलाघवम्‌।
द्रव्याणां गर्हितोऽभ्यासो येषां, येषां च शस्यते॥१०५॥
अञ्जनं धूमवर्तिश्च त्रिविधा वर्तिकल्पना।
धूमपानगुणाः कालाः पानमानं च यस्य यत्‌॥१०६॥
व्यापत्तिचिह्नं भैषज्यं धूमो येषां विगर्हितः।
पेयो यथा यन्मयं च नेत्रं यस्य च यद्विधम्‌॥१०७॥
नस्यकर्मगुणा नस्तःकार्यं यच्च यथा यदा।
भक्षयेद्दन्तपवनं यथा यद्यद्गुणं च यत्‌॥१०८॥
यदर्थं यानि चास्येन धार्याणि कवलग्रहे।
तैलस्य ये गुणा दिष्टाः शिरस्तैलगुणाश्च ये॥१०९॥
कर्णतैले तथाऽभ्यङ्गे पादाभ्यङ्गेऽङ्गमार्जने।
स्नाने वाससि शुद्धे च सौगन्ध्ये रत्नधारणे॥११०॥
शौचे संहरणे लोम्नां पादत्रच्छत्रधारणे।
गुणा मात्राशितीयेऽस्मिंस्तथोक्ता दण्डधारणे॥१११॥

Quantity of food, articles of food, quantity of food with reference to their heaviness and lightness, such of the diets which are permitted and those which are prohibited, collyrium, herbal smoking, its 3 types, the advantages of smoking, its timings and frequency of use, signs of complications and their treatment, individuals for whom smoking is prohibited, the manner of smoking, the materials which the cigar pipe is made of, different varieties of pipes for different categories of smoking, the therapeutic properties of nasal therapy, the procedure, the therapy that should be used, the manner in which it is to be used and its timings; how and what kind of tooth cleaning stick is to be used and their individual properties, the drugs that are to be kept in mouth for chewing and purpose; therapeutic utility of oil gargle, the benefits of applying oil on the head; benefits of dropping oil into ears, massage, oil massage over the feet, unction, bating, wearing of clean apparel, shaving and cutting of hair, use of foot wear, umbrella and walking stick - all these are described in this Chapter entitled "Matrasitiya, i.e. Quantitative of Dietetics ". [105-111]

इत्यग्निवेशकृते तन्त्रे चरकप्रतिसंस्कृते श्लोकस्थाने मात्राशितीयो नाम पञ्चमोऽध्यायः समाप्तः॥५॥

Thus ends the fifth chapter on "Quantitative Dietetics" of the Sutrasthana of Agnivesha's work as redacted by Charaka.

# 6

# Sutrasthana  Chapter 6
# Tasyashiteeyam

तस्याशितीयोऽध्यायः Tasyashiteeya Adhyaya

अथातस्तस्याशितीयमध्यायं व्याख्यास्यामः||१||

इति ह स्माह भगवानात्रेयः||२||

The sixth chapter of Sutrasthana of Charak Samhita explains the seasonal regimen in detail. It is called Tasyashiteeya Adhyaya. It literally means – qualitative dietetics explained based on seasons.

**Importance of the knowledge of Dietetics:**

तस्याशिताद्यादाहाराद्बलं वर्णश्च वर्धते|

यस्यर्तुसात्म्यं विदितं चेष्टाहारव्यपाश्रयम्||३||

**Importance of the knowledge of Dietetics:**

The strength and luster get improved and enhanced in people who know about the suitable diet and regimen pertaining to every season and practices them accordingly. [3]

**The two Solstices in a year:**

इह खलु संवत्सरं षडङ्गमृतुविभागेन विद्यात्|

तत्रादित्यस्योदगयनमादानं च त्रीनृतूंछिशिरादीन् ग्रीष्मान्तान् व्यवस्येत्, वर्षादीन् पुनर्हेमन्तान्तान् दक्षिणायनं विसर्गं च||४||

विसर्गे पुनर्वायवो नातिरूक्षाः प्रवान्ति, इतरे पुनरादाने; सोमश्चाव्याहतबलः शिशिराभिर्भाभिरापूरयञ्जगदाप्याययति शश्वत्, अतो विसर्गः सौम्यः|

आदानं पुनराग्नेयं; तावेतावर्कवायू सोमश्च कालस्वभावमार्गपरिगृहीताः कालर्तुरसदोषदेहबलनिर्वृत्तिप्रत्ययभूताः समुपदिश्यन्ते||५||

**The two Solstices in a year**

A year comprises six different seasons. 3 seasons each are grouped into two solstices.

**Adana Kala** – means seasons which are hot and dry. The north movement of the Sun brings about water loss in the body. This comprises seasons beginning from late winter to summer. Sun is dominant in the seasons coming under adana kala.

**Visarga Kala** – means seasons which are cold and wet. The southward movement of the Sun is coolant and forms the other seasons beginning with the rainy season to early winter. Moon is dominant in the seasons coming under visarga kala.

Hence one has to adjust his diet based on these variations. [4-5]

**Effect of Adana Kala on body:**

**Uttarayana – Adana kala – Northern Solstice – mid January – mid July**

तत्र रविर्भाभिराददानो जगतः स्नेहं वायवस्तीव्ररूक्षाश्चोपशोषयन्तः शिशिरवसन्तग्रीष्मेषु यथाक्रमं रौक्ष्यमुत्पादयन्तो रूक्षान्
रसांस्तिक्तकषायकटुकांश्चाभिवर्धयन्तो नृणां दौर्बल्यमावहन्ति||६||

**Effect of Adana Kala on body:**
During this, strong sun rays and fast paced winds bring about dryness and absorb moisture from the earth.
The three seasons of this period are –
**Shishira Rutu** – includes Magha and Phalguna months (Mid January – Mid March) – and includes late winter. This
season enhances Bitter taste. The body strength in this season is low.
**Vasanta Rutu** – includes Chaitra and Vaishakha months (Mid-March – Mid May) – and include spring season. This
season enhances astringent taste. The body strength in this season is lower.
**Greeshma** – includes Jyeshta and Ashadha months (Mid May to Mid-July) –and includes summer season. This season
enhances the pungent taste. The body strength in this season is the lowest.Due to increased dryness, the body
becomes weak. [6]

**Effect of Visarga Kala on body:**
**Dakshinayana – Visarga Kala – Southern Solstice – mid July – mid January**
वर्षाशरद्धेमन्तेषु तु दक्षिणाभिमुखेऽर्कं कालमार्गमेघवातवर्षाभिहतप्रतापे, शशिनि चाव्याहतबले, माहेन्द्रसलिलप्रशान्तसन्तापे जगति,
अरूक्षा रसाः प्रवर्धन्तेऽम्ललवणमधुरा यथाक्रमं तत्र बलमुपचीयते नृणामिति||७||

**Visarga Kala** has three seasons.

**Varsha Ritu** (Rainy Season) – includes Shravana and Bhadrapada months – Mid July – mid September – and includes
rainy/monsoon season. This season enhances sour taste. The body strength in this season is mild.

**Sharath Ritu** (Autumn season) – includes Ashvayuja and Karthika months – Mid September to Mid November – and
includes autumn season. This season enhances the salt taste. The body strength in this season is moderate.

**Hemantha Ritu** (Winter season) – includes Margashira and Pushya months – Mid November to Mid January – and
includes winter season. This season enhances the sweet taste. The body strength in this season is high. The oiliness/
unctuousness in the body grows in these periods and dryness is relieved. Hence body strength increases in this
period. [7-8]

**Dietetics and Regimen for winter (Hemanta Rutu):**
भवति चात्र-
आदावन्ते च दौर्बल्यं विसर्गादानयोर्नृणाम्|
मध्ये मध्यबलं, त्वन्ते श्रेष्ठमग्रे च निर्दिशेत्||८||
शीते शीतानिलस्पर्शसंरुद्धो बलिनां बली|
पक्ता भवति हेमन्ते मात्राद्रव्यगुरुक्षमः||९||
स यदा नेन्धनं युक्तं लभते देहजं तदा|
रसं हिनस्त्यतो वायुः शीतः शीते प्रकुप्यति||१०||
तस्मात्तुषारसमये स्निग्धाम्ललवणान् रसान्|
औदकानूपमांसानां मेद्यानामुपयोजयेत्||११||
बिलेशयानां मांसानि प्रसहानां भृतानि च|
भक्षयेन्मदिरां शीधुं मधु चानुपिबेन्नरः||१२||
गोरसानिक्षुविकृतीर्वसां तैलं नवौदनम्|
हेमन्तेऽभ्यस्यतस्तोयमुष्णं चायुर्न हीयते||१३||

अभ्यङ्गोत्सादनं मूर्ध्नि तैलं जेन्ताकमातपम्|
भजेद्भूमिगृहं चोष्णमुष्णं गर्भगृहं तथा||१४||
शीतेषु संवृतं सेव्यं यानं शयनमासनम्|
प्रावाराजिनकौषेयप्रवेणीकुथकास्तृतम्||१५||
गुरूष्णवासा दिग्धाङ्गो गुरुणाऽगुरुणा सदा|
शयने प्रमदां पीनां विशालोपचितस्तनीम्||१६||
आलिङ्ग्यागुरुदिग्धाङ्गीं सुप्यात् समदमन्मथः|
प्रकामं च निषेवेत मैथुनं शिशिरागमे||१७||
वर्जयेदन्नपानानि वातलानि लघूनि च|
प्रवातं प्रमिताहारमुदमन्थं हिमागमे||१८||

**Dietetics and Regimen for winter (Hemanta Rutu):**
During winter, the strength of digestion is so much improved that it is capable of digesting any food irrespective of its heaviness and the quantity. During winter, if proper quantity of food is not taken, it affects the quality of Rasa Dhatu (nutritious fluid generated as a product of digestion). This in turn leads to Vata imbalance.

Therefore, during the winter one should take foods having below mentioned qualities.
Snigdha – oily – unctuous,
Amla – sour and
Lavana – Salt.
Audaka mamsa – meat of the aquatic animals
Anupa mamsa – meat of animals from marshy place
Medya – meet with fat.
Bileshaya Mamsa – meat of burrow- dwelling animals and
Prasaha – animals which catch food by teeth, tear it and eat it
Madira – wine
Seedhu – fermented liquid prepared with ripened fruit should be consumed with honey.
Gorasa Vikruti – cow milk and its products
Ikshu Vikruti – sugarcane and its juice, products like sugar
Vasa – fat of animals
Taila – sesame oil
Nava Odana – fresh rice and grains
Ushna toya – hot water

One should follow below regimen during winter –
Abhyanga – oil massage
Utsadana – palm massage
Murdhni taila – oil application to head
Jentaka Sweda – a type of sweating therapy where one resides in an underground home
Atapa – exposure to sunlight.

- One should ensure that conveyance, bedding and seats are well covered with heavy wrappers, skin, silk cloth, ropes and blankets. One should wear heavy and warm clothes.
- One should smear his body with Agaru – Aquilaria Agallocha.
- One should embrace a healthy woman with big breasts, who has anointed her body with Agaru (Aquilaria agallocha Linn); then he should lie down on the bed, intoxicated, with strong passion.
- One may indulge in excessive sexual intercourse during the winter.

- One should avoid food and drink which are light and are known to cause Vata vitiation.
- One should not expose himself to cold wave.
- One should avoid eating less food and intake of Yavagu (gruel) [9-18]

## Late winter regimen – (Shishira Rutu)

हेमन्तशिशिरौ तुल्यौ शिशिरेऽल्पं विशेषणम्|
रौक्ष्यमादानजं शीतं मेघमारुतवर्षजम्||१९||
तस्माद्धैमन्तिकः सर्वः शिशिरे विधिरिष्यते|
निवातमुष्णं त्वधिकं शिशिरे गृहमाश्रयेत्||२०||
कटुतिक्तकषायाणि वातलानि लघूनि च|
वर्जयेदन्नपानानि शिशिरे शीतलानि च||२१||

## Late winter regimen – (Shishira Rutu)

The Hemanta (early winter) and Shishira (late winter) seasons are similar. But the dryness of Adana kala (shishira falls in Adana Kala) and cold caused by cloud, wind and rain intensifies. So the entire prescription for Hemanta (winter) is to be followed in the Sisira as well. One should stay in a windless and warm home. One should avoid taking diets and drinks which are rich in pungent, bitter and astringent tastes which cause Vata imbalance. One should avoid foods that are light to digest, foods having coolant property and cold drinks. [19-21]

## Spring healthy regimen (Vasanta Rutu)

वसन्ते निचितः श्लेष्मा दिनकृद्भाभिरीरितः|
कायाग्निं बाधते रोगांस्ततः प्रकुरुते बहून्||२२||
तस्माद्वसन्ते कर्माणि वमनादीनि कारयेत्|
गुर्वम्लस्निग्धमधुरं दिवास्वप्नं च वर्जयेत्||२३||
व्यायामोद्वर्तनं धूमं कवलग्रहमञ्जनम्|
सुखाम्बुना शौचविधिं शीलयेत् कुसुमागमे||२४||
चन्दनागुरुदिग्धाङ्गो यवगोधूमभोजनः|
शारभं शाशमैणेयं मांसं लावकपिञ्जलम्||२५||
भक्षयेन्निर्गदं सीधुं पिबेन्माध्वीकमेव वा|
वसन्तेऽनुभवेत् स्त्रीणां काननानां च यौवनम्||२६||

## Spring healthy regimen (Vasanta Rutu)

During spring, Kapha that is accumulated in winters gets liquefied by the heat of the sun and disturbs the power of digestion. It leads to many diseases. So, one should undergo therapies like Vamana (vomiting therapy).

One should avoid

Guru – heavy to digest foods

Snigdha – oily, unctuous foods

Amla and Madhura – sour and sweet foods

One should not sleep during day time

At the advent of spring season, one should habitually resort to

- Vyayama – exercise,
- Mardana – Palm massage/unction,
- Dhumapana – smoking,
- Gandusha – gargling and

- Anjana – collyrium

The excretory orifices should be regularly washed with lukewarm water.
One should smear his body with Chandana (Sandalwood) and Aguru (Aquilaria agallocha)

One should take following foods –

- Yava – barley
- Godhuma – wheat
- Meat of Sarabha (Wapiti), Shasha (Rabbit), Ena (Antelope), Lava (common quail) and Kapinjala and Mridvika (raisins) types of wine.
- One can have sex. [22-26]

**Summer regimen – Greeshma Rutu:**
मयूखैर्जगतः स्नेहं ग्रीष्मे पेपीयते रविः|
स्वादु शीतं द्रवं स्निग्धमन्नपानं तदा हितम्||२७||
शीतं सशर्करं मन्थं जाङ्गलान्मृगपक्षिणः|
घृतं पयः सशाल्यन्नं भजन् ग्रीष्मे न सीदति||२८||
मद्यमल्पं न वा पेयमथवा सुबहूदकम्|
लवणाम्लकटूष्णानि व्यायामं च विवर्जयेत् ||२९||
दिवा शीतगृहे निद्रां निशि चन्द्रांशुशीतले|
भजेच्चन्दनदिग्धाङ्गः प्रवाते हर्म्यमस्तके||३०||
व्यजनैः पाणिसंस्पर्शैश्चन्दनोदकशीतलैः|
सेव्यमानो भजेदास्यां मुक्तामणिविभूषितः||३१||
काननानि च शीतानि जलानि कुसुमानि च|
ग्रीष्मकाले निषेवेत मैथुनादिवरतो नरः||३२||

**Summer regimen – Greeshma Rutu:**
During the summer, the sun rays evaporate moisture from the earth. One should have

- Madhura – sweet tasting foods
- Sheeta – coolant foods
- Drava – liquid foods
- Snigdha – oily, unctuous foods and drinks.
- Cold Mantha (mashed fruits with sugar)
- Jangala Mriga Pakshi – meat of the animals or birds of windy climate,
- ghee and milk along with rice.

**Avoid alcohol during summer :**
One should either drink alcohol in little quantities or should not drink at all. Even if someone consumes alcohol, it should be diluted with plenty of water.

One should avoid taking

- Lavana, Amla, Katu and Ushna – foods having salt, sour, pungent tastes and hot qualities.
- Vyayama – Physical exercise should be avoided

During day time one should sleep in an air-cooled apartment. During the night, after smearing the body with sandalwood paste, one should sleep on an open airy roof, which is cooled by moon rays.

- One should wear pearls
- One should avoid sex and should enjoy gardens, cold water and flowers during summer. [27-32]

**Dietetics and Regimen for rainy season (Varsha Rutu):**
आदानदुर्बले देहे पक्ता भवति दुर्बलः|
स वर्षास्वनिलादीनां दूषणैर्बाध्यते पुनः||३३||
भूबाष्पान्मेघनिस्यन्दात् पाकादम्लाज्जलस्य च|
वर्षास्वग्निबले क्षीणे कुप्यन्ति पवनादयः||३४||
तस्मात् साधारणः सर्वो विधिर्वर्षासु शस्यते|
उदमन्थं दिवास्वप्नमवश्यायं नदीजलम्||३५||
व्यायाममातपं चैव व्यवायं चात्र वर्जयेत्|
पानभोजनसंस्कारान् प्रायः क्षौद्रान्वितान् भजेत्||३६||
व्यक्ताम्ललवणस्नेहं वातवर्षाकुलेऽहनि|
विशेषशीते भोक्तव्यं वर्षास्वनिलशान्तये||३७||
अग्निसंरक्षणवता यवगोधूमशालयः|
पुराणा जाङ्गलैर्मांसैर्भोज्या यूषैश्च संस्कृतैः||३८||
पिबेत् क्षौद्रान्वितं चाल्पं माध्वीकारिष्टमम्बु वा|
माहेन्द्रं तप्तशीतं वा कौपं सारसमेव वा||३९||
प्रघर्षोद्वर्तनस्नानगन्धमाल्यपरो भवेत्|
लघुशुद्धाम्बरः स्थानं भजेदक्लेदि वार्षिकम्||४०||

**Dietetics and Regiment for rainy season (Varsha Rutu):**
During the rainy season, the body is weakened due to weak digestion strength. It is further weakened due to Vata imbalance, which vitiates body tissues. The water acquires a sour taste due to clouds, cold wind and mist. One should avoid the below mentioned during rainy season

- Udamantha (beverage prepared with flour of corns mixed with ghee)
- Divasvapna – day sleep,
- Nadi Jala – water from river,
- Vyayama – exercise,
- Atapa – exposure to sunlight
- Vyavaya – sex.

One should generally use honey in preparing diets, drinks and other kinds of foods. If the days are cooler due to heavy rains with storms, one should take diets which are predominantly sour, salty and unctuous. This serves as an effective antidote to the vitiation of Vata during this season.

In order to maintain normal digestion strength, one should take :

- Purana Yava – old barley,
- Godhuma – wheat and
- Shali – rice
- Jangala Mamsa – meat of animals from arid regions. It should be processed with Yusha (vegetable soup).
- Madhvika or Aristhta (alcoholic preparation) along with honey and water should be consumed.
- Pure rain water or water from the well or pond- boiled and cooled, mixed with little honey should be consumed.
- Pragharshana – massage body with palm
- Udvartana – powder massage
- Snana – bathing
- Gandhamala – wear fragrant garlands during the season.

One should wear light and clean cloth and should reside in a house devoid of humidity. [33-40]

**Healthy regimen for autumn – Sharath Rutu:**
वर्षाशीतोचिताङ्गानां सहसैवार्करश्मिभिः|
तप्तानामाचितं पित्तं प्रायः शरदि कुप्यति||४१||
तत्रान्नपानं मधुरं लघु शीतं सतिक्तकम्|
पित्तप्रशमनं सेव्यं मात्रया सुप्रकाङ्क्षितैः||४२||
लावान् कपिञ्जलानेणानुरभ्राञ्छरभान् शशान्|
शालीन् सयवगोधूमान् सेव्यानाहुर्घनात्यये||४३||
तिक्तस्य सर्पिषः पानं विरेको रक्तमोक्षणम्|
धाराधरात्यये कार्यमातपस्य च वर्जनम्||४४||
वसां तैलमवश्यायमौदकानूपमामिषम्|
क्षारं दधि दिवास्वप्नं प्राग्वातं चात्र वर्जयेत्||४५||
दिवा सूर्यांशुसन्तप्तं निशि चन्द्रांशुशीतलम्|
कालेन पक्वं निर्दोषमगस्त्येनाविषीकृतम्||४६||
हंसोदकमिति ख्यातं शारदं विमलं शुचि|
स्नानपानावगाहेषु हितमम्बु यथाऽमृतम्||४७||
शारदानि च माल्यानि वासांसि विमलानि च|
शरत्काले प्रशस्यन्ते प्रदोषे चन्दुरश्मयः||४८||

The body parts adapted for the rains and cold of the rainy season are suddenly exposed to the heat of the sun with the beginning of autumn. The Pitta accumulated during the rainy season gets imbalanced/aggravated. In this season, sweet, light, cold, and bitter foods and drinks should be taken so as to tackle Pitta. One should consume the below mentioned

- Lava – meat of common quail,
- Kapinjala (grey partridge),
- Ena (Antelope),
- Urabhara (sheep),
- Sharabha (Wapiti), and
- Shasha (Rabbit),
- Rice, barley and wheat
- Tiktasha Sarpisha Pana – Intake of ghee processed with bitter herbs,
- Virechana – Purgation therapy,
- Raktamokshana – bloodletting are advised.

One should avoid

- Atapa – sun bath,
- fat, oil and meat of aquatic and marshy animals and
- Kshara – alkaline and Lavana (salt) preparation and
- Dadhi – curds.

One should not sleep during day time and one should not expose himself to frost and east wind.

**Hamsodaka :**
The water is exposed to the heat during the day and moonlight during night. It is also purified and detoxified by Agastya star. Such water is known as Hansodaka. It is very clear and is good for bathing, swimming and drinking. Use of garlands made of autumnal flowers and clean cloth and also the rays of the moon in the evenings are very beneficial. [41-48].
Thus the seasonal regimen and diet has been explained.

Satmya – Habit forming:
इत्युक्तमृतुसात्म्यं यच्चेष्टाहारव्यपाश्रयम्|
उपशेते यदौचित्यादोकःसात्म्यं तदुच्यते||४९||
When a person indulges in wrong food/lifestyle habits for a long period of time, that wrong habit becomes habitual to the person. This is called as Oka Satmya. Though it is wrong, it might not cause much harm to the person, like the poison in a snake. [49]

देशानामामयानां च विपरीतगुणं गुणैः|
सात्म्यमिच्छन्ति सात्म्यज्ञाश्चेष्टितं चाद्यमेव च||५०||
One should consciously resort to food and lifestyle habits that are opposite to the nature of the season and of the disease. [50]

तत्र श्लोकः:-
ऋतावृतौ नृभिः सेव्यमसेव्यं यच्च किञ्चन|
तस्याशितीये निर्दिष्टं हेतुमत् सात्म्यमेव च||५१||
As per season, the good and avoidable diet and lifestyle, considering Satmya (congeniality) of the person, is explained in the chapter of Tasyashiteeya Adhyaya.
इत्यग्निवेशकृते तन्त्रे चरकप्रतिसंस्कृते श्लोकस्थाने तस्याशितीयो नाम षष्ठोऽध्यायः||६||
Thus ends the sixth chapter on Tasyashiteeya chapter of Sutrasthana of Agnivesha, as redacted by Charaka.

# 7

# Sutrasthana Chapter 7 Na Vegandharaneeyam

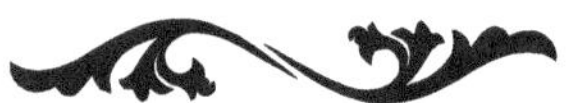

**Na Vegan Dharaneeya Adhyaya - Do Not Suppress Body Urges**

अथातो नवेगान्धारणीयमध्यायं व्याख्यास्यामः||१||

इति ह स्माह भगवानात्रेयः||२||

As per Ayurveda, natural body urges like the urge to defecate, to urinate etc. should not be suppressed. The 7th chapter of Charak Samhita Sutrasthana explains in detail about various diseases caused due to suppression of natural body urges and line of treatment for each.

**Natural body urges that should not be suppressed :**

न वेगान् धारयेद्धीमाञ्जातान् मूत्रपुरीषयोः|

न रेतसो न वातस्य न छर्द्याः क्षवथोर्न च||३||

नोद्गारस्य न जृम्भाया न वेगान् क्षुत्पिपासयोः|

न बाष्पस्य न निद्राया निःश्वासस्य श्रमेण च||४||

**Natural body urges that should not be suppressed :**

One should not suppress the following natural urges:

- Mutra Vega – urge to urinate
- Pureesha Vega – urge to defecate
- Retas – Urge to ejaculate
- Vata – urge to fart,
- Chardi – Urge to vomit
- Kshavatu – Urge to sneeze
- Udagara – urge to belch
- Jrumbha – urge to yawn
- Kshut – hunger
- Pipasa – thirst
- Vashpa – urge to weep
- Nidra – urge to sleep
- Nishwasa – breath caused by overexertion [3-4]

एतान् धारयतो जातान् वेगान् रोगा भवन्ति ये|

पृथक्पृथक्चिकित्सार्थं तान्मे निगदतः शृणु||५||

Various types of diseases occur by the suppression of these urges. Such diseases and lines of treatment are explained below. [5]

**Symptoms caused by suppressing urge to urinate :**

बस्तिमेहनयोः शूलं मूत्रकृच्छ्रं शिरोरुजा |
विनामो वङ्क्षणानाहः स्याल्लिङ्गं मूत्रनिग्रहे||६||
स्वेदावगाहनाभ्यङ्गान् सर्पिषश्चावपीडकम् |
मूत्रे प्रतिहते कुर्यात्त्रिविधं बस्तिकर्म च||७||

**Suppression of urge to urinate causes**
Basti Mehanayo shoolam – pain in bladder and phallus,
Mutrakruchra – dysuria, pain while passing urine,
Shiro Ruja – headache,
Vinamo – bending of the body
Vamkshana anaaha – distension, fullness of lower abdomen

**Treatment for symptoms of suppressing urge to urinate**
Sveda – sweating therapy
Avagahana – tub bath therapy
Abhyanga – oil massage,
Sarpisha Avapidana – nasal drops of ghee
Three types of Basti – urethral / vaginal / rectal enema. [6-7]

**Urge to defecate – symptoms of avoidance**

पक्वाशयशिरःशूलं वातवर्चोऽप्रवर्तनम् |
पिण्डिकोद्वेष्टनाध्मानं पुरीषे स्यादिवधारिते||८||
स्वेदाभ्यङ्गावगाहाश्च वर्तयो बस्तिकर्म च|
हितं प्रतिहते वर्चस्यन्नपानं प्रमाथि च||९||

**Urge to defecate – symptoms of avoidance**
If one holds the urge for defecation, it causes

- Pakvashaya Shula – abdominal colic pain,
- Shirashula – headache,
- Vata, Varcha Pravartana – involuntary defecation and release of flatus
- Pindikodveshtana – cramps in the calf muscles
- Adhmana – distension, fullness of abdomen.

**Treatment**
In such cases, the below mentioned treatments should be done as and when required

- Sveda – sweating therapy
- Abhyanga – oil massage,
- Avagaha – sitz bath,
- Varti – rectal suppositories
- Basti Karma – rectal enema

- Pramathi Annapana – intake of foods and drinks that are laxative in nature [8-9]

**Urge for Seminal discharge / ejaculation of semen – Shukra Vega Avarodha Janya Vyadhi**
मेढ्रे वृषणयोः शूलमङ्गमर्दो हृदि व्यथा।
भवेत् प्रतिहते शुक्रे विबद्धं मूत्रमेव च॥१०॥
तत्राभ्यङ्गोऽवगाहश्च मदिरा चरणायुधाः।
शालिः पयो निरूहश्च शस्तं मैथुनमेव च॥११॥

**Urge for seminal discharge – Shukra Vega Avarodha Janya Vyadhi**
Suppressing 'urge to ejaculation' leads to –

- Medhra Vrushana shoola – Pain in phallus and testicles,
- Angamarda – malaise, body ache,
- Hrudi Vyatha – pain and discomfort in chest region
- Mutra Vibandha – retention of urine

**Treatment**
Abhyanga – oil massage to groin region
Avagaha – sitz bath
Madira - wine
Charanayudha – chicken,
Shali – rice
Paya – milk
Niruha type of basti (made with Kashayam)
Maithuna – sexual intercourse [10-11]

**Suppression of urge to fart – Adhovata Vega Nirodha**
सङ्गो विण्मूत्रवातानामाध्मानं वेदना क्लमः।
जठरे वातजाश्चान्ये रोगाः स्युर्वातनिग्रहात्॥१२॥
स्नेहस्वेदविधिस्तत्र वर्तयो भोजनानि च।
पानानि बस्तयश्चैव शस्तं वातानुलोमनम्॥१३॥
If one suppresses the urge for passing flatus / fart, this causes

- Sango Vit Mutra Vatanaam – retention of feces, urine and flatus,
- Adhmana – distension, fullness of abdomen,
- Vedana – pain,
- Klama – exhaustion, tiredness
- Diseases of Vata imbalance in stomach

**Treatment**
Snehana – oil massage
Sveda – sweating treatment
Varti – rectal suppositories,
Vatanulomana Bhojana, Pana – intake of foods and drinks that enables normal downward movement of flatus

Basti – rectal enema [12-13]

## Suppression of urge for vomiting – Chardi Vega Avarodha:

कण्डूकोठारुचिव्यङ्गशोथपाण्ड्वामयज्वराः|
कुष्ठहृल्लासवीसर्पाश्छर्दिनिग्रहजा गदाः||१४||
भुक्त्वा प्रच्छर्दनं धूमो लङ्घनं रक्तमोक्षणम्|
रूक्षान्नपानं व्यायामो विरेकश्चात्र शस्यते||१५||

## Suppression of urge for vomiting – Chardi Vega Avarodha

Kandu – itching, pruritus, urticaria,

Kota – black pigmentation of face,

Aruchi – Anorexia,

Shotha – oedema,

Pandu – anaemia,

Jvara – fever,

Kushta – skin diseases,

Hrullasa – nausea

Visarpa – erysipelas, a spreading type of skin disease.

## Treatment

Prachardanam – induction of vomiting,

Dhumapana – herbal smoking,

Langhana – fasting,

Raktamokshana – bloodletting (useful in skin diseases),

Rooksha Annapana – food and drink that are dry in nature,

Vyayama – physical exercise and

Virechana – purgation treatment [14-15]

## Diseases caused by suppression of urge to sneeze – Kshavatu vega Avarodha

मन्यास्तम्भः शिरःशूलमर्दितार्धावभेदकौ|
इन्द्रियाणां च दौर्बल्यं क्षवथोः स्यादिवधारणात्||१६||
तत्रोर्ध्वजत्रुकेऽभ्यङ्गः स्वेदो धूमः सनावनः|
हितं वातघ्नमाद्यं च घृतं चौत्तरभक्तिकम्||१७||

## Diseases caused by suppression of urge to sneeze are

Manyasthamba – neck stiffness – torticollis,

Shirashoola – headache,

Ardita – facial paralysis,

Ardhavabhedaka – hemicrania, migraine and

Indriyanam Daurbalyam – weakness of the sense organs.

## Treatment

Urdhwa Jatru Abhyanga – oil massage to head and neck

Svedana – sweating therapy

Dhumapana – herbal smoking

Navana – nasal drops

Food that pacifies Vata

Ghrita – intake of ghee after meals [16-17]

## Diseases caused by suppression of belching / eructation reflex: - Udgara Vega

Hikka – hiccups

Shwasa – breathing difficulties

Aruchi – anorexia

Kampa – tremors

Vibandho Hrudaya uraso – feeling of obstruction in chest and heart region.

## Treatment:

हिक्का श्वासोऽरुचिः कम्पो विबन्धो हृदयोरसोः|

उद्गारनिग्रहात्तत्र हिक्कायास्तुल्यमौषधम्||१८||

**Treatment:** Similar to the treatment for suppression of hiccups. [18]

## Diseases caused by suppression of yawning reflex: Jrmbha Vega Avarodha

विनामाक्षेपसङ्कोचाः सुप्तिः कम्पः प्रवेपनम्|

जृम्भाया निग्रहात्तत्र सर्वं वातघ्नमौषधम्||१९||

Vinama – forward bending of the body

Akshepa – convulsion,

Samkocha – contractions,

Supti – numbness,

Kampa – tremor and

Pravepana – shaking of the body.

**Treatment:** All the measures to balance Vata Dosha should be considered / taken up. [19]

## Diseases caused by suppression of hunger – Kshut Vega Avarodha

कार्श्यदौर्बल्यवैवर्ण्यमङ्गमर्दाऽरुचिर्भ्रमः|

क्षुद्वेगनिग्रहात्तत्र स्निग्धोष्णं लघु भोजनम्||२०||

Karshya – weight loss, emaciation,

Dourbalya – weakness,

Vaivarnya – change in skin complexion,

Angamarda – Malaise, body ache,

Aruchi – Anorexia

Bhrama – dizziness.

Treatment – Intake of oily (unctuous), hot and light-to-digest foods [20]

## Diseases caused by suppression of thirst – Trushna Vega Avarodha

कण्ठास्यशोषो बाधिर्यं श्रमः सादो हृदि व्यथा|

पिपासानिग्रहात्तत्र शीतं तर्पणमिष्यते||२१||

Kanta Asya shosha – dryness of throat and mouth,

Badhirya – deafness,

Shrama – tiredness,

Sada – weakness, body ache and

Hrudi Vyatha – discomfort in heart.

**Treatment** – Coolant drinks that bring about satiation [21]

**Diseases caused by suppression of Tears – Bashpa Vega Avarodha**

प्रतिश्यायोऽक्षिरोगश्च हृद्रोगश्चारुचिर्भ्रमः|
बाष्पनिग्रहणात्तत्र स्वप्नो मद्यं प्रियाः कथाः||२२||

Pratishyaya – rhinitis, running nose,

Akshi roga – eye diseases,

Hrudroga – heart diseases,

Aruchi – anorexia

Bhrama – dizziness

Treatment – sleep, intake of wine and pleasing talks [22]

**Diseases caused by suppression of Sleep: - Nidra Vega Avarodha:**

जृम्भाऽङ्गमर्दस्तन्द्रा च शिरोरोगोऽक्षिगौरवम्|
निद्राविधारणात्तत्र स्वप्नः संवाहनानि च||२३||

**Diseases caused by suppression of Sleep:**

Jrumbha – yawning,

Angamarda – malaise, body ache,

Tandra – drowsiness,

Shiroroga – headache, diseases of head,

Akshi Gourava – heaviness in the eyes.

**Treatment** – havingsound sleep and body massage [23]

**Diseases caused by suppression of exertional breathing: Shramashwasa**

गुल्महृद्रोगसम्मोहाः श्रमनिःश्वासधारणात्|
जायन्ते तत्र विश्रामो वातघ्न्यश्च क्रिया हिताः||२४||

Gulma – bloating

Hrudroga – heart diseases and

Sammoha – fainting, unconsciousness.

**Treatment –** Rest and following of regimen prescribed for Vata Dosha balance [24]

वेगनिग्रहजा रोगा य एते परिकीर्तिताः|
इच्छंस्तेषामनुत्पतिं वेगानेतान्न धारयेत्||२५||

These are the diseases caused by the suppression of the various natural body urges. One who wants to prevent diseases should not suppress these urges. [25] We learnt about Adharaneeya Vega – the urges that should not be suppressed / withheld.

Now Charaka explains about Dharaneeya Vegas – the urges that should be suppressed

**Dharaneeya Vega – Suppressible urges:**

इमांस्तु धारयेद्वेगान् हितार्थी प्रेत्य चेह च|
साहसानामशस्तानां मनोवाक्कायकर्मणाम्||२६||

One, who is desirous of his well-being during his lifetime and after death, should suppress urges of rashness and evil deeds – of mental, oral and physical nature. [26]

**Mental suppressible urges**

लोभशोकभयक्रोधमानवेगान् विधारयेत्|

नैर्लज्ज्येर्ष्यातिरागाणामभिध्यायाश्च बुद्धिमान्||२७||

A wise person should suppress mental urges pertaining to

Lobha – greed,

Shoka – grief,

Bhaya – fear,

Krodha – anger,

Mana – vanity,

Nairlajja – shamelessness,

Irshya – jealousy,

Atiraga – excessive desire

Abhidhyaya – ill will, malice [27]


**Speech related suppressible urges**

परुषस्यातिमात्रस्य सूचकस्यानृतस्य च|

वाक्यस्याकालयुक्तस्य धारयेद्वेगमुत्थितम्||२८||

One should suppress the urges of

Parusha – speaking extremely harsh words,

Atimatra – speaking excessively,

Soochaka – back-biting

Anruta – lies

Akala Vakya – use of untimely words [28]


**Suppressible urges related to deeds**

देहप्रवृत्तिर्या काचिद्विद्यते परपीडया|

स्त्रीभोगस्तेयहिंसाद्या तस्यावेगान्विधारयेत्||२९||


**Suppressible urges related to deeds**

Stribhoga – desire towards other women

Astheya – theft,

Himsa – Violence, hostility,

Parapeeda – ill-treatment / harming others are to be restrained [29]


पुण्यशब्दो विपापत्वान्मनोवाक्कायकर्मणाम्|

धर्मार्थकामान् पुरुषः सुखी भुङ्क्ते चिनोति च||३०||


The virtuous person who suppresses all the above bad urges relating to mind, speech and physical actions, is happy and he alone enjoys the fruits of

Dharma – good deeds,

Artha – wealth, prosperity

Kama – desire, wish [30]


**Definition of exercise**

शरीरचेष्टा या चेष्टा स्थैर्यार्था बलवर्धिनी|

देहव्यायामसङ्ख्याता मात्रया तां समाचरेत्||३१||

The physical activity done with the purpose of improving body strength and immunity is called as Exercise – Vyayama. Exercise should always be done in moderation. [31]

## Good effects of exercise:

लाघवं कर्मसामर्थ्यं स्थैर्यं दुःखसहिष्णुता |
दोषक्षयोऽग्निवृद्धिश्च व्यायामादुपजायते||३२||

Right amount of exercise brings about

Laghavam – lightness to the body (and mind)

Karmasaamrthyam – increases work capacity

Sthairyam – increases body stability,

Dukha sahishunta – improves body and mind resistance to discomfort / tolerance to hardships and pain

Doshakshaya – balances the Tridosha

Agnivruddhi – improves digestion strength. [32]

## Bad effect of excessive exercise:

श्रमः क्लमः क्षयस्तृष्णा रक्तपित्तं प्रतामकः|
अतिव्यायामतः कासो ज्वरश्छर्दिश्च जायते||३३||
(स्वेदागमः श्वासवृद्धिर्गात्राणां लाघवं तथा|
हृदयाद्युपरोधश्च इति व्यायामलक्षणम्||१||)|

## Bad effect of excessive exercise:

Shrama – tiredness,

Klama – exhaustion

Kshaya – depletion of body tissues

Trushna – excessive thirst

Raktapitta – bleeding disorders – such as nasal bleeding, worsening of menorrhagia in women etc.

Pratamaka – breathing difficulties,

Kasa – cough,

Jwara – fever,

Chardi – vomiting. [33]

## Features of right amount of exercise:

Svedagama – sweating, perspiration,

Shvasa vruddhi – enhanced breathing,

Gaatranaam laghavam – lightness of the body parts,

Hrudayadi Uparodha – feeling of inhibition / resistance in the heart and such other organs of the body are indication that it is time to stop exercising.

## Avoid excess indulgence in the following:

व्यायामहास्यभाष्याध्वग्राम्यधर्ममप्रजागरान्|
नोचितानपि सेवेत बुद्धिमानतिमात्रया||३४||
एतानेवंविधांश्चान्यान् योऽतिमात्रं निषेवते|
गजं सिंह इवाकर्षन् सहसा स विनश्यति||३५||
(अतिव्यवायभाराध्वकर्मभिश्चातिकर्शिताः |
क्रोधशोकभयायासैः क्रान्ता ये चापि मानवाः||१||
बालवृद्धप्रवाताश्च ये चोच्चैर्बहुभाषकाः|
ते वर्जयेयुर्व्यायामं क्षुधितास्तृषिताश्च ये||२||) |

## Avoid excess indulgence in the following:

Vyayama – exercise

Hasya – laughing,

Bhashya – speaking,

Adhva – travelling on foot / walking

Gramya Dharma – sexual activities and

Prajagara – staying awake till late night. [34]

One who indulges excessively in these and such other activities, perishes like a lion trying to fight a huge elephant. [35]

**Who should quit exercise**

Ativyavaya – who indulges in excessive sexual activity

Bhara – who lifts heavy weight

Adhva – who walks long distances

Karmabhi atikarshita – who is weakened by excessive work

Bala – children

Vruddha – elderly

Pravata – who have Vata imbalance

Ucchai Bahu Bhashaka – who speak loudly and who speak too much

Kshudhita – who is hungry

Trushita – who is thirsty

**Schedule for giving up bad habits:**

उचितादहितादद्धीमान् क्रमशो विरमेन्नरः|

हितं क्रमेण सेवेत क्रमश्चात्रोपदिश्यते||३६||

प्रक्षेपापचये ताभ्यां क्रमः पादांशिको भवेत्|

एकान्तरं ततश्चोर्ध्वं द्व्यन्तरं त्र्यन्तरं तथा||३७||

**Schedule for giving up bad habits:**

A wise person should give up unwholesome and unhealthy practices to which he is addicted and should gradually adopt wholesome and healthy practices. This process of shifting to healthy practices should be gradual.

- On the first day one should give up a quarter of the unhealthy practice (shall maintain ¾ of it) and correspondingly adopt a quarter of healthy and wholesome practice.
- On the second and third days, half of the bad habit should be given up and half of the wholesome practice is to be continued.
- On the 4th, 5th and 6th days, ¾ of the good habits should be adopted.
- On the 7th day, switch fully to the good habit. [36-37]

क्रमेणापचिता दोषाः क्रमेणोपचिता गुणाः|

सन्तो यान्त्यपुनर्भावमप्रकम्प्या भवन्ति च||३८||

By slowly and gradually giving up the bad habits and by slowly cultivating the good habit, the body becomes accustomed well to the new habit without any complication. [38]

**Dosha Body types**

समपित्तानिलकफाः केचिद्गर्भादि मानवाः|

दृश्यन्ते वातलाः केचित्पित्तलाः श्लेष्मलास्तथा||३९||

तेषामनातुराः पूर्वं वातलाद्याः सदातुराः|

दोषानुशयिता ह्येषां देहप्रकृतिरुच्यते||४०||

## Dosha Body types

Some persons maintain perfect balance of Vata, Pitta and Kapha Dosha from the very time of conception; some are dominated by Vata, some by Pitta and some others by Kapha. Those with perfect balance of Tridosha are not prone to diseases. They are called Anatura i.e. *not diseased*. Those with single Dosha body types, like Vata body type, Pitta body type etc. are called Sadatura 'always have or always prone to diseases' and are very much susceptible to diseases. The persons having dominance of two doshas i.e. Vata-Pitta, Pitta-Kapha, Vata-Kapha are less prone to diseases, than those with single Dosha body types. [39-40]

विपरीतगुणस्तेषां स्वस्थवृत्तेर्विधिर्हितः|
समसर्वरसं सात्म्यं समधातोः प्रशस्यते||४१||

In case of 'Single Dosha body types', diet and regimen with qualities opposite to the Dosha should be followed. For individuals having 'Tridosha balance body type', habitual intake of diets consisting of all Rasas (tastes) in proportionate quantity is prescribed. [41]

## Excretory orifices:

द्वे अधः सप्त शिरसि खानि स्वेदमुखानि च|
मलायनानि बाध्यन्ते दुष्टैर्मात्राधिकैर्मलैः||४२||
मलवृद्धिं गुरुतया लाघवान्मलसङ्क्षयम्|
मलायनानां बुध्येत सङ्गोत्सर्गादतीव च||४३||

## Excretory orifices:

There are two orifices in the lower part of the body (rectum and urethra), seven orifices in head (two eyes, two ears, two nostrils and mouth) and there are multiple openings of sweat glands, i.e. hair roots serving the purpose of excretion. These orifices may get vitiated by excessive production of waste products. If there is heaviness in the excretory orifices or there is excessive excretion, it is indicative of an increase in excreta (waste products). Similarly, if there is lightness in the excretory orifices or three is no excretion it indicates the decrease in excreta. [42-43]

## Principle of treatment for disorders of excretory orifices:

तान् दोषलिङ्गैरादिश्य व्याधीन् साध्यानुपाचरेत्|
व्याधिहेतुप्रतिद्वन्द्वैर्मात्राकालौ विचारयन्||४४||

One should decide on the exact nature of the disease with the help of signs and symptoms indicated above. One should ascertain the extent of increase or vitiation of excreta and then should treat the curable ones. The treatment shall be done with therapies which are having opposite qualities as those of the diseases and their causes. The treatment should also be done paying due regard to the dose of medicine and time. [44]

## Importance of following the regimen for healthy persons:

विषमस्वस्थवृत्तानामेते रोगास्तथाऽपरे|
जायन्तेऽनातुरस्तस्मात् स्वस्थवृत्तपरो भवेत्||४५||

Those who do not follow healthy daily and seasonal habits are prone to diseases. Hence, a healthy person should follow proper daily and seasonal regimens for the maintenance of good health. [45]

## Time for Panchakarma purification procedures:

माधवप्रथमे मासि नभस्यप्रथमे पुनः|
सहस्यप्रथमे चैव हारयेद्दोषसञ्चयम्||४६||

स्निग्धस्विन्नशरीराणामूर्ध्वं चाधश्च नित्यशः|
बस्तिकर्म ततः कुर्यान्नस्यकर्म च बुद्धिमान्||४७||
यथाक्रमं यथायोग्यमत ऊर्ध्वं प्रयोजयेत्|
रसायनानि सिद्धानि वृष्ययोगांश्च कालवित्||४८||
रोगास्तथा न जायन्ते प्रकृतिस्थेषु धातुषु|
धातवश्चाभिवर्धन्ते जरा मान्द्यमुपैति च||४९||
विधिरेष विकाराणामनुत्पत्तौ निदर्शितः|
निजानामितरेषां तु पृथग्गेवोपदेक्ष्यते||५०||

## Time for Panchakarma purification procedures

One should administer purification procedures on

Madhava Prathame Maasi – Chaitra (Mid-March – Mid April)

Nabhasya Prathame Maasi – Shravana (Mid July – Mid August)

Sahasya Prathame Maasi – Margashira (Mid November – Mid December)

After the oleation (Sneha karma) and sweating therapies (Svedana), one should administer emetics (Vamana) and purgatives (Virechana). Then one should administer enema (Basti) and inhalation therapies (Nasya) in proper sequences according to the requirement. After that, one should administer rejuvenation and aphrodisiac therapies (Rasayana and Vajikarana) based on the patient's requirement. By this, the body tissues get good nourishment. This delays the ageing process.

Thus, the ways and means of preventing diseases due to endogenous factors (Nija vyadhis) have been described. Those with exogenous causes (Agantuja Vyadhis) are explained further. [45-50]

## Exogenous diseases – Agantuja Roga

ये भूतविषवाय्वग्निसम्प्रहारादिसम्भवाः|
नृणामागन्तवो रोगाः प्रज्ञा तेष्वपराध्यति||५१||
ईर्ष्याशोकभयक्रोधमानद्वेषादयश्च ये|
मनोविकारास्तेऽप्युक्ताः सर्वे प्रज्ञापराधजाः||५२||

## Exogenous diseases – Agantuja Roga

- These disorders are caused by
- Bhuta – evil spirits,
- Visha – poison,
- Vayu – wind,
- Agni – fire,
- Samprahaara – assault / external injury

These diseases are caused by Prajnaparadha – acting against one's right conscience.

Even the bad emotions such as

- Irshya – malice, jealous
- Shoka – despair, grief
- Bhaya – fear
- Krodha – anger
- Mana – vanity and
- Dvesha – hatred, etc mental disorders are due to Prajnaparadha. [51-52]

**Prevention of exogenous diseases- Agantuja Roga:**

त्यागः प्रज्ञापराधानामिन्द्रियोपशमः स्मृतिः|
देशकालात्मविज्ञानं सद्वृत्तस्यानुवर्तनम्||५३||
आगन्तूनामनुत्पत्तावेष मार्गो निदर्शितः|
प्राज्ञः प्रागेव तत् कुर्यादिधितं विद्याद्यदात्मनः||५४||

**Prevention of exogenous diseases- Agantuja Roga:**
These Agantu rogas can be prevented by

- Avoiding Prajnaparadha – acting as per one's right conscience,
- Indriyopashama – control over sense organs,
- Smruti – Keeping God in memory,
- Desha, Kala Atma Vijnana – knowledge of the place, time and one's own soul and
- Sadvrutta – good conduct.

One desirous of his own well-being should follow this, in advance. [53-54]

आप्तोपदेशप्रज्ञानं प्रतिपत्तिश्च कारणम्|
विकाराणामनुत्पत्तावुत्पन्नानां च शान्तये||५५||
Aptopadesha (Knowledge about the prescription and advice of ancient authority sages),
Prajnana – having superior knowledge, are the means to prevent and to treat diseases. [55]

**Unsuitable persons for company:**

पापवृत्तवचःसत्वाः सूचकाः कलहप्रियाः|
मर्मोपहासिनो लुब्धाः परवृद्धिद्विषः शठाः||५६||
परापवादरतयश्चपला रिपुसेविनः|
निर्घृणास्त्यक्तधर्माणः परिवर्ज्या नराधमाः||५७||

**Unsuitable persons for company:**
Below mentioned kinds of people are unsuitable for company and hence need to be disowned –

- those who have sinful conduct,
- tension seekers,
- backbiters,
- sadists,
- greedy,
- those who envy the property of others,
- cruel,
- those who indulge in defaming others,
- the fickle minded,
- those who serve the enemy,
- those without any compassion and
- those who do not follow the virtuous course of life [56-57]

**Suitable persons for company:**
बुद्धिविद्यावयःशीलधैर्यस्मृतिसमाधिभिः|

वृद्धोपसेविनो वृद्धाः स्वभावज्ञा गतव्यथाः||५८||
सुमुखाः सर्वभूतानां प्रशान्ताः शंसितव्रताः|
सेव्याः सन्मार्गवक्तारः पुण्यश्रवणदर्शनाः||५९||

**Suitable persons for company:**

Below mentioned kinds of people are suitable for company and hence should be accompanied –

- those who are experienced, intellectuals, knowledgeable,
- those having good character, are courageous, having good memory,
- those who take care of elders
- aged,
- those who understands your nature,
- those who are devoid of anxieties,
- those who are sweet spoken
- those who are peaceful,
- those who follow righteous course of action;
- those who advocate good conduct and
- those whose very name and sight are auspicious [58-59]

आहाराचारचेष्टासु सुखार्थी प्रेत्य चेह च|
परं प्रयत्नमातिष्ठेद्बुद्धिमान् हितसेवने||६०||

One desirous of health in this world and the world beyond, should try his level best to follow the principles of health relating to diet, conduct and action.[60]

**Rules for using curd:**

न नक्तं दधि भुञ्जीत न चाप्यघृतशर्करम्|
नामुद्गयूषं नाक्षौद्रं नोष्णं नामलकैर्विना ||६१||
ज्वरासृक्पित्तवीसर्पकुष्ठपाण्ड्वामयभ्रमान्|
प्राप्नुयात्कामलां चोग्रां विधिं हित्वा दधिप्रियः||६२||
न नक्तं दधि भुञ्जीत न चाप्यघृतशर्करम्|
नामुद्गयूषं नाक्षौद्रं नोष्णं नामलकैर्विना ||६१||
ज्वरासृक्पित्तवीसर्पकुष्ठपाण्ड्वामयभ्रमान्|
प्राप्नुयात्कामलां चोग्रां विधिं हित्वा दधिप्रियः||६२||

**Rules for using curd:**

- One should not take curd at night;
- If one desires to take curd at night, it can be taken along with ghee, sugar, green gram soup, honey or Amalaka (Amla – Indian Gooseberry)
- It should not be taken hot.
- If one does not follow these rules he is likely to suffer from diseases like fever, Raktapitta (bleeding disorders), Visarpa (Erysipelas), Kushta (skin diseases), Pandu (Anemia), Bhrama (dizziness) and Kamala (Jaundice).[61-62]

**Summary:**

तत्र श्लोकाः:-

वेगा वेगसमुत्थाश्च रोगास्तेषां च भेषजम्|
येषां वेगा विधार्याश्च यदर्थं यदिद्धिताहितम्||६३||
उचिते चाहिते वर्ज्ये सेव्ये चानुचिते क्रमः|
यथाप्रकृति चाहारो मलायनगदौषधम्||६४||
भविष्यतामनुत्पत्तौ रोगाणामौषधं च यत्|
वर्ज्याः सेव्याश्च पुरुषा धीमताऽऽत्मसुखार्थिना||६५||
विधिना दधि सेव्यं च येन यस्मात्तदत्रिजः|
नवेगान्धारणेऽध्याये सर्वमेवावदन्मुनिः||६६||
इत्यग्निवेशकृते तन्त्रे चरकप्रतिसंस्कृते श्लोकस्थाने नवेगान्धारणीयो नाम सप्तमोऽध्यायः||७||

**Summary**

In this chapter, Acharya Atreya has explained, all about natural urges, diseases caused due to suppressing them, urges that are to be suppressed, what is wholesome, what is unwholesome; how to leave a bad habit and replace it with a good habit, diet rules, prevention of diseases, persons who should be accompanied and who should not be and rules regarding intake of curd. [63-64].

इत्यग्निवेशकृते तन्त्रे चरकप्रतिसंस्कृते श्लोकस्थाने नवेगान्धारणीयो नाम सप्तमोऽध्यायः||७||

Thus ends the seventh chapter.

# 8

# Sutrasthana Chapter 8 Indriyopakramaneeyam

**Indriyopakramaneeya Adhyaya - Mind, Sense Organs**

अथात इन्द्रियोपक्रमणीयमध्यायं व्याख्यास्यामः||१||

इति ह स्माह भगवानात्रेयः||२||

The 8th chapter of Charaka Samhita Sutrasthana is called Indriyopakramaneeya Adhyaya. It explains in detail regarding the mind and sense organs, their qualities, functions and ways of protecting them etc.

**Pancha Panchaka**

इह खलु पञ्चेन्द्रियाणि, पञ्चेन्द्रियद्रव्याणि, पञ्चेन्द्रियाधिष्ठानानि, पञ्चेन्द्रियार्थाः, पञ्चेन्द्रियबुद्धयो भवन्ति, इत्युक्तमिन्द्रियाधिकारे||३||

Panchendriya – 5 sense faculties

Panchendriya Dravya – 5 fundamental materials

Panchendria Adhistana – 5 sense organs

Panchendriya Artha – 5 sense objects

Panchendriya Buddhi – 5 sense perceptions

This set of '5 fives' form Panchapanchaka. The concept of gaining knowledge has been explained with the help of these factors

**Qualities of mind:**

अतीन्द्रियं पुनर्मनः सत्त्वसञ्ज्ञकं, 'चेतः' इत्याहुरेके, तदर्थात्मसम्पदायत्तचेष्टं चेष्टाप्रत्ययभूतमिन्द्रियाणाम्||४||

**Qualities of mind:**

Mind is Atindriya – cannot be perceived by sense organs.

Mind connects sense organs with the intellect. It is known as Satva or Chetas.

Mind's action is determined by the quality of Atma (soul), like happiness, misery etc.

Mind acts as the driving force for all the sense faculties. [4]

**Mind is one, not many:**

स्वार्थेन्द्रियार्थसङ्कल्पव्यभिचरणाच्चानेकमेकस्मिन् पुरुषे सत्त्वं,
रजस्तमःसत्त्वगुणयोगाच्च; न चानेकत्वं, नह्येकं ह्येककालमनेकेषु प्रवर्तते;
तस्मान्नैककाला सर्वेन्द्रियप्रवृत्तिः||५||

**Mind is one, not many:**

In an individual, the mind appears to have multiple characters due to its various actions like

- Sva Artha – perception of its objects,
- Indriya Artha – perception of the objects of the sense faculties,
- Sankalpa Vyabhicharana – its disposition, determination, swift association with sense organs to receive knowledge,

Its association with Rajas, Tamas and Satva qualities. Though the mind does so many actions so swiftly, there is no multiplicity of mind. It is one and only one. Hence the mind does not get associated with multiple sense organs at a single point of time. [5]

## Quality determination of mind:

यद्गुणं चाभीक्ष्णं पुरुषमनुवर्तते सत्त्वं तत्सत्त्वमेवोपदिशन्ति मुनयो बाहुल्यानुशयात्||६||

## Quality determination of mind:

The mind of a person is qualified on the basis of the type of his repeated action; As one indulges in a particular type of good or bad deeds, his mind gets the qualities based on one's actions over a period of time.

## The role of mind in perception of knowledge:

मनःपुरःसराणीन्द्रियाण्यर्थग्रहणसमर्थानि भवन्ति||७||

The sense faculties are capable of perceiving their respective objects only when they are connected to Buddhi (Intellect) by mind. Mind acts as connecting point between sense organs and intellect. [7]

## Pancha Panchaka

**Panchendriya - 5 sense faculties**

Ghranendriya – Olfactory system

Rasanendriya – Gustatory perception system

Chakshurendriya – Ocular system

Sparshanendriya– Somatosensory system

Shravanendriya – Auditory system.

**Panchendriya Dravyani – 5 basic materials**

Prithvi – earth

Ap – water

Teja – fire

Vayu – air

Akasha – ether

**Panchendriya Adhishtana – 5 sense organs**

Ghraana – Nose

Rasana – tongue

Chakshu – eyes

Twak – skin

Karna – ears

**Panchendriya Artha – 5 sense objects**

Gandha – smell

Rasa – taste

Roopa – shape

Sparsha – touch sensation

Shabda – sound

## Panchendriya Buddhi – 5 sense perceptions

तत्र चक्षुः श्रोत्रं घ्राणं रसनं स्पर्शनमिति पञ्चेन्द्रियाणि||८||

पञ्चेन्द्रियद्रव्याणि- खं वायुर्ज्योतिरापो भूरिति||९||

पञ्चेन्द्रियाधिष्ठानानि- अक्षिणी कर्णौ नासिके जिह्वा त्वक् चेति||१०||

पञ्चेन्द्रियार्थाः- शब्दस्पर्शरूपरसगन्धाः||११||

पञ्चेन्द्रियबुद्धयः- चक्षुर्बुद्ध्यादिकाः; ताः पुनरिन्द्रियेन्द्रियार्थसत्त्वात्मसन्निकर्षजाः, क्षणिका, निश्चयात्मिकाश्च, इत्येतत् पञ्चपञ्चकम्||१२||

## Panchendriya Buddhi – 5 sense perceptions

Ghranendriya buddhi – Intellect obtained by smell

Rasanendriya Buddhi – Intellect obtained by tasting

Chakshurendriya Buddhi – Intellect obtained by seeing

Sparshanendriya Buddhi – Intellect obtained by touching

Shravanendriya Buddhi – Intellect obtained by hearing

These 25 form Pancha Panchaka (Five pentads).

The knowledge is the product of combination of objects (Indriya Artha), sense faculties (Indriya), mind (Manas), intellect (Buddhi), and the soul (Atma); they are momentary and determinative. [12]

## Spiritual elements and their actions:

मनो मनोर्थो बुद्धिरात्मा चेत्यध्यात्मद्रव्यगुणसङ्ग्रहः

शुभाशुभप्रवृत्तिनिवृत्तिहेतुश्च, द्रव्याश्रितं च कर्म; यदुच्यते क्रियेति||१३||

## Spiritual elements and their actions:

The mind, the object of the mind, intellect and soul – these four factors constitute spiritual elements and qualities; They serve as factors for promoting an individual to indulge or refrain from virtuous and sinful acts. Like every object (Dravya) has its own Karma (function), the functions of human beings are dependent on the above 4 factors. [13]

## Correlation of Panchabhutika elements with five sense faculties:

तत्रानुमानगम्यानां पञ्चमहाभूतविकारसमुदायात्मकानामपि

सतामिन्द्रियाणां तेजश्चक्षुषि, खं श्रोत्रे, घ्राणे क्षितिः,

आपो रसने, स्पर्शनेऽनिलो विशेषेणोपपद्यते|

तत्र यद्यदात्मकमिन्द्रियं विशेषात्तत्तदात्मकमेवार्थमनुगृह्णाति, तत्स्वभावादिविभुत्वाच्च||१४||

## Correlation of Pancabhutika elements with five sense faculties:

The sense faculties (Indriya) are to be inferred. They cannot be perceived directly. They consist of all the five Mahabhutas (5 basic elements). The olfactory, gustatory, visual, tactile and auditory faculties are specially dominated by Prithvi (earth), Ap (water), Tejas (fire) Vayu (Air) and Akasha (Ether) respectively. The sense faculties perceive only such objects as dominated faculties. This is so, because, the very nature of sense faculties is determined by the particular Mahabhuta it (sense faculty) is specially made of. Sense faculties are capable of perceiving only the objects having the same qualities. [14] For example, the Olfactory system can only perceive smell, the tactile system can only perceive the touch sensation and so on.

## How do sense organs get hurt? How do sense organs gain knowledge?

तदर्थातियोगायोगमिथ्यायोगात् समनस्कमिन्द्रियं विकृतिमापद्यमानं यथास्वं

बुद्ध्युपघाताय सम्पद्यते, सामर्थ्ययोगात् पुनः प्रकृतिमापद्यमानं यथास्वं बुद्धिमाप्याययति॥१५॥

**How do sense organs get hurt? How do sense organs gain knowledge?**

The sense faculties, together with the mind get vitiated by

- Atiyoga – excessive utilisation or indulgence / association of a sense organ with its object (example: seeing at one object for a long period of time)
- Ayoga – non- utilistion or indulgence / association of a sense organ with its object (Eg: sitting in darkness, not seeing anything for a long period of time) and
- Mithya Yoga – or indulgence / association of a sense organ with its object wrong utilisation of the objects concerned. E.g.: seeing very bright objects, gazing at the Sun etc.

These types of contacts cause vitiation of respective sense organs. When the sense organs are utilised properly, they help in acquiring respective knowledge. [15]

**Object of Manas (mind):**

मनसस्तु चिन्त्यमर्थः।

तत्र मनसो मनोबुद्धेश्च त एव समानातिहीनमिथ्यायोगाः

प्रकृतिविकृतिहेतवो भवन्ति॥१६॥

Object (Artha) of Manas (Mind) is Chintana (thinking). The proper or excessive / wrong utilization of mind is responsible for normal or abnormal mental conditions respectively. [16]

**Principles of preventing psychological disturbances:**

तत्रेन्द्रियाणां समनस्कानामनुपतप्तानामनुपतापाय प्रकृतिभावे प्रयतितव्यमेभिर्हेतुभिः; तद्यथा- सात्म्येन्द्रियार्थसंयोगेन बुद्ध्या सम्यगवेक्ष्यावेक्ष्य कर्मणां सम्यक् प्रतिपादनेन, देशकालात्मगुणविपरीतोपासनेन चेति।

तस्मादात्महितं चिकीर्षता सर्वेण सर्वं सर्वदा स्मृतिमास्थाय सद्वृत्तमनुष्ठेयम्॥१७॥

**Principles of preventing psychological disturbances:**

In a healthy state (Prakruti), mind and sense faculties are not disturbed and they perform their duties in a healthy way. In order to maintain mental health, one should make all positive efforts. This can be achieved by the performance of duties after duly considering their pros and cons, with the help of the intellect (Buddhi), together with the sense faculties (Indriya) applied to their respective objects (Indriya Artha). Hence, person, who is desirous of his own well-being should always perform Nobel acts (Sadvritta) with proper care. [17]

**Sadvritta – noble deeds**

तदध्यनुतिष्ठन् युगपत् सम्पादयत्यर्थद्वयमारोग्यमिन्द्रियविजयं चेति; तत् सद्वृत्तमखिलेनोपदेक्ष्यामोऽग्निवेश! तद्यथा- देवगोब्राह्मणगुरुवृद्धसिद्धाचार्यानर्चयेत्, अग्निमुपचरेत्, ओषधीः प्रशस्ता धारयेत्, द्वौ कालावुपस्पृशेत्, मलायनेष्वभीक्ष्णं पादयोश्च वैमल्यमादध्यात्, त्रिःपक्षस्य केशश्मश्रुलोमनखान् संहारयेत्, नित्यमनुपहतवासाःसुमनाः सुगन्धिः स्यात्, साधुवेशः, प्रसिद्धकेशः, मूर्धश्रोत्रघ्राणपादतैलनित्यः, धूमपः, पूर्वाभिभाषी, सुमुखः, दुर्गेष्वभ्युपपत्ता, होता, यष्टा, दाता, चतुष्पथानां नमस्कर्ता, बलीनामुपहर्ता, अतिथीनां पूजकः, पितृभ्यः पिण्डदः, काले हितमितमधुरार्थवादी, वश्यात्मा, धर्मात्मा, हेतावीर्ष्युः, फले नेर्ष्युः, निश्चिन्तः, निर्भीकः, ह्रीमान्, धीमान्, महोत्साहः, दक्षः, क्षमावान्, धार्मिकः, आस्तिकः, विनयबुद्धिविद्याभिजनवयोवृद्धसिद्धाचार्याणामुपासिता, छत्री दण्डी मौली सोपानत्को युगमात्रदृग्विचरेत्, मङ्गलाचारशीलः, कुचेलास्थिकण्टकामेध्यकेशतुषोत्करभस्मकपालस्नानबलिभूमीनां परिहर्ता, प्राक् श्रमाद् व्यायामवर्जी स्यात्, सर्वप्राणिषु बन्धुभूतः स्यात्, क्रुद्धानामनुनेता, भीतानामाश्वासयिता, दीनानामभ्युपपत्ता, सत्यसन्धः, सामप्रधानः, परपरुषवचनसहिष्णुः, अमर्षघ्नः, प्रशमगुणदर्शी, रागद्वेषहेतूनां हन्ता च॥१८॥

**Sadvritta – noble deeds**

One who acts after due analysis of pros and cons simultaneously fulfils both the objectives of maintenance of positive health and control of sense faculties. Such Sadvritta (noble deeds) are explained further.

One should pay respects to the

- Deva – Gods,
- Go – Cows,
- Brahmins,
- Guru – Teacher
- Vruddha – elderly,
- Siddha Acharyas- higher spiritual experts and spiritual teachers

One should give due respects to fire.
One should wear / consume good herbs
One should perform Sandhya Vandana (a vedic ritual aimed at cleansing mind and body) during dawn and dusk, twice a day;
One should clean excretory orifices and feet frequently;
One should have a haircut, shave and nail cut thrice every fortnight;
One should wear good apparel; be happy, apply scent, wear good dress, comb the hair,
One should always apply oil to the head, ears, nostrils and feet,
Dhumapa – do herbal smoking,
Purva Abhibhashi – One should not wait for the others to wish him, in fact one should try to wish first.
Sumukha – One should have a delightful face,
One should protect people in affliction, offer oblation, perform religious ceremonies, donate,
One should pay respect to cross roads, offer bali (a religious oblation), honor the guests, offer pinda (rice and sesame seed lump, offered in memory of the departed souls of the family (Shraaddha),
One should be envy in action, competition and cause but should not be envy in the results,
Nishchinta – do not worry much,
Nirbheeka – be fearless,
Be bashful and wise, have enormous enthusiasm, be clever, forbearing, virtuous, having faith in God,
Be devoted to higher spiritual teachers and those who are advanced in modesty, intellect, learning, heredity and age;
Use an umbrella, a stick, a turban, shoes and see only six feet forward while walking;
Behave auspiciously and display good manners;
Avoid places with dirty apparel, bones, thorns, impure hair, chaff, garbage, ash, fragments of earthen vessels, and the places of bath and worship,
Stop exercise before getting tired excessively,
Be friendly to all creatures, reconcile the angry, console the frightened, be merciful to the poor, be truthful
Have compromising nature, be tolerant towards unpleasant words uttered by others, be controller of intolerance,
Be peaceful and conquer the very roots of attachment and hatred. [18]

## General ethics

नानृतं ब्रूयात्, नान्यस्वमाददीत, नान्यस्त्रियमभिलषेन्नान्यश्रियं, न वैरं रोचयेत्, न कुर्यात् पापं, न पापेऽपि पापी स्यात्, नान्यदोषान् ब्रूयात्, नान्यरहस्यमागमयेन्, नाधार्मिकैर्न नरेन्द्रद्विष्टैः सहासीत नोन्मत्तैर्न पतितैर्न भ्रूणहन्तृभिर्न क्षुद्रैर्न दुष्टैः, न दुष्टयानान्यारोहेत्, न जानुसमं कठिनमासनमध्यासीत, नानास्तीर्णमनुपहितमविशालमसमं वा शयनं प्रपद्येत, न गिरिविषममस्तकेष्वनुचरेत्, न द्रुममारोहेत्, न जलोग्रवेगमवगाहेत्, न कुलच्छायामुपासीत , नाग्न्युत्पातमभितश्चरेत्, नोच्चैर्हसेत्, न शब्दवन्तं मारुतं मुञ्चेत्, नानावृतमुखो जृम्भां क्षवथुं हास्यं वा प्रवर्तयेत्, न नासिकां कुष्णीयात्, न दन्तान् विघट्टयेत्, न नखान् वादयेत्, नास्थीन्यभिहन्यात्, न भूमिं विलिखेत्, न छिन्द्यात्तृणं, न लोष्टं मृद्नीयात्, न विगुणमङ्गैश्चेष्टेत, ज्योतींष्यनिष्टममेध्यमशस्तं च नाभिवीक्षेत, न हुङ्कुर्याच्छवं , न

चैत्यध्वजगुरुपूज्याशस्तच्छायामाक्रामेत्, न क्षपास्वमरसदनचैत्यचत्वरचतुष्पथोपवनश्मशानाघातनान्यासेवेत , नैकः शून्यगृहं न चाटवीमनुप्रविशेत्, न पापवृत्तान् स्त्रीमित्रभृत्यान् भजेत, नोत्तमैर्विरुध्येत, नावरानुपासीत, न जिह्मं रोचयेत्, नानार्यमाश्रयेत्, न भयमुत्पादयेत्, न साहसातिस्वप्नप्रजागरस्नानपानाशनान्यासेवेत, नोर्ध्वजानुश्चिरं तिष्ठेत्, न व्यालानुपसर्पेन्न दंष्ट्रिणो न विषाणिनः, पुरोवातातपावश्यायातिप्रवाताञ्जह्यात्, कलिं नारभेत, नासुनिभृतोऽग्निमुपासीत नोच्छिष्टः, नाधः कृत्वा प्रतापयेत्, नाविगतक्लमो नानाप्लुतवदनो न नग्न उपस्पृशेत्, न स्नानशाट्या स्पृशेदुत्तमाङ्गं, न केशाग्राण्यभिहन्यात्, नोपस्पृश्य ते एव वाससी बिभृयात्, नास्पृष्ट्वा रत्नाज्यपूज्यमङ्गलसुमनसोऽभिनिष्क्रामेत्, न पूज्यमङ्गलान्यपसव्यं गच्छेन्नेतराण्यनुदक्षिणम्||१९||

## General ethics

Do not tell lies.

Do not take over others properties.

Do not long for others wives or property.

Do not indulge in hatred or sinful activities. Never be vice.

Do not disclose other's secrets;

Ditch un-virtuous, traitors, lunatics, fallen persons, abortionists, mean and crooked people

Do not ride dangerous vehicles

Do not sit on a hard seat of knee height.

Do not sleep on a cover-less and pillow-less bed.

Do not sleep or walk on uneven slopes of mountains.

Do not climb an uneven tree.

Do not take a bath in a river having turbulent flow.

Do not sit in the shadow of people of noble families.

Do not move around place of fire.

Do not laugh loudly or release flatus / fart with sound.

Do not yawn / sneeze / laugh without covering your mouth.

Do not itch the nostrils, grind the teeth, produce sound with the nails or knuckles, strike the bones, scrape or dig the earth with nails, cut the straw / grass with nails, mix or break the masses of mud,

Do not maintain improper position of different parts of the body;

Do not see the planets or undesirable, impure or condemned objects.

Do not frown before a corpse nor produce sounds of disgust like 'hum' after seeing the dead body;

Do not cross the shadow of a sacred tree, a flag, teacher, a respectable person or an undesirable person;

During nights, do not enter the premises of a temple, a sacred tree, public courtyard, crossroad, garden, cemetery and slaughter house;

Do not enter a solitary house or forest alone;

Do not have relations with women, friends or servants of bad conduct;

Do not be an enemy of good men. Do not be a friend of bad men.

Do not keep doing crooked things as a choice of action.

Do not indulge in ignoble or frightening acts.

Do not take undue, unnecessary courage.

Do not sleep, vigil, bath, drink or food in excess quantity;

Do not sit for a long time with your knees up.

Do not approach snakes or animals with dangerous teeth and horns;

Avoid easterly wind, sun, snowfall and storms.

Do not provoke a quarrel;

Do not come close to the fire without concentration of mind or without a wash after taking food;

Do not heat the body by keeping fire below;

Do not take a bath unless free from exertion.

Do mouth gargling before bath.

Do not take a bath while naked.

Do not touch your head with the apparel worn at the time of bath or strike the tip of the hair.

After taking bath do not wear the same cloth

Do not go out without touching gems, ghee, feet of respectable persons, auspicious objects and flowers;

Do not pass through by the right side of respectable persons or auspicious objects. [19]

## Healthy Diet Practices

नारत्नपाणिर्नास्नातो नोपहतवासा नाजपित्वा नाहुत्वा देवताभ्यो नानिरूप्य पितृभ्यो नादत्वा गुरुभ्यो नातिथिभ्यो नोपाश्रितेभ्यो नापुण्यगन्धो नामाली नाप्रक्षालितपाणिपादवदनो नाशुद्धमुखो नोदङ्मुखो न विमना नाभक्ताशिष्टाशुचिक्षुधितपरिचरो न पात्रीष्वमेध्यासु नादेशे नाकाले नाकीर्णे नादत्वाऽग्रमग्नये नाप्रोक्षितं प्रोक्षणोदकैर्न मन्त्रैरनभिमन्त्रितं न कुत्सयन्न कुत्सितं न प्रतिकूलोपहितमन्नमाददीत, न पर्युषितमन्यत्र मांसहरितकशुष्कशाकफलभक्ष्येभ्यः, नाशेषभुक् स्यादन्यत्र दधिमधुलवणसक्तुसर्पिभ्यः, न नक्तं दधि भुञ्जीत, न सक्तूनेकानश्नीयान्न निशि न भुक्त्वा न बहून्न द्विर्नोदकान्तरितात्, न छित्वा द्विजैर्भक्षयेत्||२०||

## Healthy Diet Practices

Do not take food –

* without wearing precious stones in hand or without taking bath
* wearing torn apparel or without reciting mantras or
* without offering oblations to the Gods or
* without making offerings to the departed ancestors, teachers, guest and dependents or
* without applying sacred scents or without garlands or
* without washing hands, feet and face or
* without cleaning the mouth
* with face turned towards to the north or
* with disturbed mind or
* surrounded by the insincere, uncultured, dirty or hungry persons
* which is unknown
* at improper place and time or
* in a place surrounded by many persons or
* without first offering food to the fire or
* without sprinkling with sacred waters or
* without sanctifying the food with sacred mantras
* that you hate
* which is dirty or
* which has been served by the opponents

  Also –

* One should consume meat, rhizomes, dry vegetables, fruits and sweets, and avoid any kinds of stale foods
* Do not consume the entire food except in the case of curd, honey, salt and roasted grain flour and ghee.
* Do not take curd at night.
* Do not take roasted- grain flour without mixing it with ghee and sugar or at night or after meals or in large quantities or twice daily or interrupted with water intake. Do not eat by chewing it with your teeth. [20]

नानृजुः क्षुयान्नाद्यान्न शयीत, न वेगितोऽन्यकार्यः स्यात्, न वाय्वग्निसलिलसोमार्कद्विजगुरुप्रतिमुखं निष्ठीविका(वात)वर्चोमूत्राण्युत्सृजेत्, न पन्थानमवमूत्रयेन्न जनवति नान्नकाले, न जपहोमाध्ययनबलिमङ्गलक्रियासु श्लेष्मसिङ्घाणकं मुञ्चेत्||२१||

- Do not sneeze or eat or sleep in a prone position (lying upside down, tummy facing downwards, sleeping on tummy).
- Do not attend to any other work while under the pressure of natural urge;
- Do not let out sputum, excreta or urine in front of the wind, fire, water, the moon, the sun, the Brahmans and the teachers.
- Do not take water on the roadside or in a public place.
- Do not drink water at the time when you are supposed to have food.
- Do not let out nasal excreta during the course of recitation, religious rites, studies, religious offerings and auspicious acts. [21]


न स्त्रियमवजानीत, नातिविश्रम्भयेत्, न गुह्यमनुश्रावयेत्, नाधिकुर्यात्।
न रजस्वलां नातुरां नामेध्यां नाशस्तां नानिष्टरूपाचारोपचारां नादक्षां नादक्षिणां नाकामां नान्यकामां नान्यस्त्रियं नान्ययोनिं नायोनौ
न चैत्यचत्वरचतुष्पथोपवनश्मशानाघातनसलिलौषधिद्विजगुरुसुरालयेषु न सन्ध्ययोर्नातिथिषु नाशुचिर्नाजग्धभेषजो नाप्रणीतसङ्कल्पो
नानुपस्थितप्रहर्षो नाभुक्तवान्नात्यशितो न विषमस्थो न मूत्रोच्चारपीडितो न श्रमव्यायामोपवासक्लमाभिहतो नारहसि व्यवायं
गच्छेत्॥२२॥

Do not insult women.
Do not have too much reliance on them, do not confide secrets to them. Do not authorise them indiscriminately.
Do not indulge in sex with a woman during her menses or with a woman who is suffering from a disease or is impure or is having infection, or a woman with an ugly appearance, or with bad conducts or manners, or with the one devoid of skill.
Do not indulge in sexual intercourse with a woman who is not friendly or has not passionate desire or is passionately attached to somebody else or is married to somebody else or a woman of another caste.
Do not indulge in sex in any organ other than the genital organ.
Avoid sex under religious trees, in a public courtyard, on a cross- road, in a garden, at cemetery, at slaughter house, in water, in clinics or in the houses of Brahmans or teachers or in temples.
Avoid sex during dawn and dusk and on inauspicious days.
Avoid sex being impure, without aphrodisiacs, without intense desire or without erection or without having taken food or with excessive intake of food or in an uneven place or while under the pressure of the urge for urination, after exertion, after physical exercise, in fasts, having exhaustion or in a place having no privacy. [22]


न सतो न गुरून् परिवदेत्, नाशुचिरभिचारकर्मचैत्यपूज्यपूजाध्ययनमभिनिर्वर्तयेत्॥२३॥
Do not speak ill of noble persons and teachers. Do not perform spells, worship of sacred trees and superiors, and studies while being impure. [23]


**How to study properly?**
न विद्युत्स्वनार्तवीषु नाभ्युदितासु दिक्षु नाग्निसम्प्लवे न भूमिकम्पे न महोत्सवे नोल्कापाते न महाग्रहोपगमने न नष्टचन्द्रायां तिथौ
न सन्ध्ययोर्नामुखाद्गुरोर्नावपतितं नातिमात्रं न तान्तं न विस्वरं नानवस्थितपदं नातिद्रुतं न विलम्बितं नातिक्लीबं नात्युच्चैर्नातिनीचैः
स्वरैरध्ययनमभ्यस्येत्॥२४॥
Do not study during un-seasonal lightning, when there is excessive brightness, when there is outbreak of fire, during earthquake, during important festivals, during fall of meteors, during solar or lunar eclipse during new moon day or during dawn or dusk.
Do not study without being initiated by a teacher.
While studying, do not recite words incompletely in sounds nor in high / coarse voice, with improper accent, without sitting symmetrically. Do not recite very fast or very slowly. Do not delay in between recitation. Do not recite in high or low pitch. [24]

नातिसमयं जह्यात्, न नियमं भिन्द्यात्, न नक्तं नादेशे चरेत्, न सन्ध्यास्वभ्यवहाराध्ययनस्त्रीस्वप्नसेवी स्यात्, न बालवृद्धलुब्धमूर्खक्लिष्टक्लीबैः सह सख्यं कुर्यात्, न मद्यद्यूतवेश्याप्रसङ्गरुचिः स्यात्, न गुह्यं विवृणुयात्, न कञ्चिदवजानीयात्, नाहम्मानी स्यान्नादक्षो नादक्षिणो नासूयकः, न ब्राह्मणान् परिवदेत्, न गवां दण्डमुद्यच्छेत्, न वृद्धान्न गुरून्न गणान्न नृपान् वाऽधिक्षिपेत्, न चातिब्रूयात्, न बान्धवानुरक्तकृच्छ्रद्वितीयगुह्यज्ञान् बहिष्कुर्यात्||२५||

Do not deviate from generally approved principles. Do not break code of conduct and ethics.

Do not walk during night or in an inappropriate place.

Do not indulge in eating, studies, sex or sleep during dawn or dusk.

Do not make friends with children, the old, greedy, the fools, persons under affliction or eunuchs.

Do not be attracted towards wine, gambling and prostitutes.

Do not expose secret parts of the body.

Do not insult anyone.

Do not be conceited, unfriendly.

Do not back bite.

Do not insult Brahmans, do not beat cows.

Do not use harsh words towards elders, teachers, persons grouped together or kings.

Do not speak too much.

Do not oust kin, folk, persons attached or persons who had helped you during the time of misery and those who know secrets. [25]

नाधीरो नात्युच्छ्रितसत्त्वः स्यात्, नाभृतभृत्यः, नाविश्रब्धस्वजनः, नैकः सुखी,
न दुःखशीलाचारोपचारः, न सर्वविश्रम्भी, न सर्वाभिशङ्की, न सर्वकालविचारी||२६||

Do not be impatient or over-bold. Do not neglect servants. Do not doubt your kin. Do not enjoy alone. Do not have uncomfortable character, conduct, manners and diseases. Do not rely / suspect everyone. Do not be over-meticulous. [26]

### Self-restraint

न कार्यकालमतिपातयेत्, नापरीक्षितमभिनिविशेत्, नेन्द्रियवशगः स्यात्, न चञ्चलं मनोऽनुभ्रामयेत्, न बुद्धीन्द्रियाणामतिभारमादध्यात्, न चातिदीर्घसूत्री स्यात्, न क्रोधहर्षावनुविदध्यात्, न शोकमनुवसेत्, न सिद्धावुत्सेकं यच्छेन्नासिद्धौ दैन्यं, प्रकृतिमभीक्ष्णं स्मरेत्, हेतुप्रभावनिश्चितः स्याद्धेत्वारम्भनित्यश्च, न कृतमित्याश्वसेत्, न वीर्यं जह्यात्, नापवादमनुस्मरेत्||२७||

Do not have the habit of procrastination and postponing things. Do not do anything without proper examination. Do not be a slave to senses. Do not let lose fickle mind. Do not inflict too much burden over the intellect or senses. Do not act on anger / rejoicing. Do not grieve continuously. Do not be over-happy about achievements or overly depressed about the loss. Always remember your nature and act accordingly. Have faith in correlation of cause and effect. Have faith that good deeds bring good results. Do not be complacent. Do not lose spirit. Do not contemplate on your insults. [27]

### Practices regarding fire worship:

नाशुचिरुतमाज्याक्षततिलकुशसर्षपैरग्निं जुहुयादात्मानमाशीर्भिराशासानः, अग्निर्मे नापगच्छेच्छरीराद्वायुर्मे प्राणानादधातु विष्णुर्मे बलमादधातु इन्द्रो मे वीर्यं शिवा मां प्रविशन्त्वाप आपोहिष्ठेत्यपः स्पृशेत्, दिवः परिमृज्योष्ठौ पादौ चाभ्युक्ष्य मूर्धनि खानि चोपस्पृशेदद्भिरात्मानं हृदयं शिरश्च||२८||

### Practices regarding fire worship:

Do not offer oblations to the fire with cow ghee, intact grains, sesame seeds, Kusha grass and mustard seeds while in impure condition. One should touch water, reciting- Apo hi stha (Rgveda X.9.1) with the following invocation:-
"Let not fire go away from my body",
"May the Wind- God bring life",

"May Lord Vishnu give me strength (Bala)",
"May Lord Indra give me Energy (Veerya)",
"May the benevolent waters enter my body".
After cleaning his lips and feet twice, one should touch with water all the orifices of the head. [28]

**Social good deeds:**
ब्रह्मचर्य ज्ञान दान मैत्रीकारुण्य हर्षोपेक्षा प्रशमपरश्च स्यादिति||२९||
One should keenly follow the path of Brahmacharya knowledge, charity, friendship, compassion, happiness, detachment and peace.[29]

**Summary:**
तत्र श्लोकाः-
पञ्चपञ्चकमुद्दिष्टं मनो हेतुचतुष्टयम्|
इन्द्रियोपक्रमेऽध्याये सद्वृत्तमखिलेन च||३०||
स्वस्थवृत्तं यथोद्दिष्टं यः सम्यगनुतिष्ठति|
स समाः शतमव्याधिरायुषा न वियुज्यते||३१||
नृलोकमापूरयते यशसा साधुसम्मतः|
धर्मार्थावेति भूतानां बन्धुतामुपगच्छति||३२||
परान् सुकृतिनो लोकान् पुण्यकर्मा प्रपद्यते|
तस्माद्वृत्तमनुष्ठेयमिदं सर्वेण सर्वदा||३३||
In this chapter on" the Description of Sense Organs", five pentads, mind, four causative factors and good conduct are explained in detail. One who keenly follows these prescriptions for maintenance of positive health will be devoid of all diseases and lives for hundred years, without meeting an untimely death. He will be praised by the good. He will earn fame all over the world. He will attain virtue and wealth and will become a friend of all living beings. The one with virtuous acts attains the divine abode of good souls, after death. So this code of conduct should always be followed. [30-33]

यच्चान्यदपि किञ्चित् स्यादनुक्तमिह पूजितम्|
वृत्तं तदपि चात्रेयः सदैवाभ्यनुमन्यते||३४||
Even if something is not stated here but that is prescribed elsewhere as a virtuous act, that should also be followed. [35]
इत्यग्निवेशकृते तन्त्रे चरकप्रतिसंस्कृते श्लोकस्थाने इन्द्रियोपक्रमणीयो नामाष्टमोऽध्यायः||८|| इति स्वस्थचतुष्को द्वितीयः||२||
Thus ends the eighth chapter of Sutrasthana of Charaka Samhita, called Indriyopakramaneeya Adhyaya. Thus ends Svastha Chatushka.

# 9

# Sutrasthana Chapter 9 Khuddaka Chatushpadam

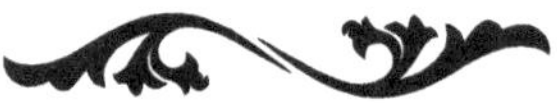

**Khuddaka Chatushpada Adhyaya**
**4 Basic Elements of Ayurvedic Treatment :**
अथातः खुड्डाकचतुष्पादमध्यायं व्याख्यास्यामः||१||
इति ह स्माह भगवानात्रेयः||२||

The 9th chapter of Sutrasthana of Charaka Samhita explains in brief regarding the 4 basic elements of Ayurvedic treatment. This chapter is called Khuddaka Chatushpada Adhyaya. These four elements are essential to fulfil the purpose of treatment.

**4 elements of Ayurvedic treatment**
भिषग्द्रव्याण्युपस्थाता रोगी पादचतुष्टयम्|
गुणवत् कारणं ज्ञेयं विकारव्युपशान्तये||३||

The four aspects of treatment are –
1. Bhishak – Physician,
2. Dravya – Medicine
3. Upasthata – Attendant / nurse
4. Rogi – Patient.
They are responsible for the cure of diseases, provided they have the requisite qualities. [3]

**Definition of health and disease:**
विकारो धातुवैषम्यं, साम्यं प्रकृतिरुच्यते|
सुखसञ्ज्ञकमारोग्यं, विकारो दुःखमेव च||४||

Any disturbance in the equilibrium of Dhatus (Tridosha, body tissues and waste products) is known as disease. The state of their equilibrium is health. Happiness signals towards health and pain signals disease. [4]

**Definition of treatment:**

चतुर्णां भिषगादीनां शस्तानां धातुवैकृते|
प्रवृत्तिर्धातुसाम्यार्था चिकित्सेत्यभिधीयते||५||

The combined efforts of Physician, medicine, attendant and patient, who possess requisite qualities, for restoration of the equilibrium of Dhatus (Tridosha, body tissues and waste products) is known as treatment. [5]

## 4 essential qualities of physician:

श्रुते पर्यवदातत्वं बहुशो दृष्टकर्मता|
दाक्ष्यं शौचमिति ज्ञेयं वैद्ये गुणचतुष्टयम्||६||

Shrute Paryavadatatvam – excellent medical knowledge, sound knowledge of text books / health literature
Bahusho Drushtakarmata – extensive practical knowledge and experience
Dakshya – Dakshata – dexterity, discipline
Shaoucha – Shuchi – cleanliness, clarity, purity [6]

## 4 essential qualities of medicine / herb:

बहुता तत्रयोग्यत्वमनेकविधकल्पना|
सम्पच्चेति चतुष्कोऽयं द्रव्याणां गुण उच्यते||७||

Bahuta – availability in abundance. Ideally the herb or the herbal medicine should be easily and extensively / abundantly available everywhere, all over the world.
Yogyatvam – means suitability. The herb / medicine should be suitable for the particular disease.
Aneka Vidha Kalpana – The herb should be usable in different forms / formulations and doses.
Sampat – the herb / medicine should be so prepared that it has all the desired therapeutic qualities. [7]

## 4 essential qualities of nurse / attendant:

उपचारज्ञता दाक्ष्यमनुरागश्च भर्तरि|
शौचं चेति चतुष्कोऽयं गुणः परिचरे जने||८||

Upachaarajnata – Knowledge of nursing
Daakshya – Dakshata – dexterity, discipline
Anuraga – affection and compassion towards patient
Shaucham – cleanliness, hygiene and purity [8]

## 4 essential qualities of patient:

स्मृतिनिर्देशकारित्वमभीरुत्वमथापि च|
ज्ञापकत्वं च रोगाणामातुरस्य गुणाः स्मृताः||९||

Smruti - Good memory power to learn about instructions about medicine intake.
Nirdeshakaritva – obedience, ability to follow instructions properly
Abhirutva – fearlessness, courage
Jnapakatvam cha roganaam – good memory about list of health complaints / diseases that he is suffering with and uninhibited expressing - these are the four qualities of a patient.[9]

## Importance of physician:

कारणं षोडशगुणं सिद्धौ पादचतुष्टयम्|

विज्ञाता शासिता योक्ता प्रधानं भिषगत्र तु||१०||

These are the 4 factors in treatment, each with 4 essential qualities. These sixteen qualities are responsible for success in treatment. But the physician, by the virtue of his knowledge, administrative power and prescribing knowledge and capacity, is the most important among the four. [10]

**Simile regarding physician:**

पक्तौ हि कारणं पक्तुर्यथा पात्रेन्धनानलाः|
विजेतुर्विजये भूमिश्चमूः प्रहरणानि च||११||
आतुराद्यास्तथा सिद्धौ पादाः कारणसञ्ज्ञिताः|
वैद्यस्यातश्चिकित्सायां प्रधानं कारणं भिषक्||१२||

Vessels, fuel and fire are helping factors for the cook to prepare food;
Favourable topographical position, army and weapons are needed for a king to win the war;
Similarly in the success of treatment the patient, attendant and medicament are only the helpers to the physician. Thus the physician plays the most prominent role in treatment. [11-12]

मृद्दण्डचक्रसूत्राद्याः कुम्भकारादृते यथा|
नावहन्ति गुणं वैद्यादृते पादत्रयं तथा||१३||

In making a mud pot, the cold earth, the wheel, the thread, etc. are of no use without the help of the potter. Without the physician, other three factors, (viz, a patient, the attendant and the herbs) do not serve the purpose. [13]

गन्धर्वपुरवन्नाशं यद्विकाराः सुदारुणाः|
यान्ति यच्चेतरे वृद्धिमाशूपायप्रतीक्षिणः||१४||

If the qualities of patient, attendant and herbs are kept constant, in the most difficult-to-treat diseases, the disease may vanish or may get aggravated very quickly, like the city of Gandharvas, depending on the quality of the physician. [14]

**Condemnation of quackery / bad clinical practices of the doctor:**

सति पादत्रये ज्ञाज्ञौ भिषजावत्र कारणम्
वरमात्मा हुतोऽज्ञेन न चिकित्सा प्रवर्तिता||१५||
पाणिचाराद्यथाऽचक्षुर्ज्ञानाद्भीतभीतवत्|
नौर्मारुतवशेवाज्ञो भिषक् चरति कर्मसु||१६||

It is better to die than to be treated by an ignorant physician. Because, like a blind person moving with help of his hands or like a boat being driven by the wind, a quack physician applies the course of treatment with anxiety and fear because of his ignorance. [15-16]

यद्दृच्छया समापन्नमुतार्य नियतायुषम्|
भिषङ्मानी निहन्त्याशु शतान्यनियतायुषाम्||१७||

Such an inefficient physician may cure a few patients by chance, whose ailments might get cured automatically, but he is likely to kill patients in quick time, who would have otherwise survived if treated properly. [17]

**Qualities of Royal Physician:**

तस्माच्छास्त्रेऽर्थविज्ञाने प्रवृत्तौ कर्मदर्शने|
भिषक् चतुष्टये युक्तः प्राणाभिसर उच्यते||१८||

A good Ayurvedic doctoris the one, who is duly engaged in the study of the science, mastering the actual implications of the disease and the right application of the treatment with practical experience. Such a doctor is known as Pranabhisara Vaidya (saviour of life) [18]

हेतौ लिङ्गे प्रशमने रोगाणामपुनर्भवे|
ज्ञानं चतुर्विधं यस्य स राजार्हो भिषक्तमः||१९||
शस्त्रं शास्त्राणि सलिलं गुणदोषप्रवृत्तये|
पात्रापेक्षीण्यतः प्रज्ञां चिकित्सार्थं विशोधयेत्||२०||

One who possesses the knowledge of the below four factors is fit to become a Royal physician. Those factors are –
Hetu – causative factors for diseases
Linga – characteristic features of diseases
Prashamana – treatment methods for diseases
Rogaanaam Apunarbhave – preventive measures for disease and to maintain health / to treat the diseases in such a way that there would be no recurrence. [19]

A weapon, scripture and water have merits and demerits, depending upon who uses it for what. So, a physician should always have pure thoughts and intellect for the sake of giving proper treatment. [20]

**Six qualities of physician –**
विद्या वितर्को विज्ञानं स्मृतिस्तत्परता क्रिया|
यस्यैते षड्गुणास्तस्य न साध्यमतिवर्तते||२१||
विद्या मतिः कर्मदृष्टिरभ्यासः सिद्धिराश्रयः|
वैद्यशब्दाभिनिष्पत्तावलमेकैकमप्यतः||२२||
यस्य त्वेते गुणाः सर्वे सन्ति विद्यादयः शुभाः|
स वैद्यशब्दं सद्भूतमर्हन् प्राणिसुखप्रदः||२३||

For a physician who possesses below six qualities, no disease is incurable. Those six qualities are –

Vidya – Education,
Vitarka – critical approach, analytical mind
Vijnana – insightful understanding, special knowledge
Smruti – good memory
Tatparata – perseverance
Kriya – practical knowledge

Also,

Vidya – education, knowledge,
Mati – intellect,
Karmadrushti – practical experience,
Abhyasa – knowledge

Siddhi – expertise
Ashraya – accommodating mindset
– these words explains the qualities of "Vaidya – physician" - the one who combines in him all these good qualities will distribute happiness and comfort to all living beings.[21-23]

**Simile about relation of intellect and literature:**

शास्त्रं ज्योतिः प्रकाशार्थं दर्शनं बुद्धिरात्मनः|
ताभ्यां भिषक् सुयुक्ताभ्यां चिकित्सन्नापराध्यति||२४||
चिकित्सिते त्रयः पादा यस्माद्वैद्यव्यपाश्रयः|
तस्मात् प्रयत्नमातिष्ठेद्भिषक् स्वगुणसम्पदि||२५||

Knowledge of medical science = light, which illuminates the room and relieves darkness.
Intellect of the physician can also be likened to light, which enlightens the patient about disease and treatment. Such a physician having good knowledge and intellect will never commit mistakes in treatment. As the remaining three factors (patient, medicine and nurse) of treatment depend on the quality of the physician, a physician should always thrive hard to have all the required good qualities. [24-25]

**4 principles for physician**

मैत्री कारुण्यमार्तेषु शक्ये प्रीतिरुपेक्षणम्|
प्रकृतिस्थेषु भूतेषु वैद्यवृत्तिश्चतुर्विधेति||२६||

Doctor should be
Maitri – friendly,
Karunyam artheshu – sympathetic and kind to patients
Shakye preetihi – should concentrate on the diseases that could be cured
Upekshanam prakrutishteshu – should neglect the incurable diseases
These are the four disciplines for physician.[26]

**Summary:**

तत्र श्लोकौ-
भिषग्जितं चतुष्पादं पादः पादश्चतुर्गुणः|
भिषक् प्रधानं पादेभ्यो यस्माद्वैद्यस्तु यद्गुणः||२७||
ज्ञानानि बुद्धिर्ब्राह्मी च भिषजां या चतुर्विधा|
सर्वमेतच्चतुष्पादे खुड्डाके सम्प्रकाशितमिति||२८||

In this brief chapter on 4 elements of treatment, all the four factors of therapeutics and their respective qualities, the importance and qualities of the physician, his knowledge and fourfold spiritual disposition in profession – all these are explained. [27-28]
इत्यग्निवेशकृते तन्त्रे चरकप्रतिसंस्कृते श्लोकस्थाने खुड्डाकचतुष्पादो नाम नवमोऽध्यायः||९||
Thus ends the ninth chapter of Sutrasthana of Charaka Samhita.

# 10

# Sutrasthana Chapter 10 Maha Chatushpadam

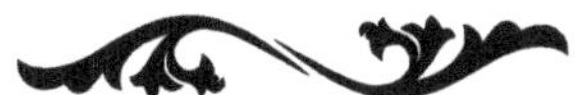

**Maha Chatushpada Adhyaya**

*42 Different Criteria for Ayurvedic Prognosis*

अथातो महाचतुष्पादमध्यायं व्याख्यास्यामः||१|| इति ह स्माह भगवानात्रेयः||२||

There are different parameters considered in Ayurvedic prognosis, to decide if a particular disease in a specific stage in a specific patient is curable, easily curable, not curable, just maintainable etc. Before committing to treat the patient, the doctor has to make this critical decision. There are 42 and more criteria explained for this purpose in the 10th chapter of Sutrasthana of Charaka Samhita. The 10th chapter is called Maha Chatushpada Adhyaya.

Chatushpada means the 4 basic elements of treatment that were covered in the last chapter. This chapter further elaborates on the subject of the last chapter.

**What is the role of therapeutics in treating diseases?**

चतुष्पादं षोडशकलं भेषजमिति भिषजो भाषन्ते, यदुक्तं पूर्वाध्याये षोडशगुणमिति, तद्भेषजं युक्तियुक्तमलमारोग्यायेति भगवान् पुनर्वसुरात्रेयः||३||

नेति मैत्रेयः, किं कारणं? दृश्यन्ते ह्यातुराः केचिदुपकरणवन्तश्च परिचारकसम्पन्नाश्चात्मवन्तश्च कुशलैश्च भिषग्भिरनुष्ठिताः समुत्तिष्ठमानाः, तथायुक्ताश्चापरे म्रियमाणाः; तस्माद्भेषजमकिञ्चित्करं भवति, तद्यथा- श्वभ्रे सरसि च प्रसिक्तमल्पमुदकं, नद्यां वा स्यन्दमानायां पांसुधाने वा पांसुमुष्टिः प्रकीर्ण इति; तथाऽपरे दृश्यन्तेऽनुपकरणाश्चापरिचारकाश्चानात्मवन्तश्चाकुशलैश्च भिषग्भिरनुष्ठिताः समुत्तिष्ठमानाः, तथायुक्ता म्रियमाणाश्चापरे|

यतश्च प्रतिकुर्वन् सिध्यति, प्रतिकुर्वन् म्रियते; अप्रतिकुर्वन् सिध्यति, अप्रतिकुर्वन् म्रियते; ततश्चिन्त्यते भेषजमभेषजेनाविशिष्टमिति ||४||

**What is the role of therapeutics in treating diseases?**

Sage Maitreya puts a query – Some patients get cured easily from diseases, when they are treated with proper medicines, attendants, and well qualified physicians, who also have self-control. On the other hand, in spite of all this being done, some people die. What is the cause?

So, therapeutics are of no value in the eradication of diseases. This is just like a drop of water thrown into a ditch or pond or a handful of dust thrown in a flowing river or on a heap of dust.

To sum up: with the same therapeutic measures, some patients get healed and some die. Similarly, when no therapeutic measures are undertaken, then also some patients recover and some die. So, what is the significance of treatment at all? When the outcomes are totally unpredictable? [4]

**Answer by Sage Atreya**

मैत्रेय ! मिथ्या चिन्त्यत इत्यात्रेयः; किं कारणं, ये ह्यातुराः षोडशगुणसमुदितेनानेन भेषजेनोपपद्यमाना म्रियन्त इत्युक्तं तदनुपपन्नं, न हि भेषजसाध्यानां व्याधीनां भेषजमकारणं भवति; ये पुनरातुराः केवलाद्भेषजादृते समुत्तिष्ठन्ते, न तेषां सम्पूर्णभेषजोपपादनाय समुत्थानविशेषो नास्ति; यथा हि पतितं पुरुषं समर्थमुत्थानायोत्थापयन् पुरुषो बलमस्योपादध्यात्, स क्षिप्रतरमपरिक्लिष्ट एवोत्तिष्ठेत्, तद्वत् सम्पूर्णभेषजोपलम्भादातुराः; ये चातुराः केवलाद्भेषजादपि म्रियन्ते, न च सर्व एव ते भेषजोपपन्नाः समुत्तिष्ठेरन्, नहि सर्वे व्याधयो भवन्त्युपायसाध्याः, न चोपायसाध्यानां व्याधीनामनुपायेन सिद्धिरस्ति, न चासाध्यानां व्याधीनां भेषजसमुदायोऽयमस्ति , न ह्यलं ज्ञानवान् भिषङ्मुमूर्षुमातुरमुत्थापयितुं; परीक्ष्यकारिणो हि कुशला भवन्ति, यथा हि योगज्ञोऽभ्यासनित्य इष्वासो धनुरादायेषुमस्यन्नातिविप्रकृष्टे महति काये नापराधवान् भवति, सम्पादयति चेष्टकार्यं, तथा भिषक् स्वगुणसम्पन्न उपकरणवान् वीक्ष्य कर्मारभमाणः साध्यरोगमनपराधः सम्पादयत्येवातुरमारोग्येण; तस्मान्न भेषजमभेषजेनाविशिष्टं भवति||५||

**Answer by Sage Atreya :**

Oh, Maitreya! The conclusion derived by you is incorrect. Because, it is far from fact to tell that the patients die in spite of adopting therapeutic measures adorned by sixteen best qualities (of the four limbs of treatment). Therapeutic measures can never be ineffective in curable diseases. Similarly, even in such cases where patients are cured without proper medicines, etc. it should be understood that, had there been proper administration of therapeutic measures the process of cure would have been quicker and better. This can be likened to the lifting of a person who has fallen. He can no doubt get up himself but if he is helped and lifted by another person, he would get up sooner without much difficulty. Such is the case with patients who get cured without any treatment.

Regarding cases where patients die even by taking adequate treatment, it is not that all patients taking sufficient treatment are necessarily cured because all diseases are not curable.

The diseases that are curable can only be cured by proper treatment. Those which are not curable will certainly not respond to treatment. Not even the most able and wisest physician is capable of curing a patient with an incurable disease.

Able physicians always proceed with their treatment after proper examination. An archer having the knowledge and practice of archery shoots arrows with the help of his bow and does not commit mistakes in hitting the target. Similarly, a physician endowed with his own qualities and other accessories proceeding with the treatment after proper examination will certainly cure a curable patient without fail. So, application of therapeutic measures has its own special significance. [5]

**Examples of therapeutic principles, to prove the role of therapeutics:**
इदं च नः प्रत्यक्षं- यदनातुरेण भेषजेनातुरं चिकित्सामः, क्षाममक्षामेण, कृशं च दुर्बलमाप्याययामः, स्थूलं मेदस्विनमपतर्पयामः, शीतेनोष्णाभिभूतमुपचरामः, शीताभिभूतमुष्णेन, न्यूनान् धातून् पूरयामः, व्यतिरिक्तान् ह्रासयामः, व्याधीन् मूलविपर्ययेणोपचरन्तः सम्यक् प्रकृतौ स्थापयामः; तेषां नस्तथा कुर्वतामयं भेषजसमुदायः कान्ततमो भवति||६||

**Examples of therapeutic principles, to prove the role of therapeutics:**

And we see with our eyes that we cure a weak patient by providing nourishment, obese and over-nourished patients with Apatarpana (depletion of nourishment, cleansing), a patient who has been afflicted with cold with hot remedies, a patient who has been afflicted with heat with cold remedies, an emaciated patient with nourishment, etc. We treat the patient with principles that are opposite to the qualities of the disease. By this, we restore the natural balance (Prakruti) of the patient. Thus, the groups of therapeutic measures are the best tools in managing diseases. [6]

## Why is the right prognosis very important in treatment?

भवन्ति चात्र-
साध्यासाध्यविभागज्ञो ज्ञानपूर्वं चिकित्सकः|
काले चारभते कर्म यत्तत् साधयति ध्रुवम्||७||
अर्थविद्यायशोहानिमुपक्रोशमसङ्ग्रहम् |
प्राप्नुयान्नियतं वैद्यो योऽसाध्यं समुपाचरेत्||८||

## Why is the right prognosis very important in treatment?

('Prognosis' means judging if a disease is treatable / curable or not or how easy / difficult it is to treat a disease)

A physician who can distinguish between curable and incurable diseases and initiates treatments in time with the full knowledge of therapeutics can certainly accomplish his objective of curing the disease.

On the other hand, a physician who undertakes the treatment of an incurable disease would undoubtedly subject himself to

Arthahaani – loss of wealth

Vidyahaani – loss of knowledge

Yashohaani – loss of fame and he will also earn bad reputations, sanctions or punishments. [7-8]

## Classification of diseases according to prognosis:

सुखसाध्यं मतं साध्यं कृच्छ्रसाध्यमथापि च|
द्विविधं चाप्यसाध्यं स्याद्याप्यं यच्चानुपक्रमम् ||९||
साध्यानां त्रिविधश्चाल्पमध्यमोत्कृष्टतां प्रति|
विकल्पो, न त्वसाध्यानां नियतानां विकल्पना||१०||

Sadhya Vyadhi – Curable diseases are of two types:

- Sukha Sadhya Vyadhi – easily curable diseases
- Krichra Sadhya Vyadhi – difficult-to-cure disease

  Similarly, Asadhya Vyadhi – incurable diseases are two types, viz

- Yapya – maintainable, the symptoms of which can be kept under check till death
- Anupakrama / Pratyakhyeya – impossible to treat. [9-10]

  Sadhya Vyadhi – easy-to cure diseases can also be classified as

- easy to cure,
- moderately easy to cure and
- curable with difficulty.

## Features of Sukha Sadhya Vyadhi – easy-to-treat disease:

हेतवः पूर्वरूपाणि रूपाण्यल्पानि यस्य च|
न च तुल्यगुणो दूष्यो न दोषः प्रकृतिर्भवेत्||११||
न च कालगुणस्तुल्यो न देशो दुरुपक्रमः|

गतिरेका नवत्वं च रोगस्योपद्रवो न च||१२||
दोषश्चैकः समुत्पत्तौ देहः सर्वौषधक्षमः|
चतुष्पादोपपत्तिश्च सुखसाध्यस्य लक्षणम्||१३||

**Features of Sukha Sadhya Vyadhi – easy-to-treat disease:**

1. Alpa Hetu – mild / few causative factors
2. Alpa Purvaroopa – very few premonitory symptoms are manifested
3. Alpa Roopa – very few symptoms of the disease are manifested
4. Na Cha Tulyaguno Dushyo – If the disease causing Dosha and the Dhatu (tissues) are not similar; for example, Vata usually causes diseases in Asthi (bones). But if it causes disease in Meda (fatty tissue), which is the site of Kapha, such a Vata disorder is easy to treat.
5. Na Doshaha Prakrutirbhavet – If the body type of the person does not match with the disease-causing Dosha. For example, if a Vata body type person gets Kapha dominant disease, it is easy to treat.
6. Na Cha Kala Guna: Tulyo – if the season and the qualities of disease do not match; E.g.: if cough and cold happens in summer, then it is easy to treat
7. Ne Desho Durupakramaha – if the place of the patient is ideal, and if the site of disease manifestation is harmless,
8. Gati: Eka – if the disease occurs in a single path / direction
9. Navatvam – disease of recent onset
10. Upadrava Na Cha – disease with no complications.
11. Doshashcha ekaha – if the disease is caused by a single Dosha,
12. Dehaha Sarva Aushadha Kshamaha – patient's body is capable of tolerating all types of treatments and medicines
13. Chatushpaada Upapattishcha – availability of good doctor, nurse and medicines


**Features of difficult-to-cure disease: Krichra Sadhya Vyadhi –**

निमित्तपूर्वरूपाणां रूपाणां मध्यमे बले|
कालप्रकृतिदूष्याणां सामान्येऽन्यतमस्य च||१४||
गर्भिणीवृद्धबालानां नात्युपद्रवपीडितम्|
शस्त्रक्षाराग्निकृत्यानामनवं कृच्छ्रदेशजम्||१५||
विद्यादेकपथं रोगं नातिपूर्णचतुष्पदम्|
द्विपथं नातिकालं वा कृच्छ्रसाध्यं द्विदोषजम्||१६||

**Features of difficult-to-cure disease: Krichra Sadhya Vyadhi –**

1. Madhyama Bala Nimitta – moderate causative factors
2. Madhyama Purvaroopa – moderate number and strength of premonitory symptoms
3. Madhyama Roopa – moderate number and strength of characteristic features / signs and symptoms of disease
4. Kala Prakruti Dushyanaam Saamanya Anyatama – Any one among seasons / body type / body tissue involved is similar to the disease-causing Dosha.
5. Garbhini Vruddha Baalaanaam – disease afflicting pregnant / elderly / children
6. Na Ati Upadrava – not excess complications
7. Shastra Kshara Agnikrutyaanaam – if the treatment involves use of Shastra – Surgery, Ksharakarma – alkali (as in piles and fistula) and Agnikarma (fire / heat treatment / cautery).
8. Anavam – if the disease is not new (neither too old)
9. Kruchra Deshajam – if the patient belongs to a difficult place or if the disease involves a complicated body part

10. Ekapatham rogam, Naati Poorna Chatushtayam - disease afflicting a single body channel / single system, but if the doctor, nurse / proper medicines are not fully available / not of good quality
11. Dvipatham, Naati Kaalam – involves two body channels but disease is not very old
12. Dvidoshajam – two Doshas are involved in the disease [14-16]

## Features of maintainable diseases – Yapya Vyadhi Lakshana

शेषत्वादायुषो याप्यमसाध्यं पथ्यसेवया|
लब्धाल्पसुखमल्पेन हेतुनाऽऽशुप्रवर्तकम्||१७||
गम्भीरं बहुधातुस्थं मर्मसन्धिसमाश्रितम्|
नित्यानुशायिनं रोगं दीर्घकालमवस्थितम्||१८||
विद्यादिद्दवदोषजं...|१९|

## Features of maintainable diseases – Yapya Vyadhi Lakshana

1. Pathya Sevaya Alpa Sukham -The patient can survive by following Pathya – wholesome regimen and enjoys a little relief.
2. Alpena Hetuna Ashu Pravartakam – disease gets quickly exacerbated with simple and mild causative factors
3. Gambheeram – disease afflicting deep seated body tissues
4. Bahu Dhatustham – disease involves many body tissues
5. Marma Sandhi Samashritam – disease involves Marma (vital points of body, such as heart), bones and joints (joining part of different body tissues and organs)
6. Nitya Anushayi – Symptoms manifest everyday
7. Deerghakaalam – chronic disease, long standing disorders
8. Dvidoshajam – involves 2 Doshas. [17-18]

## Features of incurable diseases – prathyakhyeya / Anupakrama

...तद्वत् प्रत्याख्येयं त्रिदोषजम्|
क्रियापथमतिक्रान्तं सर्वमार्गानुसारिणम्||१९||
औत्सुक्यारतिसम्मोहकरमिन्द्रियनाशनम्|
दुर्बलस्य सुसंवृद्धं व्याधिं सारिष्टमेव च||२०||

## Features of incurable diseases – prathyakhyeya / Anupakrama

1. Tridoshajam – involves all the three Doshas – Vata, Pitta and Kapha
2. Kriyaapatham Atikraantam – the disease has grown beyond the abilities of all possible treatment modalities
3. Sarva Marganusarinam – disease involves all the body channels / multiple systems
4. Autsukya – sudden excitement in patient
5. Arati – restlessness
6. Sammoha – unconsciousness
7. Indriyanasha – loss of functions of sense organs
8. Durbalasya Susamvruddham – in a weak patient, the disease is well manifested
9. Sa Arishtam – having bad prognostic signs

## Importance of thorough patient examination

भिषजा प्राक् परीक्ष्यैवं विकाराणां स्वलक्षणम्‌|
पश्चात्कर्मसमारम्भः कार्यः साध्येषु धीमता||२१||
साध्यासाध्यविभागज्ञो यः सम्यक्प्रतिपत्तिमान्‌
न स मैत्रेयतुल्यानां मिथ्याबुद्धिं प्रकल्पयेत्‌||२२||

## Importance of thorough patient examination

A wise physician should examine the distinctive features of the diseases beforehand and then only he should start his treatment for only those diseases that are curable. So a physician who can distinguish between curable and incurable diseases, he with his right applications will not subscribe to the wrong notions like sage Maitreya. [21-22]

तत्र श्लोकौ-
इहौषधं पादगुणाः प्रभवो भेषजाश्रयः|
आत्रेयमैत्रेयमती मतिद्वैविध्यनिश्चयः||२३||
चतुर्विधविकल्पाश्च व्याधयः स्वस्वलक्षणाः|
उक्ता महाचतुष्पादे येष्वायत्तं भिषग्जितम्‌||२४||

Therapies, qualities of each of the four aspects of therapeutics, their effects, views (in this connection) of Atreya and Maitreya, two different views, conclusion, features of all types of curable and incurable diseases – all these are described in this chapter. [23-24]
इत्यग्निवेशकृते तन्त्रे चरकप्रतिसंस्कृते श्लोकस्थाने महाचतुष्पादो नाम दशमोऽध्यायः||१०||
Thus ends the tenth chapter – Maha Chatushpada Adhyaya of Sutrasthana section of Agnivesha's Charaka Samhita, as redacted by Charaka.

# 11

# Sutrasthana Chapter 11
# Tisraishaneeyam

**Tris Eshaneeya Adhyaya - 3 Basic Desires of Life**

अथातस्तिस्रैषणीयमध्यायं व्याख्यास्यामः||१|| इति ह स्माह भगवानात्रेयः||२||

Ayurveda explains in detail about three basic desires of human beings, four means of knowledge, three types of human strengths, three methods of usage of sense organs, three types of diseases, three channels of diseases, three types of physicians and treatment. All these are explained in 11th chapter of Sutrasthana of Charaka Samhita, called Tris Eshaniya Adhyaya.

**The three basic pursuits:**

इह खलु पुरुषेणानुपहतसत्त्वबुद्धिपौरुषपराक्रमेण हितमिह चामुष्मिंश्च
लोके समनुपश्यता तिस्र एषणाः पर्येष्टव्या भवन्ति|
तद्यथा- प्राणैषणा, धनैषणा, परलोकैषणेति||३||

A person of normal mental faculty, intelligence, strength and energy, desirous of his well-being pertaining to this world and the world beyond has to seek three basic desires, viz.,

Praneshana – desire to live,

Dhaneshana – desire to earn and

Paralokeshana – desire to have superior position after-death / to obtain salvation or freedom from the vicious cycle of life and death. [3]

**Desire for longevity: Praneshana**

आसां तु खल्वेषणानां प्राणैषणां तावत् पूर्वतरमापद्येत|
कस्मात्? प्राणपरित्यागे हि सर्वत्यागः|
तस्यानुपालनं- स्वस्थस्य स्वस्थवृत्तानुवृत्तिः, आतुरस्य विकारप्रशमनेऽप्रमादः, तदुभयमेतदुक्तं वक्ष्यते च; तद्यथोक्तमनुवर्तमानः
प्राणानुपालनाद्दीर्घमायुरवाप्नोतीति प्रथमैषणा व्याख्याता भवति||४||

**Desire for longevity: Praneshana**

Out of all these desires, one should, give priority to the desire for longevity. Why? Because, end of life means end of everything. A good life can be achieved by

- Swasthasya Swastha anuvrutti – observance of healthy rules by healthy person
- Aturasya vikara prashamana – treatment of the diseased

Both these have already been described and will be described further, in detail. [4]

## Desire for wealth: Dhaneshana

अथ द्विवतीयां धनैषणमापद्येत, प्राणेभ्यो ह्यनन्तरं धनमेव पर्येष्टव्यं भवति;
न ह्यतः पापात् पापीयोऽस्ति यदनुपकरणस्य दीर्घमायुः, तस्मादुपकरणानि पर्येष्टुं यतेत|
तत्रोपकरणोपायाननुव्याख्यास्यामः; तद्यथा- कृषिपाशुपाल्यवाणिज्यराजोपसेवादीनि,
यानि चान्यान्यपि सतामविगर्हितानि कर्माणि वृतिपुष्टिकराणि विद्यात्तान्यारभेत कर्तुं;
तथा कुर्वन् दीर्घजीवितं जीवत्यनवमतः पुरुषो भवति |
इति द्विवतीया धनैषणा व्याख्याता भवति||५||

## Desire for wealth:

Thereafter comes the second desire – the desire for wealth. One must have a desire for wealth because there is nothing as miserable as a long life without wealth. So, one must try to tap in various sources of wealth. These sources of wealth are – farming, cattle breeding, trade, government service, etc. One can adopt any other means of livelihood that is not disapproved by good men. Doing so, one lives a long life, without suffering any loss of prestige. [5]

## Desire for good position in after-life: Paralokeshana

## Doubts regarding rebirth

अथ तृतीयां परलोकैषणामापद्येत|
संशयश्चात्र, कथं? भविष्याम इतश्च्युता नवेति; कुतः पुनः संशय इति, उच्यते- सन्ति ह्येके प्रत्यक्षपराः परोक्षत्वात् पुनर्भवस्य
नास्तिक्यमाश्रिताः, सन्ति चागमप्रत्ययादेव पुनर्भवमिच्छन्ति; श्रुतिभेदाच्च-
'मातरं पितरं चैके मन्यन्ते जन्मकारणम् |
स्वभावं परनिर्माणं यदृच्छां चापरे जनाः' || इति |
अतः संशयः- किं नु खल्वस्ति पुनर्भवो न वेति||६||

## Desire for good position in after-life: Paralokeshana

## Doubts regarding rebirth :

Then comes the third desire – the desire to attain the happiness in after-life. This desire arises some doubts. There is doubt, whether one will have a life (rebirth) after death at all? But why should one doubt on this? There are people who believe only in things which are perceived and as such do not believe in rebirth because of its imperceptibility. On the other hand people believing in rebirth simply rely upon the evidence of scriptures. There are contradictory opinions with different theories like parent theory, nature theory, impersonal soul, free will theory etc. These theories try to explain cause of birth. So the question remains whether there is rebirth after death. [6]

## Evidence against perception theory:

तत्र बुद्धिमान्नास्तिक्यबुद्धिं जह्यादिवचिकित्सां च|
कस्मात्? प्रत्यक्षं ह्यल्पम्; अनल्पमप्रत्यक्षमस्ति, यदागमानुमानयुक्तिभिरुपलभ्यते;
यैरेव तावदिन्द्रियैः प्रत्यक्षमुपलभ्यते, तान्येव सन्ति चाप्रत्यक्षाणि||७||

## Evidence against perception theory:

A wise man should however give up these unreasonable theories and doubts. Why? Because,

- Prathyaksham hi alpam – scope of perception is limited
- Analpam Apratyaksham – those that cannot be perceived by sense organs are huge

  Those un-observable things can only be perceived by

- Aagama – ancient scriptures
- Anumana – by inference
- Yukti – by special inference, intelligence and reasoning

Even the method of perception of knowledge by sense organs itself cannot be perceived by sense organs. [7]

सतां च रूपाणामतिसन्निकर्षादतिविप्रकर्षादावरणात् करणदौर्बल्यान्मनोनवस्थानात् समानाभिहारादभिभवादतिसौक्ष्म्याच्च प्रत्यक्षानुपलब्धिः; तस्मादपरीक्षितमेतदुच्यते- प्रत्यक्षमेवास्ति, नान्यदस्तीति||८||

Moreover, it is not correct to say that only things which can be directly perceived exist, and others do not. There are things, which though existent, cannot be directly perceived due to the below mentioned reasons:

- Ati sannikarshat – a thing that is too close to eyes cannot be perceived
- Ati viprakarshaat – a thing that is too far, cannot be perceived
- Avaranaat – if a thing is covered by another object, then it cannot be perceived
- Karana daurbalyaat – if sense organs are weak, then nothing can be perceived,
- Mano Anavasthaanaat- if mind is not in place, even if a person is seeing an object, he cannot see it,
- Samaana Abhiharat – confusion with other similar objects,
- Abhibhaavat – over shadowing and
- Ati saukshmaat – very minute object [8]

**Evidences against parent theory of birth:**

श्रुतयश्चैता न कारणं, युक्तिविरोधात्|
आत्मा मातुः पितुर्वा यः सोऽपत्यं यदि सञ्चरेत्|
द्विविधं सञ्चरेदात्मा सर्वोवाऽवयवेन वा||९||
सर्वश्चेत् सञ्चरेन्मातुः पितुर्वा मरणं भवेत्|
निरन्तरं, नावयवः कश्चित्सूक्ष्मस्य चात्मनः||१०||

Even the critical view of scriptures cannot stand against the theory of transmigration (presence of after-life) as these are not based on proper reasoning. If the soul of mother or father enters in her/his progeny, it may be whole or a part of it. If it is transferred wholly, then certainly, the father or mother should die instantaneously. On the other hand, transformation of the subtle self in part is not possible. [9-10]

बुद्धिर्मनश्च निर्णीते यथैवात्मा तथैव ते|
येषां चैषा मतिस्तेषां योनिर्नास्ति चतुर्विधा||११||

On the same principle neither the mind nor the intellect of parents can be regarded as the sole causative factor for progeny. If this theory is accepted, then the fourfold classification of species will not be possible. [11]

**Evidence against natural theory of birth:**

विद्यात् स्वाभाविकं षण्णां धातूनां यत् स्वलक्षणम्|
संयोगे च वियोगे च तेषां कर्मैव कारणम्||१२||

Five basic elements and Atman (soul, life principle) possess specific qualities. (Thus, the five elements are incapable of imbibing consciousness of their own even if combined together. Consciousness is the distinctive feature of Atman alone.) Their combination and separation are conditioned by the past action of Atman. [12]

**Views regarding soul in the creation of universe:**

अनादेश्चेतनाधातोर्नेष्यते परनिर्मितिः|
पर आत्मा स चेद्धेतुरिष्टोऽस्तु परनिर्मितिः||१३||

Atman, the abode of consciousness is without any beginning. So it cannot be created. Universe is not the creator of

Atman. It is the place where Atman exhibits itself. [13]

**Views against the theory of accidental creation of universe:**
न परीक्षा न परीक्ष्यं न कर्ता कारणं न च|
न देवा नर्षयः सिद्धाः कर्म कर्मफलं न च||१४||
नास्तिकस्यास्ति नैवात्मा यदृच्छोपहतात्मनः|
पातकेभ्यः परं चैतत् पातकं नास्तिकग्रहः||१५||

Nihilism constitutes the worst of the sinful. For a Nihilist, everything happens accidentally. So for him there is no existence of the soul and he does not believe in examination or in a thing to be examined; for him there is no efficient or material cause of a thing, and in his view there is no existence of Gods, sages and Siddhas (those who have attained salvation/perfection) and there is no theory of cause and effect or action and results, with a nihilist. [14-15]

तस्मान्मतिं विमुच्यैताममार्गप्रसृतां बुधः|
सतां बुद्धिप्रदीपेन पश्येत्सर्वं यथातथम्||१६||

So, a wise person should get rid of the contempt way of thinking of a nihilist and should see things properly with the lamp of wisdom offered by good men. [16]

**Pramanas – The four means for getting correct knowledge:**
द्विविधमेव खलु सर्वं सच्चासच्च; तस्य चतुर्विधा परीक्षा- आप्तोपदेशः, प्रत्यक्षम्, अनुमानं, युक्तिश्चेति||१७||

All things of the universe can be divided into two.

* Sat – true / existent
* Asat – untrue / nonexistent

   These can be examined by means of –

* Aptopadesha – scriptural testimony (words of enlightened, realized souls),
* Pratyaksha – direct perception using sense organs
* Anumana – inference, guessing with reasoning
* Yukti – reasoning with intelligence. [17]

**Definition of Authority:**
**Sages, enlightened souls – Apta Lakshana**
आप्तास्तावत्-
रजस्तमोभ्यां निर्मुक्तास्तपोज्ञानबलेन ये|
येषां त्रिकालममलं ज्ञानमव्याहतं सदा||१८||
आप्ताः शिष्टा विबुद्धास्ते तेषां वाक्यमसंशयम्|
सत्यं, वक्ष्यन्ति ते कस्मादसत्यं नीरजस्तमाः ||१९||

Enlightened and pure persons are those who are completely free from Rajas and Tamas attributes (and influence of these mental qualities). Such people always possess uninterrupted knowledge of the past, present and future events by the strength of penance (deep meditation) and knowledge. These persons are known as Apta or authorities. They are also known as disciplined (Shishta) and enlightened persons (vibuddha). Their words are true beyond doubt. How could such persons, being free from Rajas and Tamas lie? [18-19]

**Pratyaksha – Definition of Perception or observation:**
आत्मेन्द्रियमनोर्थानां सन्निकर्षात् प्रवर्तते|
व्यक्ता तदात्वे या बुद्धिः प्रत्यक्षं स निरुच्यते||२०||

The knowledge / intelligence acquired by the unison of Atma (soul), Indriya (sense organs), Manas (mind) and artha (object of sense organs) is called as Pratyaksha (perception or direct observation, with the help of sense organs). [20]

## Anumana – Definition of Inference (guessing with reasoning):

प्रत्यक्षपूर्वं त्रिविधं त्रिकालं चानुमीयते|

वह्निर्निगूढो धूमेन मैथुनं गर्भदर्शनात्||२१||

एवं व्यवस्यन्त्यतीतं बीजात् फलमनागतम्|

दृष्ट्वा बीजात् फलं जातमिहैव सदृशं बुधाः||२२||

Inference is dependent on perception. It is of three types, related to the present, past and future.

For example,

Inference of present thing – fire is inferred from the smoke

Inference of past thing – sexual intercourse is inferred by pregnancy

Inference of future – inference of future-tree by looking at the seed, on the basis of the frequent observation about the production of fruits from seeds through direct perception. [21-22]

## Example of Yukti:

जलकर्षणबीजर्तुसंयोगात् सस्यसम्भवः|

युक्तिः षड्धातुसंयोगाद्गर्भाणां सम्भवस्तथा||२३||

मथ्यमन्थन(क)मन्थानसंयोगादग्निसम्भवः|

युक्तियुक्ता चतुष्पादसम्पद्व्याधिनिबर्हणी||२४||

Yukti is the fourth means of knowledge. It comprises of skilful / intellectual application of knowledge of combining right things in right time so as to obtain right results or action done through the process of reasoning. Example: Growth of crops from the combination of irrigation, land, seed and seasons;

Formation of embryo from the combination of six Dhatus (five Mahabhutas and Atman): Production of fire from the combination of the lower-fire-drill, upper-fire-drill and the act of drilling; Cure of diseases by fourfold efficient therapeutic measures. [23-24]

### Yukti – Definition of intellect-based reasoning:

बुद्धिः पश्यति या भावान् बहुकारणयोगजान्|

युक्तिस्त्रिकाला सा ज्ञेया त्रिवर्गः साध्यते यया||२५||

The intellect which perceives things as outcome of combination of multiple causative factors, valid for the past, present and future, is known as Yukti (reasoning). This helps in the fulfillment of the three objects of human life, i.e., righteousness (Dharma), wealth (Artha) and desire (Kama). [25]

एषा परीक्षा नास्त्यन्या यया सर्वं परीक्ष्यते|

परीक्ष्यं सदसच्चैवं तया चास्ति पुनर्भवः||२६||

This is how all things-existent or non-existence can be examined and not otherwise. Such an examination establishes the theory of rebirth. [26]

## Aptopadesha – Scriptural testimony in favour of rebirth:

तत्राप्तागमस्तावद्वेदः, यश्चान्योऽपि कश्चिद्वेदार्थादविपरीतः परीक्षकैः प्रणीतः शिष्टानुमतो लोकानुग्रहप्रवृत्तः शास्त्रवादः, स चाऽऽप्तागमः; आप्तागमादुपलभ्यतेदानतपोय ज्ञसत्याहिंसाब्रह्मचर्याण्यभ्युदयनिःश्रेयसकराणीति||२७||

## Aptopadesha – Scriptural testimony in favor of rebirth:

Scriptural testimony is based on the Vedas or other scriptural material in agreement with the Vedas which is approved by the experts, gentlemen and initiated with a view to bringing about happiness to the mankind. It is derived from the words of authoritative people. It has been stated that donation, penance, sacred rituals, truthfulness, non-violence and Brahmacharya are supposed to provide heaven and to help in liberation. (This establishes the theory of continuation of soul after death and thus of rebirth). [27]

न चानतिवृत्तसत्त्वदोषाणामदोषैरपुनर्भवो धर्मद्वारेषूपदिश्यते॥२८॥

Ancient sages, devoid of all human weaknesses, have clearly stated in the religious scriptures that those who could not conquer their mental defects are not eligible for salvation (they are liable to be reborn). [28]

धर्मद्वारावहितैश्च व्यपगतभयरागद्वेषलोभमोहमानैर्ब्रह्मपरैराप्तैः कर्मविद्भिरनुपहतसत्त्वबुद्धिप्रचारैः पूर्वैः पूर्वतरैर्महर्षिभिर्दिव्यचक्षुभिर्दृष्ट्वोपदिष्टः पुनर्भव इति व्यवस्येदेवम्॥२९॥

The theory of rebirth has been approved after careful observation by ancient sages endowed with divine faculty. These sages were devoted to the path of virtue; they were devoid of fear, attachment, hatred, greed, confusion and vanity; they were in tune with the Almighty; they were reliable par excellence and were conversant with the principles of 'Karman' or action; their mental and intellectual faculties were never tarnished. So, one should not doubt this theory. [29]

**Proving rebirth by means of Pratyaksha (direct perception):**
प्रत्यक्षमपि चोपलभ्यते- मातापित्रोर्विसदृशान्यपत्यानि, तुल्यसम्भवानां वर्णस्वराकृतिसत्त्वबुद्धिभाग्यविशेषाः, प्रवरावरकुलजन्म, दास्यैश्वर्य, सुखासुखमायुः, आयुषो वैषम्यम्, इह कृतस्यावाप्तिः, अशिक्षितानां च रुदितस्तनपानहासत्रासादीनां प्रवृत्तिः, लक्षणोत्पत्तिः, कर्मसादृश्ये फलविशेषः, मेधा क्वचित् क्वचित् कर्मण्यमेधा, जातिस्मरणम्- इहागमनमितश्च्युतानामिति, समदर्शने प्रियाप्रियत्वम्॥३०॥

In spite of the parentage and other factors being the same, the birth of children dissimilar to their parents, and having difference in complexion, voice, shape, mind, intellect and fate.

Birth in high and low family; slavery and sovereignty; happy and miserable life;

Difference in the span of life; enjoyment of results without the corresponding action in this life;

Actions of a newborn like crying, sucking breast, laughing, fear etc., even without training,

Appearance of marks in the body indicating good or bad fortunes;

Difference in its results, in spite of the action being the same,

Intuitive interest in certain types of work in some persons and not in others;

Jatismarana – Preservation of memory of previous life in some persons;

People having similar external appearance but being favored / hated,

All these confirm the theory of re-birth. [30]

**Theory of rebirth confirmed by Anumana (Inference):**
अत एवानुमीयते- यत्- स्वकृतमपरिहार्यमविनाशि पौर्वदेहिकं देवसञ्ज्ञकमानुबन्धिकं कर्म,
तस्यैतत् फलम्; इतश्चान्यद्भविष्यतीति; फलद्बीजमनुमीयते, फलं च बीजात्॥३१॥

The action performed in the previous life which is unavoidable, eternal and having continuity is known as fate. Its results are enjoyable in this life. Action performed in this life will bring about its results in its future life. The seed is from the fruit and the fruit from the seed. [31]

**Theory of rebirth confirmed by Yukti (intellect based reasoning) :**
युक्तिश्चैषा- षड्धातुसमुदयाद्गर्भजन्म, कर्तृकरणसंयोगात् क्रिया; कृतस्य कर्मणः फलं नाकृतस्य,
नाङ्कुरोत्पत्तिरबीजात्; कर्मसदृशं फलं, नान्यस्माद्बीजादन्यस्योत्पत्तिः; इति युक्तिः॥३२॥

The embryo is formed out of the combination of the six Dhatus (5 basic elements plus Atman). Actions are manifested by the combination of the agent (Katru) and the instrument (Karana); the results come out of the action performed. There can be no germination without a seed. The result always corresponds to action. A seed cannot bring out heterogeneous products. [32]

## Conclusion regarding the theory of rebirth:

एवं प्रमाणैश्चतुर्भिरुपदिष्टे पुनर्भवे धर्मद्वारेष्ववधीयेत; तद्यथा- गुरुशुश्रूषायामध्ययने व्रतचर्यायां दारक्रियायामपत्योत्पादने भृत्यभरणेऽतिथिपूजायां दानेऽनभिध्यायां तपस्यनसूयायां देहवाङ्मानसे कर्मण्यक्लिष्टे देहेन्द्रियमनोर्थबुद्ध्यात्मपरीक्षायां मनःसमाधाविति; यानि चान्यान्यप्येवंविधानि कर्माणि सतामविगर्हितानि स्वर्ग्याणि वृत्तिपुष्टिकराणि विद्यातान्यारभेत कर्तुं;

तथा कुर्वन्निह चैव यशो लभते प्रेत्य च स्वर्गम्‌|

इति तृतीया परलोकैषणा व्याख्याता भवति||३३||

So, all the four means of knowledge establish the theory of rebirth. One should, therefore, have faith in religious scriptures; one should attend to the services of the teacher, studies, performance of religious acts, marriage, production of children, maintenance of servants, respect to guests, donations, abstinence from selfish motives, penance, avoidance of backbiting, good physical, verbal and mental acts, introspection with regard to body, sense faculties, mind objects (of senses), intellect and self, and meditation, and other similar acts recommended by virtuous persons which are conducive for doing good in the life, and after death are known as the accepted means of livelihood. A person, attending to these acts, earns fame in this world and attains heaven after death. Thus the third basic desire relating to the life-beyond is explained. [33]

## Seven Triads:

अथ खलु त्रय उपस्तम्भाः, त्रिविधं बलं, त्रीण्यायतनानि, त्रयो रोगाः,

त्रयो रोगमार्गाः, त्रिविधा भिषजः, त्रिविधमौषधमिति||३४||

There are

1. Trayopasthambha – three factors supporting life,
2. Trividha Bala – Three types of strength,
3. Tri Ayatana – three types of causes,
4. Tri Roga – three types of diseases,
5. Trayo Rogamarga – three channels of disease manifestation
6. Trividha Bhishaja – three types of physicians and
7. Trividha Aushadha – three types of medicine / treatment. [34]

## 1. Trayopasthambha – three factors supporting life:

त्रय उपस्तम्भा इति- आहारः, स्वप्नो, ब्रह्मचर्यमिति; एभिस्त्रिभिर्युक्तियुक्तैरुपस्तब्धमुपस्तम्भैः शरीरं बलवर्णोपचयोपचितमनुवर्तते यावदायुःसंस्कारात् संस्कारमहितमनुपसेवमानस्य, य इहैवोपदेक्ष्यते||३५||

The three supports of life are

Ahara – food

Nidra – sleep and

Brahmacharya - Celibacy

Healthy habits pertaining to food, sleep and celibacy lead to good complexion and growth, full health till the full span of life. [35]

## Trividha Bala – Three types of strength:

त्रिविधं बलमिति- सहजं, कालजं, युक्तिकृतं च|

सहजं यच्छरीरसत्त्वयोः प्राकृतं, कालकृतमृतुविभागजं वयःकृतं च,

युक्तिकृतं पुनस्तद्यदाहारचेष्टायोगजम्‌||३६||

Sahaja – constitutional, based on one's body type. It exists in the mind and body from the very birth.

Kalaja – due to seasons (in winter, one has more strength) / Age (like youth having more energy)

Yuktikruta – acquired (say, by having Panchakarma, rejuvenation treatment), by combination of diet and regimen. [36]

## Tri Ayatana – three types of causes and types of sensory stress:

त्रीण्यायतनानीति- अर्थानां कर्मणः कालस्य चातियोगायोगमिथ्यायोगाः|
तत्रातिप्रभावतां दृश्यानामतिमात्रं दर्शनमतियोगः, सर्वशोऽदर्शनमयोगः,
अतिश्लिष्टातिविप्रकृष्टरौद्रभैरवाद्भुतद्विष्टबीभत्सनविकृतवित्रासनादिरूपदर्शनं मिथ्यायोगः; तथाऽतिमात्रस्तनितपटहोत्कृष्टादीनां
शब्दानामतिमात्रं श्रवणमतियोगः, सर्वशोऽश्रवणमयोगः, परुषेष्टविनाशोपघातप्रधर्षणाभीषणादिशब्दश्रवणं मिथ्यायोगः;
तथाऽतितीक्ष्णोग्राभिष्यन्दिनां गन्धानामतिमात्रं घ्राणमतियोगः, सर्वशोऽघ्राणमयोगः, पूतिद्विष्टामेध्यक्लिन्नविषपवनकुणपगन्धादिघ्राणं
मिथ्यायोगः; तथा रसानामत्यादानमतियोगः, सर्वशोऽनादानमयोगः, मिथ्यायोगो राशिवर्ज्येष्वाहारविधिविशेषायतनेष्पदेक्ष्यते;
तथाऽतिशीतोष्णानां स्पृश्यानां स्नानाभ्यङ्गोत्सादनादीनां चात्युपसेवनमतियोगः, सर्वशोऽनुपसेवनमयोगः, स्नानादीनां शीतोष्णादीनां च
स्पृश्यानामनानुपूर्व्योपसेवनं विषमस्थानाभिघाताशुचिभूतसंस्पर्शादयश्चेति मिथ्यायोगः||३७||

**Tri Ayatana – three types of causes and types of sensory stress:**
These are the three types of causes (of diseases) – i.e. Atiyoga – excessive utilization, Ayoga – non-utilisation and Mithya Yoga – wrong utilization of the below mentioned –

- Kala – time,
- Artha – objects of sense organs and
- Karma – acts /deeds

For example, excessive gazing at very bright substance would constitute excessive utilization of the vision in seeing the visual objects.
Not looking at anything at all would amount to its non-utilization.
Seeing things that are too close or too far away, looking at awful, terrifying, surprising, contemptuous, frightful, deformed and alarming things is wrong / perverted utilization of sense organ.

Excessive utilization of sense organ of hearing in perceiving auditory objects / sounds would be to hear uproarious noise coming out of thunder and kettle drum, loud cries, etc.; its non-utilization would be not to hear anything at all; hearing of harsh words, news about the death of friends, assaulting, insulting and terrifying sounds constitute the wrong utilization. Smell of exceedingly sharp, acute and intoxicating odors constitute Ati yoga – excessive utilization of olfactory sense faculties, not to smell at all is its Ayoga – non-utilization; Smell of exceedingly putrid, unpleasant, dirty and cadaverous odor and poisonous gas is Mithya yoga (wrong utilization). Similarly excessive intake of various substances having various tastes would amount to Atiyoga of tongue, Not tasting anything – is Ayoga and tasting obnoxious things Mithya yoga.

Excessive use of exceedingly cold and hot bath, massage and unction etc., amounts to Atiyoga of the tactile sense faculty;
Not to use it at all is Ayoga;
Use of bath, massage and unction and other hot and cold substances without observing the prescribed order, touch of uneven place, dirty objects, microbes and injurious touch constitute Mithya Yoga. [37]

**Mode of operation of sensory stress:**

तत्रैकं स्पर्शनमिन्द्रियाणामिन्द्रियव्यापकं, चेतः- समवायि, स्पर्शनव्याप्तेर्व्यापकमपि च चेतः;
तस्मात् सर्वेन्द्रियाणां व्यापकस्पर्शकृतो यो भावविशेषः,
सोऽयमनुपशयात् पञ्चविधस्त्रिविधविकल्पो भवत्यसात्म्येन्द्रियार्थसंयोगः; सात्म्यार्थो ह्युपशयार्थः||३८||

The sense organ of touch pervades all other organs. It is spread all over the body. It is continuously associated with the mind. The mind again pervades the sense of touch. So the unfavorable reaction of all the senses caused by the all pervasive sense of touch is known as the unwholesome conjunction (sensory stress). The objects of sense faculties which are of five types are further sub-divided into three each (Ati yoga – excessive utilization, Ayoga – non-utilisation, and Mithya yoga – wrong utilization). The favorable reaction of the senses is regarded as the wholesome conjunction of the senses with their objects. [38]

## Types of unwholesome action:

कर्म वाङ्मनःशरीरप्रवृत्तिः|

तत्र वाङ्मनःशरीरातिप्रवृत्तिरतियोगः; सर्वशोऽप्रवृत्तिरयोगः; वेगधारणोदीरणविषमस्खलनपतनाङ्गप्रणिधानाङ्गप्रदूषणप्रहारमर्दनप्राणोपरोधसङ्क्लेशनादिः शारीरो मिथ्यायोगः, सूचकानृताकालकलहाप्रियाबद्धानुपचारपरुषवचनादिर्वाङ्मिथ्यायोगः, भयशोकक्रोधलोभमोहमानेर्ष्यामिथ्यादर्शनादिर्मानसो मिथ्यायोगः||३९||

Action includes speech, thoughts and deeds.

The examples of wrong utilization of the body are

Vegadhaarana – suppression of natural urges.

Vega Udeerana – forceful initiation of natural urges,

unbalanced slipping, falling and posture; excessive itching of the body, bodily assault, excessive massage, excessive holding of breath and exposing oneself to excessive torture.

Examples of wrong utilization with regard to speech are back-biting, lying, useless quarrels, unpleasant talk, irrelevant unfavorable talks and harsh expressions.

Those relating to mind are fear, anxiety, anger, greed, confusion, vanity, envy and misconception. [39]

सङ्ग्रहेण चातियोगायोगवर्जं कर्म वाङ्मनःशरीरजमहितमनुपदिष्टं यत्तच्च मिथ्यायोगं विद्यात्||४०||

In brief, any action relating to speech, mind and body which is not included either in the categories of excessive utilization or non-utilization, and which is harmful for the health in the present life and which is against the religious prescriptions comes under the category of wrong utilization of speech, mind and body. [40]

इति त्रिविधविकल्पं त्रिविधमेव कर्म प्रज्ञापराध इति व्यवस्येत्||४१||

So three-fold actions (i.e. relating to speech, mind and body) further divided into three categories (in the form of non-utilization, excessive utilization and wrong utilization) constitute intellectual misuse. [41]

## Unhealthy season:

शीतोष्णवर्षलक्षणाः पुनर्हेमन्तग्रीष्मवर्षाः संवत्सरः, स कालः|

तत्रातिमात्रस्वलक्षणः कालः कालातियोगः, हीनस्वलक्षणः (कालः) कालायोगः,

यथास्वलक्षणविपरीतलक्षणस्तु (कालः) कालमिथ्यायोगः|

कालः पुनः परिणाम उच्यते||४२||

A year is the unit of time which is further sub-divided into winter (Hemanta), summer (Grisma) and rains (Varsa) characterized by cold, heat and rainfall respectively.

If a particular season manifests itself excessively, this should be regarded as Atiyoga; example, extremely heavy rains during rainy season.

If the season manifests itself in lesser measure, it would be its Ayoga. Eg: less rains in rainy season

If characteristics of a season are contrary to the normal ones, this would be wrong utilization (for example rainfall in winter, cold in the rainy season, etc.). [42]

## Three causes of Disease

इत्यसात्म्येन्द्रियार्थसंयोगः, प्रज्ञापराधः, परिणामश्चेति त्रयस्त्रिविधविकल्पा हेतवो विकाराणां; समयोगयुक्तास्तु प्रकृतिहेतवो भवन्ति||४३||

Asatma Indriyartha Samyoga – unwholesome conjunction of the sense organs with their objects,

Prajnaparadha – doing wrong deeds even with the knowledge

Parinama – transformation / conversion / effect or impact of time – these are the threefold causes of diseases.

Proper utilization of the objects, action and time is beneficial to the maintenance of normal health. [43]

सर्वेषामेव भावानां भावाभावौ नान्तरेण योगायोगातियोगमिथ्यायोगान् समुपलभ्येते; यथास्वयुक्त्यपेक्षिणौ हि भावाभावौ||४४||

Proper maintenance or otherwise of various items of creation depends on proper utilization, non-utilization, excessive utilization and wrong utilization of certain conditions because both proper maintenance as well as abnormality depend on the conjunction (of wholesome or unwholesome nature). [44]

**Three types of diseases:**

त्रयो रोगा इति- निजागन्तुमानसाः|

तत्र निजः शारीरदोषसमुत्थः, आगन्तुर्भूतविषवार्य्वग्निसम्प्रहारादिसमुत्थः, मानसः पुनरिष्टस्य लाभाल्लाभाच्चानिष्टस्योपजायते||४५||

There are three types of diseases-

Nija – endogenous, due to imbalance of the internal factors of the body, caused by Dosha imbalance

Agantuja – exogenous, due to external causes like injury, fire, poison etc

Manasa – mental disorders / psychic disorders [45]

**Principles of treatment of mental diseases:**

तत्र बुद्धिमता मानसव्याधिपरीतेनापि सता बुद्ध्या हिताहितमवेक्ष्यावेक्ष्य धर्मार्थकामानामहितानामनुपसेवने हितानां चोपसेवने प्रयतितव्यं, न ह्यन्तरेण लोके त्रयमेतन्मानसं किञ्चिन्निष्पद्यते सुखं वा दुःखं वा; तस्मादेतच्चानुष्ठेयं- तद्विद्यानां चोपसेवने प्रयतितव्यम्, आत्मदेशकुलकालबलशक्तिज्ञाने यथावच्चेति||४६||

So, a wise person (even if) suffering from the mental diseases should very carefully and repeatedly analyze what is useful and what is harmful to health. He should strive for discarding the harmful or unwholesome regimens and adopt the wholesome ones in regard to righteousness (Dharma), wealth (Artha) and desire (Kama). No happiness or unhappiness can occur in this world without these three elements. So, one should try to serve persons well versed in the nature and cure of psychic diseases. One should also try to acquire knowledge of the self (Atman), the place, family, time, strength and the capacity. [46]

**Thus, it is said:**

भवति चात्र-

मानसं प्रति भैषज्यं त्रिवर्गस्यान्ववेक्षणम्|

तद्विद्यसेवा विज्ञानमात्मादीनां च सर्वशः||४७||

The following are be attended for the treatment of psychic diseases:

(i) To attend the course of conduct relating to virtue, wealth and desire;

(ii) To render service to the persons well versed in the nature and cure of psychic diseases;

(iii) To obtain all round knowledge about the self etc. [47]

**Three paths of diseases in body:**

त्रयो रोगमार्गा इति- शाखा, मर्मास्थिसन्धयः, कोष्ठश्च|

तत्र शाखा रक्तादयो धातवस्त्वक् च, स बाह्यो रोगमार्गः; मर्माणि पुनर्बस्तिहृदयमूर्धादीनि, अस्थिसन्धयोऽस्थिसंयोगास्त्रोपनिबद्धाश्च स्नायुकण्डराः, स मध्यमो रोगमार्गः; कोष्ठः पुनरुच्यते महास्रोतः शरीरमध्यं महानिम्नमामपक्वाशयश्चेति पर्यायशब्दैस्तन्त्रे, स रोगमार्ग आभ्यन्तरः||४८||

The three courses of the disease are

Shakha (peripheral system) – diseases afflicting the 7 dhatus (lymph, blood, muscles, fat, bone, marrow and reproductive system). They are also called as Bahya roga marga, (peripheral system)

**Marmasthisandhi** (vital organs and joints of bones), – diseases involving vital organs (marmas) like Basti – bladder, heart, bone joints and related tendons and ligaments etc. This path is called as Madhyama roga marga.

Kostha (gastro intestinal system) – diseases caused in digestive tract – stomach, intestines etc., from mouth to anus. [48] This is known as internal path (Abhyantara rogamarga)

**Example of diseases of Shakha, Koshta and Marma :**

तत्र, गण्डपिडकालज्यपचीचर्मकीलाधिमांसमषककुष्ठव्यङ्गादयो विकारा बहिर्मार्गजाश्च विसर्पश्वयथुगुल्मार्शोविद्रध्यादयः शाखानुसारिणो भवन्ति रोगाः; पक्षवधग्रहापतानकार्दितशोषराजयक्ष्मास्थिसन्धिशूलगुदभ्रंशादयः शिरोहृद्बस्तिरोगादयश्च मध्यममार्गानुसारिणो भवन्ति रोगाः; ज्वरातीसारच्छर्द्यलसकविसूचिकाकासश्वासहिक्कानाहोदरप्लीहादयोऽन्तर्मार्गजाश्च विसर्पश्वयथुगुल्मार्शोविद्रध्यादयः कोष्ठानुसारिणो भवन्ति रोगाः||४९||

**Example of diseases of Shakha, Koshta and Marma :**

Diseases afflicting the shakha / peripheral system include –
Ganda (goiter), Pidaka (pimple), Alaji (boil), Apachi (scrofula), Charmakeela (wart), Adhimamsa (granuloma), Mashaka (moles), Kushta (skin diseases) and Vyanga (freckles), Visarpa (herpes), Shvayathu (oedema), Gulma (abdominal tumour), Arshas (piles) and Vidradhi (abscess)

Usual diseases occurring in the marma asthi sandhis i.e. vital organs and joints of bones include –
Pakshavadha (hemiplegia), Pakshagraha (stiffness), Apatanaka (convulsion), Ardita (facial paralysis), Shosha (consumption), Rajayakshma (tuberculosis), Asthi-sandhisula (pain in the bone joints), Gudobhramsha (prolapse rectum) and the diseases of the head, heart and bladder.

Ailments occurring in the koshta i.e. central system include - like Jvara (fever), Atisara (diarrhea), Chardi (vomiting), Alasaka (intestinal torper), Visuchika (cholera, Kasa (cough), Shvasa (dyspnoea), Hikka (hiccough), Anaha (constipation), Udara (diseases of the abdomen), and Pliha (splenic disorders) and the internal variety of Visarpa (skin diseases characterized by an acute spread), Shvayathu (oedema), Gulma (abdominal tumour), Arshas (piles) and Vidradhi (internal abscess). [49]

**Three types of Physicians:**

त्रिविधा भिषज इति-
भिषक्छद्मचराः सन्ति सन्त्येके सिद्धसाधिताः|
सन्ति वैद्यगुणैर्युक्तास्त्रिविधा भिषजो भुवि||५०||
वैद्यभाण्डौषधैः पुस्तैः पल्लवैरवलोकनैः|
लभन्ते ये भिषक्शब्दमज्ञास्ते प्रतिरूपकाः||५१||
श्रीयशोज्ञानसिद्धानां व्यपदेशादतद्विधाः|
वैद्यशब्दं लभन्ते ये ज्ञेयास्ते सिद्धसाधिताः||५२||
प्रयोगज्ञानविज्ञानसिद्धिसिद्धाः सुखप्रदाः|
जीविताभिसरास्ते स्युर्वैद्यत्वं तेष्ववस्थितमिति||५३||

**Chadmachara** – quacks, pseudo physicians. They pose themselves as doctors by exhibiting a few medical books, medicine box etc. They are ignorant about medical science.

**Siddhisadhita** – feigned physicians, who practice just with the help of experience. They claim to have wealth, fame and knowledge. But they do not have any of these.

**Vaidya Guna Yukta** – Good ones, endowed with all the qualities.

Those who are accomplished in the administration of therapies, insight and knowledge of therapeutics are endowed with infallible success and can bring out happiness to the patient are saviors of life. [50-53]

**Three types of treatments:**

त्रिविधमौषधमिति- दैवव्यपाश्रयं, युक्तिव्यपाश्रयं, सत्त्वावजयश्च|

तत्र देवव्यपाश्रयं- मन्त्रौषधिमणिमङ्गलबल्युपहारहोमनियमप्रायश्चित्तोपवासस्वस्त्ययनप्रणिपातगमनादि, युक्तिव्यपाश्रयं- पुनराहारौषधद्रव्याणां योजना, सत्त्वावजयः- पुनरहितेभ्योऽर्थेभ्यो मनोनिग्रहः||५४||

### Daiva Vyapashraya – Spiritual treatment :

Mantra (holy recitations), Mani (gem therapy), Mangala Bali, Homa – good deeds, Fire rituals, Niyama – Self restrictions like fasting, reconciliation, holy chanting,

**Yukti Vyapashraya** - therapy based on reasoning and planning. Administration of proper diet and medicinal drugs comes under the second category.

**Satva Avajaya** - , Withdrawal of mind from harmful objects constitutes psychic therapy. [54]

### Three types of therapies:

शरीरदोषप्रकोपे खलु शरीरमेवाश्रित्य प्रायश्चिविधमौषधमिच्छन्ति- अन्तःपरिमार्जनं, बहिःपरिमार्जनं, शस्त्रप्रणिधानं चेति|
तत्रान्तःपरिमार्जनं यदन्तःशरीरमनुप्रविश्यौषधमाहारजातव्याधीन् प्रमार्ष्टि,
यत्पुनर्बहिःस्पर्शमाश्रित्याभ्यङ्गस्वेदप्रदेहपरिषेकोन्मर्दनाद्यैरामयान् प्रमार्ष्टि तद्बहिःपरिमार्जनं, शस्त्रप्रणिधानं पुनश्छेदनभेदनव्यधनदारणलेखनोत्पाटनप्रच्छनसीवनैषणक्षारजलौकसश्चेति||५५||

When there is Dosha imbalance (=disease) in the body, generally three types of therapies are required. viz.,

**Antah Parimarjana** – internal-cleansing, useful in diseases caused by improper diet.

**Bahi Parimarjana** – external-cleansing. Like Abhyanga (massage),Sveda (fomentation), Pradeha (unction), Parisheka (dripping), Mardana (kneading) etc.

**Shastra Pranidhana** – surgical therapy. Chedana (excision), Bhedana (incision), Vyadhana (puncturing), Darana (rupturing), Lekhana (scraping), Utpatana (uprooting), Pracchanna (multiple puncturing), Seevana (rupturing), Eshana (probing), application of (Kshara) alkalies and Jalauka (leeches). [55]

### Importance of management of diseases:

भवन्ति चात्र-
प्राज्ञो रोगे समुत्पन्ने बाह्येनाभ्यन्तरेण वा|
कर्मणा लभते शर्म शस्त्रोपक्रमणेन वा||५६||
बालस्तु खलु मोहाद्वा प्रमादाद्वा न बुध्यते|
उत्पद्यमानं प्रथमं रोगं शत्रुमिवाबुधः||५७||
अणुर्हि प्रथमं भूत्वा रोगः पश्चाद्विवर्धते|
स जातमूलो मुष्णाति बलमायुश्च दुर्मतेः||५८||
न मूढो लभते सञ्ज्ञां तावद्यावन्न पीड्यते|
पीडितस्तु मतिं पश्चात् कुरुते व्याधिनिग्रहे||५९||
अथ पुत्रांश्च दारांश्च ज्ञातींश्चाह्वय भाषते|
सर्वस्वेनापि मे कश्चिदिभषगानीयतामिति||६०||
तथाविधं च कः शक्तो दुर्बलं व्याधिपीडितम्|
कृशं क्षीणेन्द्रियं दीनं परित्रातुं गतायुषम्||६१||
स त्रातारमनासाद्य बालस्त्यजति जीवितम्|
गोधा लाङ्गूलबद्धेवाकृष्यमाणा बलीयसा||६२||
तस्मात् प्रागेव रोगेभ्यो रोगेषु तरुणेषु वा|
भेषजैः प्रतिकुर्वीत य इच्छेत् सुखमात्मनः||६३||

### Importance of management of diseases:

In the event of a disease, a wise person regains his health by administering external and internal cleansing therapies and also by surgical procedures. However, as an incompetent king neglects his enemy, so also an ignorant person does not realize the need to take care of the disease in its primary stage because of his negligence. This disease, in its early stage appears to be insignificant, but it grows and thereafter gaining a strong hold on the body. It takes away the strength and life of the fool. The fool is never conscious of any defect unless he is seriously afflicted. After he is actually afflicted seriously, he thinks about disease eradication. Then he calls his children, wives and kins and requests them to call in a physician and says, "I am prepared to pay him my entire earnings." But then, who can save such a weak, emaciated, wretched and moribund person afflicted with diseases and with his sense organs losing all the strength. Having failed to find a savior of his health, the fool is deprived of his life (in spite of his efforts to preserve it) like an iguana with her tail bound by a rope being dragged by a strong person. Therefore, a wise person desirous of his well-being should take recourse to the appropriate therapies before the occurrence of the diseases or even while the diseases are in their primary stage of manifestation. [56-63]

**To sum up :**
तत्र श्लोकौ-
एषणाः समुपस्तम्भा बलं कारणमामयाः|
तिस्रैषणीये मार्गाश्च भिषजो भेषजानि च||६४||
त्रित्वेनाष्टौ समुद्दिष्टाः कृष्णात्रेयेण धीमता|
भावा, भावेष्वसक्तेन येषु सर्वं प्रतिष्ठितम्||६५||
Basic desires, supporters, strength, causes (of diseases), diseases themselves, paths, physicians and therapies – all these eight factors – each classified into three groups have been described in this chapter by the sage Krushnatreya who is wise and free from worldly attachments. Everything (virtue, wealth and desire) is based on these eight factors. [64-65]
इत्यग्निवेशकृते तन्त्रे चरकप्रतिसंस्कृते श्लोकस्थाने तिस्रैषणीयो नामैकादशोऽध्यायः||११||
Thus, ends Tris Eshaniya Chapter of Shloka section of Charaka Samhita, written by Acharya Agnivesha, redated by Acharya Charaka.

# 12

# Sutrasthana Chapter 12 Vata Kalakaleeyam

**Vata Kalakaleeya Adhyaya**

**Vata Dosha – Qualities, Functions, Imbalance :**

अथातो वातकलाकलीयमध्यायं व्याख्यास्यामः||१||

इति ह स्माह भगवानात्रेयः||२||

Master Charaka has explained about qualities of Vata Dosha, its normal functions, causes and features of Vata Dosha imbalance, how to restore Vata Dosha balance etc in 12th chapter of Charaka Samhita Sutrasthana – Vata Kalakaliya Adhyaya. This chapter was written as per the discussions held in a symposium, conducted by Sage Atreya. The symposium was attended by many leading Ayurveda sages and scholars of ancient times.

**Symposium on the properties of Vata, Topics for discussion:**

वातकलाकलाज्ञानमधिकृत्य परस्परमतानि जिज्ञासमानाः समुपविश्य महर्षयः पपर्च्छुरन्योऽन्यं- किङ्गुणो वायुः, किमस्य प्रकोपणम्, उपशमनानि वाऽस्य कानि, कथं चैनमसङ्घातवन्तमनवस्थितमनासाद्य प्रकोपणप्रशमनानि प्रकोपयन्ति प्रशमयन्ति वा, कानि चास्य कुपिताकुपितस्य शरीराशरीरचरस्य शरीरेषु चरतः कर्माणि बहिःशरीरेभ्योवेति||३||

The Ancient sages, desirous of knowledge about good and bad properties of Vata, assembled and proposed the following topics for discussion among themselves.

I. What are the qualities of Vata?

II. What causes Vata Dosha imbalance (aggravation)?

III. What are the factors for Vata Balance?

IV. How do the aggravating and balancing factors respectively act on Vata, which is inaccessible to sense organs?

V. What are the actions in normal and imbalanced states of Vata which are situated both within and outside the body?

**Six physical qualities of Vata by Kusha:**

अत्रोवाच कुशः साङ्कृत्यायनः- रूक्षलघुशीतदारुणखरविशदाः षडिमे वातगुणा भवन्ति||४||

Kusha, descendant of Sankruti says –

Rooksha – Dryness

Laghu – Lightness

Sheeta – coldness,

Daruna – instability,

Khara – coarseness, roughness and

Vishada – non-sliminess, clarity – are the six qualities of Vata. [4]

**Causes of Aggravation of Vata by Kumaras Shira Bharadwaj:**

तच्छुत्वा वाक्यं कुमारशिरा भरद्वाज उवाच- एवमेतद्यथा भगवानाह, एत एव वातगुणा भवन्ति,

स त्वेवङ्गुणैरेवन्द्रव्यैरेवम्प्रभावैश्च कर्मभिरभ्यस्यमानैर्वायुः प्रकोपमापद्यते,
समानगुणाभ्यासो हि धातूनां वृद्धिकारणमिति||५||

Having heard this, Kumarashira Bharadwaj said, "these, as explained by you, sir, are the six qualities of Vata. Vata Dosha gets aggravated by use of diet, medicines and activities that are similar to these six qualities. Because, diet and activities of similar properties lead to increase of Dosha of similar qualities. [5]

## Cause of Dosha Balance by Kankayana:
तच्छ्रुत्वा वाक्यं काङ्कायनो बाह्लीकभिषगुवाच- एवमेतद्यथा भगवानाह, एतान्येव वातप्रकोपणानि भवन्ति;
अतो विपरीतानि वातस्य प्रशमनानि भवन्ति, प्रकोपणविपर्ययो हि धातूनां प्रशमकारणमिति||६||

Having heard this, Kankayana, a physician from Bahilka said, "what you said, Sir, is correct". These are very much the aggravating factors of Vata Dosha. Diet and activities having opposite qualities of a Dosha, leads to mitigation (balancing) of that aggravated Dosha. [6]

## Mode of action of aggravating and alleviating factors by Badisa Dhamargava:
तच्छ्रुत्वा वाक्यं बडिशो धामार्गव उवाच- एवमेतद्यथा भगवानाह, एतान्येव वातप्रकोपप्रशमनानि भवन्ति|
यथा ह्येनमसङ्घातमनवस्थितमनासाद्य प्रकोपणप्रशमनानि प्रकोपयन्ति प्रशमयन्ति वा, तथाऽनुव्याख्यास्यामः- वातप्रकोपणानि खलु रूक्षलघुशीतदारुणखरविशदशुषिरकराणि शरीराणां, तथाविधेषु शरीरेषु वायुराश्रयं गत्वाऽप्यायमानः प्रकोपमापद्यते; वातप्रशमनानि पुनःस्निग्धगुरूष्णश्लक्ष्णमृदुपिच्छिलघनकराणि शरीराणां,
तथाविधेषु शरीरेषु वायुरसज्यमानश्चरन् प्रशान्तिमापद्यते||७||

## Mode of action of aggravating and alleviating factors by Badisa Dhamargava:
Badisha Dhamargava says, "what you have said is correct, Sir! These are very much the aggravating and alleviating factors of Vata". We shall now explain how the aggravating and alleviating factors respectively aggravate and alleviate the Vata, which is Asanghata (unquantifiable) and Anavasthita (unstable) – thereby inaccessible. The aggravating factors of Vata are those which bring about

Rooksha – dryness
Laghu – lightness,
Sheeta – coldness,
Daruna – coarseness,
Khara – rough,
Vishada – clarity, non-sliminess,
Sushira – hollowness.
By these qualities, Vata gets situated in one / any susceptible part of the body and attains increase. Following this it gets aggravated. The alleviating factors of Vata, on the other hand, are those which bring about

Snigdha – unctuousness, oiliness
Guru – heaviness,
Ushna – heat,
Shlakshna – smoothness,
Mrudu – softness,
Picchila – sliminess and
Ghana – compactness.
By the use of these qualities, Vata gets dislodged from the affected place and gets alleviated. [7]

## Functions of normal and abnormal Vata by Vayorvida:
Having heard the scientific explanation of Badisha, which was approved by the sages, the royal sage Vayorvida said, "All that you have said, Sir, is true and free from any contradiction".

Let us explore the functions (normal and aggravated) of Vata Dosha, which is present inside and outside the body (=air). The below-mentioned functions are understood by means of

- Pratyaksha – direct observation, with the help of sense organs
- Anumana – inference and
- Aptopadesha – scriptural testimony.

Let us pay obeisance to Lord Vayu and explore his functions.

**Functions of normal vata of body:**
Vayuhu Tantra Yantra Dharaha – The Vata Dosha, when it is normal, sustains the functioning of all the organs of the body.
Prana Udana, Samana, Vyana Apana – These are the five types of Vata Dosha.
Pravartaka Cheshtanam Ucchavachanam – Vata initiates all the actions and speech.
Niyanta Praneta Cha Manasaha – Vata controls and directs the mind.
Sarva Indriyanam Udyojakaha – it coordinates and stimulates all the sense organs.
Sarva Indriya Arthanam Abhivoda – it controls all the objects of sense faculties.
Sarva Sharira Dhatu Vyuhakaraha – it maintains the compactness and unison of all the body organs.
Sandhanakaraha Shareerasya – it maintains body compactness.
Pravartako Vacha – it initiates speech.
Prakruti Sparsha Shabdayoho shrotra Sparshanayoho moolam – It is the root for touch, sound, ears and sensation of touch.
Harsha Utsahayoho Yonihi – it is the root cause for happiness and enthusiasm.
Sameerano Agnehe – it controls Agni – digestion strength (air is necessary for the fire to stay on).
Dosha Samshoshanaha – it dries up Pitta and Kapha.
Kshepta Bahirmalanam – it evacuates waste products out of the body.
Sthula Anu srotasaam Bhetta – it forms all the body channels – minute and large.
Karta Garbhakrutinam – Vata is responsible for growth of the foetus. Vata moulds and shapes embryos.
Ayusho anuvrutti – it is the cause for continuity of life.

**Function of imbalanced Vata in the body:**
Vata, when aggravated, afflicts the body with various types of diseases and affects the strength, skin complexion, happiness and the span of life. It perturbs the mind: affects all the sense organs and sense faculties; destroys, deforms the embryo or delays delivery of the fetus. Vata causes fear, anxiety, bewilderment, humility and delirium. It shortens life span.

**Normal functions of air:**
The following are the actions of the Vayu (air), moving in the world, outside the body:-

- Maintenance and sustenance of the earth,
- kindling of fire,
- bringing about compactness and movement in the sun, moon, stars and planets,
- creation of clouds, showering of rains, flowing of rivers, bringing about maturity of flowers and fruits, shooting forth the plants, classification of seasons as well as five Mahabhutas (five basic elements):
- Air manifests the shape and the size of the products of the five Mahabhutas,
- Air is responsible for germination of seeds, growth of plants, brings about hardness and dryness to the grains. Air is the cause for transformation.

**Abnormal functions of air or wind:**

तच्छ्रुत्वा बडिशवचनमवितथमृषिगणैरनुमतमुवाच वार्योविदो राजर्षिः- एवमेतत् सर्वमनपवादं यथा भगवानाह|

यानि तु खलु वायोः कुपिताकुपितस्य शरीराशरीरचरस्य शरीरेषु चरतः कर्माणि बहिःशरीरेभ्यो वा भवन्ति, तेषामवयवान् प्रत्यक्षानुमानोपदेशैः साधयित्वा नमस्कृत्य वायवे यथाशक्ति प्रवक्ष्यामः- वायुस्तन्त्रयन्त्रधरः, प्राणोदानसमानव्यानापानात्मा, प्रवर्तकश्चेष्टानामुच्चावचानां, नियन्ता प्रणेता च मनसः, सर्वेन्द्रियाणामुद्योजकः, सर्वेन्द्रियार्थानामभिवोढा, सर्वशरीरधातुव्यूहकरः, सन्धानकरः शरीरस्य, प्रवर्तको वाचः, प्रकृतिः स्पर्शशब्दयोः, श्रोत्रस्पर्शनयोर्मूलं, हर्षोत्साहयोर्योनिः, समीरणोऽग्नेः, दोषसंशोषणः, क्षेप्ता बहिर्मलानां, स्थूलाणुस्रोतसां भेत्ता, कर्तागर्भाकृतीनाम्, आयुषोऽनुवृत्तिप्रत्ययभूतो भवत्यकुपितः|

कुपितस्तु खलु शरीरे शरीरं नानाविधैर्विकारैरुपतपति बलवर्णसुखायुषामुपघाताय, मनो व्याहर्षयति, सर्वेन्द्रियाण्युपहन्ति, विनिहन्ति गर्भान् विकृतिमापादयत्यतिकालं वा धारयति, भयशोकमोहदैन्यातिप्रलापाञ्जनयति, प्राणांश्चोपरुणद्धि|

प्रकृतिभूतस्य खल्वस्य लोके चरतः कर्माणीमानि भवन्ति; तद्यथा- धरणीधारणं, ज्वलनोज्ज्वालनम्, आदित्यचन्द्रनक्षत्रग्रहगणानां सन्तानगतिविधानं, सृष्टिश्च मेघानाम्, अपां विसर्गः, प्रवर्तनं स्रोतसां, पुष्पफलानां चाभिनिर्वर्तनम्, उद्भेदनं चौषिभदानाम्, ऋतूनां प्रविभागः, विभागो धातूनां, धातुमानसंस्थानव्यक्तिः, बीजाभिसंस्कारः, शस्याभिवर्धनमविक्लेदोपशोषणे, अवैकारिकविकारश्चेति|

प्रकुपितस्य खल्वस्य लोकेषु चरतः कर्माणीमानि भवन्ति; तद्यथा- शिखरिशिखरावमथनम्, उन्मथनमनोकहानाम्, उत्पीडनं सागराणाम्, उद्वर्तनं सरसां, प्रतिसरणमापगानाम्, आकम्पनं च भूमेः, आधमनमम्बुदानां , नीहारनिर्ह्रादपांशुसिकतामत्स्यभेकोरगक्षाररुधिराश्माशनिविसर्गः, व्यापादनं च षण्णामृतूनां, शस्यानामसङ्घातः, भूतानां चोपसर्गः, भावानां चाभावकरणं, चतुर्युगान्तकराणां मेघसूर्यानलानिलानां विसर्गः; स हि भगवान् प्रभवश्चाव्ययश्च, भूतानां भावाभावकरः, सुखासुखयोर्विधाता, मृत्युः, यमः, नियन्ता, प्रजापतिः, अदितिः, विश्वकर्मा, विश्वरूपः, सर्वगः, सर्वतन्त्राणां विधाता, भावानामणुः, विभुः, विष्णुः, क्रान्ता लोकानां, वायुरेव भगवानिति||८||

**Abnormal functions of air or wind:**

The following are the actions of the aggravated Vata (air) moving in the world outside the body:-

Breaking though the peak of mountains, uprooting trees, disturbing the oceans, overflowing of the lakes, changing the course of rivers, bringing about earthquakes, causing thunders in the clouds, release of dew, thunder without cloud, dust, and fish, frog, serpents, alkaline water, blood, stone and thunder storm, disturbance of the six seasons; disturbance in the productivity of plants; spread of epidemics in humans,

Doing away with the positive factors of creation; bringing about cloud, sun, fire and wind which could destroy all the four ages.

**Other qualities of Vata:** The God Vayu (Vata) is the eternal cause of the universe: He brings existence as well as destruction to all living beings. He causes happiness and misery. He is the God of death, controller, Lord of creatures, Aditi and Visvakarman (creator of the universe). He possesses innumerable forms. He can move everywhere, and is responsible for all actions and thoughts. He is subtle and omnipresent. He is Lord Vishnu. He has created and is maintaining the whole universe. The God Vayu alone has the above distinctive features.[8]

**Question by Marichi on Vayorvida's observation:**

तच्छ्रुत्वा वार्योविदवचो मरीचिरुवाच- यद्यप्येवमेतत्, किमर्थस्यास्य वचने विज्ञाने वा सामर्थ्यमस्ति भिषग्विद्यायां; भिषग्विद्यामधिकृत्येयं कथा प्रवृत्तेति ||९||

After listening to the sage Vayorvida, Marichi inquires, "The present symposium is related to the science of medicine. Even though what has been stated about the qualities of Vayu is correct, is this exposition or understanding of such qualities of Vayu is applicable to the science of medicine?" [9]

**Answer by Vayorvida:**

वार्योविद उवाच- भिषक् पवनमतिबलमतिपरुषमतिशीघ्रकारिणमात्ययिकं चेन्नानुनिशम्येत्, सहसा प्रकुपितमतिप्रयतः कथमग्रेऽभिरक्षितुमभिधास्यति प्रागेवैनमत्ययभयात्; वायोर्यथार्था स्तुतिरपि भवत्यारोग्याय बलवर्णविवृद्धये वर्चस्वित्वायोपचयाय ज्ञानोपपत्तये परमायुःप्रकर्षाय चेति||१०||

**Sage Varyovida answered**, "If a physician does not understand the Vayu which excels in strength, roughness, quickness and destructive power, how would he be able to forewarn a patient about the ill-effects of Vata, well in advance, before it affects the body? How would he advise about the normal qualities of Vayu conducive to good health, improvement of strength and complexion, luster, growth, attainment of knowledge and longevity? [10]

### Normal and abnormal functions of pitta by Marichi:

मरीचिरुवाच- अग्निरेव शरीरे पित्तान्तर्गतः कुपिताकुपितः शुभाशुभानि करोति; तद्यथा- पक्तिमपक्तिं दर्शनमदर्शनं मात्रामात्रत्वमूष्मणः प्रकृतिविकृतिवर्णौ शौर्यं भयं क्रोधं हर्षं मोहं प्रसादमित्येवमादीनि चापराणि द्वन्द्वानीति||११||

Marichi said; "it is Agni alone represented by Pitta in the body which brings about good or bad effects according to its normal or imbalanced state, e.g. digestion or indigestion, vision or loss of vision, normalcy or imbalance of body heat, of skin complexion, valour and fear, anger and joy, bewilderment and happiness and such other pairs of opposite qualities.[11]

### Normal and abnormal functions of Kapha by Kapya:

तच्छ्रुत्वा मरीचिवचः काप्य उवाच- सोम एव शरीरे श्लेष्मान्तर्गतः कुपिताकुपितः शुभाशुभानि करोति;
तद्यथा- दार्ढ्यं शैथिल्यमुपचयं कार्श्यमुत्साहमालस्यं वृषतां क्लीबतां ज्ञानमज्ञानं बुद्धिं मोहमेवमादीनि चापराणि द्वन्द्वानीति||१२||

Having listened to Marichi, Kapya said, "Soma (the God of water or the moon) which is represented by Kapha in the body brings about good or bad effects according to this normal or abnormal state.
E.g. sturdiness and brittleness, good nourishment and emaciation, enthusiasm and laziness, potency and impotency, knowledge, wisdom and ignorance and such other pairs of qualities.[12]

### Presidential remark by Punarvasu Atreya:

तच्छ्रुत्वा काप्यवचो भगवान् पुनर्वसुरात्रेय उवाच- सर्व एव भवन्तः सम्यगाहुरन्यत्रैकान्तिकवचनात्; सर्व एव खलु वातपित्तश्लेष्माणः प्रकृतिभूताः पुरुषमव्यापन्नेन्द्रियं बलवर्णसुखोपपन्नमायुषा महतोपपादयन्ति सम्यगेवाचरिता धर्मार्थकामा इव निःश्रेयसेन महता पुरुषमिह चामुष्मिंश्च लोके; विकृतास्त्वेनं महता विपर्ययेणोपपादयन्ति ऋतवस्त्रय इव विकृतिमापन्ना लोकमशुभेनोपघातकाल इति||१३||

After having listened to Kapya, Lord Punarvasu Atreya said, "All of you have dealt with the subject quite well except that you have not made any general statement on this topic. In fact, all the three Doshas viz. Vata, Pitta and kapha while they are in their natural state,
**Avyapannam Indriyam** – maintain proper functioning of sense organs without any abnormality,
**Bala Varna Sukha Ayusha** – maintains strength, complexion, happiness and long-life span.

In life, if one follows good aspects of Dharma (righteousness), Artha (wealth), Kama (desire, lust) he will have a successful life. But if he or she follows bad aspects of Dharma, Artha and Kama, then one will have a bad quality of life. Likewise, if one maintains Tridosha in good condition, he will have good health, or else suffer from diseases. [13]

### Opinion of the house:

तद्दृषयः सर्व एवानुमेनिरे वचनमात्रेयस्य भगवतोऽभिननन्दुश्चेति||१४||

All the sages concurred in and welcomed the exposition of Lord Atreya.[14]

भवति चात्र-
तदात्रेयवचः श्रुत्वा सर्व एवानुमेनिरे|
ऋषयोऽभिननन्दुश्च यथेन्द्रवचनं सुराः||१५||

Thus, it is said: -
Having listened to the exposition of Lord Atreya, all the sages concurred in and welcomed it as the Gods did on hearing the words of Indra. [15]

**Summary:**

तत्र श्लोकौ-

गुणाः षड् द्विविधो हेतुर्विविधं कर्म यत् पुनः|

वायोश्चतुर्विधं कर्म पृथक् च कफपित्तयोः||१६||

महर्षीणां मतिर्या या पुनर्वसुमतिश्च या|

कलाकलीये वातस्य तत् सर्वं सम्प्रकाशितम्||१७||

The six qualities of Vata, two types of causes (relating to the aggravation and vitiation of Vata), several functions of Vata, its four aspects (normalcy and aggravation within and without the body); functions of Kapha and Pitta, views of the sages and conclusion by Lord Atreya- all this about Vata has been explained in this chapter on "Merits and Demerits of Vata" [16-17]

इत्यग्निवेशकृते तन्त्रे चरकप्रतिसंस्कृते श्लोकस्थाने वातकलाकलीयो नाम द्वादशोऽध्यायः समाप्तः||१२|| इति निर्देशचतुष्कः||३||

Thus, ends the twelfth chapter of the Sutra section on "the Merits and Demerits of Vata" of Agnivesha's work as redacted by Charaka.

# 13

# Sutrasthana Chapter 13 Snehadhyayam

**Snehakarma – preparation For Panchakarma**

अथातः स्नेहाध्यायं व्याख्यास्यामः||१||

इति ह स्माह भगवानात्रेयः||२||

Before administration of Panchakarma treatment, Snehakarma (oiling treatment) and Swedana (sweating treatment) are done as preparatory procedures. Panchakarma comprises 5 major therapies of Ayurveda and comprises methods of expelling the imbalanced Doshas out of the body. Before they are expelled either by oral or anal route, the imbalanced Doshas needs to be softened, mobilized and brought into the gastro-intestinal tract. This is achieved by Snehakarma and Swedakarma. This chapter, the 13th of Sutrasthana of Charak Samhita explains Snehakarma in full detail.

साङ्ख्यैः सङ्ख्यातसङ्ख्येयैः सहासीनं पुनर्वसुम्|

जगद्धितार्थं पप्रच्छ वह्निवेशः स्वसंशयम्||३||

Once upon a time, Lord Punaravasu was sitting with scholars. Agnivesha put forth a few doubts before Punarvasu, for the sake of the well-being of the universe. [3]

**Questions regarding oils and fats:**

किंयोनयः कति स्नेहाः के च स्नेहगुणाः पृथक्|

कालानुपाने के कस्य कति काश्च विचारणाः||४||

कति मात्राः कथम्मानाः का च केषूपदिश्यते|

कश्च केभ्यो हितः स्नेहः प्रकर्षः स्नेहने च कः||५||

स्नेह्याः के के न च स्निग्धास्निग्धातिस्निग्धलक्षणम्|

किं पानात् प्रथमं पीते जीर्णे किञ्च हिताहितम्||६||

के मृदुक्रूरकोष्ठाः का व्यापदः सिद्धयश्च काः|

अच्छे संशोधने चैव स्नेहे का वृत्तिरिष्यते||७||

विचारणाः केषु योज्या विधिना केन तत् प्रभो!|

स्नेहस्यामितविज्ञान ज्ञानमिच्छामि वेदितुम्||८||

**Questions regarding oils and fats:**

- What are the sources of Snehadravya – unctuous (oily) substances?
- What are the types of unctuous substances?
- What are the qualities of different oily substances?

- What are the appropriate times and Anupana (substance to be taken with or after the intake of medicine) for administering different types of oily substances?
- What and how many are the recipes of unctuous substances?[4]
- What are the different types of dosage and
- What are the measures?
- Which specific dose is prescribed for whom?
- Which oily substance is beneficial for whom?
- What are the maximum and minimum durations of Snehakarma (oleation)?[5]
- What are the indications and contra-indications for oleation?
- What are the features of proper oleation, non-oleation and excessive oleation?
- What is beneficial and what is harmful before and after the intake of fats, and also after its complete digestion?[6]
- What are the features of Mrdukostha (laxed bowel / soft bowel) and Krurakostha (hard bowel)?
- What are the complications of oleation therapy and what are their managements?
- What is the regimen prescribed during oleation therapy of both types administered for elimination or as palliative measure?[7]
- What recipes should be given to whom and how are they to be prepared?
- I want to know all these about oils and fats, O my Lord![8]

**Sneha Yoni – Sources of oils and fats:**

अथ तत्संशयच्छेता प्रत्युवाच पुनर्वसुः|

स्नेहानां द्विविधा सौम्य योनिः स्थावरजङ्गमा||९||

Lord Punarvasu replied, "There are two sources of oils and fats viz, vegetable and animal [9]

**Vegetable sources – Sthavara Yoni of Sneha :**

तिलः प्रियालाभिषुकौ बिभीतकश्चित्राभयैरण्डमधूकसर्षपाः|

कुसुम्भबिल्वारुकमूलकातसीनिकोचकाक्षोडकरञ्जशिग्रुकाः||१०||

स्नेहाशयाः स्थावरसञ्ज्ञितास्तथा स्युर्जङ्गमा मत्स्यमृगाः सपक्षिणः|

तेषां दधिक्षीरघृतामिषं वसा स्नेहेषु मज्जा च तथोपदिश्यते||११||

**Vegetable sources – Sthavara Yoni of Sneha :**

Tila – Sesame (Sesamum indicum), Priyala (Buchanania lanzan Spreng), Abhishuka (Pistacia vera Linn),

Bibhitaki (Terminalia belerica Roxb), Chitra – Baliospermum montanum,

Abhaya – Terminalia chebula, Eranda – castor (Ricinus communis Linn),

Madhuka – Licorice – Glycyrrhiza glabra, Sarshapa – mustard (Brassica nigra Koch),

Kusumbha (Carthamus tinctorius Linn), Bilva – (Aegle marmelos Corr),

Aruka (Prunus persica Linn) Mulaka – Radish – (Raphanus sativus Linn),

Atasi – Linseed (Linum usitatissimum Linn), Mikocaka (Artocarpus lakoocha Roxb),

Akshoda (Aleurites moluccana Willd), Karanja (Pongamia pinnata Merr), and

Shigruka (Moringa oleifera Lam).

These are the vegetable sources of oil.

**Animal fat – Jangama Yoni of Sneha :**

is contributed by – The fish, quadrupeds and birds.

Curd, milk, ghee, meat, muscle fat and bone marrow of these animals and birds are administered as oily substances. [10-11]

**Properties of Sesamum oil and castor oil:**

सर्वेषां तैलजातानां तिलतैलं विशिष्यते।
बलार्थे स्नेहने चाग्र्यमैरण्डं तु विरेचने॥१२॥
(कटूष्णं तैलमैरण्डं वातश्लेष्महरं गुरु।
कषायस्वादुतिक्तैश्च योजितं पित्तहन्त्रपि ॥१॥)।

Of all the varieties, Tila taila – Sesame oil is the most efficacious for the purpose of strength and oiling the body; Eranda – castor oil is the best oil for purgation.
Castor oil is Katu (pungent), hot and heavy to digest.
Castor oil balances Vata and Kapha. But when mixed up with herbs possessing astringent, sweet and bitter tastes, it alleviates pitta as well. [12]

**Types of Sneha Dravya – Unctuous substances:**
सर्पिस्तैलं वसा मज्जा सर्वस्नेहोत्तमा मताः।
एषु चैवोत्तमं सर्पिः संस्कारस्यानुवर्तनात्॥१३॥
Ghrita – Ghee,

Taila – oil,

Meda (Vasa) – muscle fat and

Majja – Bone marrow

These are the best fatty substances of all. Among them ghee is the best oily substance / fat, because of its power to assimilate effectively the properties of other substances. (Samskara Anuvartana)

**Medicinal Properties of ghee:**
घृतं पित्तानिलहरं रसशुक्रौजसां हितम्।
निर्वापणं मृदुकरं स्वरवर्णप्रसादनम्॥१४॥
Ghee balances Pitta and Vata,

It is conducive to Rasadhatu, Shukra Dhatu (semen) and Ojas. It has a cooling and softening effect on the body. It adds to the clarity of the voice and complexion. [14]

**Properties of Taila – oils:**
मारुतघ्नं न च श्लेष्मवर्धनं बलवर्धनम्।
त्वच्यमुष्णं स्थिरकरं तैलं योनिविशोधनम्॥१५॥
Oil alleviates Vata, it does not aggravate Kapha, it promotes body strength.
It controls the morbidity of the female genital organs. [15]

**Properties of Vasa – fat:**
विद्धभग्नाहत भ्रष्टयोनिकर्णशिरोरुजि।
पौरुषोपचये स्नेहे व्यायामे चेष्यते वसा॥१६॥
The fat is prescribed for the treatment of injury, fracture, trauma, uterine prolapse, earache and headache. It enhances the virility of a person. It helps in oleation and is ideal for those who do daily exercise. [16]

**Properties of bone marrow:**
बलशुक्ररस श्लेष्ममेदोमज्जविवर्धनः।
मज्जा विशेषतोऽस्थ्नां च बलकृत् स्नेहने हितः॥१७॥
The (bone) marrow enhances strength, Shukra (male and female reproductive system), Rasadhatu, Kapha Dosha, Medo Dhatu (fat) and Majja (marrow). It improves strength, especially of the bones and is useful for oleation. [17]

**Seasonal indications for different types of unctuous substances:**

**Time for consumption of fats:**

सर्पिः शरदि पातव्यं वसा मज्जा च माधवे|
तैलं प्रावृषि नात्युष्णशीते स्नेहं पिबेन्नरः||१८||

Ghee is to be used in autumn (Sharath Rutu),
Vasa and Majja (Fat and marrow) in the month of Vaishakha (April- may) and
Taila – oil during the rainy (Pravrit) season.
One should not take any of the oily substance when it is extremely hot or cold. [18]


**Time for the administration of fats:**

वातपित्ताधिको रात्रावुष्णे चापि पिबेन्नरः|
श्लेष्माधिको दिवा शीते पिबेच्चामलभास्करे||१९||

In case of Vata and Pitta imbalance, oleation therapy should be administered in the evening.
When the Kapha is vitiated it is administered in mid-day. [19]


**Complications of untimely administration of fats:**

अत्युष्णे वा दिवा पीतो वातपित्ताधिकेन वा|
मूर्च्छां पिपासामुन्मादं कामलां वा समीरयेत्||२०||
शीते रात्रौ पिबन् स्नेहं नरः श्लेष्माधिकोऽपि वा|
आनाहमरुचिं शूलं पाण्डुतां वा समृच्छति||२१||

If oleation therapy is administered during the day time in summer or to patients suffering from diseases dominated by the vitiation of Vata or Pitta, this may cause fainting, thirst, insanity or jaundice. If one suffering from diseases of Kapha imbalance or from a disease during the course of the winter, if he is administered with oleation during evening, he will suffer from anaha (bloating), anorexia (aruchi), colic pain and anemia. [20-21]


**Anupana for unctuous substances:**

जलमुष्णं घृते पेयं यूषस्तैलेऽनु शस्यते|
वसामज्ज्ञोस्तु मण्डः स्यात् सर्वेषूष्णमथाम्बु वा||२२||

Ghee is to be taken with the Anupana of hot water,
oil with anupana of Yusha (vegetable soup),
muscle fat and bone marrow with Anupana of Manda (thin gruel) or all these oily substances may be taken with the Anupana of hot water. [22]


**Sneha Pravicharana – Twenty-four recipes of oils and fats:**

ओदनश्च विलेपी च रसो मांसं पयो दधि|
यवागूः सूपशाकौ च यूषः काम्बलिकः खडः||२३||
सक्तवस्तिलपिष्टं च मद्यं लेहास्तथैव च|
भक्ष्यमभ्यञ्जनं बस्तिस्तथा चोतरबस्तयः||२४||
गण्डूषः कर्णतैलं च नस्तःकर्णाक्षितर्पणम्|
चतुर्विंशतिरित्येताः स्नेहस्य प्रविचारणाः ||२५||


**Sneha Pravicharana – Twenty four recipes of oils and fats:**

The following are the 24 forms of preparation of unctuous substances:-
Odana (porridge),Vilepi (a type of gruel prepared with four times of water),
Mamsarasa (meat soup), meat, milk, curd,
Yavagu (a type of gruel prepared with six times of water), pulse, curry, vegetable soup,
Kambalika (sour milk mixed with whey and vinegar),

Khada (butter milk boiled with acid vegetables and spices),
Saktu (roasted grain flour),
pastry prepared of sesame , Liquor, Linctus,
Bhakshya (foods that require hard chewing)
Massage, Enema, Douche, Gandusha -Gargle, Karna taila – ear drop, Dhumapana – Inhalation,
preparation soothing to the ears and eyes. [23-25]

**Importance of Acchapeya – pure-fat administration:**
अच्छपेयस्तु यः स्नेहो न तामाहुर्विचारणाम्|
स्नेहस्य स भिषग्दृष्टः कल्पः प्राथमकल्पिकः||२६||
The intake of simple (unmixed) oily substance is regarded by physicians as the best oleation therapy.[26]

**Sneha Pravicharana – Classification of fat preparation combinations:**
रसैश्चोपहितः स्नेहः समासव्यासयोगिभिः|
षड्भिस्त्रिषष्टिधा सङ्ख्यां प्राप्नोत्येकश्च केवलः||२७||
एवमेताश्चतुःषष्टिः स्नेहानां प्रविचारणा |
ओकर्तुव्याधिपुरुषान् प्रयोज्या जानता भवेत्||२८||

**Sneha Pravicharana – Classification of fat preparation combinations:**
Oily preparations are of 63 types depending on their association with the drugs having six rasas (tastes) in isolation or variant combination. Together with the simple (unmixed) ones, these substances are of sixty four types. A physician, being expert with the habit, seasons, diseases and individual requirements should accordingly administer these sixty four types of preparations of fats and oils. [27-28]

Note: the term Sneha Pravicharana is used both for different forms of oil and fat administration and also for different types of oil and fat administration.

**Dose schedule for fat administration:**
अहोरात्रमहः कृत्स्नमर्धाहं च प्रतीक्षते|
प्रधाना मध्यमा ह्रस्वा स्नेहमात्रा जरां प्रति||२९||
इति तिस्रः समुद्दिष्टा मात्राः स्नेहस्य मानतः|
The dose of the oleation therapy is of three types, depending upon the time taken for its digestion.
**Superior quantity** - The dose of oils and fats that require 24 hours for its digestion is of the first type (superior).
**Moderate quantity** - The one requiring the whole day (12 hours) for digestion is of the second type (moderate) and
**Inferior quantity** - The one requiring six hours for digestion is of the third type (inferior).

**Administration of oils and fats based on individual needs :**
**Indication for maximum dose of fats and oils** (which digests in 24 hours)
तासां प्रयोगान् वक्ष्यामि पुरुषं पुरुषं प्रति||३०||
प्रभूतस्नेहनित्या ये क्षुत्पिपासासहा नराः|
पावकश्चोत्तमबलो येषां ये चोत्तमा बले||३१||
गुल्मिनः सर्पदष्टाश्च विसर्पोपहताश्च ये|
उन्मत्ताः कृच्छ्रमूत्राश्च गाढवर्चस एव च||३२||
पिबेयुरुत्तमां मात्रां तस्याः पाने गुणाञ्छृणु|
विकाराञ्छमयत्येषां शीघ्रं सम्यक्प्रयोजिता||३३||
दोषानुकर्षिणी मात्रा सर्वमार्गानुसारिणी|

बल्या पुनर्नवकरी शरीरेन्द्रियचेतसाम्||३४||

The below mentioned patients should use the first (superior) type of dose of oleation therapy (which would get digested in 24 hours duration) –

- those who are in the habit of taking adequate quantity of oils and fats and
- those having resistance to hunger and thirst,
- those whose digestion power is high,
- those who are themselves very strong,
- those suffering from Gulma (abdominal tumor), snake bite, Visarpa (skin diseases characterized with spread), insanity, dysuria, constipation

The following are the effects of its intake. If properly administered, it alleviates all ailments instantaneously; it eliminates the Doshas, it strengthens all the systems of the body; it rejuvenates the body, sense organs and mind.

**Indication for moderate dose of fats and oils** (which digests in 12 hours)

अरुष्कस्फोटपिडकाकण्डूपामाभिरर्दिताः|
कुष्ठिनश्च प्रमीढाश्च वातशोणितिकाश्च ये||३५||
नातिबहुवाशिनश्चैव मृदुकोष्ठास्तथैव च|
पिबेयुर्मध्यमां मात्रां मध्यमाश्चापि ये बले||३६||
मात्रैषा मन्दविभ्रंशा न चातिबलहारिणी|
सुखेन च स्नेहयति शोधनार्थे च युज्यते||३७||

Fats and oils of moderate dose i.e., the quantity which gets digested in 12 hours is indicated in –

- those suffering from eruptions, boils, pimples, itching, papules, spreading type of skin disease, chronic urinary disorders and gout (Vatarakta).
- those who cannot eat much.
- those who are of laxed bowels.
- those with moderate strength.

The oleation therapy, in this dosage, does not create much complications nor does it affect the strength too much.

**Indication for low dose of fats and oils** (which digests in 6 hours)

ये तु वृद्धाश्च बालाश्च सुकुमाराः सुखोचिताः|
रिक्तकोष्ठत्वमहितं येषां मन्दाग्नयश्च ये||३८||
ज्वरातीसारकासाश्च येषां चिरसमुत्थिताः|
स्नेहमात्रां पिबेयुस्ते ह्रस्वां ये चावरा बले||३९||
परिहारे सुखा चैषा मात्रा स्नेहनबृंहणी|
वृष्या बल्या निराबाधा चिरं चाप्यनुवर्तते||४०||

Low dose of oils and fats (that quantity which gets digested in six hours' time) is prescribed in the below mentioned –

- the old people and the children,
- those with tender health,
- those who have been brought up in luxury,
- those for whom evacuation of bowel is not good,
- those with weak digestion, chronic fever, diarrhoea and cough, and

- those who are very weak,

**Benefits:** This stimulates libido and gives strength. This is least harmful and can be administered for a long time. [29-40]

## Indications for the administration of Ghee:

वातपित्तप्रकृतयो वातपित्तविकारिणः|
चक्षुःकामाः क्षताः क्षीणा वृद्धा बालास्तथाऽबलाः||४१||
आयुःप्रकर्षकामाश्च बलवर्णस्वरार्थिनः|
पुष्टिकामाः प्रजाकामाः सौकुमार्यार्थिनश्च ये||४२||
दीप्त्योजःस्मृतिमेधाग्निबुद्धीन्द्रियबलार्थिनः|
पिबेयुः सर्पिरार्तांश्च दाहशस्त्रविषाग्निभिः||४३||

Intake of herbal ghee is prescribed for those with

- Vata Pitta body type
- those suffering from Vata and Pitta imbalance disorders,
- those desiring good eyesight
- those with chest injury
- for the old, children and weak
- those desirous of longevity, of strength, good complexion, voice, nourishment, progeny, tenderness, luster, Ojas, memory, intelligence, power of digestion, wisdom, proper functioning of sense organs and
- those afflicted with injuries due to burns, by weapons, poisons and fire. [41-43]

## Indications for the administration of oils:

प्रवृद्धश्लेष्ममेदस्काश्चलस्थूलगलोदराः|
वातव्याधिभिराविष्टा वातप्रकृतयश्च ये||४४||
बलं तनुत्वं लघुतां दृढतां स्थिरगात्रताम्|
स्निग्धश्लक्ष्णतनुत्वक्तां ये च काङ्क्षन्ति देहिनः||४५||
कृमिकोष्ठा क्रूरकोष्ठास्तथा नाडीभिरर्दिताः|
पिबेयुः शीतले काले तैलं तैलोचिताश्च ये||४६||

Intake of oil is prescribed even in the winter for those –

- having Kapha in excess,
- having excess fat in throat and abdomen,
- suffering from Vata imbalance diseases and
- those desirous of strength, slimness, lightness, sturdiness, steadiness, tenderness and smoothness of the skin,
- those having worms and other infection in their bowels,
- those having Krura koshta (unpredictable bowel – sometime soft, most of the times hard)
- those afflicted with wound sinuses and those who are accustomed to the intake of oil. [44-46]

## Indications for the administration of muscle fat:

वातातपसहा ये च रूक्षा भाराध्वकर्शिताः|
संशुष्करेतोरुधिरा निष्पीतकफमेदसः||४७||
अस्थिसन्धिसिरास्नायुर्मर्मकोष्ठमहारुजः|
बलवान्मारुतो येषां खानि चावृत्य तिष्ठति||४८||
महच्चाग्निबलं येषां वसासात्म्याश्च ये नराः|

तेषां स्नेहयितव्यानां वसापानं विधीयते||४९||

Intake of muscle fat is prescribed for –

- those who can stand the wind and the sun,
- those with rough skin,
- those who are emaciated due to the bearing of heavy loads or exertion from long walks
- those with depleted semen and blood,
- those with less Kapha and Medas (fat),
- those having excruciating pain, in bone joints, veins, ligaments, vital organs, abdominal viscera,
- those whose channels of circulation are affected by strong Vata,
  those with excellent digestion strength and those who are accustomed to the intake of fats.

This is, however, to be administered only to such patients as are required to be given oleation therapy. [47-49]

**Indications for the administration of bone marrow:**

दीप्ताग्नयः क्लेशसहा घस्मराः स्नेहसेविनः|
वातार्ताः क्रूरकोष्ठाश्च स्नेह्या मज्जानमाप्नुयुः||५०||

The intake of bone marrow is prescribed for –

- those who have strong digestive power
- those who can withstand stress and strain, greedy eaters
- those accustomed to the intake of oils and fats
- those afflicted with Vata and those with a hard bowel.

This is, however, to be administered only to such patients who are required to be given oleation therapy.
Thus, the indications for different types of oleation therapy useful for different types of patients have been explained. [50]

**Course for fat administration before Panchakarma:**

येभ्यो येभ्यो हितो यो यः स्नेहः स परिकीर्तितः|५१|

Minimum period is 3 days.
Maximum period is 7 days. [51]

**General indications for fat / oil therapy:**

स्वेद्याः शोधयितव्याश्च रूक्षा वातविकारिणः|
व्यायाममद्यस्त्रीनित्याः स्नेह्याः स्युर्ये च चिन्तकाः||५२||

Oleation therapy in general is prescribed for –

- those who are to be given Swedana (sweating treatment) or Panchakarma therapy
- those who have roughness in the skin
- those suffering from diseases due to Vata imbalance
- those who indulge in physical exercise, wine and women
- those who suffer from mental strain [52]

**Contra- indications for fat administration:**

संशोधनाद्दते येषां रूक्षणं सम्प्रवक्ष्यते|

न तेषां स्नेहनं शस्तमुत्सन्नकफमेदसाम्||५३||
अभिष्यण्णाननगुदा नित्यमन्दाग्नयश्च ये|
तृष्णामूर्च्छापरीताश्च गर्भिण्यस्तालुशोषिणः||५४||
अन्नद्विषश्छर्दयन्तो जठरामगरादिताः|
दुर्बलाश्च प्रतान्ताश्च स्नेहग्लाना मदातुराः||५५||
न स्नेह्या वर्तमानेषु न नस्तो बस्तिकर्मसु|
स्नेहपानात् प्रजायन्ते तेषां रोगाः सुदारुणाः||५६||

## Contra-indications for fat administration:

Oleation therapy should not be administered to such of the patients who are

- eligible for Rukshana (drying therapy)
- to those in whom Kapha and Medas (fat) are aggravated
- those with Kapha symptoms like excess mucus secretion from mouth and anus
- those whose power of digestion is continuously weak
- those suffering from thirst and fainting
- the pregnant women
- those with dry palate
- those having aversion to food
- those suffering from vomiting, abdominal diseases, diseases due to improper digestion as well as metabolism
- those afflicted with Gara type of poison (chronic diet-poison)
- the weak, emaciated, those having aversion to the intake of unctuous substances
- those intoxicated and those being administered inhalation and enema therapies.

If Oleation therapy is administered to such persons, they are likely to fall victims of disastrous complications. [53-56]

## Signs and symptoms of incomplete oleation:

पुरीषं ग्रथितं रूक्षं वायुरप्रगुणो मृदुः|
पक्ता खरत्वं रौक्ष्यं च गात्रस्यास्निग्धलक्षणम्||५७||

Hard and dry stool, derangement of Vayu, weak digestion power, roughness and dryness of the skin- these are the signs of under oleation [57]

## Signs and symptoms of proper oleation:

वातानुलोम्यं दीप्तोऽग्निर्वर्चः स्निग्धमसंहतम्|
मार्दवं स्निग्धता चाङ्गे स्निग्धानामुपजायते||५८||

Evacuation of the flatus, good digestive power, unctuous and soft stool, tenderness and smoothness of the body- these are the signs of proper oleation.[58]

## Signs and symptoms of over oleation:

पाण्डुता गौरवं जाड्यं पुरीषस्याविपक्वता|
तन्द्रीररुचिरुत्केशः स्यादतिस्निग्धलक्षणम्||५९||

Paleness, heaviness, stiffness, stool indicative of indigestion, drowsiness, anorexia are the signs of over oleation.[59]

## Pre-oleation management:

द्रवोष्णमनभिष्यन्दि भोज्यमन्नं प्रमाणतः|
नातिस्निग्धमसङ्कीर्ण श्वः स्नेहं पातुमिच्छता||६०||

पिबेत् संशमनं स्नेहमन्नकाले प्रकाङ्क्षितः|
शुद्ध्यर्थं पुनराहारे नैशे जीर्णे पिबेन्नरः||६१||

A day preceding the administration of Oleation therapy, one should take food in proper quantity. The food should be liquid, hot and Anabhisyandi (that does not obstruct the channel of circulation / that which does not leave a coating on body channels). It should neither be too unctuous nor a mixture of two opposite qualities (hot and cold). When hungry, one should take alleviation (samshamana) type of oleation therapy in low doses, during lunch hours. Samsodhana type of oleation therapy should be administered when the food taken in the preceding night has been well digested. [60-61]

## Management during Oleation :

उष्णोदकोपचारी स्याद्ब्रह्मचारी क्षपाशयः |
शकृन्मूत्रानिलोद्गारानुदीर्णांश्च न धारयेत्||६२||
व्यायाममुच्चैर्वचनं क्रोधशोकौ हिमातपौ|
वर्जयेदप्रवातं च सेवेत शयनासनम्||६३||
स्नेहं पीत्वा नरः स्नेहं प्रतिभुञ्जान एव च|
स्नेहमिथ्योपचारादिध जायन्ते दारुणा गदाः||६४||

While under the oleation therapy, one should –

- always use hot water,
- observe Brahmacharya
- not sleep during day time
- not suppress urges of motion, urination, flatus eructation, etc.
- avoid physical exercise, loud speech, anger, anxiety, cold and sun,
- lie down or sit in a place well protected from wind

Even after the completion of the course of oleation therapy one might be required to take some more unctuous substance of homologous qualities. Adoption of wrong regimen during the course of oleation therapy will result in serious complications [62-64]

## Therapeutic test for the diagnosis of Koshta (bowel):

मृदुकोष्ठस्त्रिरात्रेण स्निह्यत्यच्छोपसेवया|
स्निह्यति क्रूरकोष्ठस्तु सप्तरात्रेण मानवः||६५||
गुडमिक्षुरसं मस्तु क्षीरमुल्लोडितं दधि|
पायसं कृशरां सर्पिः काश्मर्यत्रिफलारसम्||६६||
द्राक्षारसं पीलुरसं जलमुष्णमथापि वा|
मद्यं वा तरुणं पीत्वा मृदुकोष्ठो विरिच्यते||६७||
विरेचयन्ति नैतानि क्रूरकोष्ठं कदाचन|
भवति क्रूरकोष्ठस्य ग्रहण्यत्युल्बणानिला||६८||
उदीर्णपित्ताऽल्पकफा ग्रहणी मन्दमारुता|
मृदुकोष्ठस्य तस्मात् स सुविरेच्यो नरः स्मृतः||६९||

## Therapeutic test for the diagnosis of Koshta (bowel):

A person with Mridu Koshta (laxed bowel), is properly oleated by taking an unctuous substance for three consecutive nights and one with Krura Koshta (costive bowels) for seven consecutive nights.

People with mridu koshta would have purgation with following :

Sugar candy, sugarcane juice, mastu (whey), milk cream from the curd, curd, payasa (milk preparation), gruel made from sesame, rice and black gram, ghee, juice of Kashmarya (Gmelina arborea Linn), Haritaki – (Chebulic myrobalan), Amla, Bibhitaki (Terminalia belerica Roxb), raisins and Pilu (Salvadora persica Linn), even hot water or fresh wine.

But these cannot produce purgative effect for those with Krura Koshta (costive bowel) because their intestine is too much dominated by Vata, Purgation is easy for those with laxed bowel, because their Grahani i.e. intestine is dominated by Pitta and is least affected by Kapha and Vata. [65-69]

**Side effects of oleation and its management:**
उदीर्णपित्ता ग्रहणी यस्य चाग्निबलं महत्।
भस्मीभवति तस्याशु स्नेहः पीतोऽग्नितेजसा॥७०॥
स जग्ध्वा स्नेहमात्रां तामोजः प्रक्षारयन् बली।
स्नेहाग्निरुत्तमां तृष्णां सोपसर्गामुदीरयेत्॥७१॥
नालं स्नेहसमृद्धस्य शमायान्नं सुगुर्वपि।
स चेत् सुशीतं सलिलं नासादयति दह्यते।
यथैवाशीविषः कक्षमध्यगः स्वविषाग्निना॥७२॥
अजीर्णे यदि तु स्नेहे तृष्णा स्याच्छर्दयेद्भिषक्।
शीतोदकं पुनः पीत्वा भुक्त्वा रूक्षान्नमुल्लिखेत्॥७३॥
न सर्पिः केवलं पित्ते पेयं सामे विशेषतः।
सर्वं ह्यनुरजेद्देहं हत्वा सञ्ज्ञां च मारयेत्॥७४॥
तन्द्रा सोत्क्लेश आनाहो ज्वरः स्तम्भो विसञ्ज्ञता।
कुष्ठानि कण्डूः पाण्डुत्वं शोफार्शास्यरुचिस्तृषा॥७५॥
जठरं ग्रहणीदोषाः स्तैमित्यं वाक्यनिग्रहः।
शूलमामप्रदोषाश्च जायन्ते स्नेहविभ्रमात्॥७६॥
तत्राप्युल्लेखनं शस्तं स्वेदः कालप्रतीक्षणम्।
प्रति प्रति व्याधिबलं बुद्ध्वा संसनमेव च॥७७॥
तक्रारिष्टप्रयोगश्च रूक्षपानान्नसेवनम्।
मूत्राणां त्रिफलायाश्च स्नेहव्यापत्तिभेषजम्॥७८॥

**Side effects of oleation and its management:**

Unctuous substances taken by a person with Pitta imbalance in duodenum and having strong digestive power, gets digested quickly by virtue of the power of the digestive fire. Strong digestive fire, having consumed the heavy dose of unctuous substance displaces the Ojas and aggravates the thirst with complications. Even very heavy food is not enough to satisfy the digestive fire excited by oleation.

In the circumstances, unless he takes recourse to cold water, the patient may die as a serpent lying in the midst of a heap of wood dies with the fire of its own poisonous breath.

If a patient gets thirst due to indigestion of the unctuous substances taken, the physician should administer vomiting treatment (Vamana) The patient should again be given Vamana after being given cold water and unctuous food.

Unmixed ghee should not be taken in the event of the domination of Pitta especially when Pitta is associated with Ama. Ghee taken in this condition brings about paleness (Jaundice) in the body and may prove to be fatal by impairing the consciousness.

If Oleation therapy is not administered properly, drowsiness, nausea, acute constipation, fever, stiffness, unconsciousness, spreading type of skin disease, pruritus, paleness, edema, piles, anorexia, thirst, obstinate abdominal diseases due to the malfunctioning of the intestine including duodenum, stillness, suppression of speech, colic pain and diseases due to improper digestion and metabolism will occur.

In that case Vamana, Swedana (sweating) or fasting (till the previous intake of unctuous substance gets digested) is prescribed. Purgation should also be administered with due regard to the strength of the disease depending on individual cases. Complications arising out of the inappropriate oleation may also be neutralized by the intake of Takrarista (Charaka Chikitsa 14:72-75), unctuous drink and food, urine, Triphala Churna [70-78]

अकाले चाहितश्चैव मात्रया न च योजितः|
स्नेहो मिथ्योपचाराच्च व्यापद्येतातिसेवितः||७९||

The Oleation Therapy gives rise to many complications, if it is administered at inappropriate times or is not taken in the proper dose or taken in excess or (even if taken properly but) followed by improper regimen. [79]

स्नेहात् प्रस्कन्दनं जन्तुस्त्रिरात्रोपरतः पिबेत्|
स्नेहवद्द्रवमुष्णं च त्र्यहं भुक्त्वा रसौदनम्||८०||

Virechana (Purgation) is to be administered three days after the completion of the oleation therapy. During this interval of three days, the patient should take unctuous liquid and hot porridge together with meat juice. [80]

एकाहोपरतस्तद्वद्भुक्त्वा प्रच्छर्दनं पिबेत्
स्यात्वसंशोधनार्थीये वृत्तिः स्नेहे विरिक्तवत्||८१||
The Vamana (vomiting treatment) is to be administered one day after the completion of the oleation therapy. The food prescribed during this interval of one day is the same as indicated in the preceding verse. The regimen prescribed in connection with the purgation is to be followed with regard to the alleviation type of oleation therapy also.

If oleation is being given for the purpose of shamana i.e. palliative purpose (the follow up in relation to) the dietetic regimen and activities as adviced for those who have undergone purgation therapy shall be adopted. [81]

**Indications for the administration of fat preparation:**
स्नेहद्विषः स्नेहनित्या मृदुकोष्ठाश्च ये नराः|
क्लेशासहा मद्यनित्यास्तेषामिष्टा विचारणा||८२||
लावतैत्तिरमायूरहांसवाराहकौक्कुटाः|
गव्याजौरभ्रमात्स्याश्च रसाः स्युः स्नेहने हिताः||८३||
यवकोलकुलत्थाश्च स्नेहाः सगुडशर्कराः|
दाडिमं दधि सव्योषं रससंयोगसङ्ग्रहः||८४||
स्नेहयन्ति तिलाः पूर्वं जग्धाः सस्नेहफाणिताः|
कृशराश्च बहुस्नेहास्तिलकाम्बलिकास्तथा||८५||
फाणितं शृङ्गवेरं च तैलं च सुरया सह|
पिबेद्रूक्षो भृतैर्मांसैर्जीर्णेऽश्नीयाच्च भोजनम्||८६||
तैलं सुराया मण्डेन वसां मज्जानमेव वा|
पिबन् सफाणितं क्षीरं नरः स्निह्यति वातिकः||८७||
धारोष्णं स्नेहसंयुक्तं पीत्वा सशर्करं पयः|
नरः स्निह्यति पीत्वा वा सरं दध्नः सफाणितम्||८८||

पाञ्चप्रसृतिकी पेया पायसो माषमिश्रकः|
क्षीरसिद्धो बहुस्नेहः स्नेहयेदचिरान्नरम्||८९||
सर्पिस्तैलवसामज्जातण्डुलप्रसृतैः शृ(कृ)ता|
पाञ्चप्रसृतिकी पेया पेया स्नेहनमिच्छता||९०||
(शौकरो वा रसः स्निग्धः सर्पिर्लवणसंयुतः |
पीतो द्विर्वासरे यत्नात् स्नेहयेदचिरान्नरम् )|

Unctuous preparations rather than pure unctuous substances are to be prescribed for persons who have aversion of taking unctuous substance, those who are in the habit or regularly taking unctuous substances, wine, those with Mridu Koshta (laxed bowels) and those who cannot resist to physical strain. [82]

The meat juice of Lava (Common quail), Tittira (black partridge), Mayura (peacock), Hamsa (swan), Varaha (Pig), Kukkuta (red squrfowl), Go (Cow), Aja (Goat), Aurabhra (wild sheep) and fish are useful in oleation.

The drugs required to be mixed with meat juice are
Yava – Barley (Hordeum vulgare), Kola (Zizyphus jujuba Lam), Kulattha (Dolichos biflorus Linn), Sugar candy, Crystal sugar, Dadima – Pomegranate, Curd, Sunthi (Zingiber officinale Rosc), Pippali – Long pepper fruit – (Piper longum Linn) and Maricha – Black pepper fruit – (Piper nigrum Linn).

If sesame seeds together with unctuous substances, Phanita (a preparation of sugar cane), Krishara (a type of gruel) added with sufficient quantity of unctuous substance and Kambalika (sour milk mixed with whey and vinegar) prepared with sesame seed, are taken before meals, they are useful in oleation.

One who is having dryness should take Phanita (a preparation of sugar cane), ginger juice and oil together with wine. After they have been digested he should take his meal with minced meat.

A person with Vata body type can be oleated by taking oil, together with the upper portion of wine, muscle fat, marrow milk and Phanita (a preparation of sugar cane).

One gets oleated by taking warm milk fresh from the cow mixed up with sugar and unctuous substance or cream of the curd along with Phanita. Pancha prasritaki Peya – type of gruel prepared with milk and black gram and added with unctuous substance in sufficient quantity oleates immediately.

Pancha prasritaki Peya is prepared with ghee, oil, muscle fat, marrow and rice - Prarita (96 g) of each. This is prescribed for one in need of oleation therapy. Juice of pork made unctuous by adding ghee and salt, if taken properly twice a day, oleates immediately. [83-90]

**Specific Contra-Indications of Substances used in oleation Therapy:**
ग्राम्यानूपौदकं मांसं गुडं दधि पयस्तिलान्|
कुष्ठी शोथी प्रमेही च स्नेहने न प्रयोजयेत्||९१||
स्नेहैर्यथार्हं तान् सिद्धैः स्नेहयेदविकारिभिः|
पिप्पलीभिर्हरीतक्या सिद्धैस्त्रिफलयाऽपि वा||९२||
द्राक्षामलकयूषाभ्यां दध्ना चाम्लेन साधयेत्|
व्योषगर्भं भिषक् स्नेहं पीत्वा स्निह्यति तं नरः||९३||
यवकोलकुलत्थानां रसाः क्षारः सुरा दधि|
क्षीरसर्पिश्च तत् सिद्धं स्नेहनीयं घृतोतमम्||९४||

**Specific Contra- Indications of Substances used in oleation Therapy:**

One suffering from spreading type of skin disease, oedema and obstinate urinary disorders should not use meat juice of domestic, marshy and aquatic animals, sugar candy, curd, and milk and sesame seeds.

If necessary, such patients should be oleated by means of ghee duly prepared with therapeutically useful drugs or with Pippali – Long pepper, Haritaki and Triphala.

A physician should prepare an unctuous drink with the juice of raisin, and Amalaki (Emblica officinalis Gaertn), sour curd, ginger, long pepper and black pepper. By taking this, one gets oleated.

The medicated ghee best suited for the purpose of oleation therapy is to be prepared with the decoction of Barley, jujube, horse gram, alkalies, wine, curd and ghee prepared out of milk. [91-94]

**Oleation therapy in genital disorders:**

तैलमज्जवसासर्पिर्बदरत्रिफलारसैः|

योनिशुक्रप्रदोषेषु साधयित्वा प्रयोजयेत्||९५||

Therapeutic preparation for oleation in the treatment of diseases of the female genital tract and semen is to be made with oil, marrow, muscle fat, ghee and the decoction of Badara – Ziziphus jujuba, Lam, Triphala. [95]

**Sadya Snehana – Simile regarding the effect of quick oleation:**

गृह्णात्यम्बु यथा वस्त्रं प्रस्रवत्यधिकं यथा|

यथाग्नि जीर्यति स्नेहस्तथा स्रवति चाधिकः||९६||

यथा वाऽऽक्लेद्य मृत्पिण्डमासिक्तं त्वरया जलम्|

स्रवति संसते स्नेहस्तथा त्वरितसेवितः||९७||

As a cloth absorbs certain amount of water but oozes out the water in excess, so the oleation therapy used just in proportion with the digestive power gets digested (that is, it is ineffective for the purpose of oleation); It oleates only when it is administered in excess. Or as water poured on a cold earth pot in quick succession oozes out after slightly saturating the latter, so, oleation therapy administered in quick succession in a day, goes waste without oleating properly. [96-97]

**Role of salt in Sadyo Snehana – quick oleation:**

लवणोपहिताः स्नेहाः स्नेहयन्त्यचिरान्नरम्|

तद्ध्यभिष्यन्द्यरूक्षं च सूक्ष्ममुष्णं व्यवायि च||९८||

Unctuous drink prepared with salt oleates an individual instantaneously because salt is by nature Abhisyandi (that obstructs the channel of circulation), unctuous, Sukshma (that passes though subtle channels), hot, Vyavayi (which gets digested only after its absorption and pervasion in the whole body). [98]

**Routine for the administration of different therapeutic measures:**

स्नेहमग्रे प्रयुञ्जीत ततः स्वेदमनन्तरम्|

स्नेहस्वेदोपपन्नस्य संशोधनमथेतरत्||९९||

Oleation therapy is required to be administered first; then sweating therapy is to be applied; finally elimination therapy is to be administered after the administration of oleation and fomentation.[99]

**To sum up:**

तत्र श्लोकः:-

स्नेहाः स्नेहविधिः कृत्स्नव्यापत्सिद्धिः सभेषजा|

यथाप्रश्नं भगवता व्याहृतं चान्द्रभागिना||१००||

Lord Punarvasu has described in response to the question, the various types of oleation, the procedure for oleation, all the related complications and the preparations of various drugs useful for this therapy.[100]

इत्यग्निवेशकृते तन्त्रे चरकप्रतिसंस्कृते श्लोकस्थाने स्नेहाध्यायो नाम त्रयोदशोऽध्यायः समाप्तः||१३||

Thus, ends the thirteenth Chapter on "Oleation" of the Sutra section of Agnivesha's work as redacted by Charaka.

# 14

# Sutrasthana Chapter 14 Swedadhyayam

**Sweating Treatment – Swedana Types and Methods**

अथातः स्वेदाध्यायं व्याख्यास्यामः||१||

इति ह स्माह भगवानात्रेयः||२||

Sweating treatment (Swedana) is usually given after fat administration (oleation – Snehana) therapy. These two are administered as preparation for Panchakarma therapy. In some cases, sweating treatment is administered as a standalone treatment for diseases of Vata and Kapha treatment. The 14th chapter of Charaka Samhita Sutrashana explains in detail about Sweating Therapy.

**A simile for the effect of fomentation therapy:**

अतः स्वेदाः प्रवक्ष्यन्ते यैर्यथावत्प्रयोजितैः|

स्वेदसाध्याः प्रशाम्यन्ति गदा वातकफात्मकाः||३||

स्नेहपूर्वं प्रयुक्तेन स्वेदेनावजितेऽनिले|

पुरीषमूत्ररेतांसि न सज्जन्ति कथञ्चन||४||

शुष्काण्यपि हि काष्ठानि स्नेहस्वेदोपपादनैः|

नमयन्ति यथान्यायं किं पुनर्जीवतो नरान्||५||

Now the different types of Sweating Therapy (fomentation) will be explained. If properly administered, diseases of Vata and kapha imbalance can surely be treated with fomentation. If administered after Snehakarma (oleation), fomentation brings Vata under control. It cleanses feces, urine and semen.

Even dry pieces of wood can be bent by oiling and heating. Similarly, Doshas can be balanced with oleation and fomentation. [3-5]

**Extent of fomentation:**

रोगर्तुव्याधितापेक्षो नात्युष्णोऽतिमृदुर्न च|

द्रव्यवान् कल्पितो देशे स्वेदः कार्यकरो मतः||६||

**Sweating therapy** – is very effective if done neither too hot nor too mild-combined with proper herbs and applied by taking the diseases, the season, the individual patient and organ affected by the disease into account. [6]

**Grades of fomentation:**

व्याधौ शीते शरीरे च महान् स्वेदो महाबले|

दुर्बले दुर्बलः स्वेदो मध्यमे मध्यमो हितः||७||

वातश्लेष्मणि वाते वा कफे वा स्वेद इष्यते|

स्निग्धरूक्षस्तथा स्निग्धो रूक्षश्चाप्युपकल्पितः||८||

"

If the disease is of serious type, if the season is very cold and if the body of the patient is quite strong, then very strong fomentation is prescribed. If the disease is mild, the season is moderately cold and the body is weak, mild fomentation is prescribed. If all are of moderate nature, then moderate fomentation is prescribed.

In Vata – Kapha imbalance disorder, Snighda-Rooksha sweda is administered i.e., oiling and drying type of sweating.
In Vata imbalance disorder, Snigdha sweda – an oiling type of sweating is administered.
In Kapha imbalance disorder, Rooksha Sweda – dry type of sweating is administered. [7-8]

### Treatment for Vata in Amashaya (Stomach) and Pakvashaya (Large intestine)
आमाशयगते वाते कफे पक्वाशयाश्रिते|
रूक्षपूर्वो हितः स्वेदः स्नेहपूर्वस्तथैव च||९||
If the Vata is accumulated in Amashaya (stomach) then Rooksha sweda (dry fomentation) is preferred. This is because Amashaya is the site of Kapha. (Read more – Kapha Dosha dominant body parts). If the Vata is accumulated in Pakwashaya – intestines, then Snigdha Sweda (oily fomentation) is preferred. [9] Because Pakwashaya is dominated by Vata.

### Body parts Contra-Indicated for fomentation:
वृषणौ हृदयं दृष्टी स्वेदयेन्मृदु नैव वा|
मध्यमं वङ्क्षणौ शेषमङ्गावयवमिष्टतः||१०||
Fomentation should be avoided over testicles, heart and eyes. Even if it is very necessary to administer, it should be of mild type. Over groins it should be moderate. Fomentation on other parts of the body could be according to the individual needs. [10]

### Rules for Swedana near eye and heart regions:
सुशुद्धैर्नक्तकैः पिण्ड्या गोधूमानामथापि वा|
पद्मोत्पलपलाशैर्वा स्वेद्यः संवृत्य चक्षुषी||११||
मुक्तावलीभिः शीताभिः शीतलैर्भाजनैरपि|
जलार्द्रैर्जलजैर्हस्तैः स्विद्यतो हृदयं स्पृशेत्||१२||

### Rules for Swedana near eye and heart regions:
Before sweating therapy, eyes should be covered with very clean clothes, a ball of wheat flour or leaves of Kamala (lotus) and Utpala (Nymphaea alba) or Palasha (Butea monosperma). Similarly, Heart is to be covered with cool pearl necklaces, cool utensils, Lotuses, wet water or simply by the touch of cold hands. [11-12]

### Signs of Ideal fomentation – Samyak Swinna Lakshana
शीतशूलव्युपरमे स्तम्भगौरवनिग्रहे|
सञ्जाते मार्दवे स्वेदे स्वेदनादिवरतिर्मता||१३||

Fomentation is to be administered until there is
**Sheeta Shoola Vyuparama** – complete recovery from coldness and pain,
**Sthambha Gaurava Nigraha** – relief from stiffness and heaviness of the body
**Mardava** – softness or tenderness of body parts.
After observing these signs, the sweating process should be stopped. [13]

### Signs of excessive sweating treatment – Ati Sweda Lakshana
पित्तप्रकोपो मूर्च्छा च शरीरसदनं तृषा|

दाहः स्वराङ्गदौर्बल्यमतिस्विन्नस्य लक्षणम्||१४||
उक्तस्तस्याशितीये यो ग्रैष्मिकः सर्वशो विधिः|
सोऽतिस्विन्नस्य कर्तव्यो मधुरः स्निग्धशीतलः||१५||

Below mentioned are the symptoms of excessive sweating :

- Aggravation of Pitta,
- fainting,
- fatigue,
- excessive thirst,
- burning sensation,
- weakness of the voice and limbs

Such a person should be treated with summer season regimen (cooling therapies). Sweet, unctuous and cold principles should be used in treatment. [14-15]

## Contra-Indications for fomentation: Swedaha Anarha / Aswedya

कषायमद्यनित्यानां गर्भिण्या रक्तपित्तिनाम्|
पित्तिनां सातिसाराणां रूक्षाणां मधुमेहिनाम्||१६||
विदग्धभ्रष्टब्रध्नानां विषमद्यविकारिणाम्|
श्रान्तानां नष्टसञ्ज्ञानां स्थूलानां पित्तमेहिनाम्||१७||
तृष्यतां क्षुधितानां च क्रुद्धानां शोचतामपि|
कामल्युदरिणां चैव क्षतानामाढ्यरोगिणाम्||१८||
दुर्बलातिविशुष्काणामुपक्षीणौजसां तथा|
भिषक् तैमिरिकाणां च न स्वेदमवतारयेत्||१९||

## Contra-Indications for fomentation: Swedaha Anarha / Aswedya

It is contraindicated in
Kashaya Madya Nitya – those who take excessive astringent foods and alcohol on a regular basis,
Garbhini – the pregnant woman,
Raktapitta – bleeding disorders, such as menorrhagia, nasal bleeding etc.
People with Pitta body type
diarrhoea, people with excessive dryness,
chronic urinary disorders, diabetes,
Vidagdha-Bhrasta-Bradhna – inflammation and prolapsed of the rectum, burn injuries, toxic conditions, Alcoholism;
Those who are fatigued, unconscious,
very obese people, who are very thirsty, hungry,
who are suffering from anger and anxiety,
those suffering from jaundice, abdominal diseases, Vatarakta (gout), Timira (fainting);
those who are weak and dried up and whose Ojas has been reduced. [16-19]

## Indications for Sweating Therapy:

तिश्याये च कासे च हिक्काश्वासेष्वलाघवे|
कर्णमन्याशिरःशूले स्वरभेदे गलग्रहे||२०||
अर्दितैकाङ्गसर्वाङ्गपक्षाघाते विनामके|
कोष्ठानाहविबन्धेषु मूत्राघाते विजृम्भके||२१||

पार्श्वपृष्ठकटीकुक्षिसङ्ग्रहे गृध्रसीषु च|
मूत्रकृच्छ्रे महत्त्वे च मुष्कयोरङ्गमर्दके||२२||
पादजानूरुजङ्घार्तिसङ्ग्रहे श्वयथावपि|
खल्लीष्वामेषु शीते च वेपथौ वातकण्टके||२३||
सङ्कोचायामशूलेषु स्तम्भगौरवसुप्तिषु |
सर्वाङ्गेषु विकारेषु स्वेदनं हितमुच्यते||२४||

**Indications for sweating therapy:**
Fomentation is useful for
Pratisyaya (coryza) – running nose,
Kasa – cough, cold,
Hikka – hiccup,
Shwasa – dyspnea, asthma,
Alaghava – heaviness of the body,
Karna, Manya Shira Shula – pain in the ear, neck and head,
Svarabheda – hoarseness of voice,
Galagraha – obstruction in the throat,
Ardita – facial paralysis,
Ekanga Sarvanga Pakshaghata – paralysis of one limb, whole body or half of the body,
Vinamaka – bending of the body,
Anaha, Vibandha – bloating, constipation,
Mutraghata – dysuria, urinary obstruction,
Vijrumbhaka – Pendiculation, excessive yawning,
Parshva Prushta Kati Kukshi sangraha – stiffness of sides, back, waists and abdomen,
Grudhrasi – sciatica,
Mutrakrichra – dysuria,
enragement of scrotum, malaise,
pain and stiffness of feet, knee, calf, oedema,
Khalli – spondylosis,
Ama – diseases due to impaired digestion and metabolism,
in chills and shivering,
affliction of the ankle joint by Vata (Vata Kantaka),
in contraction, extension or colic pain, stiffness, excessive heaviness, numbness an in diseases affecting the whole body.[20-24]

**Pinda Sveda:**
तिलमाषकुलत्थाम्लघृततैलामिषौदनैः|
पायसैः कृशरैर्मांसैः पिण्डस्वेदं प्रयोजयेत्||२५||
गोखरोष्ट्रवराहाश्वशकृद्भिः सतुषैर्यवैः|
सिकतापांशुपाषाणकरीषायसपूटकैः||२६||
श्लैष्मिकान् स्वेदयेत् पूर्वैर्वातिकान् समुपाचरेत्|
द्रव्याण्येतानि शस्यन्ते यथास्वं प्रस्तरेष्वपि||२७||

Pinda means bolus. In Pinda sweda, a bolus or paste is prepared and used as a source of heat to induce sweating. One should prepare a bolus for fomentation with Tila – Sesame (Sesamum indium), Masha – black gram, Kulattha – horse gram, sour preparations, ghee, oil, meat porridge, Payasa (milk preparations), and flesh. This is indicated for Vata imbalance disorders.

Feces of cow, ass, camel, pig and horse along with the barley grains with chaff, sand, dust, stone dried cow-dung and iron powder in a bolus form is useful for fomentation in diseases of Kapha imbalance. These very drugs may be used for Prastara Sveda (fomentation by a hot stone) depending upon the nature of diseases. [25-27]

## Jentaka and Nadi Sveda:

भूगृहेषु च जेन्ताकेषूष्णगर्भगृहेषु च|
विधूमाङ्गारतप्तेषु स्वभ्यक्तः स्विद्यते सुखम्||२८||
ग्राम्यानूपौदकं मांसं पयो बस्तशिरस्तथा|
वराहमध्यपितासृक् स्नेहवत्तिलतण्डुलाः||२९||
इत्येतानि समुत्क्वाथ्य नाडीस्वेदं प्रयोजयेत्|
देशकालविभागज्ञो युक्त्यपेक्षो भिषक्तमः||३०||

## Jentaka Sveda:

The person should be well massaged. Then he is taken into a heated underground cellar, which is heated with charcoal, without smoke. This leads to comfortable sweating.

## Nadi Sveda:

Nadi means a tube. In Nadi Sweda, the steam is generated by boiling specific liquids in a pot. The pot is attached with a pipe and through that pipe the steam is directed towards the desired body part that requires sweating treatment.

**For Vata disorders** - The steam is generated by boiling the flesh of domestic, marshy and aquatic animals, milk, head of goat, blood, bile and the flesh of middle part of pig, unctuous substances like castor seeds, sesame seeds and rice. [28-30]

## Material for tub fomentation:

वारुणामृतकैरण्डशिगुमूलकसर्षपैः|
वासावंशकरञ्जार्कपत्रैरश्मन्तकस्य च||३१||
शोभाञ्जनकसैरेयमालतीसुरसार्जकैः |
पत्रैरुत्क्वाथ्य सलिलं नाडीस्वेदं प्रयोजयेत्||३२||
भूतीकपञ्चमूलाभ्यां सुरया दधिमस्तुना|
मूत्रैरम्लैश्च सस्नेहैर्नाडीस्वेदं प्रयोजयेत्||३३||
एत एव च निर्यूहाः प्रयोज्या जलकोष्ठके|
स्वेदनार्थं घृतक्षीरतैलकोष्ठांश्च कारयेत्||३४||

**For Kapha disorders**, the steam is generated by boiling leaves of Varuna (Crataeva religiosa Frorst), Amritaka – Giloya, Eranda – castor root, Shigru (Moringa oleifera Lam), Mulaka – radish, Sarshapa – mustard, Vasa (Adhatoda vasica Nees), Vamsha (Bambusa arundinacea Retz), Karanja (Pongamia pinnata), Arka – Calotropis gigantea, Ashmantaka (Bauhinia racemosa Lam), Shobhanjana (seed of moringa), Saireya (Barleria prionitis Linn), Malati (Jasminum grandiflorum), Surasa – Tulsi and Arjaka (Ocimum gratissimum Linn).

**For Vata-Kaphaja disorders**, Nadi Sveda should be given by boiling Bhutika (Trachyspermum ammi Sprague), Panchamula (roots of Aegle Marmelos Corr, Oroxylum indicum Vent, Gmelina arborea Linn Stereospermum suaveolens DC. and Clerodendrum phlomidis Linn.f) added with wine, dadhi mastu (Whey), cow urine and sour preparations. The Kashaya (decoction) prepared using above-mentioned herbs are to be used in a big water-tub for fomentation. Wherever necessary, tub fomentation is also administered with ghee, milk or oils. [31-34]

## Ingredients of Upanaha Sveda:

गोधूमशकलैश्चूर्णैर्यवानामम्लसंयुतैः|
सस्नेहकिण्वलवणैरुपनाहः प्रशस्यते||३५||
गन्धैः सुरायाः किण्वेन जीवन्त्या शतपुष्पया|
उमया कुष्ठतैलाभ्यां युक्तया चोपनाहयेत्||३६||
चर्मभिश्चोपनद्धव्यः सलोमभिरपूतिभिः|
उष्णवीर्यैरलाभे तु कौशेयाविकशाटकैः||३७||

### Ingredients of Upanaha Sveda:

Upanaha means pack, bandage or poultice. Here, sweating is induced by making a pack / bandage of ingredients, heating it and bandaging the body parts with such hot packs. Poultice should be prepared with wheat chips, barley mixed with acidic preparations, unctuous substance, yeast and salt, or with fragrant substance, yeast, Jivanti – Leptadenia reticulata, Dill (Shatapuspa), Linseed (Uma), Kushta (Saussurea lappa.G.B Clarke) mixed with Oil.

Leather with hair, devoid of bad smell and of hot potency animals (like antelope etc., whose meat produces heat) is to be used as bandage. In cases of their non-availability, silk or woolen blankets may be used for this purpose. [35-37]

### Period for Upanaha Sveda:

रात्रौ बद्धं दिवा मुञ्चेन्मुञ्चेद्रात्रौ दिवा कृतम्|
विदाहपरिहारार्थं, स्यात् प्रकर्षस्तु शीतले||३८||

In order that the burning sensation may be prevented, normally, the bandage applied in the night should be removed in the morning and that applied during the day, should be removed in the evening: the duration of bandage may be prolonged in the winter.[38]

### Thirteen types of Swedana – fomentation:

सङ्करः प्रस्तरो नाडी परिषेकोऽवगाहनम्|
जेन्ताकोऽश्मघनः कर्षूः कुटी भूः कुम्भिकैव च||३९||
कूपो होलाक इत्येते स्वेदयन्ति त्रयोदश|
तान् यथावत् प्रवक्ष्यामि सर्वानेवानुपूर्वशः||४०||

The thirteen varieties of fomentation are Sankara, Prastara, Nadi, Pariseka, avagahana, Jentaka, Ashmaghana, Karshu, Kuti, Bhu, Kumbhika, Kupa and Holaka. They are described below. [39-40]

### Sankara Sveda:

तत्र वस्त्रान्तरितैरवस्त्रान्तरितैर्वा पिण्डैर्यथोक्तैरुपस्वेदनं सङ्करस्वेद इति विद्यात्||४१||

Sankara Sveda: Fomentation by means of bolus containing prescribed drugs with or without being wrapped with cloths. [41]

### Prastara Sveda: – bed fomentation:

शूकशमीधान्यपुलाकानां वेशवारपायसकृशरोत्कारिकादीनां वा प्रस्तरे
कौशेयाविकोत्तरप्रच्छदेपञ्चाङ्गुलोरुबूकार्कपत्रप्रच्छदे वा
स्वभ्यक्तसर्वगात्रस्य शयानस्योपस्वेदनं प्रस्तरस्वेद इति विद्यात्||४२||

### Prastara Sveda: – bed fomentation

A bed is to be prepared of the size of the individual with corn, pulse and Pulaka (an inferior type of grain) or vesavara (a preparation of meat without bones together with long-pepper, black pepper, ginger, sugar-candy and ghee), Payasa (sweet milk preparation), Krushara (thick gruel), Utkarika (pudding), etc.

The bed is covered with silk, wool or with the leaves of Panchangula (Ricinus communis Linn), Urubuka (castor leaves) and Arka – (Calotropis gigantea R.Br . ex Ait) the individual, well-massaged all over the body, should be made to lie down over this bed. This process is known as Prastara Sveda. [42]

## Nadi Sveda – Tube fomentation:

स्वेदनद्रव्याणां पुनर्मूलफलपत्रशुङ्गादीनां मृगशकुनपिशितशिरस्पदादीनामुष्णस्वभावानां वा यथार्हमम्ललवणस्नेहोपसंहितानां मूत्रक्षीरादीनां वा कुम्भ्यां बाष्पमनुद्वमन्त्यामुत्क्वथितानां नाडिया शरेषीकावंशदलकरञ्जार्कपत्रान्यतमकृतया गजाग्रहस्तसंस्थानया व्यामदीर्घया व्यामार्धदीर्घया वा व्यामचतुर्भागाष्टभागमूलाग्रपरिणाहस्रोतसा सर्वतो वातहरपत्रसंवृतच्छिद्रया द्विस्त्रिर्वा विनामितया वातहरसिद्धस्नेहाभ्यक्तगात्रो बाष्पमुपहरेत्; बाष्पो ह्यनृजुगामी [१] विहतचण्डवेगस्त्वचमविदहन् सुखं स्वेदयतीति नाडीस्वेदः||४३||

## Nadi Sveda – Tube fomentation:

Drugs for fomentation like roots, fruits, leaves, buds etc. or flesh and head etc. of hot animals and birds are mixed with sour, salt or unctuous substances and urine, milk etc. depending on the nature of the disease. They are then heated in a mud pot, connected to a pipe. Pipe is made of Sareyaka or leaves of Vamsa (Bambusa arundinacea R etz), Karanja – Indian Beech (bark / seed) –(Pongama Pinnata Merr). or Arka – (Calotropis gigantea R.Br.ex Ait) with its fore part having the shape of the trunk of an elephant. The pipe is required to be one Vyama (91.44cm) or half a Vyama (45.72cm) long at its proximal end, and one eighth of Vyama (11.43 cm) in the distal end. All the clefts in the pipe should be well covered with the leaves that alleviate Vata (like castor Leaves, Dasha Moola etc.). The pipe should be curved in 2 or 3 places. The individual well massaged with unctuous substances that alleviate Vata should get this vapour through the curved pipe. Curvatures of the pipe help to lessen the intensity of vapour so as to avoid burning sensation. [43]

## Parisheka – sprinkling :

वातिकोत्तरवातिकानां पुनर्मूलादीनामुत्क्वाथैः सुखोष्णैः कुम्भीर्वर्षणिकाः प्रनाडीर्वा पूरयित्वा यथार्हसिद्धस्नेहाभ्यक्तगात्रं वस्त्रावच्छन्नं परिषेचयेदिति परिषेकः||४४||

## Parisheka – sprinkling – showering:

Here, hot liquids are sprinkled over the body parts or whole body. Pots with small holes at the bottom, bamboo pipes, Nala (Phragmites karka Trin etc.) are to be filled up with luke warm decoctions (Kashaya) of roots, etc. of drugs which can cure Vata / Vata-Kapha diseases where Vata is predominant. Showers are then to be taken by an individual after he has been well-massaged with suitable unctuous substance and has been covered with cloth. [44]

## Avagaha: Tub fomentation:

वातहरोत्क्वाथक्षीरतैलघृतपिशितरसोष्णसलिलकोष्ठकावगाहस्तु यथोक्त एवावगाहः||४५||
A tub should be filled up with Kashaya, milk, oil, ghee, meat juice or hot water that balances Vata and the patient should take bath in it. [45]

## Jentaka Sveda – fomentation in a house:

अथ जेन्ताकं चिकीर्षुर्भूमिं परीक्षेत- तत्र पूर्वस्यां दिश्युत्तरस्यां वा गुणवति प्रशस्ते भूमिभागे कृष्णमधुरमृत्तिके सुवर्णमृत्तिके वा परीवापपुष्करिण्यादीनां जलाशयानामन्यतमस्य कूले दक्षिणे पश्चिमे वा सूपतीर्थे समसुविभक्तभूमिभागे सप्ताष्टौ वाऽरत्नीरुपक्रम्योदकात् प्राङ्मुखमुदङ्मुखं वाऽभिमुखतीर्थं कूटागारं कारयेत्, उत्सेधविस्तारतः परमरत्नीः षोडश, समन्तात् सुवृत्तं मृत्कर्मसम्पन्नमनेकवातायनम्; अस्य कूटागारस्यान्तः समन्ततो भित्तिमरत्निविस्तारोत्सेधां पिण्डिकां कारयेदाकपाटात्, मध्ये चास्य कूटागारस्य चतुष्किष्कुमात्रं पुरुषप्रमाणं मृन्मयं कन्दुसंस्थानं बहुसूक्ष्मच्छिद्रमङ्गारकोष्ठकस्तम्भं सपिधानं कारयेत्; तं च खादिराणामाश्वकर्णादीनां वा काष्ठानां पूरयित्वा प्रदीपयेत्; स यदा जानीयात् साधु दग्धानि काष्ठानि गतधूमान्यवतप्तं च केवलमग्निना तदग्निगृहं स्वेदयोग्येन चोष्मणा युक्तमिति, तत्रैनं पुरुषं वातहराभ्यक्तगात्रं वस्त्रावच्छन्नं प्रवेशयेत्, प्रवेशयंश्चैनमनुशिष्यात्- सौम्य! प्रविश कल्याणायारोग्याय चेति, प्रविश्य चैनां पिण्डिकामधिरुह्य पार्श्वापरपार्श्वाभ्यां यथासुखं शयीथाः, न च त्वया स्वेदमूर्च्छापरीतेनापि सता पिण्डिकैषा

विमोक्तव्याऽऽप्राणोच्छ्वासात्, भ्रश्यमानो ह्यतः पिण्डिवकावकाशाद्द्वारमनधिगच्छन् स्वेदमूच्छोपरीततया सद्यः प्राणाञ्जह्या:, तस्मात् पिण्डिकामेनां न कथञ्चन मुञ्चेथा:; त्वं यदा जानीया:- विगताभिष्यन्दमात्मानं सम्यक्प्रसुतस्वेदपिच्छं सर्वस्रोतोविमुक्तं लघूभूतमपगतविबन्धस्तम्भसुप्तिवेदनागौरवमिति, ततस्तां पिण्डिकामनुसरन् द्वारं प्रपद्येथा:, निष्क्रम्य च न सहसा चक्षुषो: परिपालनार्थं शीतोदकमुपस्पृशेथा:, अपगतसन्तापक्लमस्तु मुहूर्तात् सुखोष्णेन वारिणा यथान्यायं परिषिक्तोऽश्नीया:; इति जेन्ताकस्वेद:||४६||

### Jentaka Sveda – fomentation in a house:

One should construct a circular building facing the east or north side having a pond in front, at a suitable place. This should be done in the east or in the north direction. The building is to be erected on the southern or eastern bank of a water reservoir like a small or big pond.

- The level of the land should be plain and it should be situated at a distance of 7 – 8 Aratnis (320 cm to 365.76 cm) from the water reservoir.
- The height and diameter of the building should be sixteen aratnis (731.52 cm) each.
- The building should be uniformly circular, well plastered with mud and should have many windows.
- A bench one Artani (45.72 cm) wide is then to be prepared all around the wall up to the door.
- An oven of clay should be prepared in the center of the room. Its diameter should be four Hastas (1.8 m) and height should be equal to that of an individual.
- It should be circular in shape and should have many fine holes. The pillar-like oven should have a lid. This should be filled up with the fuel of Khadira – Black Catechu and Ashvakarna (Dipterocarpus alatus Roxb), etc. and should be ignited.
- When the physician is sure that the fuel is burnt nicely and the smoke has completely disappeared and the room is heated by fire alone, and the hot temperature is achieved, he should ask the patient who is well-massaged with oils of Vata curing herbs and covered with a cloth, to enter the room.
- The patient is asked to go over the bench and lie down on the cot (which is constructed along the circular wall from end to end). He should not leave the bench. He should move along the bench so as to finish a circle in the room. When he feels that he is free from all obstructions, the sweat along with its sticking portion is completely drained out of the body, when his body is very light, and free from all obstructions, devoid of stiffness, numbness, pain, heaviness, then he should move towards the door following the bench. The patient should not sprinkle eyes with cold water immediately after coming out of the room. After heat and exertions are relieved, he should take a bath with Lukewarm water after about three-fourth of an hour and then he can have meals. [46]

### Ashmaghana Sveda – Stone Bed fomentation:

शयानस्य प्रमाणेन घनामश्ममयीं शिलाम्|
तापयित्वा मारुतघ्नैर्दारुभि: सम्प्रदीपितै:||४७||
व्यपोज्झ्य सर्वानङ्गारान् प्रोक्ष्य चैवोष्णवारिणा|
तां शिलामथ कुर्वीत कौषेयाविकसंस्तराम्||४८||
तस्यां स्वभ्यक्तसर्वाङ्ग: स्वपन् स्विद्यति ना सुखम्|
कौरवाजिनकौषेयप्रावाराद्यै: सुसंवृत: ||४९||

### Ashmaghana Sveda – Stone Bed fomentation:

A compact slab of stone of the measurement of a man, is to be heated with the fuel of trees having Vata curing properties. All fire brands are then to be removed and the stone slab to be sprinkled with hot water. The slab then should be covered with silk or wool sheets. The person after being massaged should be covered with cotton / silk and should be made to lie down on the slab. By doing so, he will be comfortably fomented. [47-49]

### Karshu Sveda: – bed fomentation inside a room :

कर्षूस्वेद: प्रवक्ष्यते|

खानयेच्छयनस्याधः कर्षूं स्थानविभागवित्||५०||
दीप्तैरधूमैरङ्गारैस्तां कर्षूं पूरयेततः|
तस्यामुपरि शय्यायां स्वपन् स्विद्यति ना सुखम्||५१||

## Karshu Sveda: – bed fomentation inside a room :

The physician knowing about geology, should get a flask shaped trench dug below the bed stead. This trench should be filled up with smokeless fire substances. The person lying on the bed over this gets comfortable sweating treatment.

## Kuti Sweda: Sweating treatment in a hut / cottage:

अनत्युत्सेधविस्तारां वृत्ताकारामलोचनाम्|
घनभित्तिं कुटीं कृत्वा कुष्ठाद्यैः सम्प्रलेपयेत्||५२||
कुटीमध्ये भिषक् शय्यां स्वास्तीर्णामुपकल्पयेत्|
प्रावाराजिनकौशेयकुथकम्बलगोलकैः||५३||
हसन्तिकाभिरङ्गारपूर्णाभिस्तां च सर्वशः|
परिवार्यान्तरारोहेदभ्यक्तः स्विद्यते सुखम्||५४||

## Kuti Sweda: Sweating treatment in a hut / cottage:

A thick-walled cottage, round in shape, should be constructed. It should neither be too high nor too wide. There should not be any window in it. The (inner wall of this) cottage should be plastered with drugs like Kushta – Saussurea lappa etc. In the center of the cottage, there should be well-covered sheets prepared of cotton, silk, Kusha grass, blanket or Golaka (a variety of Woolen cloth). The bed should be surrounded with furnaces filled up with fire-brands. The person well-massaged should lie over this bed. Thus, he will get comfortably fomented. [52-54]

## Bhu Sveda:

य एवाश्मघनस्वेदविधिर्भूमौ स एव तु|
प्रशस्तायां निवातायां समायामुपदिश्यते||५५||

Bhu type of fomentation should be carried out on the same principle as "Ashmaghana Sveda" on the floor (instead of lying down on a bed, here, the patient lies down on the floor). An auspicious area, which is free from excessive wind, should be selected for this purpose. [55]

## Kumbhi Sveda:

कुम्भीं वातहरक्वाथपूर्णां भूमौ निखानयेत्|
अर्धभागं त्रिभागं वा शयनं तत्र चोपरि||५६||
स्थापयेदासनं वाऽपि नातिसान्द्रपरिच्छदम्|
अथ कुम्भ्यां सुसन्तप्तान् प्रक्षिपेदयसो गुडान्||५७||
पाषाणान् वोष्मणा तेन तत्स्थः स्विद्यति ना सुखम्|
सुसंवृताङ्गः स्वभ्यक्तः स्नेहैरनिलनाशनैः||५८||

## Kumbhi Sveda:

A pitcher / pot is to be filled up with Kashaya of drugs that alleviate Vata and buried in earth up to one half or one-third part. Hot iron balls or stones should be put into the pitcher. A bed or seat covered with a thin sheet should be kept over it and the patient should either lie down or sit over it. Before administering this type of Sweda, the patient should undergo massage and his body should be covered with cloth. [56-58]

## Kupa Sveda – well fomentation:

कूपं शयनविस्तारं द्विगुणं चापि वेधतः|
देशे निवाते शस्ते च कुर्यादन्तःसुमार्जितम्||५९||
हस्त्यश्वगोखरोष्ट्राणां करीषैर्दग्धपूरिते|
स्ववच्छन्नः सुसंस्तीर्णोऽभ्यक्तः स्विद्यति ना सुखम्||६०||

### Kupa Sveda – well fomentation:

A well-like pit of the width of a bed and twice as deep as the width should be dug out in an auspicious place which is not exposed to wind. Inner portion of this should be cleaned up. It should be filled with the dung of elephants, horses, cows, asses or camels and then ignited. A bed should then be placed over this well. The person well- massaged and well-covered, lying on this bed gets comfortably fomented. [59-60]

### Holaka Sveda:

धीतीकां तु करीषाणां यथोक्तानां प्रदीपयेत्|
शयनान्तःप्रमाणेन शय्यामुपरि तत्र च||६१||
सुदग्धायां विधूमायां यथोक्तामुपकल्पयेत्|
स्ववच्छन्नः स्वपंस्तत्राभ्यक्तः स्विद्यति ना सुखम्||६२||
होलाकस्वेद इत्येष सुखः प्रोक्तो महर्षिणा|
इति त्रयोदशविधः स्वेदोऽग्निगुणसंश्रयः||६३||

A heap of dung (of elephants, horses, cows, asses or camels) the size of a bed is to be ignited. When it is well burnt, and has become smokeless, a bed covered with a thin sheet is to be kept over it. The patient with his body well-covered after massage should lie over it to get fomentation comfortably. [61-62] The above are the thirteen types of fomentation involving the direct application of fire – Agni Sweda. [63]

### Niragni sweda – Fomentation without fire:

व्यायाम उष्णसदनं गुरुप्रावरणं क्षुधा|
बहुपानं भयक्रोधावुपनाहाहवातपाः||६४||

The ten methods of fomentation without direct source of heat are called as Niragni Sweda. They are:

Vyayama – exercise,

Ushma Sadana – residing in a warm chamber,

Guru Pravarana – wearing of heavy clothing,

Kshuda – hunger,

Bahupana – excessive drinking,

Bhaya – fear,

Krodha – anger,

Upanaha – application of poultice,

Aha – wrestling and

Atapa – exposure to sunlight. [64]

### Classification of fomentation techniques:

स्वेदयन्ति दशैतानि नरमग्निगुणादृते|इत्युक्तो
द्विविधः स्वेदः संयुक्तोऽग्निगुणैर्न च||६७||
एकाङ्गसर्वाङ्गगतः स्निग्धो रूक्षस्तथैव च|
इत्येतत्त्रिविधं द्वन्द्वं स्वेदमुद्दिश्य कीर्तितम्||६६||

### Classification of fomentation techniques:

Agni Sweda – direct heat application

Niragni Sweda – without heat source
Ekanga Sweda – fomentation only to a particular body part
Sarvanga Sweda – fomentation to the whole-body part.
Snigdha sweda – fomentation using oily and fat substances (in Vata disorders)
Rooksha sweda – fomentation using dry substances (In Kapha disorders) [65-66]

**Pre- fomentation and post fomentation managements:**
स्निग्धः स्वेदैरुपक्रम्यः स्विन्नः पथ्याशनो भवेत्|
तदहः स्विन्नगात्रस्तु व्यायामं वर्जयेन्नरः||६७||
After the Oleation therapy, the patient should be kept on a wholesome diet. After fomentation, the patient should abstain from exercise on that day. [67]

**Summing up the contents:**
तत्र श्लोकाः:-
स्वेदो यथा कार्यकरो हितो येभ्यश्च यद्विधः|
यत्र देशे यथा योग्यो देशो रक्ष्यश्च यो यथा||६८||
स्विन्नातिस्विन्नरूपाणि तथाऽतिस्विन्नभेषजम्|
अस्वेद्याः स्वेदयोग्याश्च स्वेदद्रव्याणि कल्पना||६९||
त्रयोदशविधः स्वेदो विना दशविधोऽग्निना|
सङ्ग्रहेण च षट् स्वेदाः स्वेदाध्याये निदर्शिताः||७०||
स्वेदाधिकारे यद्वाच्यमुक्तमेतन्महर्षिणा |
शिष्यैस्तु प्रतिपत्तव्यमुपदेष्टा पुनर्वसुः||७१||

The procedure for the effective administration of fomentation, patients for whom it is beneficial, different types of sweating techniques, signs and symptoms of proper, excess fomentation, drugs useful in fomentation, general principles guiding fomentation, thirteen types of fomentation involving the direct application of fire- the ten types without it – all these are described in this chapter on fomentation. [68-70]
इत्यग्निवेशकृते तन्त्रे चरकप्रतिसंस्कृते श्लोकस्थाने स्वेदाध्यायो नाम चतुर्दशोऽध्यायः||१४||
Thus, ends the fourteenth chapter on "fomentation" of the Sutra section of Agnivesha's work as redacted by Charaka.

# 15

# Sutrasthana Chapter 15
# Upakalpaneeyam

**Rules For Vamana and Virechana Treatment**

अथात उपकल्पनीयमध्यायं व्याख्यास्यामः||१||

इति ह स्माह भगवानात्रेयः||२||

Requirements of a doctor to carry out proper Ayurvedic treatment includes a good hospital, availability of medical attendants, instruments and medicines related with the treatment. These requirements are very essential in case of administration of Panchakarma treatments like Vamana (emesis) and Virechana (purgation). The 15th chapter of Sutrasthana of Charaka Samhita is Upakalpaneeya Adhyaya. It explains about the facilities required for treatment and also about rules for Vamana and Virechana.

**Preparation for Vamana and Virechana**

इह खलु राजानं राजमात्रमन्यं वा विपुलद्रव्यं वमनं विरेचनं वा पाययितुकामेन
भिषजा प्रागेवौषधपानात् सम्भारा उपकल्पनीया भवन्ति सम्यक्चैव हि गच्छत्यौषधे प्रतिभोगार्थाः,
व्यापन्ने चौषधे व्यापदः परिसङ्ख्याय प्रतीकारार्थाः; न हि सन्निकृष्टे काले प्रादुर्भूतायामापदि
सत्यपि क्रयाक्रये सुकरमाशु सम्भरणमौषधानां यथावदिति||३||
एवंवादिनं भगवन्तमात्रेयमग्निवेश उवाच- ननु भगवन्! आदावेव ज्ञानवता तथा
प्रतिविधातव्यं यथा प्रतिविहिते सिध्येदेवौषधमेकान्तेन, सम्यक्प्रयोगनिमित्ता हि सर्वकर्मणां सिद्धिरिष्टा,
व्यापच्चासम्यक्प्रयोगनिमित्ता; अथ सम्यगसम्यक् च समारब्धं
कर्म सिद्ध्यति व्यापद्यते वाऽनियमेन, तुल्यं भवति ज्ञानमज्ञानेनेति||४||

**Preparation for Vamana and Virechana**

The physician who is going to administer Vamana (emesis) or Virechana (purgation) treatment to people of higher order, like king, should collect all requirements well in advance. If such collected materials are left over, after the treatment, those can be used in treating other patients. During treatment, if the procedures go wrong, then these important materials and medicines can be utilized to handle the treatment complications. Hence, to avoid panic during treatment procedure, a wise physician should collect all the medicines and equipment of the treatment well in advance, though they may be available locally for sale. Thus said Lord Atreya.

Agnivesha seeks a clarification – "O Lord! A wise physician at the outset should administer the therapy in such a way that it is always accurate, without any mistakes. Effectiveness of the treatment is defined as "always infallibly effective". Effectiveness of all actions depends on proper administration. Conversely, failure is the result of improper administration. If the physician is not sure of the success of his treatment, and if he is anticipating a failure, then would it not indicate lack of knowledge? [3-4]

**Minuteness of the factors determining the result of the treatment:**

तमुवाच भगवानात्रेयः- शक्यं तथा प्रतिविधातुमस्माभिरस्मद्विधैर्वाऽप्यग्निवेश! यथा प्रतिविहिते सिध्येदेवौषधमेकान्तेन, तच्च प्रयोगसौष्ठवमुपदेष्टुं यथावत्; नहि कश्चिदस्ति य एतदेवमुपदिष्टमुपधारयितुमुत्सहेत, उपधार्य वा तथा प्रतिपत्तुं प्रयोक्तुं वा; सूक्ष्माणि हि दोषभेषजदेशकालबलशरीराहारसात्म्यसत्त्वप्रकृतिवयसामवस्थान्तराणि, यान्यनुचिन्त्यमानानि विमलविपुलबुद्धेरपि बुद्धिमाकुलीकुर्युः किं पुनरल्पबुद्धेः; तस्मादुभयमेतद्यथावदुपदेक्ष्यामः- सम्यक्प्रयोगं चौषधानां, व्यापन्नानां च व्यापत्साधनानि सिद्धिधषूतरकालम्||५||

Lord Atreya replied, :O Agnivesha! Some able doctors can certainly administer therapy in such a flawless way. It is within our competence to impart instructions for the proper administration of therapy. But how many are there who would fully comprehend our instructions or act on them or use them properly.

The difference in variations of the following factors is very subtle.
Dosha – the imbalanced Dosha causing disease in the treatment
Bheshaja – medicines used in the treatment,
Kala – time, season,
Bala – strength and immunity of the patient,
Shareera – nature of the body of the patient
Ahara – diet habits of the patient,
Satmya – congenial habits of the patient,
Satva – ability of the patient to tolerate the disease / treatment
Prakruti – nature, Dosha body type of the patient.

Variation of these factors in causing disease is very subtle. Hence, even a brilliant physician can sometimes err in judging the disease or the line and quantity of treatment. So, subsequently signs of a good treatment, bad treatment and antidotes are explained further. [5]

**Hospital building:**

इदानीं तावत् सम्भारान् विविधानपि समासेनोपदेक्ष्यामः; तद्यथा- दृढं निवातं प्रवातैकदेशं सुखप्रविचारमनुपत्यकं धूमातपजलरजसामनभिगमनीयमनिष्ठानां च शब्दस्पर्शरसरूपगन्धानां सोदपानोदूखलमुसलवर्चःस्थानस्नानभूमिमहानसं वास्तुविद्याकुशलः प्रशस्तं गृहमेव तावत् पूर्वमुपकल्पयेत्||६||

**Hospital building:**

The hospital building should not only be well equipped with all facilities but should satisfy the below mentioned conditions –

- Should have been designed by an expert architect
- It should be strong and well built
- It should not be exposed to winds
- There should be only one passage to allow wind in a metered way
- It shall provide comfortable space to move around
- It shall not be constructed over a mountain or hilltop or place surrounded by mountains and hills
- It should not be located near a bigger building

- It shall not be exposed to smoke, extreme heat of the Sun, rushing water, dust or any undesirable noise
- It should not have an undesirable touch, sight, taste or smell
- It should be well equipped with water reservoir or water pot, pestle, mortar, latrine, bathroom and kitchen [6]

**Medical attendants and other general requirements of a hospital:**

ततः शीलशौचाचारानुरागदाक्ष्यप्रादक्षिण्योपपन्नानुपचारकुशलान् सर्वकर्मसु पर्यवदातान् सूपौदनपाचकस्नापकसंवाहकोत्थापकसंवेशकौषधपेषकांश्च परिचारकान् सर्वकर्मस्वप्रतिकूलान्, तथा गीतवादित्रोल्लापकश्लोकगाथाख्यायिकेतिहासपुराणकुशलानभिप्रायज्ञाननुमतांश्च देशकालविदः पारिषद्यांश्च, तथा लावकपिञ्जिलशशहरिणैणकालपुच्छकमृगमातृकोरभ्रान्, गां दोग्ध्रीं शीलवतीमनातुरां जीवद्वत्सां सुप्रतिविहिततृणशरणपानीयां, पात्र्याचमनीयोदकोष्ठमणिकघटपिठरपर्योगकुम्भीकुम्भकुण्डशराव- दर्वीकटोदञ्चनपरिपचनमन्थानचर्मचेलसूत्रकार्पासोर्णादीनि च, शयनासनादीनि चोपन्यस्तभृङ्गारप्रतिग्रहाणि सुप्रयुक्तास्तरणोतरप्रच्छदोपधानानि सोपाश्रयाणि [१] संवेशनोपवेशनस्नेहस्वेदाभ्यङ्गप्रदेहपरिषेकानुलेपनवमनविरेचनास्थापनानुवासन- शिरोविरेचनमूत्रोच्चारकर्मणामुपचारसुखानि, सुप्रक्षालितोपधानाश्च सुश्लक्ष्णखरमध्यमा दृषदः, शस्त्राणि चोपकरणार्थानि, धूमनेत्रं च, बस्तिनेत्रं चोतरबस्तिकं च, कुशहस्तकं च, तुलां च, मानभाण्डं च, घृततैलवसामज्जक्षौद्रफाणितलवणेन्धनोदकमधुसीधुसुरासौवीरकतुषोदक- मैरेयमेदकदधिदधिमण्डोदस्विद्धान्याम्लमूत्राणि च, तथा शालिषष्टिकमुद्गमाषयवतिलकुलत्थबदरमृद्वीकाकाश्मर्यपरूषकाभयामलकबिभीतकानि, नानाविधानि च स्नेहस्वेदोपकरणानि द्रव्याणि, तथैवोर्ध्वहरानुलोमिकोभयभाञ्जि, सङ्ग्रहणीयदीपनीयपाचनीयोपशमनीयवातहरादिसमाख्यातानि चौषधानि; यच्चान्यदपि किञ्चिद्व्यापदः परिसङ्ख्याय प्रतीकारार्थमुपकरणं विद्यात्, यच्च प्रतिभोगार्थं, तत्तदुपकल्पयेत्॥७॥

There should be attendants who are endowed with good conduct, cleanliness, character, devotion, dexterity and sympathy. They should also be well versed with the art of nursing and good in administering therapies.

Several such attendants are required for various purposes like cooking soup, porridge, etc. bathing, massaging, lifting, and seating the patients and also for grinding the drugs (in preparing herbal powders, Kashayam etc.). These attendants should be those who would work willingly and not by force. People well-versed with vocal and instrumental music, panegyrics, recitation of verses, ancient lores, short stories, epics and Purana (Mythology), those who can grasp the inner desires, who are obedient, and who have knowledge of the time and place should also be arranged (as attendants).

**Birds and animals** – Presence of Lava (common quail), Kapinijala (Grey partridge), Shasha (Rabbit), Harina (Black Buck), Ena (Antelope), Kalapucchaka (Black Tailed deer), Mrigamatruka (red deer), Urabhra (wild sheep) is necessary. There should be a milch-cow of good temper and free from diseases with her calf alive. Proper arrangement should be made for her fodder, dwelling and water.

**Basic amenities:** Provision should also be made for water vessel (Patra), spoon (Achamaniya), water tub (Udakostha), big and small earthen jars (Manika and Ghata), frying pan (Pithara), Bowl (Kunda), saucer (Sharava), Ladle (darvi), Mat (kata), Cover plate (Udanchana), cooking pan (Paripachana), Churning stick (manthana), Leather, cloth, thread, cotton, wool etc.

**Facilities for Panchakarma treatment** – Arrangements are to be made for beds, seats, golden vase and spittoon, bed sheet, towel, pillow and cushion. These should facilitate lying flat and sitting, for oleation (Snehana), fomentation (Swedana), massage (Abhyanga), unction (Pradeha), effusion (Parisheka), anointment (Lepa), emesis (Vamana), purgation (Virechana), Asthapana type of enema, Anuvasana type of enema, elimination of Doshas from head (Shiro Virechana) and passing of stool and urine.

**Herbs to manage complications of Panchakarma :**

There should also be smooth, hard and medium sized, along with well cleared pestles, sharp instruments, accessories, smoking pipe, tube for enema and douche, broom, scales and measuring vessels, ghee, oil, muscle fat, marrow, honey, Phanita (a semisolid sugarcane preparation), salt, fuel, various types of wine like the one prepared of honey, Sidhu, Sura, Sauviraka, Maireya, Tushodaka, Curd, whey, Udashvita (a mixture of water and butter milk in equal parts), Dhanyamla (Sour gruel), Shali (rice), Shastika (a variety of rice harvested in 60 days), Mudga (green gram), Masha (black gram), Yava (Barley), Tila (Sesame seeds), Kulattha (Horse gram), Badara (Ber fruit), Mridveeka (raisins), Kashmarya (Gmelina arborea inn), Parushaka (Grewia asiatica Linn), Abhaya (Haritaki), Amalaki (Emblica officinalis Gaertn), Bibhitaki (Terminalia billirica Roxb) and other drugs employed in oleation, fomentation, emesis, purgation, those having the combined action of emesis and purgation, those which can cause constipation (to treat excess purgation or loose motion which might occur as a complication of excessively administered purgation therapy) and appetizers, those which digest ama, those which pacify the aggravated doshas, those which balance / suppress aggravated Vata etc. and such other medicines as are conducive to the treatment of complications, if any, and also those which are useful in and after-treatment should also be collected. [7]

**Hospitalization and general plan for the treatment:**

ततस्तं पुरुषं यथोक्ताभ्यां स्नेहस्वेदाभ्यां यथार्हमुपपादयेत्, तं चेदस्मिन्नन्तरे मानसः शारीरो वा व्याधिः कश्चित्तीव्रतरः सहसाऽभ्यागच्छेतमेव तावदस्योपावर्तयितुं यतेत, ततस्तमुपावर्त्य तावन्तमेवैनं कालं तथाविधेनैव कर्मणोपाचरेत्||८||

The patient who is to be administered with shodhana i.e. cleansing therapies should then be treated by means of oleation (snehana) and fomentation (Swedana) therapies as required. In the event of a sudden attack of a more serious psychic or somatic disease during the course of treatment, the physician should try to correct the newly arrived complications first. Even after it has been corrected the corrective therapy should be continued for an equivalent duration.

**Administering medicine for Vamana – emesis therapy :**

ततस्तं पुरुषं स्नेहस्वेदोपपन्नमनुपहतमनसमभिसमीक्ष्य सुखोषितं सुप्रजीर्णभक्तं शिरःस्नातमनुलिप्तगात्रं स्रग्विणमनुपहतवस्त्रसंवीतं देवताग्निद्विजगुरुवृद्धवैद्यानर्चितवन्तमिष्टे नक्षत्रतिथिकरणमुहूर्ते कारयित्वा ब्राह्मणान् स्वस्तिवाचनं प्रयुक्ताभिराशीर्भिरभिमन्त्रितां मधुमधुकसैन्धवफाणितोपहितां मदनफलकषायमात्रां पाययेत्||९||

**Administering medicine for Vamana – emesis therapy :**

After successful administration of oleation and fomentation therapies and on ensuring that the patient's mind has come to a balance, he has taken bath, anointed his body, worn a garland and an un-torn clean cloth and has offered worship to the Deity, fire, Brahmana, preceptor, elderly persons and physician – the Brahmanas should be requested to recite auspicious Mantras and bestow their blessing on the patient on an auspicious day with auspicious constellation, Date, Karana, And Muhurta (astrologically important moments in a day). Thereafter, the physician should administer a dose of the decoction of the fruit of Madana (Randia dumetorum Lam) along with Honey, Rock salt, Phanita ( a preparation of Sugar cane juice) and the powder of Madhuka (Licorice – Glycyrrhiza glabra) [8-9]

**Dose of emetics (Vamana Dravya) :**

मदनफलकषायमात्राप्रमाणं तु खलु सर्वसंशोधनमात्राप्रमाणानि च प्रतिपुरुषमपेक्षितव्यानि भवन्ति; यावदिध यस्य संशोधनं पीतं वैकारिकदोषहरणायोपपद्यते न चातियोगायोगाय, तावदस्य मात्राप्रमाणं वेदितव्यं भवति||१०||

The Dosage of the Kashayam of the fruit of Madana (Randia dumetorum Lam) and of all the other drugs used in elimination therapy should be determined according to the individual needs. In other words, that quantity of medicine shall be regarded as the proper dose for the patient which when taken (by mouth) –

- brings about the desired effect - in the form of elimination of the vitiated Doshas,
- does not cause over-elimination or inadequate elimination of doshas, [10]


**Signs and symptoms indicating the proper action of the drug:**

पीतवन्तं तु खल्वेनं मुहूर्तमनुकाङ्क्षेत, तस्य यदा जानीयात् स्वेदप्रादुर्भावेण दोषं प्रविलयनमापद्यमानं, लोमहर्षेण च स्थानेभ्यः प्रचलितं, कुक्षिसमाध्मापनेन च कुक्षिमनुगतं, हृल्लासास्यस्रवणाभ्यामपि चोर्ध्वमुखीभूतम्, अथास्मै जानुसममसम्बाधं सुप्रयुक्तास्तरणोत्तरप्रच्छदोपधानं सोपाश्रयमासनमुपवेष्टुं प्रयच्छेत्, प्रतिग्रहांश्चोपचारयेत्, लालाटप्रतिग्रहे पार्श्वोपग्रहणे नाभिप्रपीडने पृष्ठोन्मर्दने चानपत्रपणीयाः सुहृदोऽनुमताः प्रयतेरन्||११||

अथैनमनुशिष्यात्- विवृतोष्ठतालुकण्ठो नातिमहता व्यायामेन वेगानुदीर्णानुदीरयन् किञ्चिदवनम्य ग्रीवामूर्ध्वशरीरमुपवेगमप्रवृत्तान् प्रवर्तयन् सुपरिलिखितनखाभ्यामङ्गुलिभ्यामुत्पलकुमुदसौगन्धिकनालैर्वा कण्ठमभिस्पृशन् सुखं प्रवर्तयस्वेति, स तथाविधं कुर्यात्; ततोऽस्य वेगान् प्रतिग्रहगतानवेक्षेतावहितः, वेगविशेषदर्शनादिध कुशलो योगायोगातियोगविशेषानुपलभेत, वेगविशेषदर्शी पुनः कृत्यं यथार्हमवबुध्येत लक्षणेन; तस्माद्वेगानवेक्षेतावहितः||१२||

**Signs and symptoms indicating the proper action of the drug:**


After the administration of decoction, the patient should be watched for some time.

The first effect of the administration of decoction would be **perspiration** which indicates that the Dosha has started melting. After that, the patient would have **horripilation** (Romaharsha) which shows that the Dosha has started moving from its own position. In the third stage, the patient will have **distension of the abdomen (**kuskhi adhmana) indicating that the doshas have come to (shifted to the) the intestine.

**Nausea and salivation** which occur in the fourth stage indicate that the Dosha has started moving upwards.


**Position of patient during vomiting:**

It is at this stage that the patient should be asked to sit on a bed of knee height, comfortable, well covered and equipped with a bed-sheet, towel, pillow and cushion. A spittoon should be kept nearby. The caretaker of the patient should support his head, sides, press the navel and massage the back of the patient.

The patient should then be instructed as follows, "Keep your lips, Palate and throat open: do not exert too much but allow the vomiting urge to be fully manifested. In case the urge is not well apparent, its manifestation will be facilitated if you slightly bend the neck and upper part of the body and touch your throat by means of two fingers whose nails have been well clipped off. You may touch your throat with the lotus stalk or Saugandhika".

The patient should act on this advice. The physician should very carefully observe the vomit in the spittoon, and ascertain the number of urges. He should later conclude as to whether the therapy has been well administered, inadequately administered or administered in excess. It is from this observation that the physician can determine the further line of action. So he should very carefully observe the vomiting urges. [12]


**Features of proper and improper administration of emetics:**

तत्रामून्ययोगयोगातियोगविशेषज्ञानानि भवन्ति; तद्यथा- अप्रवृत्तिः कुतश्चित् केवलस्य वाऽप्यौषधस्य विभ्रंशो विबन्धो वेगानामयोगलक्षणानि भवन्ति; काले प्रवृत्तिरनतिमहती व्यथा यथाक्रमं दोषहरणं स्वयं चावस्थानमिति योगलक्षणानि भवन्ति, योगेन तु दोषप्रमाणविशेषेण तीक्ष्णमृदुमध्यविभागो ज्ञेयः; योगाधिक्येन तु फेनिलरक्तचन्द्रिकोपगमनमित्यतियोगलक्षणानि भवन्ति|
तत्रातियोगायोगनिमित्तानिमानुपद्रवान् विद्यात्- आध्मानं परिकर्तिका परिस्रावो हृदयोपसरणमङ्गग्रहो जीवादानं विभ्रंशः स्तम्भः क्लमश्चेत्युपद्रवाः||१३||

## Inadequate administration of Vamana therapy:

Absence of vomiting or occasional vomiting
Vomiting of the drug material only, without the elimination of the vitiated Dosha
Excretion of the drug material through purgation (instead of through emesis)
Obstruction to the vomiting urges

## Signs of proper administration of Vamana therapy:

Manifestation of the vomiting urges in time
Absence of too much pain
Elimination of Doshas in proper order.
The urge for vomiting will recede on its own, after the Doshas are properly eliminated.
Proper administration is of three types, viz, sharp / intense / severe (Teekshna), mild and moderate depending on the quantity of Dosha eliminated.

## Over administration of Vamana :

Appearance of foam in the vomit
Appearance of blood-stained vomit.

## Complications of Vamana treatment :

The following complications arise out of over administration or inadequate administration of the therapy;
Adhmana – distension of abdomen,
Parikartika – sawing type of pain,
Parisrava – salivation,
Hrudaya Upasarana – palpitation,
Angagraha – rigidity, and
Jeevadana – blood vomiting,
Vibhramsha – displacement of viscera of the body,
Sthamba – stiffness,
and Shrama – exhaustion. [13]

## Post emesis management:

योगेन तु खल्वेनं छर्दितवन्तमभिसमीक्ष्य सुप्रक्षालितपाणिपादास्यं मुहूर्तमाश्वास्य, स्नैहिकवैरेचनिकोपशमनीयानां धूमानामन्यतमं सामर्थ्यतः पाययित्वा, पुनरेवोदकमुपस्पर्शयेत्||१४||
उपस्पृष्टोदकं चैनं निवातमागारमनुप्रवेश्य संवेश्य चानुशिष्यात्- उच्चैर्भाष्यमत्याशनमतिस्थानमतिचङ्क्रमणं क्रोधशोकहिमातपावश्यायातिप्रवातान् यानयानं ग्राम्यधर्ममस्वपनं निशि दिवा स्वप्नं विरुद्धाजीर्णासात्म्याकालप्रमितातिहीनगुरुविषमभोजनवेगसन्धारणोदीरणमिति भावानेतान्मनसाऽप्यसेवमानः सर्वमहो गमयस्वेति | स तथा कुर्यात्||१५||

## Post emesis management:

After the therapy has been well-administered, the hands, feet and face of the patient should be washed and he should be consoled. He should then be asked to smoke unctuous type (Snehana Dhoomapana), eliminative type (Shodhana Dhoomapana) or alleviating type of cigar (Shamana Dhoomapana) as it suits him. He should then enter a room which is not exposed to the wind and should lie down there.

Then he should be instructed, 'You should abstain from the following for the whole day-

Ucchair Bhashana – speaking aloud,

Atyashana – excess eating,

Atisthana – sitting at one place for long time,

Atichankramana – walking long distances,

Krodha, Shoka – anger and grief,

Hima, Atapa, Pravata – exposure to sun, dew and stormy wind,

Yana – travelling,

Gramya Dharma – indulging in sexual intercourse,

Asvapanam nishi – Vigil during night,

Diva Swapna – sleeping during day time,

Viruddha Ahara, Asatmya Ahara – foods with opposite qualities, wrong food combinations and

Ajirna Ahara – foods that may cause indigestion,

Pramita, Ati, Heena Vishama Bhojana – intake of diet exclusively having one taste, intake of diet deficient in nutritive value, or heavy or irregularly / improperly mixed up

Vega Sandharana, Udeerana – suppression or forcible initiation of natural urges. [14-15]

## Diet regimen after Vamana treatment:

अथैनं सायाह्ने परे वाह्नि सुखोदकपरिषिक्तं पुराणानां लोहितशालितण्डुलानां स्वक्क्लिन्नां मण्डपूर्वां सुखोष्णां यवागूं पाययेदग्निबलमभिसमीक्ष्य, एवं द्विवतीये तृतीये चान्नकाले, चतुर्थे त्वन्नकाले तथाविधानामेव शालितण्डुलानामुत्स्विन्नां विलेपीमुष्णोदकद्विवतीयामस्नेहलवणामल्पस्नेहलवणां वा भोजयेत्, एवं पञ्चमे षष्ठे चान्नकाले, सप्तमे त्वन्नकाले तथाविधानामेव शालीनां दिवप्रसृतं सुस्विन्नमोदनमुष्णोदकानुपानं तनुना तनुस्नेहलवणोपपन्नेन मुद्गयूषेण भोजयेत्, एवमष्टमे नवमे चान्नकाले, दशमे त्वन्नकले लावकपिञ्जलादीनामन्यतमस्य मांसरसेनौदकलावणिकेन नातिसारवता भोजयेदुष्णोदकानुपानम्; एवमेकादशे द्वादशे चान्नकाले; अत ऊर्ध्वमन्नगुणान् क्रमेणोपभुञ्जानः सप्तरात्रेण प्रकृतिभोजनमागच्छेत्||१६||

## Diet regimen after Vamana treatment:

In the same evening or the next day after Vamana, the patient should take a bath in lukewarm water.

He should be given warm gruel (Manda) prepared with well-cooked old rice. The gruel should be very thin. This is to be given with due regard to the power of digestion, for three meal-times. For the fourth meal- time, gruel prepared with rice (Vilepi), well-cooked, warm and devoid of oil / ghee and salt altogether or with oil / ghee and salt in small quantities is to be given. Warm water is to be taken after the intake of gruel. The same type of diet is to be continued for the fifth and sixth meal-times.

For the seventh meal-time again, well-cooked porridge (odana) prepared with the same type of rice of two Prasruta along with a very thin green gram soup (Mudga yusha), added with oil / ghee and salt in small quantities is to be given. Warm water should be taken after the intake of the porridge. The same diet is to be repeated for the eighth and ninth meal-times. For the tenth meal-time, thin meat-soup (Mamsarasa) of common quail (Lava), grey partridge, (Kapinjala) etc, prepared with water and salt should be given. Warm water is to be taken after this. This is again to be repeated for the eleventh and twelfth meal times. Thereafter, the patient should take food having different tastes and he should start taking his normal diet from the seventh night. [16]

## Virechana – Purgation therapy:

अथैनं पुनरेव स्नेहस्वेदाभ्यामुपपाद्यानुपहतमनसमभिसमीक्ष्य सुखोषितं सुप्रजीर्णभक्तं कृतहोमबलिमङ्गलजपप्रायश्चित्तमिष्टे तिथिनक्षत्रकरणमुहूर्ते ब्राह्मणान् स्वस्ति वाचयित्वा त्रिवृत्कल्कमक्षमात्रं यथार्हालोडनप्रतिविनीतं पाययेत् प्रसमीक्ष्य दोषभेषजदेशकालबलशरीराहारसात्म्यसत्त्वप्रकृतिवयसामवस्थान्तराणि विकारांश्च, सम्यक् विरिक्तं चैनं वमनोक्तेन धूमवर्जेन विधिनोपपादयेदाबलवर्णप्रकृतिलाभात्, बलवर्णोपपन्नं चैनमनुपहतमनसमभिसमीक्ष्य सुखोषितं सुप्रजीर्णभक्तं शिरःस्नातमनुलिप्तगात्रं स्रग्विणमनुपहतवस्त्रसंवीतमनुरूपालङ्कारालङ्कृतं सुहृदां दर्शयित्वा ज्ञातीनां दर्शयेत्, अथैनं कामेष्ववसृजेत्||१७||

**Virechana – Purgation therapy:**

After the post- therapeutic dietetic program, after Vamana, oleation (Snehana) and fomentation therapies (Swedana) should be administered again. After the patient has come to normalcy, has rested for a while and the food taken by him has been digested, he should be asked to offer oblations, chants and worships and to recite auspicious chants and expiatory verses. The Brahmanas should then be invited to recite the auspicious Svasthivachanas on an auspicious day with auspicious constellations, Karana and Muhurta. The patient should thereafter be given the drink of the paste of Trivrit (Operculina turpethum R.B) in one aksha (12 g) dose after stirring and mixing up. The difference in the variation of Dosha, medicinal drugs, location, time, strength, body, diet, wholesomeness, mind, constitution and age should be kept in view while administering this therapy.

After the patient has been administered purgation therapy, the entire regimen (prescribed to be followed after Vamana therapy (except smoking) should be followed till he regains the normal strength, complexion and health. After he has regained mental and physical balance and has rested for a while and the food taken by him is fully digested, he should take a full bath, apply unction, wear garlands, clean clothes and favourite ornaments and thus appear before friends and kinds. Thereafter, he should be free to lead a normal life.[17]

भवन्ति चात्र-
अनेन विधिना राजा राजमात्रोऽथवा पुनः|
यस्य वा विपुलं द्रव्यं स संशोधनमर्हति||१८||

The above-mentioned process is to be followed while administering elimination to resourceful persons like kings and others of an equivalent status. [18]

**Plan for emergency management:**
दरिद्रस्त्वापदं प्राप्य प्राप्तकालं विशोधनम्|
पिबेत् काममसम्भृत्य सम्भारानपि दुर्लभान्||१९||
न हि सर्वमनुष्याणां सन्ति सर्वे परिच्छदाः|
न च रोगा न बाधन्ते दरिद्रानपि दारुणाः||२०||
यद्यच्छक्यं मनुष्येण कर्तुमौषधमापदि|
तत्तत् सेव्यं यथाशक्ति वसनान्यशनानि च||२१||

**Plan for emergency management:**
A poor man, in the event of an emergency necessitating the administration of the elimination therapy should take the prescribed medicines available without caring for collecting all the rare medicines in advance. All the prescribed medicines are not available to all human beings. At the same time diseases can attack even the poor. So in the case of an emergency, whatever drugs, clothes, diets are easily available should be used by patients according to their capacity. [19-21]

**Good effects of elimination therapy:**
मलापहं रोगहरं बलवर्णप्रसादनम्|

पीत्वा संशोधन सम्यगायुषा युज्यते चिरम्||२२||

**Good effects of elimination therapy:**
Elimination therapy eliminates the Doshas, eradicates diseases and restores normal strength and complexion. If administered properly, it ensures longevity.

**To sum up:**
तत्र श्लोकाः-
ईश्वराणां वसुमतां वमनं सविरेचनम्|
सम्भारा ये यदर्थं च समानीय प्रयोजयेत्||२३||
यथा प्रयोज्या मात्रा या यदयोगस्य लक्षणम्|
योगातियोगयोर्यच्च दोषा ये चाप्युपद्रवाः||२४||
यदसेव्यं विशुद्धेन यश्च संसर्जनक्रमः|
तत् सर्वं कल्पनाध्याये व्याजहार पुनर्वसुः||२५||

All the requirements for administration of elimination therapy to resourceful persons like kings, etc. their utility, the dose, signs and symptoms of inadequate administration, proper administration, and over administration, the afflicted Doshas, the complication, regimen prescribed during the therapy and those prescribed in the course of the post-therapeutic program- these has all been explained by the lord Punarvasu in this Chapter. [23-25]

इत्यग्निवेशकृते तन्त्रे चरकप्रतिसंस्कृते श्लोकस्थाने उपकल्पनीयो नाम पञ्चदशोऽध्यायः||१५||

Thus, ends the fifteenth chapter on "requirements of a Physician "of the Sutra section of Agnivesha's work as redacted by Charaka.

# 16

# Sutrasthana Chapter 16 Chikitsa Prabhruteeyam

**Chikitsa Prabhuteeya Adhyaya**

**Benefits of Vamana and Virechana Treatment:**

अथातश्चिकित्साप्राभृतीयमध्यायं व्याख्यास्यामः॥१॥

इति ह स्माह भगवानात्रेयः॥२॥

The necessity of timely Panchakarma treatment, signs and symptoms of excessive and inadequate administration of Vamana and Virechana procedure, and their management etc. are explained in 16th chapter of Charaka Samhita Sutrasthana.

**Effect of the quality of physician on the result of treatment:**

चिकित्साप्राभृतो धीमान् शास्त्रवान् कर्मतत्परः।

नरं विरेचयति यं स योगात् सुखमश्नुते॥३॥

यं वैद्यमानी त्वबुधो विरेचयति मानवम्।

सोऽतियोगादयोगाच्च मानवो दुःखमश्नुते॥४॥

**Effect of the quality of physician on the result of treatment:**

A qualified physician is the one, who is

- well acquainted with the principles of treatment,
- who is wise,
- is well-versed in textual knowledge and is prompt in initiating action.

The patient, who is administered with proper Vamana (emesis) and Virechana (purgation) treatments by such a physician attains happiness and becomes free from diseases.

On the other hand, if these therapies are administered by a person who only claims to be a physician but doesn't have any practical knowledge of Ayurveda, the patients treated by such a person would face many complications caused due to excessive or inadequate administration of Panchakarma treatment.

**Signs and symptoms of proper Virechana treatment (purgation) :**

दौर्बल्यं लाघवं ग्लानिर्व्याधीनामणुता रुचिः।

हृद्वर्णशुद्धिः क्षुत्तृष्णा काले वेगप्रवर्तनम्॥५॥

बुद्धीन्द्रियमनःशुद्धिर्मारुतस्यानुलोमता|
सम्यग्विरिक्तलिङ्गानि कायाग्नेश्चानुवर्तनम्||६||
ष्ठीवनं हृदयाशुद्धिरुत्क्लेशः श्लेष्मपित्तयोः|
आध्मानमरुचिश्छर्दिरदौर्बल्यमलाघवम्||७||
जङ्घोरुसदनं तन्द्रा स्तैमित्यं पीनसागमः|
लक्षणान्यविरिक्तानां मारुतस्य च निग्रहः||८||
विट्पित्तकफवातानामागतानां यथाक्रमम्|
परं स्रवति यद्रक्तं मेदोमांसोदकोपमम्||९||
निःश्लेष्मपित्तमुदकं शोणितं कृष्णमेव वा|
तृष्यतो मारुतार्तस्य सोऽतियोगः प्रमुह्यतः||१०||

**Signs and symptoms of proper Virechana treatment (purgation) :**

Samyak Virechana Lakshana
Dourbalya – tiredness, slimness,
Laghava – lightness of the body
Glani – tiredness of sense organs
Vyadheenaam anuta – recession of diseases,
Hrit Shuddhi – Feeling of clarity in heart,
Varna Shuddhi – feeling of clarity in skin, restoration of normal skin complexion,
Kshut Trishna – timely hunger and thirst
Kaale Vega Pravartanam – timely initiation of natural urges – like defecation, urination etc.
Buddhi Indriya Mano shuddhi – clarity in intellect, sense faculties and mind,
Marutasya Anulomana – Movement of Vata in downward direction (its normal direction) in the body.
Kayagneshcha anuvartanam – proper digestion and metabolic activities.

**Signs and symptoms of inadequate purgation – Virechana Heena Yoga Lakshana :**

Shteevana – spitting,
Hrudaya Ashuddhi – chest discomfort, lack of clarity
Utklsehaha shleshma Pittayo – nausea, feeling of increase (overflowing) of Kapha and Pitta
Adhmana – bloating, feeling of distention
Aruchi – anorexia, lack of taste
Chardi – vomiting
Daurbalya – weakness
Alaghava – lack of lightness
Jangha Uru Sadana – stiffness of hip and thighs
Tandra – sleepiness / stupor / drowsiness, sense organ tiredness,
Staimitya – stiffness
Peenasa – rhinitis
Marutasya Nigraha – Obstruction of Vata

**Signs and symptoms of excessive purgation – Virechana Atiyoga Lakshana :**
Excretion of faeces, Pitta, Kapha and Vata
Excretion of liquid resembling a mixture of water with blood, fat and muscle tissue, through the anus
Excretion of black colored blood without Shleshma (Kapha) and Pitta
The patient will be afflicted with thirst and he may faint due to vitiated Vata [5-10]

**Signs and symptoms of over-emesis – Vamana Atiyoga Lakshana**
वमनेऽतिकृते लिङ्गान्येतान्येव भवन्ति हि|
ऊर्ध्वगा वातरोगाश्च वाग्ग्रहश्चाधिको भवेत्||११||
चिकित्साप्राभृतं तस्मादुपेयाच्छरणं नरः|
युञ्ज्याद् य एनमत्यन्तमायुषा च सुखेन च||१२||

They are the same as signs of excessive purgation. Over-emesis may cause the diseases of the head and neck due to the vitiation of Vata and disturbance of speech. Hence one should consult only such physicians who are well-qualified for the administration of the therapy and who can ensure longevity and happiness. [11-12]

**Indications for Vamana and Virechana Panchakarma treatment:**

अविपाकोऽरुचिः स्थौल्यं पाण्डुता गौरवं क्लमः|
पिडकाकोठकण्डूनां सम्भवोऽरतिरेव च||१३||
आलस्यश्रमदौर्बल्यं दौर्गन्ध्यमवसादकः|
श्लेष्मपित्तसमुत्क्लेशो निद्रानाशोऽतिनिद्रता||१४||
तन्द्रा क्लैब्यमबुद्धित्वमशस्तस्वप्नदर्शनम्|
बलवर्णप्रणाशश्च तृप्यतो बृंहणैरपि||१५||
बहुदोषस्य लिङ्गानि तस्मै संशोधनं हितम्|
ऊर्ध्वं चैवानुलोमं च यथादोषं यथाबलम्||१६||

**Indications for Vamana and Virechana Panchakarma treatment :**

Panchakarma treatment should be done whenever there is excessive aggravation of doshas.
    Signs and symptoms of excessive aggravation of Doshas (Bahudosha) are :
Avipaka -indigestion,
Aruchi – Anorexia, lack of taste,
Sthoulya – obesity
Panduta – Anaemia
Gaurava – heaviness
Klama – exhaustion,
Pidaka, Kota, Kandu – eruption of pimples, urticaria, itching
Arati – lack of inclination for work, lack of co-ordination in sense organs,
Alasya – Laziness,
Shrama, Daurbalya – Fatigue, Weakness,
Daurgandhya – foul smell of the body,
Avasaadaka – lassitude,
Vitiation / aggravation (Utklesa) of Kapha and Pitta,
Nidranasha / Atinidrata – sleeplessness or excessive sleep,
Tandra – drowsiness, weak sense organs,
Kalibya – impotency,
Abuddhitvam – impediment to intelligence,
Ashasta swapna darshana – inauspicious dreams,
Bala Varna Pranasha -loss of strength and complexion in spite of the intake of nutritious diet.
In the event of such signs and symptoms, the patient should be administered with emesis and purgation treatment with due regard to the vitiated Dosha and strength of the patient. [13-16]

## Advantages of Shodhana (elimination therapy):

एवं विशुद्धकोष्ठस्य कायाग्निरभिवर्धते|
व्याधयश्चोपशाम्यन्ति प्रकृतिश्चानुवर्तते||१७||
इन्द्रियाणि मनोबुद्धिर्वर्णश्चास्य प्रसीदति|
बलं पुष्टिरपत्यं च वृषता चास्य जायते||१८||
जरां कृच्छ्रेण लभते चिरं जीवत्यनामयः|
तस्मात् संशोधनं काले युक्तियुक्तं पिबेन्नरः||१९||

## Advantages of Shodhana (elimination therapy):

By the administration of these therapies the vitiated Doshas are eliminated through the alimentary tract,
Kayagni Vardhana – the digestion and metabolism power gets enhanced,
Vyadhi upashamana – diseases are cured and
Prakruti anuvartana – normal health is restored;
The sense faculties, mind, intelligence, and complexion becomes clear and gains strength;
The person gains
Bala – strength and immunity,
Pushti – plumpness, body nourishment
Apatya – off-springs (for those seeking infertility treatment) and
Vrushata – Virlity, good sexual power.
Jaram krichrena labhate – aging process slows down,
Chiram jeevati – one can live healthily for a long time.
Therefore, one should take proper elimination therapy in time. [17-19]

## Simile regarding the lasting effect of elimination therapy:

दोषाः कदाचित् कुप्यन्ति जिता लङ्घनपाचनैः|
जिताः संशोधनैर्ये तु न तेषां पुनरुद्भवः||२०||
दोषाणां च द्रुमाणां च मूलेऽनुपहते सति|
रोगाणां प्रसवानां च गतानामागतिर्ध्रुवा||२१||

## Simile regarding the lasting effect of elimination therapy:

The vitiated Doshas that are balanced out by fasting and digestive drugs, at times get aggravated once again. But those eliminated by elimination therapies (Panchakarma treatment) do not recur. Doshas can be compared with trees. Unless the tree is uprooted from its root, it will grow in spite of branches being chopped off. Such is the case with the vitiated Doshas. They go on causing diseases unless they are eliminated from their very roots. [20-21]

## Restorative measures after elimination therapy:

भेषजक्षपिते पथ्यमाहारैरेव बृंहणम्|
घृतमांसरसक्षीरहृद्ययूषोपसंहितैः||२२||
अभ्यङ्गोत्सादनैः स्नानैर्निरूहैः सानुवासनैः|
तथा स लभते शर्म युज्यते चायुषा चिरम्||२३||

**Restorative measures after elimination therapy:**

Elimination therapy reduces Dhatus (body tissues) as well. Hence, after Shodhana treatment, restorative treatment is needed. One should take a nourishing diet along with ghee, meat soup, milk and vegetable soup which are good for the heart.He should also have massage, unction, bath, Niruha (decoction enema) and Anuvasana (oil enema) types of enema. By doing so, one attains happiness and longevity. [22-23]

**Management of over and under elimination:**

अतियोगानुबद्धानां सर्पिःपानं प्रशस्यते|
तैलं मधुरकैः सिद्धमथवाऽप्यनुवासनम्||२४||
यस्य त्वयोगस्तं स्निग्धं पुनः संशोधयेन्नरम्|
मात्राकालबलापेक्षी स्मरन् पूर्वमनुक्रमम्||२५||
स्नेहने स्वेदने शुद्धौ रोगाः संसर्जने च ये|
जायन्तेऽमार्गविहिते तेषां सिद्धिषु साधनम्||२६||

**Management of over and under elimination:**

People who suffer from Atiyoga – excess of Panchakarma treatment, should drink ghee or take sweets prepared with oil and ghee.
Anuvasana (oil enema) Basti can be administered in them,
For those who suffer from Ayoga – inadequate Panchakarma, should be given Oleation treatment followed by elimination therapy, with due regard to the dose, time, strength of patient and other relevant factors.
Management of complications arising out of improper oleation, fomentation and elimination therapies as well as post-elimination dietetic program will be subsequently explained in Siddhisthana. [24-26]

**The Theory of natural homeostasis:**

जायन्ते हेतुवैषम्यादिविषमा देहधातवः|
हेतुसाम्यात् समास्तेषां स्वभावोपरमः सदा||२७||

**The Theory of natural homeostasis:**

Disturbance in the equilibrium of body tissues (Dhatus) is caused by disturbance of causative factors of health. Balancing causative factors of health leads to health. Being healthy – is the natural state of the body. Hence, the imbalance gets cured naturally and automatically [27]

**Destruction as a passive Phenomenon:**

प्रवृत्तिहेतुर्भावानां न निरोधेऽस्ति कारणम्|
केचित्तत्रापि मन्यन्ते हेतुं हेतोरवर्तनम्||२८||

**Destruction as a passive Phenomenon:**

There is a causative factor for the manifestation of beings but no causative factor as such exists for their annihilation. Some are of the view that annihilation of beings is caused by the non-effectiveness of the causative factors of health. [28]

**Questions against the theory of natural homeostasis:**

एवमुक्तार्थमाचार्यमग्निवेशोऽभ्यभाषत|
स्वभावोपरमे कर्म चिकित्साप्राभृतस्य किम्||२९||
भेषजैर्विषमान् धातून् कान् समीकुरुते भिषक्|
का वा चिकित्सा भगवन्! किमर्थं वा प्रयुज्यते||३०||

**Questions against the theory of natural homeostasis:**

After listening to those words, Agnivesha inquired, "if disease can be cured automatically then what is the necessity of a qualified physician? What are those imbalanced Dhatus that are brought to normalcy by physicians? What after all, does the treatment amount to? What is it prescribed for? When the purpose for which the treatment is prescribed, is automatically served what is the use of any treatment at all? [29-30]

**Answer in favor of the theory of natural homeostasis:**

तच्छिष्यवचनं श्रुत्वा व्याजहार पुनर्वसुः|
श्रूयतामत्र या सोम्य! युक्तिर्दृष्टा महर्षिभिः||३१||
न नाशकारणाभावाद्भावानां नाशकारणम्|
जायते नित्यगस्येव कालस्यात्ययकारणम्||३२||

**Answer in favour of the theory of natural homeostasis:**

Lord Punarvasu replied. "I shall explain to you the views of sages in this connection. The causative factors for the annihilation cannot be comprehended because such factors do not exist at all. This is based on the analogy of time. Time is always in the process of quick movement, it automatically goes on changing or destroying itself. As such, there is no causative factor which can cause movements, change or destruction of time. So, all things that are produced would perish naturally, without any cause. [31-32]

शीघ्रगत्वाद्यथा भूतस्तथा भावो विपद्यते|
निरोधे कारणं तस्य नास्ति नैवान्यथाक्रिया||३३||

So, no causative factor exists for the annihilation of a being. Therefore, there is no possibility for bringing out a change in the destruction pattern of a being. [33]

**Definition and aim of treatment:**

याभिः क्रियाभिर्जायन्ते शरीरे धातवः समाः|
सा चिकित्सा विकाराणां कर्म तद्भिषजां स्मृतम्||३४||
कथं शरीरे धातूनां वैषम्यं न भवेदिति|
समानां चानुबन्धः स्यादित्यर्थं क्रियते क्रिया||३५||
त्यागादिविषमहेतूनां समानां चोपसेवनात्|
विषमा नानुबध्नन्ति जायन्ते धातवः समाः||३६||
समैस्तु हेतुभिर्यस्माद्धातून् सञ्जनयेत् समान्|
चिकित्साप्राभृतस्तस्माद्दाता देहसुखायुषाम्||३७||

धर्मस्यार्थस्य कामस्य नृलोकस्योभयस्य च|
दाता सम्पद्यते वैद्यो दानाद्देहसुखायुषाम्||३८||

## Definition and aim of treatment:

Those processes that bring about equilibrium of body tissues and Doshas are called Chikitsa. It is the duty of a Physician. The purpose of such action is to prevent the disturbance of the equilibrium of Dhatus and maintain their equilibrium. By avoiding the causative factors (of the disease) and by adopting (following) the causative factors which are responsible for the maintenance of equilibrium, discordance of Dhatus is automatically prevented and their normal state of equilibrium is maintained. By taking recourse to disease causing factors, the physician well versed in treatment brings about equilibrium of dhatus. Therefore the physician restores and bestows physical happiness and longevity (in patients). By virtue of his ability to bestow physical happiness and longevity, a physician is regarded as a donor of virtue, wealth and desires pertaining to this world and the world beyond. [34-38]

## To sum up:

तत्र श्लोकाः-
चिकित्साप्राभृतगुणो दोषो यश्चेतराश्रयः|
योगायोगातियोगानां लक्षणं शुद्धिसंश्रयम्||३९||
बहुदोषस्य लिङ्गानि संशोधनगुणाश्च ये|
चिकित्सासूत्रमात्रं च सिद्ध्यव्यापत्तिसंश्रयम्||४०||
या च युक्तिश्चिकित्सायां यं चार्थं कुरुते भिषक्|
चिकित्साप्राभृतेऽध्याये तत् सर्वमवदन्मुनिः||४१||

The duties of a qualified physician, defects of an unqualified one, signs and symptoms of adequate, inadequate and excessive administration of elimination therapies, signs and symptoms of patients with aggravated Dosas, benefits of elimination therapy, principles of treatment of complications that arise during the administration of the elimination therapy, the propriety of treatment and duties of a physician- all this has been dealt with by the sage in this chapter on the "Duties of a Qualified Physician."[39-41]

इत्यग्निवेशकृते तन्त्रे चरकप्रतिसंस्कृते श्लोकस्थाने चिकित्साप्राभृतीयो नाम षोडशोऽध्यायः||१६|| समाप्तः कल्पनाचतुष्कः||४||

Thus ends the sixteenth chapter on the "Duties of a qualified Physician" of the Sutra Section of Agnivesa's work as redacted by Charaka.

Here ends the fourth quadrate on the 'Therapeutically Processes' - Kalpana Chatushka.

# 17

# Sutrasthana Chapter 17 Kiyanta Shiraseeyam

**Kiyanta Shiraseeya Adhyaya - Diseases of Head, Heart and Abscess:**

अथातः कियन्तःशिरसीयमध्यायं व्याख्यास्यामः||१||

इति ह स्माह भगवानात्रेयः||२||

The diseases of head, heart, carbuncle and abscesses have been explained in great detail in the 17th chapter of Sutrasthana of Charaka Samhita. This chapter also deals with symptoms of Dosha, Dhatu and Mala Kshaya (depletion of body tissues and excreta), definition of head, different ways in which Doshas move in the body, different combinations of Dosha imbalance and their symptoms, Ojas, its nature, causes of depletion and symptoms, causes for diabetes, causes and types of carbuncle, types, causes, symptoms and prognosis of abscess, etc. The chapter is titled as Kiyanta Shiraseeya Adhyaya.

**Sage Agnivesha asked:**

कियन्तः शिरसि प्रोक्ता रोगा हृदि च देहिनाम्|

कति चाप्यनिलादीनां रोगा मानविकल्पजाः||३||

क्षयाः कति समाख्याताः पिडकाः कति चानघ!|

गतिः कतिविधा चोक्ता दोषाणां दोषसूदन!||४||

हुताशवेशस्य वचस्तच्छुत्वा गुरुरब्रवीत्|

पृष्टवानसि यत् सौम्य! तन्मे शृणु सविस्तरम्||५||

दृष्टाः पञ्च शिरोरोगाः पञ्चैव हृदयामयाः|

व्याधीनां ह्यधिका षष्टिर्दोषमानविकल्पजा||६||

दशाष्टौ च क्षयाः सप्त पिडका माधुमेहिकाः|

दोषाणां त्रिविधा चोक्ता गतिर्विस्तरतः शृणु||७||

What is the number of diseases relating to the head and the heart?

What are the diseases caused due to permutation and combination of Doshas?

What are the signs and symptoms of the decrease of Doshas, Dhatus and Malas?

How many types of pidakas (carbuncles) are manifested and what are the types of the Pidakas (carbuncles)?

What are the types of the courses of Doshas?

Lord Punarvasu replied, I am answering all your questions in detail. Listen to me, O noble one! Diseases relating to the head and heart each are five in number. Diseases arising out of the permutation and combination of Vata, etc. are sixty-two. There are eighteen conditions relating to the decrease of Doshas, Dhatus and Mala; carbuncles due to Madhumeha (Diabetes) are of seven types; there are three courses of Doshas. Now I would explain their details".

**Causes of diseases of the head:**

सन्धारणादिदिवास्वप्नाद्रात्रौ जागरणान्मदात्|
उच्चैर्भाष्यादवश्यायात् प्राग्वातादतिमैथुनात्||८||
गन्धादसात्म्यादाघ्रातादद्रजोधूमहिमातपात्|
गुर्वम्लहरितादानादति शीताम्बुसेवनात्||९||
शिरोऽभिघाताद्दुष्टामाद्रोदनाद्बाष्पनिग्रहात् [१] |
मेघागमान्मनस्तापाद्देशकालविपर्ययात्||१०||
वातादयः प्रकुप्यन्ति शिरस्यसं च दुष्यति|
ततः शिरसि जायन्ते रोगा विविधलक्षणाः||११||

**Causes of diseases of the head:**

- By the suppression of natural urges
- sleeping during day time
- vigil during the night
- intoxication, speaking aloud, exposure to frost and easterly wind
- excessive sexual indulgence, inhalation of undesirable smell
- exposure to dust, smoke, snowfall and sun
- intake of heavy and sour food, and rhizomes including tubers, etc. in excessive quantity.
- excessive intake of cold water, injury to the head.
- vitiation of Ama, (a product of improper digestion and metabolism) crying in excess, suppression of tears
- advent of cloud, anxiety and adopting regimen contrary to those prescribed for the locality and season
- Doshas like Vata, etc. get aggravated in the head resulting in the vitiation of Rakta Dhatu (blood tissue). This causes diseases with various symptoms in the head.

**Definition of head:**

प्राणाः प्राणभृतां यत्र श्रिताः सर्वेन्द्रियाणि च|
यदुत्तमाङ्गमाङ्गानां शिरस्तदभिधीयते||१२||

The head is the substratum for Prana – life. All the sense faculties are situated here. It is called as Uttama Anga i.e. the best of all body parts. So it occupies the first place amongst the vital organs of the body. [12]

**Diseases of the head:**

अर्धावभेदको वा स्यात् सर्वं वा रुज्यते शिरः|
प्रतिश्यायमुखनासाक्षिकर्णरोगशिरोभ्रमाः||१३||
अर्दितं शिरसः कम्पो गलमन्याहनुग्रहः|
विविधाश्चापरे रोगा वातादिक्रिमिसम्भवाः||१४||

**Diseases of the head:**

- Ardhavabhedaka – Hemicrania continua – pain in half side of the head
- Shiroruja – headache affecting all parts of head
- Pratishyaya – coryza, running nose
- diseases of mouth, nose, eyes, and ears
- Shiro Bhrama – dizziness, giddiness
- Ardita – facial paralysis
- Shiro Kampa – trembling of the head

- Galagraha, Manyagraha, Hanugraha – stiffness of the throat, neck and jaw
- Other diseases of Vata imbalance and due to Krimi (worm / germ infestation) [13-14]

**Causes and Symptoms of Vata type of headache:**
पृथग्दिष्टास्तु ये पञ्च सङ्ग्रहे परमर्षिभिः|
शिरोगदांस्ताञ्छृणु मे यथास्वैर्हेतुलक्षणैः||१५||
उच्चैर्भाष्यातिभाष्याभ्यां तीक्ष्णपानात् प्रजागरात्|
शीतमारुतसंस्पर्शाद्व्यवायाद्वेगनिग्रहात्||१६||
उपवासादभीघातादिविरेकाद्वमनादति|
बाष्पशोकभयत्रासाद्भारमार्गातिकर्शनात्||१७||
शिरोगताः सिरा वृद्धो वायुराविश्य कुप्यति|
ततः शूलं महत्तस्य वातात् समुपजायते||१८||
निस्तुद्येते भृशं शङ्कौ घाटा सम्भिद्यते तथा|
सभ्रूमध्यं ललाटं च तपतीवातिवेदनम्||१९||
वध्येते स्वनतः श्रोत्रे निष्कृष्येते इवाक्षिणी|
घूर्णतीव शिरः सर्वं सन्धिभ्य इव मुच्यते||२०||
स्फुरत्यति सिराजालं स्तभ्यते च शिरोधरा|
स्निग्धोष्णमुपशेते च शिरोरोगेऽनिलात्मके||२१||

**Vata -disease of head:**

The five head diseases, as envisaged by the sages will be separately enumerated in the chapter on "Eight abdominal Diseases" (Sutrasthana 19th chapter). I shall now explain their causes and symptoms. Listen to me:

- Ucchair Bhashya, Ati Bhashya – By loud and excessive speech
- Teekshna Paanaat – strong pungent drinks
- Prajaagaraat – night Vigil, waking up at night
- Sheeta Maruta Samsparshaat – excessive exposure to cold wind
- Vyavaaya – excessive sexual indulgence
- Vega nigrahaat – suppression of natural urges
- Upavasa – excessive fasting
- Abhighata – trauma
- Ati Vireka and Vamana – excessive purgation and vomiting
- Bashpa shoka bhaya trasa – excessive weeping, grief, apprehension, tiredness
- Bharat, Margat - carrying heavy load, walking for long distance
- Atikarshana – excess treatment to lose weight

By these causes, Vata gets aggravated and enters the channels of the head. It gets further vitiated to cause excruciating pain in the head.

**Symptoms of Vata type of headache:**

Pricking pain in the temporal region and cracking sensation in the nape. Severe and excessive pain is experienced as if the head is burning (pain associated with burning sensation) in the forehead and in between the eyebrows. Pain and noise in the ears, and a feeling as if eyes are coming out dizziness, and a feeling as if all the joints of the head have given way i.e. separated and have become lax and excessive throbbing pain in the veins of the head. The neck is stiffened. The patient gets relief by unctuous (oily) and warm regimen. [15-21]

**Pitta related disease of head:**

कट्वम्ललवणक्षारमद्यक्रोधातपानलैः|
पित्तं शिरसि सन्दुष्टं शिरोरोगाय कल्पते||२२||
दह्यते रुज्यते तेन शिरः शीतं सुषूयते [१] |
दह्येते चक्षुषी तृष्णा भ्रमः स्वेदश्च जायते||२३||

**Pitta related disease of head:**
**Causes:**
Katu, Amla, Lavana, Kshara – excess intake of pungent, sour, salt and alkalies,
Madya – excess alcohol
Krodha, Atapa, Analaihi – anger, exposure to sun and fire.
The Pitta Dosha in the head gets vitiated and thereby produces head diseases resulting in burning and aching sensation in the head. The patient develops a liking for cold substances. There is a burning sensation in the eyes and the patient is subjected to thirst, dizziness and perspiration in excess. [22-23]

**Kapha related disease of head:**
आस्यासुखैः स्वप्नसुखैर्गुरुस्निग्धातिभोजनैः|
श्लेष्मा शिरसि सन्दुष्टः शिरोरोगाय कल्पते||२४||
शिरो मन्दरुजं तेन सुप्तं स्तिमितभारिकम्|
भवत्युत्पद्यते तन्द्रा तथाऽऽलस्यमरोचकः||२५||

**Kapha related disease of head:**
Asyasukha – eating as per one's own will
Swapna Sukha – sedentary habits,
Guru, Snigdha, Ati Bhojana – excessive intake of heavy and unctuous food,
By these causative factors, Kapha in the head gets vitiated and causes diseases.
**Symptoms** – There is dull pain and numbness. The patient feels as if he is wet and is loaded with too heavy burden. There is drowsiness, laziness and anorexia. [24-25]

**Clinical features of Tridoshaja disease of head:**
वाताच्छूलं भ्रमः कम्पः पित्ताद्दाहो मदस्तृषा|
कफाद्गुरुत्वं तन्द्रा च शिरोरोगे त्रिदोषजे||२६||
In the event of head- diseases being caused by all the three Doshas, there is
Shula, Bhrama, Kampa – pain, dizziness, shaking of head due to vitiated Vata Dosha,
Daha, Mada, Trusha – burning sensation, intoxication and thirst due to vitiated Pitta Dosha and
Gurutva, Tandra – heaviness and drowsiness due to vitiated Kapha. [26]

**Krimija disease of head: Due to microbe**
तिलक्षीरगुडाजीर्णपूतिसङ्कीर्णभोजनात्|
क्लेदोऽसृक्कफमांसानां दोषलस्योपजायते||२७||
ततः शिरसि सङ्क्लेदात् क्रिमयः पापकर्मणः|
जनयन्ति शिरोरोगं जाता बीभत्सलक्षणम्||२८||
व्यधच्छेदरुजाकण्डूशोफदौर्गत्यदुःखितम्|
क्रिमिरोगातुरं विद्यात् क्रिमीणां दर्शनेन च||२९||

**Krimija disease of head: Due to microbe**
Krimi means worm / microbe.

## Causes

By the intake of

Tila – Sesame (Sesamum indicum Linn)

Ksheera – excess milk consumption

Guda – jaggery

Pooti – impure foods

Sankeerna Bhojana – unwholesome food, incompatible foods.

Due to regular and excessive intake of the above said things, stickiness is produced in the Rakta (blood), Kapha and Mamsa Dhatu due to the excessive vitiation of Doshas. The stickiness in the head of the patients results in the diseases associated with severe symptoms.

## Symptoms:

Vyadha, Cheda Ruja – stabbing and cutting pain,

Kandu – itching,

Shopha – swelling, inflammation,

Daurgandhya – foul smell

Durgati – sense of discomfort and

Krimi Darshana – visible pathogenic organisms. [27-29]

## Diseases of Heart:

### Vata – disease of heart:

### Causes:

शोकोपवासव्यायामरूक्षशुष्काल्पभोजनैः |
वायुराविश्य हृदयं जनयत्युत्तमां रुजम्||३०||
वेपथुर्वेष्टनं स्तम्भः प्रमोहः शून्यता दरः |
हृदि वातातुरे रूपं जीर्णे चात्यर्थवेदना||३१||

## Causes

- Shoka – grief
- Upavasa – fasting
- Vyayama – excessive exercise
- Rooksha, Shushka, Alpa Bhojana – intake of un-unctuous, dry and inadequate quantities of food
- By these causes, Vata gets vitiated and effects the heart.

### Symptoms:

- Ruja – excruciating pain
- Vepathu – trembling
- Veshtana – cramps
- Sthambha – stiffness
- Pramoha – darkness
- Shunyata – feeling of sense of emptiness
- Worsening of pain after the digestion of food. [30-31]

### Pitta disease of heart:

### Causes:

उष्णाम्ललवणक्षारकटुकाजीर्णभोजनैः|
मद्यक्रोधातपैश्चाशु हृदि पित्तं प्रकुप्यति||३२||
हृद्दाहस्तिक्तता वक्त्रे तिक्ताम्लोद्गिरणं क्लमः|
तृष्णा मूर्च्छा भ्रमः स्वेदः पित्तहृद्रोगलक्षणम्||३३||

## Pitta disease of heart:
### Causes:

- Ushna, Amla, Lavana, Kshara Katu – By the intake of hot, sour, salty, alkaline (caustic) and pungent foods.
- Ajeerna Bhojana – taking food during indigestion
- Madya – excess of alcohol
- Krodha – anger
- Atapa – exposure to Sun

Because of these causes, Pitta located in the heart gets vitiated.

### Symptoms:

- Hrit Daha – heartburn
- Titkata Vaktre – bitter taste in the mouth
- Tikta Amla Udgirana – eruptions with bitter and sour taste
- Klama – exhaustion
- Trushna – thirst
- Murcha – unconsciousness
- Bhrama – dizziness
- Sweda – perspiration. [32-33]

## Kaphaja diseases of heart:
### Causes:

अत्यादानं गुरुस्निग्धमचिन्तनमचेष्टनम्|
निद्रासुखं चाभ्यधिकं कफहृद्रोगकारणम्||३४||
हृदयं कफहृद्रोगे सुप्तं स्तिमितभारिकम्|
तन्द्रारुचिपरीतस्य भवत्यश्मावृतं यथा||३५||

### Kaphaja diseases of heart: Causes:

- Atyadana – Excessive intake of food
- Guru, Snigdha – intake of heavy and unctuous food
- Achintana – inadequate mental exercise
- Acheshtana – sedentary habits
- Nidrasukha – excessive sleep.

### Symptoms:
Hrudaya Supti – bradycadia, lesser activities of heart,
Stimita – stiffness and
Bharika – heaviness of the heart,
Tandra – drowsiness and

Aruchi – anorexia.

The patient feels as if he is loaded with stones. [34-35]

**Tridoshaja heart disease:**

हेतुलक्षणसंसर्गादुच्यते सान्निपातिकः|
(हृद्रोगः कष्टदः कष्टसाध्य उक्तो महर्षिभिः)

Sannipatika type of heart disease is the one caused by the combined vitiation of all the three Doshas. This can be diagnosed by the existence of the various signs and symptoms of all the three types of heart diseases. This type of heart disease is very painful and difficult to cure.

**Krimija disease of the heart – Due to microbe**

त्रिदोषजे तु हृद्रोगे यो दुरात्मा निषेवते||३६||
तिलक्षीरगुडादीनि ग्रन्थिस्तस्योपजायते|
मर्मैकदेशे सङ्क्लेदं रसश्चास्योपगच्छति||३७||
सङ्क्लेदात् क्रिमयश्चास्य भवन्त्युपहतात्मनः|
मर्मैकदेशे ते जाताः सर्पन्तो भक्षयन्ति च||३८||
तुद्यमानं स हृदयं सूचीभिरिव मन्यते|
छिद्यमानं यथा शस्त्रैर्जातकण्डूं महारुजम्||३९||
हृद्रोगं क्रिमिजं त्वेतैर्लिङ्गैर्बुद्ध्वा सुदारुणम्|
त्वरेत जेतुं तं विद्वान् विकारं शीघ्रकारिणम्||४०||

**Krimija disease of the heart – Due to microbe –**
Intake of Tila – Sesame (Sesamum indicum Linn), milk, sugar candy, etc. in the event of the heart diseases caused by the vitiation of all the three Doshas causes nodules in the heart. Rasa becomes sticky in some parts of the heart. This stickiness produces pathogenic organisms.

**Symptoms:**
Patient feels as if his heart is being pierced or being cut into pieces by weapons. There is itching and pain in the heart. By these symptoms a wise physician should diagnose the heart diseases as caused by the presence of pathogenic organisms. Considering the seriousness of this condition, he should expedite the treatment of this acute disease. [36-40]

**Sixty two types of combinations of Doshas:**
द्व्युल्बणैकोल्बणैः षट् स्युर्हीनमध्याधिकैश्च षट्|
समैश्चैको विकारास्ते सन्निपातास्त्रयोदश||४१||
संसर्ग नव षट् तेभ्य एकवृद्ध्या समैस्त्रयः|
पृथक् त्रयश्च तैर्वृद्धैर्व्याधयः पञ्चविंशतिः||४२||
यथा वृद्धैस्तथा क्षीणैर्दोषैः स्युः पञ्चविंशतिः|
वृद्धिक्षयकृतश्चान्यो विकल्प उपदेक्ष्यते||४३||
वृद्धिरेकस्य समता चैकस्यैकस्य सङ्क्षयः|
द्वन्द्ववृद्धिः क्षयश्चैकस्यैकवृद्धिर्द्वयोः क्षयः ||४४||

**Sixty-two types of combinations of Doshas:**
Simultaneous aggravation of all the three Doshas (Sannipata) is of thirteen types. They are as follows:

(a) Two Doshas aggravated in excess and the remaining one dosha aggravated in minor volume:

1. Vata and Pitta aggravated in excess, and Kapha just aggravated.
2. Pitta and Kapha aggravated in excess, and Vaata just aggravated.
3. Kapha and Vata aggravated iin excess, and Pitta just aggravated.

(b)One Dosha aggravated in excess and the remaining two just aggravated
4.Vata aggravated in excess, and Pitta and Kapha just aggravated.
5. Pitta aggravated in excess, and Vata and Kapha just aggravated.
6. Kapha aggravated in excess, and Vata and Pitta just aggravated.
(c) Aggravation of Doshas in progressive order.
7. Vata aggravated, Pitta more aggravated and Kapha most aggravated.
8. Vata aggravated, Kapha more aggravated and Pitta most aggravated.
9. Pitta aggravated, Kapha more aggravated and Vata most aggravated.
10. Kapha aggravated, Vata more aggravated and Pitta most aggravated.
11. Pitta aggravated, Vata more aggravated and Kapha most aggravated.
12. Kapha aggravated, Pitta more aggravated and Vata most aggravated.
(d) Aggravation of all three Doshas to the same degree.
13. Vata, Pitta and Kapha aggravated to the same degree.
Simultaneous aggravation of any Dosha (Samsarga) is of nine types as follows
(e) Aggravation of only one Dosha is of three types.
14. Pitta aggravated and Vata more aggravated.
15. Pitta aggravated and Kapha more aggravated.
16. Vata aggravated and Kapha more aggravated.
17. Vata aggravated and Pitta more aggravated.
18. Kapha aggravated and Pitta more aggravated.
19. Kapha aggravated and Vata more aggravated.
(f) Aggravation of two Doshas to the same degree.
20. Vata and Pitta aggravated to the same degree.
21. Pitta and Kapha aggravated to the same degree.
22. Kapha and Vata aggravated to the same degree.
(g) Aggravation of only one Dosha is of three types.
23. Vata aggravated.
24. Pitta aggravated.
25. Kapha aggravated
The diminution of Doshas like aggravation is also of twenty five types (aggravation and diminution are in total of fifty types)
The twelve other variable conditions of Doshas occur when aggravation and diminution happen together.
(h) when one Dosha is aggravated, the second Dosha is in normal condition and the third Dosha is in the state of diminution.
51. Vata aggravated, Pitta in normal condition and Kapha in the state of diminution.
52. Vata aggravated, Kapha in normal condition and Vata in state of diminution.
53. Kapha aggravated, Pitta in normal condition and Vata in the state of diminution.
54. Vata aggravated, Kapha in the normal condition and Pitta in the state of diminution.
55. Pitta aggravated, Vata in the normal condition and Kapha in the state of diminution.
56. Kapha aggravated, Vata in the normal condition and Pitta in the state of diminution.
(i) when two Doshas are aggravated and one Dosha is in the state of diminution.

57. Vata and Pitta aggravated, and Kapha in the state of diminution.

58. Pitta and Kapha aggravated, and vata in the state of diminution.

59. Kapha and Vata aggravated Pitta in the state of diminution.

  (j) when one Dosh is aggravated and two are in a state of diminution.

  60. Vata aggravated Pitta and Kapha in the state of diminution.

61. Pitta aggravated Pitta and Kapha in the state of diminution.

62. Kapha aggravated, Vata and Pitta in the state of diminution. [41-44]

**Clinical features of different types of combination of Doshas:**

प्रकृतिस्थं यदा पित्तं मारुतः श्लेष्मणः क्षये।

स्थानादादाय गात्रेषु यत्र यत्र विसर्पति॥४५॥

तदा भेदश्च दाहश्च तत्र तत्रानवस्थितः।

गात्रदेशे भवत्यस्य श्रमो दौर्बल्यमेव च॥४६॥

प्रकृतिस्थं कफं वायुः क्षीणे पित्ते यदा बली।

कर्षेत् कुर्यात्तदा शूलं सशैत्यस्तम्भगौरवम्॥४७॥

यदाऽनिलं प्रकृतिगं पित्तं कफपरिक्षये।

संरुणद्धि तदा दाहः शूलं चास्योपजायते॥४८॥

श्लेष्माणं हि समं पित्तं यदा वातपरिक्षये।

सन्निरुन्ध्यात्तदा कुर्यात् सतन्द्रागौरवं ज्वरम्॥४९॥

प्रवृद्धो हि यदा श्लेष्मा पित्ते क्षीणे समीरणम्।

रुन्ध्यात्तदा प्रकुर्वीत शीतकं गौरवं रुजम् [४] ॥५०॥

समीरणे परिक्षीणे कफः पित्तं समत्वगम्।

कुर्वीत सन्निरुन्धानो मृद्वग्नित्वं शिरोग्रहम् [५] ॥५१॥

निद्रां तन्द्रां प्रलापं च हृद्रोगं गात्रगौरवम्।

नखादीनां च पीतत्वं ष्ठीवनं कफपित्तयोः॥५२॥

हीनवातस्य तु श्लेष्मा पित्तेन सहितश्चरन्।

करोत्यरोचकापाकौ सदनं गौरवं तथा॥५३॥

हल्लासमास्यस्रवणं पाण्डुतां दूयनं मदम्।

विरेकस्य च वैषम्यं वैषम्यमनलस्य च॥५४॥

हीनपित्तस्य तु श्लेष्मा मारुतेनोपसंहितः।

स्तम्भं शैत्यं च तोदं च जनयत्यनवस्थितम्॥५५॥

गौरवं मृदुतामग्नेर्भक्ताश्रद्धां प्रवेपनम्।

नखादीनां च शुक्लत्वं गात्रपारुष्यमेव च॥५६॥

मारुतस्तु कफे हीने पित्तं च कुपितं द्वयम्।

करोति यानि लिङ्गानि शृणु तानि समासतः॥५७॥

भ्रममुद्वेष्टनं तोदं दाहं स्फुटनवेपने।

अङ्गमर्दं परीशोषं दूयनं धूपनं तथा॥५८॥

वातपित्तक्षये श्लेष्मा स्रोतांस्यपिदधद्भृशम्।

चेष्टाप्रणाशं मूर्च्छां च वाक्सङ्गं च करोति हि॥५९॥

वातश्लेष्मक्षये पित्तं देहौजः संसयच्चरेत्।

ग्लानिमिन्द्रियदौर्बल्यं तृष्णां मूर्च्छां क्रियाक्षयम्॥६०॥

पित्तश्लेष्मक्षये वायुर्मर्माण्यतिनिपीडयन्।

प्रणाशयति सञ्ज्ञां च वेपयत्यथवा नरम्॥६१॥

**Clinical features of different types of combination of Doshas:**

When Kapha is in the state of diminution, the aggravated Vata displaces the normal Pitta and carries it to different parts of the body. Wherever this Vitiated Vata takes Pitta to, in all those places, there will be burning sensation (Daha), cracking sensation (Bheda), exhaustion (shrama) and weakness (Daurbalya) all over the body.

When the Pitta is in the state of diminution, the aggravated Vata displaces the normal Kapha, causing colic pain (Shoola), coolness (Shaitya), stiffness (Stambha) and heaviness (Gaurava).

When Kapha is in the state of diminution, the pitta obstructs the path of normal Vata causing thereby burning sensation (Daha) and colic pain (shoola).

When Vata is in the state of diminution and Pitta is normal, then Pitta may block Kapha causing thereby drowsiness (Tandra), heaviness (Gaurava) and fever (Jwara).

When Pitta is in the state of diminution, the aggravated Kapha obstructs the channel of Vata causing thereby coolness (Sheeta), heaviness (Gaurava) and pain (Ruja).

When Vata is in the state of diminution, the Kapha obstructs the path of normal Pitta causing low digestive power (Mridu Agni), stiffness of head (Shiro Graha), sleepiness (Nidra), drowsiness (Tandra), irrelevant talk (Pralapa), heart diseases (Hridroga), heaviness in the body (Gatra gourava), yellowness of the nails, etc. and expectoration of Phlegm and bile.

When Vata is in the state of diminution, the Kapha moving together with Pitta causes anorexia (Aruchi), indigestion (Apaka), tiredness (Sadana), heaviness (Gourava), nausea (Hrillasa), salivation (Asya sravana), anaemia (Pandu), burning sensation (Daha), intoxication (Mada), irregularity in purgation and digestion.

When Pitta is in the state of diminution, the Kapha together with Vata causes an unstable stiffness (Asahmita Stambha), cold (Sheeta), pain (Toda), heaviness (Gaurava), weakness of digestive power (Mrudu Agni), dislike for food (Bhakta Ashraddha), trembling (Pravepana), pallor of nails (Nakha Shuklata) and roughness in the body (Gatra Parushya).

When Kapha is in the state of diminution, the Vata and Pitta aggravated together give rise to giddiness (Bhrama), pain (Toda), cramps (Mrudveshtana), burning (Daha), cracking sensation (Sphutana), trembling (Vepana), bodyache (Angamarda), feeling of dryness (Parishosha), heating (Duyana) and steaming sensation (Dhupana)

When Vata and Pitta are in the state of diminution, the Kapha obstructs the channels and causes depression, inability to talk (Vak sangha), fainting (Murcha) and loss of action (Cheshta Pranasha).

When Vata and Kapha are in the state of diminution, Pitta causes vitiation of Ojas, leading to Glani (debility), Indriya Daurbalya (weakness of sense organs), Trushna (excessive thirst), Murcha (fainting), Kriya kshayam – depleted body functions.

When Pitta and Kapha are in the state of diminution, the Vata afflicts the vital organs, does away with consciousness and causes trembling (Vepathu) in the patient.

**Signs and symptoms of Vitiation of Dhatus (Tissues) and Malas (Excreta):**

दोषाः प्रवृद्धाः स्वं लिङ्गं दर्शयन्ति यथाबलम्|
क्षीणा जहति लिङ्गं स्वं, समाः स्वं कर्म कुर्वते||६२||

Doshas when aggravated manifest their signs and symptoms in accordance with the degree of aggravation; those in the state of diminution give up their normal signs and symptoms; and those in a state of equilibrium operate properly.

### Kshaya Lakshana – Signs of depletion:

वातादीनां रसादीनां मलानामोजसस्तथा|
क्षयास्तत्रानिलादीनामुक्तं सङ्क्षीणलक्षणम् ||६३||

### Kshaya Lakshana – Signs of depletion:

Diminution occurs in Doshas (Vata, Pitta and Kapha), Dhatus (Rasa, Rakta, Mamsa, Medas, Asthi, Majja and Sukra), Malas (excreta of three types) and Ojas. Among these, signs and symptoms of diminution of Doshas have already been explained.

### Rasa Dhatu Kshaya – depletion of Rasa (end product of digestion)

घट्टते सहते शब्दं नोच्चैर्द्रवति शूल्यते|
हृदयं ताम्यति स्वल्पचेष्टस्यापि रसक्षये||६४||

### Rasa Dhatu Kshaya – depletion of Rasa (end product of digestion)

Ghattate - patient becomes restless,
Sahate Shabdam Na – he does not stand loud sounds, becomes intolerant;
Hrudrava – palpitation,
Hrudayam Tamyati Alpa Cheshtasya Api – cardiac pain, exhaustion even with the slightest exertion.

### Rakta Dhatu Kshaya – depletion of Rakta (blood) :

परुषा स्फुटिता म्लाना त्वग्रूक्षा रक्तसङ्क्षये|
Parusha – Roughness,
Sphutita – cracks,
Mlana- dullness,
Tvak Rukshata – skin dryness.

### Mamsa Dhatu Kshaya – depletion of muscle tissue :

मांसक्षये विशेषेण स्फिग्ग्रीवोदरशुष्कता||६५||
Sphik, Greeva Udara Shushkata – emaciation of the buttocks, neck and abdomen.

### Medo Dhatu Kshaya – depletion of fat tissue :

सन्धीनां स्फुटनं ग्लानिरक्ष्णोरायास एव च|
लक्षणं मेदसि क्षीणे तनुत्वं चोदरस्य च||६६||
Sandhi sphutana – cracking of the joints,
Glani – Lassitude,
Akshno Ayasa – tired eyes,
Udara tanutva – thinness of the abdomen.

### Asthi Dhatu Kshaya – depletion of bone tissue :

केशलोमनखश्मश्रुद्विजप्रपतनं श्रमः|
ज्ञेयमस्थिक्षये लिङ्गं सन्धिशैथिल्यमेव च||६७||
Kesha, Loma, Nakha, Shmashru, Dvija prapatana – falling of hair, nails hair of the beard including moustaches and teeth,
Shrama – tiredness,

Sandhi shaithilya – looseness of joints

## Majja Dhatu Kshaya – depletion of bone marrow:

शीर्यन्त इव चास्थीनि दुर्बलानि लघूनि च|
प्रततं वातरोगीणि क्षीणे मज्जनि देहिनाम्||६८||

Asthi Sheeryata – emptiness of bones,
Durbala, Laghu Asthi – thinness, weakness, and lightness of the bones,
Vata Roga – frequent affliction with Vata imbalance disorders.

## Shukra Dhatu Kshaya – depletion of semen / female reproductive tissues :

दौर्बल्यं मुखशोषश्च पाण्डुत्वं सदनं श्रमः|
क्लैब्यं शुक्राविसर्गश्च क्षीणशुक्रस्य लक्षणम्||६९||

Daurbalya – weakness,
Mukha Shosha – dryness of mouth,
Pandutva – pallor,
Sadana – lassitude,
Shrama – tiredness,
Klaibya – impotency and
Shukra Avisarga – non-ejaculation of semen, non-ovulation.

## Pureesha Kshaya Lakshana – depletion of faeces :

क्षीणे शकृति चान्त्राणि पीडयन्निव मारुतः|
रूक्षस्योन्नमयन् कुक्षिं तिर्यग्गूर्ध्वं च गच्छति||७०||

Antrani Peedana – Vata afflicts intestines and causes dryness (Rooksha) and pain. The abdomen is swollen; the Vata moves upwards and sideways.

## Mutra Kshaya Lakshana – depletion of urine :

मूत्रक्षये मूत्रकृच्छ्रं मूत्रवैवर्ण्यमेव च|
पिपासा बाधते चास्य मुखं च परिशुष्यति||७१||

Mutra krichrata – dysuria,
Mutra vaivarnya – discoloration of the urine
Pipasa – thirst and
Mukha shosha – dryness in the mouth.

मलायनानि चान्यानि शून्यानि च लघूनि च|
विशुष्काणि च लक्ष्यन्ते यथास्वं मलसङ्क्षये||७२||

The signs and symptoms of the diminution of other Malas (Dhatu malas) are the feeling of emptiness, lightness and dryness in the excretory organs.

## Oja Kshaya Lakshana:

बिभेति दुर्बलोऽभीक्ष्णं ध्यायति व्यथितेन्द्रियः|
दुश्छायो दुर्मना रूक्षः क्षामश्चैवौजसः क्षये||७३||
हृदि तिष्ठति यच्छुद्धं रक्तमीषत्सपीतकम्|
ओजः शरीरे सङ्ख्यातं तन्नाशान्ना विनश्यति||७४||
प्रथमं जायते ह्योजः शरीरेऽस्मिञ्छरीरिणाम्|

सर्पिर्वर्णं मधुरसं लाजगन्धि प्रजायते||७५||
(भ्रमरैः फलपुष्पेभ्यो यथा सम्भ्रियते मधु|
तद्वदोजः स्वकर्मभ्यो गुणैः सम्भ्रियते नृणाम् )|

**Ojo Kshaya Lakshana** - symptoms of depleted Ojas (immunity)
Bhaya – fear complex,
Durbala – constant weakness,
Dhyayati – worry,
Vyathita Indriya – affliction of sense organs with pain,
Dushchaya – loss of complexion,
Durmana -cheerless, depressed mood,
Rooksha – dryness, roughness
Kshaama – emaciation.

### Definition of Ojas:

The one which dwells in the heart and is predominantly white, yellowish and reddish in color is known as Ojas of the body. If the Ojas is destroyed, the human being will also perish. The form in which the Ojas is produced in the body of the humanbeings for the first time has the color of ghee; taste of honey and smell of fried paddy (Laja).

As the bees collect honey from the fruits and flowers, so the Ojas is collected in the body, by the actions, qualities, habits and diet of human being.

### Causes of depletion of Dhatu (tissues):

व्यायामोऽनशनं चिन्ता रूक्षाल्पप्रमिताशनम्|
वातातपौ भयं शोको रूक्षपानं प्रजागरः||७६||
कफशोणितशुक्राणां मलानां चातिवर्तनम्|
कालो भूतोपघातश्च ज्ञातव्याः क्षयहेतवः||७७||

Vyayama – excessive physical activities,
Anashana – fasting,
Chinta – anxiety, excessive thinking,
Rooksha, Alpa, Pramita Ashana – intake of dry food, food in small quantity or habitual intake of food having one taste only,
Vata, Atapa – exposure to the wind and sun,
Bhaya – fear,
Shoka – grief,
Rooksha pana – intake of dry drinks,
Prajagara – night vigil,
excessive elimination of phlegm, blood, semen and other excreta, old age and period of Adana Kala (seasons causing exhaustion) and Bhuta (microbes).

### Etiopathology of diabetes mellitus (Madhumeha):

गुरुस्निग्धाम्ललवणान्यतिमात्रं समश्नताम्|
नवमन्नं च पानं च निद्रामास्यासुखानि च||७८||
त्यक्तव्यायामचिन्तानां संशोधनमकुर्वताम्|
श्लेष्मा पित्तं च मेदश्च मांसं चातिप्रवर्धते||७९||

तैरावृतगतिर्वायुरोज आदाय गच्छति।
यदा बस्तिं तदा कृच्छ्रो मधुमेहः प्रवर्तते॥८०॥
स मारुतस्य पित्तस्य कफस्य च मुहुर्मुहुः।
दर्शयत्याकृतिं गत्वा क्षयमाप्यायते पुनः॥८१॥

## Etiopathology of diabetes mellitus (Madhumeha):

- Guru, Snigdha, Amla, Lavana – Excess intake of heavy to digest food, unctuous, sour and salt foods
- Nava Annam, Panam cha – consuming fresh grains (freshly collected rice, wheat etc)
- Nidra Sukha, Asya Sukha – eating and sleeping frequently (and comfortably)
- Tyakta Vyayama, Chinta – lack of exercise, lack of thinking.
- Not undergoing seasonal Panchakarma treatments.
- These causes lead to vitiation of Kapha, Pitta, Medas (fat tissue), Mamsa (muscle tissue).
- The path of Vata gets obstructed. Vata together with the Ojas comes down to reach the Basti (urinary system), causing Madhumeha (Diabetes mellitus).

In this disease, signs and symptoms pertaining to Vata, Pitta and Kapha are manifested quite frequently- they vanish at times and appear again (in more vehement form). If neglected, this disease causes serious types of carbuncles in subcutaneous and muscular areas, vital parts (Marma) and joints of the body.

## Types of Diabetic Carbuncles:

उपेक्षयाऽस्य जायन्ते पिडकाः सप्त दारुणाः।
मांसलेष्ववकाशेषु मर्मस्वपि च सन्धिषु॥८२॥
शराविका कच्छपिका जालिनी सर्षपी तथा।
अलजी विनताख्या च विद्रधी चेति सप्तमी॥८३॥
अन्तोन्नता मध्यनिम्ना श्यावा क्लेदरुगन्विता।
शराविका स्यात् पिडका शरावाकृतिसंस्थिता॥८४॥
अवगाढार्तिनिस्तोदा महावास्तुपरिग्रहा।
श्लक्ष्णा कच्छपपृष्ठाभा पिडका कच्छपी मता॥८५॥
स्तब्धा सिराजालवती स्निग्धास्रावा महाशया।
रुजानिस्तोदबहुला सूक्ष्मच्छिद्रा च जालिनी॥८६॥
पिडका नातिमहती क्षिप्रपाका महारुजा।
सर्षपी सर्षपाभाभिः पिडकाभिश्चिता भवेत्॥८७॥
दहति त्वचमुत्थाने तृष्णामोहज्वरप्रदा।
विसर्पत्यनिशं दुःखाद्दहत्यग्निरिवालजी॥८८॥
अवगाढरुजाक्लेदा पृष्ठे वाऽप्युदरेऽपि वा।
महती विनता नीला पिडका विनता मता॥८९॥

## Types of Diabetic Carbuncles:
The seven types of Carbuncles are Sharvika, Kacchapika, Jalini, Sarshapi, Alaji, Vinata and Vidradhi.

**Sharavika** type of carbuncle elevated in the border and depressed in the centre, grey in colour and associated with slough and pains. Because of its appearance as a sharava (earthen saucer), it is known as Sharvavika.

**Kacchapika** type of carbuncle is deep seated and painful, combined with a splitting type of pain; it has very big base, it is smooth and resembling the back of tortoise. (Kacchapa means tortoise).

**The Jalini** type of carbuncle is hard; it has network of vessels in surface; it's sticky; it has a very big base: it is very painful with splitting type of pain having subtle openings.

**The Sarshapika** type of carbuncle which is not very big, which suppurates quickly, which is very painful and associated with carbuncles of the size of mustard seeds is known as Sarshapi.

**Alaji** type of carbuncle causes burning sensation during eruption: when fully manifested, it causes thirst, unconsciousness, fever; it always spreads and is very painful due to burning sensation like fire.

The pain in **Vinata** type of carbuncle is also deep-seated: it is associated with slough: it occurs either in the back or abdomen; it is big in size, blue in color and having depression in the center.

**Vidradhi – External and internal abscesses:**
विद्रधिं द्विविधामाहुर्बाह्यामाभ्यन्तरीं तथा|
बाह्या त्वक्स्नायुमांसोत्था कण्डराभा महारुजा||९०||
शीतकान्नविदाह्युष्णरूक्षशुष्कातिभोजनात्|
विरुद्धाजीर्णसङ्क्लिष्टविषमासात्म्यभोजनात्||९१||
व्यापन्नबहुमद्यत्वाद्वेगसन्धारणाच्छ्रमात्|
जिह्मव्यायामशयनादतिभाराध्वमैथुनात्||९२||
अन्तःशरीरे मांसासृगाविशन्ति यदा मलाः|
तदा सञ्जायते ग्रन्थिर्गम्भीरस्थः सुदारुणः||९३||
हृदये क्लोम्नि यकृति प्लीह्नि कुक्षौ च वृक्कयोः|
नाभ्यां वङ्क्षणयोर्वाऽपि बस्तौ वा तीव्रवेदनः||९४||
दुष्टरक्तातिमात्रत्वात् स वै शीघ्रं विदह्यते|
ततः शीघ्रविदाहित्वाद्विद्रधीत्यभिधीयते||९५||
व्यधच्छेदभ्रमानाहशब्दस्फुरणसर्पणैः|
वातिकीं, पैतिकीं तृष्णादाहमोहमदज्वरैः||९६||
जृम्भोत्क्लेशारुचिस्तम्भशीतकैः श्लैष्मिकीं विदुः|
सर्वासु च महच्छूलं विद्रधीषूपजायते||९७||
शस्त्रास्त्रैर्भिद्यत इव चोल्मुकैरिव दह्यते|
विद्रधी व्यम्लता याता वृश्चिकैरिव दश्यते||९८||
तनु रूक्षारुणं श्यावं फेनिलं वातविद्रधी|
तिलमाषकुलत्थोदसन्निभं पित्तविद्रधी||९९||
श्लैष्मिकी स्रवति श्वेतं पिच्छिलं बहलं बहु|
लक्षणं सर्वमेवैतद्भजते सान्निपातिकी||१००||

**Abscess is of two types**- the external and the internal. The external one arises out of the skin, ligaments and muscles. In shape and size it resembles tendons and it is exceedingly painful.

**Abhyantara Vidradhi:** The internal abscess is caused by the excessive intake of food which is staled (Sheeta), irritant (vidaaha), hot, dry, incompatible foods, indigestible, and which is Dosha aggravating and unwholesome.

By taking meals irregularly by taking excessively strong wines, suppression of natural urges, excessive physical exertion, physical exercise and sleep in wrong postures, carrying excessive load, walking long distance and excessive sexual intercourse.

These factors are responsible for the affliction of Mamsa (muscle tissue) and Rakta (blood tissue) of the body by the Doshas, thereby causing deep-seated abscesses which are very painful. This causes excessive pain in heart, liver, spleen, sides of the abdomen kidney navel and sides of the lower abdomen or bladder. Due to excessive vitiation of Rakta, these abscesses get suppressed quickly. This is called Vidradhi" because of Vidaha (burning sensation and suppuration).

**Vidradhi**(abscess) is of four types, viz. Vataja, Pittaja, Shlaishmika (Kapha) and Sannipatika.

**Vataja Vidradhi** causes piercing (Vyadha) and cutting pain (Cheda), giddiness (Bhrama), flatulence (Anaha),

**Shabda, Sphurana, Sarpana** – sounding and throbbing sensation, and spreading tendency.
The discharge is thin, unctuous, reddish, grey and foamy.

**Pittaja Vidradhi** – thirst, burning sensation, unconsciousness, intoxication and fever. Discharge looks like the decoction of Tila – Sesame (Sesamum indicum), Masha (black gram) and Kulatha (horse gram).

**Shlaishmika Vidradhi** - yawning, nausea, stiffness and cold. Discharge is white, slimy, thick and profuse.

**The Samnipatika type of Vidradhi** (influenced by all the three Doshas) is marked by excruciating pain. Discharge will have mixed colour.

In the event of the abscess being ripened the patient feels as if being assaulted by weapons, burnt by fire brands and being bitten by scorpions.

**Symptoms based on place of Vidradhi (abscess) :**
अथासां विद्रधीनां साध्यासाध्यत्वविशेषज्ञानार्थं स्थानकृतं लिङ्गविशेषमुपदेक्ष्यामः:- तत्र प्रधानमर्मजायां विद्रध्यां हृद्धट्टनतमकप्रमोहकासश्वासाः, क्लोमजायां पिपासामुखशोषगलग्रहाः, यकृज्जायां श्वासः, प्लीहजायामुच्छ्वासोपरोधः, कुक्षिजायां कुक्षिपार्श्वान्तरांसशूलं, वृक्कजायां पृष्ठकटिग्रहः, नाभिजायां हिक्का, वङ्क्षणजायां सक्थिसादः, बस्तिजायां कृच्छ्रपूतिमूत्रवर्चसत्वं चेति||१०१||
पक्वप्रभिन्नासूर्ध्वजासु मुखात् स्रावः स्रवति, अधोजासु गुदात्, उभयतस्तु नाभिजासु||१०२||
आसां हृन्नाभिबस्तिजाः परिपक्वाः सान्निपातिकी च मरणाय; शेषाः पुनः कुशलमाशुप्रतिकारिणं चिकित्सकमासाद्योपशाम्यन्ति|
तस्मादचिरोत्थितां विद्रधीं शस्त्रसर्पविद्युदग्नितुल्यां स्नेहविरेचनैराश्वेवोपक्रमेत् सर्वशो गुल्मवच्चेति||१०३||

**If it is situated in Marma (vital points, like heart, brain etc),** there will be
Hrud Ghattana – palpitation,
Tamaka – darkness in front of eyes,
Pramoha – unconsciousness,
Kasa – coughing,
Shwasa – dyspnea.

**If Vidradhi is in Kloma (inside abdomen),** there will be thirst, dryness in mouth and obstruction in throat;
If it is in the liver, there will be dyspnoea;
If in spleen, there will be obstruction to expiration;
If in the sides of the abdomen, there will be pain in the sides and middle of the abdomen and in the shoulder (referred pain).
If it is in the kidney, there will be stiffness in the back and waist.

If the abscess is in Nabhi (umbilicus), this causes hiccup (Hikka),
If in the groyne, this will impair the movement of the thighs,
If it occurs in the urinary bladder, urine and stool will pass with difficulty and there will be a bad smell.

**When ripened and ruptured**, the discharge from the internal abscess in the upper portion of the body comes out through the mouth, whereas from the lower part of the body it comes out through the anus. When the abscess in the Nabhi region ruptures, the discharge may come out through both mouth and anus.

This disease is as dangerous as a weapon, snake, lightning and fire. The principal of treatment as mentioned for Gulma (will be dealt with in future) should be adopted here.

Curability of abscess:
Prognosis of carbuncles:
भवन्ति चात्र-
विना प्रमेहमप्येता जायन्ते दुष्टमेदसः।
तावच्चैता न लक्ष्यन्ते यावद्वास्तुपरिग्रहः॥१०४॥
शराविका कच्छपिका जालिनी चेति दुःसहाः।
जायन्ते ता ह्यतिबलाः प्रभूतश्लेष्ममेदसः॥१०५॥
सर्षपी चालजी चैव विनता विद्रधी च याः।
साध्यः पित्तोल्बणास्तास्तु सम्भवन्त्यल्पमेदसः॥१०६॥
मर्मस्वंसे गुदे पाण्योः स्तने सन्धिषु पादयोः।
जायन्ते यस्य पिडिकाः स प्रमेही न जीवति॥१०७॥

Abscesses may occur due to the vitiation of Medas even without the disease Prameha (that is diabetes mellitus). They are, however, not visible until they take a definite shape and size.

Sarvika, Kacchapika and Jalini Types of Carbuncles are intolerably painful and of very serious nature. They occur in such of the patients who have excessive Kapha and Medas. Sarshapi, Alaji, Vinata and Vidradhi types of carbuncles are on the other hand dominated by Pitta and occur in the case of such patients who have Meas in less quantity. These are curable. A diabetic patient who suffers from abscesses occurring in vital organs, shoulder, anus, hands, breasts, joints and feet seldom survive.

Complications of carbuncles:
　　तथाऽन्याः पिडकाः सन्ति रक्तपीतासितारुणाः।
पाण्डुराः पाण्डुवर्णाश्च भस्माभा मेचकप्रभाः॥१०८॥
मृद्व्यश्च कठिनाश्चान्याः स्थूलाः सूक्ष्मास्तथाऽपराः।
मन्दवेगा महावेगाः स्वल्पशूला महारुजः॥१०९॥
ता बुद्ध्वा मारुतादीनां यथास्वैर्हेतुलक्षणैः।
ब्रूयादुपचरेच्चाशु प्रागुपद्रवदर्शनात्॥११०॥
तृट्श्वासमांससङ्कोथमोहहिक्कामदज्वराः।
वीसर्पमर्मसंरोधाः पिडकानामुपद्रवाः॥१११॥

Complications of carbuncles:
There are other varieties of abscesses having red, yellow, black, reddish, grey, yellowish, unctuous black and ash color. Some are of soft, some are hard, some are of big size, some are of small size, some of them develop slowly, some of them develop quickly, some of them have dull pain and some of them have excruciating pain- they should

be diagnosed based on Dosha involved, considering their causative factors, signs and symptoms. It should be treated immediately, based on Dosha, before any complication arises.

The complications of an abscess are –

Trut – thirst,

Shwasa – dyspnoea,

Mamsa Sankotha – sloughing

Moha – unconsciousness,

Hikka – hiccup,

Mada – intoxication,

Jwara – fever,

Visarpa – herpes / cellulites

impediment of the functions of the vital organs. [108-111]

## Different courses of Doshas in the pathogenesis of diseases:

क्षयः स्थानं च वृद्धिश्च दोषाणां त्रिविधा गतिः|

ऊर्ध्वं चाधश्च तिर्यक्च विज्ञेया त्रिविधाऽपरा||११२||

त्रिविधा चापरा कोष्ठशाखामर्मास्थिसन्धिषु|

इत्युक्ता विधिभेदेन दोषाणां त्रिविधा गतिः||११३||

चयप्रकोपप्रशमाः पित्तादीनां यथाक्रमम्|

भवन्त्येकैकशः षट्सु कालेष्वभ्रागमादिषु||११४||

1. Diminution, normal state and aggravation these are the three conditions of Doshas;

2. The three more types are upwards, downward and sideway movement of Doshas.

3. The Doshas have another threefold movement.

a. Movement in Kostha or alimentary tract,

b. Movement in Shakha or exterior Dhatus

c. Movement in Marma asthi sandhi or vital organs, bones and joints.

Dosha undergo Chaya (increase in their own habitat), Prakopa (flow into other places) and prashama (subside) in different seasons, due to the effect of respective seasons. [112-114]

## Physiological and Pathological Concepts of Doshas:

गतिः कालकृता चैषा चयाद्या पुनरुच्यते|११५|

गतिश्च द्विविधा दृष्टा प्राकृती वैकृती च या||११५||

पित्तादेवोष्मणः पक्तिर्नराणामुपजायते|

तच्च पित्तं प्रकुपितं विकारान् कुरुते बहून्||११६||

प्राकृतस्तु बलं श्लेष्मा विकृतो मल उच्यते|

स चैवौजः स्मृतः काये स च पाप्मोपदिश्यते||११७||

सर्वा हि चेष्टा वातेन स प्राणः प्राणीनां स्मृतः|

तेनैव रोगा जायन्ते तेन चैवोपरुध्यते||११८||

There are two aspects of the Doshas, viz natural and morbid. In the natural state, Pitta helps in the digestion and metabolism of living beings. In its morbid state, it causes various diseases.

The Kapha in its natural state promotes strength in the form of Ojas. When in a morbid condition, it takes the form of excreta and causes misery.

Similarly Vata in its natural state is responsible for all activities of the body. Vata in fact constitutes the very life of living beings. When in morbid state, it causes disease and death. [115-118]

**Preservation of health:**

नित्यं सन्निहितामित्रं समीक्ष्यात्मानमात्मवान्।
नित्यं युक्तः परिचरेदिच्छन्नायुरनित्वरम्||११९||

One desirous of ensured longevity for himself, should always make an attempt for his well being as if surrounded by opponents [119]

**To sum up:**

तत्र श्लोकौ-

शिरोरोगाः सहृद्रोगा रोगा मानविकल्पजाः।
क्षयाः सपिडकाश्चोक्ता दोषाणां गतिरेव च||१२०||
कियन्तःशिरसीयेऽस्मिन्नध्याये तत्त्वदर्शिना।
ज्ञानार्थं भिषजां चैव प्रजानां च हितैषिणा||१२१||

Head diseases, heart diseases, the states of Doshas in different permutations and combinations, diminutions, abscesses, the course of movement of Doshas have been explained by the sage in this chapter on "The Enumeration of Diseases relating to the Head". The sage has done this with a view to enlightening the physicians about it as well as for the well- being of subjects. [120-121]

इत्यग्निवेशकृते तन्त्रे चरकप्रतिसंस्कृते श्लोकस्थाने कियन्तःशिरसीयो नाम सप्तदशोऽध्यायः||१७||

Thus, ends the seventeenth chapter on "The Enumeration of diseases relating to the Head" of the Sutra section of Agnivesha's work as redacted by Charaka

# 18

# Sutrasthana Chapter 18 Tri Shotheeyam

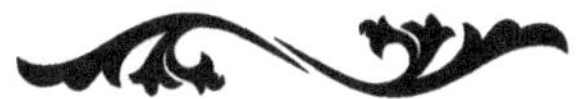

**Trishotheeya Adhyaya**

**Types Of Swelling – Ayurveda Diagnosis:**

अथातस्त्रिशोथीयमध्यायं व्याख्यास्यामः||१||

इति ह स्माह भगवानात्रेयः||२||

Inflammation or swelling is of three types as per Ayurveda. In Ayurvedic terms, swelling is called Shotha or Shopha. Charaka has explained it in the 18th chapter of Sutrasthana, called Tri-Shotheeya Adhyaya. Apart from explanation of different types of inflammation, this chapter also explains normal functions of Vata, Pitta and Kapha Dosha, what to do when perfect diagnosis cannot be achieved, how diseases are innumerable etc.

**Classification of swellings:**

त्रयः शोथा भवन्ति वातपित्तश्लेष्मनिमित्ताः, ते पुनर्द्विविधा निजागन्तुभेदेन||३||

Swellings are of three types viz;
Vatika or Vataja – arising due to Vata Dosha imbalance.
Paittika or Pittaja – arising due to Pitta Dosha imbalance.
Shlaishmika or Kaphaja – arising due to Kapha Dosha imbalance

They are again of two types -
Nija – Due to internal causes within the body, i.e. due to endogenous factors.
Agantuja – Due to external causes, such as injury, i.e. due to exogenous factors [3]

**Causes – Aetiology of exogenous swellings- Agantu Shotha Nidana:**

तत्रागन्तवश्छेदनभेदनक्षणनभञ्जनपिच्छनोत्पेषणप्रहारवधबन्धनवेष्टनव्यधनपीडनादिभिर्वा भल्लातकपुष्पफलरसात्मगुप्ताशूककृमिशूकाहितपत्रलतागुल्मसंस्पर्शनैर्वा स्वेदनपरिसर्पणावमूत्रणैर्वा विषिणां सविषप्राणिदंष्ट्रादन्तविषाणनखनिपातैर्वा सागरविषवातहिमदहनसंस्पर्शनैर्वा शोथाः समुपजायन्ते||४||

**Causes – Aetiology of exogenous swellings- Agantu Shotha Nidana:**

Chedana – excision wounds
Bhedana – incision wounds
Kshanana – comminuting,

Bhanjana – fracture,

Picchana – exposure to excessive pressure,

Utpeshana – grinding,

Prahara – assault,

Vadha – grievous hurt,

Bandhana – tight tying

Veshtana – twisting by a snake, tight wrapping etc.

Vyadhana – piercing,

Peedana – compression, squeezing,

contact of the fruit and flower of Bhallataka ( Marking nut – Semecarpus anacardium Linn), Atmagupta (Mucuna prurita Hook), bristles of poisonous insects, harmful leaves, creepers and shrubs, sweat, crawling or urine of poisonous creatures, injury by fangs, teeth, horns, nails etc. of poisonous animals and coming in contact with the sea, poisonous wind, snow and fire.[4]

**Endogenous and exogenous swellings – Nija and Agantuja Shotha :**

ते पुनर्यथास्वं हेतुव्यञ्जनैरादावुपलभ्यन्ते निजव्यञ्जनैकदेशविपरीतैः; बन्धमन्त्रागदप्रलेपप्रतापनिर्वापणादिभिश्चोपक्रमैरुपक्रम्यमाणाः
प्रशान्तिमापद्यन्ते ॥५॥

The exogenous swellings (Agantu Shotha) are diagnosed by the characteristic aetiology, signs and symptoms. Even though, ultimately the exogenous swelling may share the characteristic signs and symptoms of endogenous swelling, the difference lies in the priority or certain features common to both types of swellings.

The endogenous swelling (Nija Shotha) starts with the vitiation of Doshas and then brings about pain.
The exogenous swelling, on the other hand, starts with pain and then brings about the vitiation of Doshas. These types of swellings are cured when treated with such therapies as bandages including
Bandha – talisman, bandaging
Mantra – incantations,
Agada – administration of medicines, antidotes
Pralepa – application of ointments,
Taapa – fomentation and
Nirvapa – cold sponging. [5]

**Aetiology of endogenous swellings – Nija Shotha Nidana:**

निजाः          पुनः          स्नेहस्वेदवमनविरेचनास्थापनानुवासनशिरोविरेचनानामयथावत्प्रयोगान्मिथ्यासंसर्जनाद्वा
छर्द्यलसकविसूचिकाश्वासकासातिसारशोषपाण्डुरोगोदरज्वरप्रदरभगन्दरार्शोविकारातिकर्शनैर्वा          कुष्ठकण्डूपिडकादिभिर्वा
छर्दिक्षवथूद्गारशुक्रवातमूत्रपुरीषवेगधारणैर्वा          कर्मरोगोपवासाध्वकर्शितस्य          वा
सहसातिगुर्वम्ललवणपिष्टान्नफलशाकरागदधिहरितकमद्यमन्दकविरूढनवशूकशमीधान्यान्पौदक-
पिशितोपयोगान्मृत्पङ्कलोष्टभक्षणाल्लवणातिभक्षणाद्गर्भसम्पीडनादामगर्भप्रपतनात् प्रजातानां च मिथ्योपचारादुद्दीर्णदोषत्वाच्च शोफाः
प्रादुर्भवन्ति; इत्युक्तः सामान्यो हेतुः ॥६॥

**Aetiology of endogenous swellings – Nija Shotha Nidana:**

Endogenous swellings are caused by
Improper administration of oleation (Snehana), fomentation (Swedana), emesis (Vamana), purgation (Virechana), Asthapana and Anuvasana types of enema, elimination of Doshas from the head,

Adoption of improper post- Panchakarma dietetic program (Samsarjana Karma),
Excessive emaciation due to
Chardi – vomiting,
Alasaka – intestinal torpor,
Visuchika – Choleric diarrhoea,
Shwasa – dyspnoea,
Kasa – coughing,
Atisara – diarrhoea,
Shosha – emaciation,
Pandu – anaemia,
Udara – abdominal diseases,
Jwara – fever
Pradara – menorrhagia,
Bhagandhara – fistula in ano
Arsha – piles
Kushta – skin diseases,
Kandu – pruritus,
Vidhradi – abscess
Vega Dharana – suppression of natural urges,
When a person is emaciated due to Panchakarma therapy / due to chronic disease / due to fasting or walking long distance, suddenly starts consuming exceedingly heavy, sour and salty food , pastry, fruits pickles, salad, alcohol, immature curd, germinated and fresh corn with or without bristles, meat of marshy or aquatic animals; Intake of earth, mud, cold of earth, excessive intake of salt, Pressure on gravid uterus, abortion, adoption of improper regimen after delivery and excitation of Doshas.

These are the etiological factors for endogenous swelling (Nija shopha) [6]

**Clinical features of Vataja Shopha :**

अयं त्वत्र विशेषः- शीतरूक्षलघुविशदश्रमोपवासातिकर्शनक्षपणादिभिर्वायुः प्रकुपितस्त्वङ्मांसशोणितादीन्यभिभूय शोफं जनयति; स क्षिप्रोत्थानप्रशमो भवति, तथा श्यामारुणवर्णः प्रकृतिवर्णो वा, चलः स्पन्दनः खरपरुषभिन्नत्वग्रोमा छिद्यत इव भिद्यत इव पीड्यत इव सूचीभिरिव तुद्यते पिपीलिकाभिरिव संसृप्यते सर्षपकल्कावलिप्त इव चिमिचिमायते सङ्कुच्यत आयम्यत इवेति वातशोथः (१);

**Clinical features of Vataja Shopha :**

By the intake of cold, unctuous light and non-slimy food; exertion (Shrama), fasting (Upavasa), excessive emaciation and elimination therapy, the Vata gets aggravated and afflicts the Tvak (Skin), Mamsa (flesh) Rakta (blood) etc. and causes swellings. The swellings thus caused may appear They are either of blue or reddish colour or of the natural colour of the organ affected. The swellings thus caused may appear and disappear abruptly. They are mobile and they throb. Khara, Parusha, Bhinna Twak Roma – The skin and hair over the swellings are rough, hard and broken;

The pain due to swelling resemble:

- Chidyata Iva – cutting,
- Bhidhata iva – splitting,
- Peedyata iva – pressing,
- Soochibhiriva Tudyate – pinching by needles,

- Pipeelika sarpana - crawling by ants, etc.

There is a tingling sensation as if covered with mustard paste. They contract and expand.

**Clinical features of Pittaja Shotha :**

उष्णतीक्ष्णकटुकक्षारलवणाम्लाजीर्णभोजनैरग्न्यातपप्रतापैश्च पित्तं प्रकुपितं त्वङ्मांसशोणितान्यभिभूय शोथं जनयति; स क्षिप्रोत्थानप्रशमो भवति, कृष्णपीतनीलताम्रावभास उष्णो मृदुः कपिलताम्ररोमा उष्यते दूयते धूप्यते ऊष्मायते स्विद्यते क्लिद्यते न च स्पर्शमुष्णं च सुषूयत इति पित्तशोथः (२);

**Clinical features of Pittaja Shotha :**

By the intake of hot, pungent, bitter, alkaline, saline, sour and heavy food and exposure to heat of fire and sun, the Pitta gets aggravated and affects the Tvak (Skin), Mamsa (flesh) and Rakta (Blood) and thus swelling is caused. It appears and disappears abruptly, it is black, yellow, blue and coppery in color; it is hot and soft in touch; the hair over the swelling becomes light-gray and coppery; there is a feeling of hot sensation, pain, feeling of emission of smoke, high temperature, steaming and sloughing. Heat or hot touch will not be tolerated.

**Clinical features of Kaphaja Shopha :**

गुरुमधुर शीतस्निग्धैरतिस्वप्नाव्यायामादिभिश्च श्लेष्मा प्रकुपितस्त्वङ्मांसशोणितादीन्यभिभूय शोथं जनयति; स कृच्छ्रोत्थानप्रशमो भवति, पाण्डुश्वेतावभासो गुरुः स्निग्धः श्लक्ष्णः स्थिरः स्त्यानः शुक्लाग्ररोमा स्पर्शोष्णसहश्चेति श्लेष्मशोथः (३);

Due to the intake of heavy, sweet, cold and unctuous diet, excessive sleep, lack of exercise etc. the Kapha gets aggravated and it affects the skin, muscles, blood etc. to cause Shlaishmika type of swellings. Such swellings take a long time to manifest and also to get cured. They are of apparently pale white colour, heavy, unctuous, smooth, immobile, compact and having white hair in the border. They can tolerate pressure and heat.

According to the aetiology, signs and symptoms, there are three more types of swellings due to the combined morbidity of two Doshas (viz, Vata-Pittaja, Vata-Kaphaja and Pitta-Kaphaja). There is only one Sannipatika type of swelling arising out of the combined morbidity of all the three Doshas and it manifests the signs and symptoms of all the three Doshas. Thus there are seven varieties of swelling caused by the vitiation of Doshas.

Based on the above explanations,:

यथास्वकारणाकृतिसंसर्गादिद्वदोषजास्त्रयः शोथा भवन्ति; यथास्वकारणाकृतिसन्निपातात् सान्निपातिक एकः; एवं सप्तविधो भेदः||७||
प्रकृतिभिस्ताभिस्ताभिर्भिद्यमानो द्विविधस्त्रिविधश्चतुर्विधः सप्तविधोऽष्टविधश्च शोथ उपलभ्यते, पुनश्चैक एवोत्सेधसामान्यात्||८||

Shotha can be classified as of two types – exogenous and endogenous,

- Or of three types (vatika, Paittika and Shlaismika),
- Or of four types (Vatika, Pattika and Shlaismika and exogenous variety),
- seven types (Vatika, pattitika, Shlaismika, Vata-Pittaja, Kapha-Pittaja, Vata-Kaphaja and Sannipatika) and
- eight types (seven types of endogenous and one type of exogenous).

But on an ultimate analysis, Shotha is only of one type having the swelling as a characteristic sign in common. [7-8]

## Vataja Shotha – inflammation due to Vata :

भवन्ति चात्र-
शूयन्ते यस्य गात्राणि स्वपन्तीव रुजन्ति च|
पीडितान्युन्नमन्त्याशु वातशोथं तमादिशेत्||९||
यश्चाप्यरुणवर्णाभः शोथो नक्तं प्रणश्यति|
स्नेहोष्णमर्दनाभ्यां च प्रणश्येत् स च वातिकः||१०||

## Vataja Shotha – inflammation due to Vata :

**Vataja Shotha** is characterised by swelling, numbness and pain in the limbs and it regains its normal position immediately after it is pressed (and the pressure is withdrawn). Vatika type of swelling is also reddish in colour, disappears during the night and gets cured by the application of unctuous material during the night and also gets cured by the application of unctuous and hot massage.

## Pittaja Shotha :

यः पिपासाज्वरार्तस्य दूयतेऽथ विदह्यते|
स्विद्यति क्लिद्यते गन्धी स पैत्तः स्वयथुः स्मृतः||११||
यः पीतनेत्रवक्त्रत्वक् पूर्वं मध्यात् प्रसूयते|
तनुत्वक् चातिसारी च पित्तशोथः स उच्यते||१२||

In **Pittaja Shotha** the patient feels thirsty and feverish: there is pain and burning sensation in the swelling; there is sweating; sloughing and foul smell; the eyes, face and middle part of the body; the skin becomes thin and there is diarrhoea.

## Kaphaja Shotha :

शीतः सक्तगतिर्यस्तु कण्डूमान् पाण्डुरेव च|
निपीडितो नोन्नमति श्वयथुः स कफात्मकः||१३||
यस्य शस्त्रकुशच्छिन्नाच्छोणितं न प्रवर्तते|
कृच्छ्रेण पिच्छा स्रवति स चापि कफसम्भवः||१४||
निदानाकृतिसंसर्गाच्छ्वयथुः स्यादिद्द्वदोषजः|
सर्वाकृतिः सन्निपाताच्छोथो व्यामिश्रहेतुजः||१५||

The **Kaphaja Shotha** is cold in touch, it does not spread, it causes itching; it is pale in color; and it pits on pressure. Moreover, the Slaismika type of swelling does not bleed even if it is cut with a weapon or sharp edged grass; there is oozing after a long time. The swellings due to the combination of two doshas may be diagnosed on the basis of the combined etiology, signs and symptoms. Similarly, the Sannipatika type (due to vitiation of all three Doshas) of swelling can also be diagnosed from the combination of etiological factors. [9-15]

## Curability of Shotha Roga:

यस्तु पादाभिनिर्वृत्तः शोथः सर्वाङ्गगो भवेत्|
जन्तोः स च सुकष्टः स्यात् प्रसृतः स्त्रीमुखाच्च यः||१६||

यश्चापि गुह्यप्रभवः स्त्रिया वा पुरुषस्य वा|
स च कष्टतमो ज्ञेयो यस्य च स्युरुपद्रवाः||१७||

## Curability of Shotha Roga:

In case of male patients, if the swelling starts from the feet and spreads all over the body, and in case of female patients if it starts from the mouth (head) and spreads, it is difficult to cure. In both male and female patients if the swelling starts from the perineum and is associated with complications, it is exceedingly difficult to cure. [16-17]

## Complications of Shotha roga:

छर्दिः श्वासोऽरुचिस्तृष्णा ज्वरोऽतीसार एव च|
सप्तकोऽयं सदौर्बल्यः शोफोपद्रवसङ्ग्रहः||१८||

The seven complications of Shotha Roga are:
Chardi – vomiting
Shwasa – dyspnoea,
Aruchi – anorexia,
Trushna – thirst,
Jvara – fever,
Atisara – diarrhoea
Daurbalya – general weakness. [18]

## Localized inflammatory conditions – Sthanika Shopha

यस्य श्लेष्मा प्रकुपितो जिह्वामूलेऽवतिष्ठते|
आशु सञ्जनयेच्छोथं जायतेऽस्योपजिह्विका||१९||
यस्य श्लेष्मा प्रकुपितः काकले व्यवतिष्ठते|
आशु सञ्जनयेच्छोफं करोति गलशुण्डिकाम्||२०||
यस्य श्लेष्मा प्रकुपितो गलबाह्येऽवतिष्ठते|
शनैः सञ्जनयेच्छोफं गलगण्डोऽस्य जायते||२१||
यस्य श्लेष्मा प्रकुपितस्तिष्ठत्यन्तर्गले स्थिरः|
आशु सञ्जनयेच्छोफं जायतेऽस्य गलग्रहः||२२||
यस्य पित्तं प्रकुपितं सरक्तं त्वचि सर्पति|
शोफं सरागं जनयेद्विसर्पस्तस्य जायते||२३||
यस्य पित्तं प्रकुपितं त्वचि रक्तेऽवतिष्ठते|
शोथं सरागं जनयेत् पिडका तस्य जायते||२४||
यस्य प्रकुपितं पित्तं शोणितं प्राप्य शुष्यति|
तिलका पिप्लवो व्यङ्गा नीलिका तस्य जायते||२५||
यस्य पित्तं प्रकुपितं शङ्खयोरवतिष्ठते|
श्वयथुः शङ्खको नाम दारुणस्तस्य जायते||२६||
यस्य पित्तं प्रकुपितं कर्णमूलेऽवतिष्ठते|
ज्वरान्ते दुर्जयोऽन्ताय शोथस्तस्योपजायते||२७||
वातः प्लीहानमुद्धूय कुपितो यस्य तिष्ठति|
शनैः परितुदन् पार्श्वं प्लीहा तस्याभिवर्धते||२८||
यस्य वायुः प्रकुपितो गुल्मस्थानेऽवतिष्ठते|

शोफं सशूलं जनयन् गुल्मस्तस्योपजायते||२९||
यस्य वायुः प्रकुपितः शोफशूलकरश्चरन्|
वङ्क्षणाद्वृषणौ याति वृद्धिस्तस्योपजायते||३०||
यस्य वातः प्रकुपितस्त्वङ्मांसान्तरमाश्रितः|
शोथं सञ्जनयेत् कुक्षावुदरं तस्य जायते||३१||
यस्य वातः प्रकुपितः कुक्षिमाश्रित्य तिष्ठति|
नाधो व्रजति नाप्यूर्ध्वमानाहस्तस्य जायते||३२||
रोगाश्चोत्सेधसामान्यदधिमांसार्बुदादयः|
विशिष्टा नामरूपाभ्यां निर्देश्याः शोथसङ्ग्रहे||३३||
वातपित्तकफा यस्य युगपत् कुपितास्त्रयः|
जिह्वामूलेऽवतिष्ठन्ते विदहन्तः समुच्छ्रिताः||३४||
जनयन्ति भृशं शोथं वेदनाश्च पृथग्विधाः|
तं शीघ्रकारिणं रोगं रोहिणीति विनिर्दिशेत्||३५||
त्रिरात्रं परमं तस्य जन्तोर्भवति जीवितम्|
कुशलेन त्वनुक्रान्तः क्षिप्रं सम्पद्यते सुखी||३६||

If the aggravated Kapha is located at the root of the tongue, it causes instantaneous swelling which is known as **Upajihvika**.

When the aggravated Kapha is located in the root of the palate, it causes instantaneous swelling; this is known as **Galashundika**.

If the aggravated Kapha is located outside the throat it causes swelling. This is known as **Galaganda** (compared with cervical lymphadenitis, goiter etc.)

When the aggravated Pitta together with Rakta spreads within the skin, it causes red swelling which is known as **Visarpa** (compared with herpes). When the aggravated Pitta is located in the Tvak (skin) and Vata, this will also cause red swelling which is known as **Pidaka** (carbuncle / abscess).

When the aggravated Pitta gets dried up in combination with Rakta, this causes skin diseases like **Tilaka** (black moles), **Piplu** (port wine mark), **Vyanga** (red moles) and **Neelika** (blue moles).

When aggravated in both the temples, the Pitta causes a serious type of swelling therein which is known as **Shankhaka**.

When the aggravated Pitta localizes in the root of the ears especially after fever, it causes a swelling which is difficult to cure and may lead to death.

When the aggravated Vata disturbs the spleen and causes pain in the sides of the abdomen, it leads to the enlargement of the spleen.
    When the aggravated Vata is localised in the abdomen this causes swelling together with pain. These result in the formation of **Gulma** (tumour / fibroid) there.

When the aggravated Vata moves from the sides of the lower abdomen to testicles and thereby causes swelling and pain there, it is known as Vruddhi (hernia / hydrocele).

When the aggravated vata is localized in the abdomen but does neither move downwards nor upwards this is known as **Udararoga** (Ascites).

When the aggravated Vata is localized within the skin and muscles (in the intestines), it causes swelling in the abdomen. This is known as Anaha (constipation).

Besides such swelling as **Adhimamsa, Arrbuda** etc. though having distinctive features of their own both by their name and form, they are all to be included under Shotha because swelling is the common feature.

When Vata, Pitta and Kapha- all the three Doshas are in morbid condition, are simultaneously aggravated and they are localized in the root of the tongue causing burning sensation and swelling, this results in swelling and causes various types of pain. This acute disease is known as Rohini. The patient suffering from these diseases can hardly survive for three nights. However, if he is quickly treated by a skilled physician, he can be cured. [19-36]

**Types of diseases based on curability:**

सन्ति ह्येवंविधा रोगाः साध्या दारुणसम्मताः।
ये हन्युरनुपक्रान्ता मिथ्याचारेण वा पुनः॥३७॥
साध्याश्चाप्यपरे सन्ति व्याधयो मृदुसम्मताः।
यत्नायत्नकृतं येषु कर्म सिध्यत्यसंशयम्॥३८॥
असाध्याश्चापरे सन्ति व्याधयो याप्यसञ्ज्ञिताः।
सुसाध्वपि कृतं येषु कर्म यात्राकरं भवेत्॥३९॥
सन्ति चाप्यपरे रोगा येषु कर्म न सिध्यति।
अपि यत्नकृतं बालैर्न तान् विद्वानुपाचरेत्॥४०॥

**Progress of diseases in general:**

- There are diseases of serious type which even though curable with difficulties can cause death if not properly treated or treated wrongly.
- There are other diseases of mild nature which are definitely cured by treatment with or without any special care.
- There is another category of palliable diseases which are not curable but even the most effective treatment will only enable the patient to stand the disease.
- There are other diseases where no treatment can succeed. Only ignorant physicians will attempt to treat such cases; wise physicians will not.

**Diseases are of two types based on curability (Prognosis):**

साध्याश्चैवाप्यसाध्याश्च व्याधयो द्विविधाः स्मृताः।
मृदुदारुणभेदेन ते भवन्ति चतुर्विधाः॥४१॥

**Diseases are of two types:**

Sadhya – curable

Asadhya – incurable. Each of them is again of two types viz. mild (Mrudu) or serious (Daruna). Thus, taken together, there are four types of diseases. [37-41].

**Innumerability of diseases:**

त एवापरिसङ्ख्येया भिद्यमाना भवन्ति हि।
रुजावर्णसमुत्थानस्थानसंस्थाननामभिः॥४२॥
व्यवस्थाकरणं तेषां यथास्थूलेषु सङ्ग्रहः।
तथा प्रकृतिसामान्यं विकारेषूपदिश्यते॥४३॥

**Innumerability of diseases:**

In fact diseases are of innumerable varieties depending upon their distinctive features like pain, color (signs), etiology, site of origin and manifestation (like abdomen, Rasadatu, etc.), symptoms (like Gulma or tumor etc.) and nomenclature (like Rajayaksma, Shosha etc). Only important diseases have, however, been enumerated (in Sutrasthana 19th chapter). Other diseases are classified similarly according to the factors involved in their manifestation. [42-43]

**Correct approach to the diagnosis and treatment of diseases:**

विकारनामाकुशलो न जिह्रीयात् कदाचन।
न हि सर्वविकाराणां नामतोऽस्ति ध्रुवा स्थितिः||४४||
स एव कुपितो दोषः समुत्थानविशेषतः।
स्थानान्तरगतश्चैव जनयत्यामयान् बहून् ||४५||
तस्मादि्वकारप्रकृतीरधिष्ठानान्तराणि च।
समुत्थानविशेषांश्च बुद्ध्वा कर्म समाचरेत्||४६||
यो ह्येतत्त्रितयं ज्ञात्वा कर्माण्यारभते भिषक्।
ज्ञानपूर्वं यथान्यायं स कर्मसु न मुह्यति||४७||

**Correct approach to the diagnosis and treatment of diseases:**

If a physician is not able to name a particular disease, he should not feel ashamed on that account because it is not always possible to name all types of diseases in definite terms. When aggravated, a single Dosha may cause many fold diseases depending upon the various etiological factors and the sites of manifestation.

So a physician should try to comprehend the nature of the disease based on Dosha, the site of its manifestation and etiological factors and should then initiate the treatment, A physician who so initiates the treatment after having full knowledge of the therapeutic properties of these three aspects and paying due regard to scriptural instructions would never fail in his attempt to cure the disease. [44-47]

**Relation of Doshas with body:**

नित्याः प्राणभृतां देहे वातपित्तकफास्त्रयः।
विकृताः प्रकृतिस्था वा तान् बुभुत्सेत पण्डितः||४८||

The three Doshas, viz. Vata, Pitta and Kapha are already present in the body of all creatures. A physician should try to know whether they are in normal or morbid condition. [48]

**Functions of normal Doshas :**

उत्साहोच्छ्वासनिः श्वासचेष्टा धातुगतिः समा।
समो मोक्षो गतिमतां वायोः कर्माविकारजम्||४९||
दर्शनं पक्तिरूष्मा च क्षुत्तृष्णा देहमार्दवम्।
प्रभा प्रसादो मेधा च पित्तकर्माविकारजम्||५०||
स्नेहो बन्धः स्थिरत्वं च गौरवं वृषता बलम्।
क्षमा धृतिरलोभश्च कफकर्माविकारजम्||५१||

## Normal Functions of Vata Dosha:

When Vata is in its normal state, it reflects itself in the form of
Utsaha – enthusiasm,
Uchvasa – inspiration,
Nishvasa – expiration,
Cheshta – movements,
Vega Pravartana – expression of natural urges – like urination, etc.
Normal metabolic transformation of tissues and proper elimination of excreta

## Normal functions of Pitta Dosha :

Darshana – good vision,
Pakti – good digestion,
Ushma – normal temperature,
Kshut – normal hunger,
Trushna – thirst,
Mardava – bodily softness,
Prabha – luster,
Prasaada – happiness,
Medha - intelligence

## Normal functions of Kapha Dosha :
Effects of Kapha in its normal state are
Sneha – unctuousness, oiliness,
Bandha – cohesion, compactness,
Sthiratva – steadiness,
Gaurava – heaviness,
Vrushata – virility,
Bala – strength,
Kshama – forbearance,
Dhruti – patience, good memory and retention power
Alobha – lack of greed [49-51]

## Functions of abnormal Doshas:

वाते पित्ते कफे चैव क्षीणे लक्षणमुच्यते|
कर्मणः प्राकृताद्धानिर्वृद्धिर्वाऽपि विरोधिनाम्||५२||

The diminution of Vata, Pitta and Kapha is indicated by the decrease in their respective normal actions or increase in their respective opposite actions. [52]

दोषप्रकृतिवैशेष्यं नियतं वृद्धिलक्षणम्|
दोषाणां प्रकृतिर्हानिर्वृद्धिश्चैव परीक्ष्यते||५३||

The aggravation of Doshas is invariably indicated by something in excess of their respective normal action. Thus, one can examine the normal condition deficiency or aggravation of Doshas as the case may be. [53]

**To sum up:**

तत्र श्लोकाः-
सङ्ख्यां निमित्तं रूपाणि शोथानां साध्यतां न च|
तेषां तेषां विकाराणां शोथांस्तांस्तांश्च पूर्वजान्||५४||
विधिभेदं विकाराणां त्रिविधं बोध्यसङ्ग्रहम्|
प्राकृतं कर्म दोषाणां लक्षणं हानिवृद्धिषु||५५||
वीतमोहरजोदोषलोभमानमदस्पृहः|
व्याख्यातवांस्त्रिशोथीये रोगाध्याये पुनर्वसुः||५६||

Lord Punarvasu who is free from attachment, Rajas, greed, ego, pride and desire has explained in this chapter on" The three types of swellings" the following: types, etiology, signs and symptoms, curability or otherwise of swellings, the swelling that appear as premonitory signs of various diseases, different types of diseases, the important points which are to be kept in view during treatment, the normal functions of Doshas and signs and symptoms of diminished or aggravated Doshas. [54-56]

इत्यग्निवेशकृते तन्त्रे चरकप्रतिसंस्कृते श्लोकस्थाने त्रिशोथीयो नामाष्टादशोऽध्यायः||१८||
Thus ends the eighteenth chapter on "Trishotheeya Adhyaya - The Three Types of Swelling" of the Sutra section of Agnivesha's work as redacted by Charaka.

# 19

# Sutrasthana Chapter 19
# Ashtodareeyam

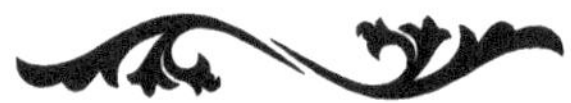

**Ashtodareeya Adhyaya**

**Ayurvedic Disease Classification :**

अथातोऽष्टोदरीयमध्यायं व्याख्यास्यामः॥१॥

इति ह स्माह भगवानात्रेयः॥२॥

The 19th chapter of Charaka Samhita Sutrasthana is called Ashtodareeya Adhyaya. This chapter deals with scientific disease classification based on Ayurvedic principles. Ashta Udareeya means eight types of Udara (ascites) disease.

**Number of the various types of diseases:**

इह खल्वष्टावुदराणि, अष्टौ मूत्राघाताः, अष्टौ क्षीरदोषाः, अष्टौ रेतोदोषाः; सप्त कुष्ठानि, सप्त पिडकाः, सप्त वीसर्पाः; षडतीसाराः, षडुदावर्ताः; पञ्च गुल्माः, पञ्च प्लीहदोषाः, पञ्च कासाः, पञ्च श्वासाः, पञ्च हिक्काः, पञ्च तृष्णाः, पञ्च छर्दयः, पञ्च भक्तस्यानशनस्थानानि, पञ्च शिरोरोगाः, पञ्च हृद्रोगाः, पञ्च पाण्डुरोगाः, पञ्चोन्मादाः, चत्वारोऽपस्माराः, चत्वारोऽक्षिरोगाः, चत्वारः कर्णरोगाः, चत्वारः प्रतिश्यायाः, चत्वारो मुखरोगाः, चत्वारो ग्रहणीदोषाः, चत्वारो मदाः, चत्वारो मूर्च्छायाः, चत्वारः शोषाः, चत्वारि क्लैब्यानि; त्रयः शोफाः, त्रीणि किलासानि, त्रिविधं लोहितपित्तं; द्वौ ज्वरौ, द्वौ व्रणौ, द्वावायामौ, द्वे गृध्रस्यौ, द्वे कामले, द्विविधमामं, द्विविधं वातरक्तं, द्विविधान्यर्शांसि; एक ऊरुस्तम्भः, एकः सन्न्यासः, एको महागदः; विंशतिः क्रिमिजातयः, विंशतिः प्रमेहाः, विंशतिर्योनिव्यापदः; इत्यष्टचत्वारिंशद्रोगाधिकरणान्यस्मिन् सङ्ग्रहे समुद्दिष्टानि॥३॥

**Number of the various types of diseases:**

There are :

8 types of Udara (Ascites – abdominal diseases),

8 types of Mutraghata (urinary obstruction),

8 types of Ksheera Dosha (breast milk vitiation),

8 types of Reto Dosha (semen vitiation),

7 types of Kushta (skin disorders)

7 types of Pidaka (carbuncles)

7 types of Visarpa (spreading type of skin disorder)

6 types of Atisara (diarrhea / dysentery)

6 types of Udavarta (reverse movement of Vata)

5 types of Gulma (abdominal tumor)

5 types of Pleeha Dosha (spleen disorders)

5 types of Kasa (cold and cough)

5 types of Shwasa (asthma, dyspnoea, difficulty in breathing)

5 types of Hikka (hiccups)

5 types of Trushna (excessive thirst)
5 types of Chardi (vomiting)
5 types of anorexia
5 types of Shiroroga (disorders of head)
5 types of Hridroga (heart disorders)
5 types of Pandu (anaemia, early stage of liver disorder)
5 types of Unmada (insanity)

4 types of Apasmara (epilepsy)
4 types of Akshi Roga (eye disorder)
4 types of Karna Roga (ear disorders)
4 types of Pratishyaya (coryza / running nose)
4 types of Mukha Roga (oral cavity disorders)
4 types of Grahani Dosha (malabsorption syndrome / IBS)
4 types of Mada (intoxication)
4 types of Murcha (Syncope / unconsciousness)
4 types of Shosha (emaciation)
4 types of Klaibya (impotency)
   3 types of Shopha (inflammation)
3 types of Kilasa (a type of leucoderma)
3 types of Raktpitta (bleeding disorder)
   2 types of Jwara (fever)
2 types of Vrana (ulcer)
2 types of Ayama (tetanus, leading to bending of body)
2 types of Gridhrasi (lumbar spondylosis / sciatica)
2 types of Kamala (jaundice)
2 types of Ama (disturbed digestion and absorption process)
2 types of Vatarakta (gout)
2 types of Arsha (haemorrhoids)
   1 type of Urusthamba (thigh stiffness)
1 type of Sanyasa (coma)
1 type of Mahagada (psycho-neurosis)
   20 types of Krimi (intestinal worms)
20 types of Prameha (urinary disorders)
20 types of Yoni Vyapat (gynaecological disorders)
   Like this, there exist 48 diseases with its types. [3]

**Classification of diseases having eight types:**

**8 types of Udara (ascites) :**

एतानि यथोद्देशमभिनिर्देक्ष्यामः-
अष्टावुदराणीति वातपित्तकफसन्निपातप्लीहबद्धच्छिद्रदकोदराणि, अष्टौ मूत्राघाता इति वातपित्तकफसन्निपाताश्मरीशर्कराशुक्रशोणितजाः, अष्टौ क्षीरदोषा इति वैवर्ण्यं वैगन्ध्यं वैरस्यं पैच्छिल्यं फेनसङ्घातो रौक्ष्यं गौरवमतिस्नेहश्च, अष्टौ रेतोदोषा इति तनु शुष्कं फेनिलमश्वेतं पूत्यतिपिच्छलमन्यधातूपहितमवसादि च (१)

**Classification of diseases having eight types:**

**8 types of Udara (ascites) :**
Vatika (because of Vata),
Paittika (because of Pitta),
Shlaishmika (because of Kapha),
Sannipatika (Due to combined influence of Vata, Pitta and Kapha),
Plihodara, (due to splenic disorder – splenomegaly),
Baddhodara – also called as Baddha Gudodara (due to intestinal obstruction),
Childrodara (Chidra means rupture, it is due to intestinal perforation),
Dakodara / Udakodara / Jalodara (ascites)

**2. Eight Mutraghatas (dysuria – difficulty in passing urine):**

Vatika (due to Vata),
Paittika (due to Pitta),
Shalismika (due to Kapha),
Sannipataja (due to combined aggravation of vata, pitta and kapha)
Ashmarija (due to stone / calculi in urinary tract),
Sharkaraja (due to gravels in urinary tract),
Shukraja (due to semen, a condition called as spermolyth),
Shonitaja (due to vitiation of blood).

**3. Eight Ksheera Dosha (Vitiation of milk)**

Vaivarnya – Discoloration,
Vaigandhya – bad smell,
Vairasya – bad taste,
Paicchilya – sliminess, highly sticky,
Phenasangata – foaminess,
Raukshya – excessively dry,
Gaurava – excess heaviness,
Atisneha – unctuousness, excessive oiliness.

**4. Eight Reto doshas(seminal disorder)**

Tanu – Thinness,
Shushka – dryness,
Phenila – foaminess,
Ashveta – absence of whiteness,
Atipoota – putrid smell,
Atipicchila – over sliminess, stickiness
Anya Dhatu Upahita – combination with other Dhatus (tissue elements), like presence of blood
Avasadi – heavy, less viscous, high specific gravity.

**Classification of diseases having seven types:**

सप्त कुष्ठानीति कपालोदुम्बरमण्डलर्ष्यजिह्वपुण्डरीकसिध्मकाकणानि, सप्त पिडका इति शराविका कच्छपिका जालिनी सर्षप्यलजी विनता विद्रधी च, सप्त विसर्पा इति वातपित्तकफाग्निकर्दमकग्रन्थिसन्निपाताख्याः (२)

5. Seven types of Kusthas (skin diseases) – Kapala, Udumbara, Mandala, Rushyajihva, Pundarika, Sidhma and

Kaakanaka.

6. Seven types of Pidakas (abscess or carbuncle) - Sharavika, Kacchapika, Jalini, Sarsapi, Alaji, Vinata and Vidradhi.

7. Seven types of Visarapa (spreading type of skin diseases) – Vatika, Paittika, Slaismika, Agnivisarpa, Kardamaka, Granthi Visarpa and Sannipatika Visarpa (due to combined influence of Vata, Pitta and Kapha).

षडतीसारा इति वातपित्तकफसन्निपातभयशोकजाः, षडुदावर्ता इति वातमूत्रपुरीषशुक्रच्छर्दिक्षवथुजाः (३)

## Classification of diseases having six types:

8. Six types of Atisara (diarrhoea) – Vatika, Pittika, Slaismika, Sannipatika, Bhayaja (due to fear) and Shokaja (due to grief).

9. Six types of Udavartas (abdominal diseases characterized by retention of feces) - Vataja (due to flatus), Mutraja (due to urine), Pureeshaa (due to faeces), Shukraja (due to semen), Chardija (due to vomiting) and Kshavathuja (due to sneezing).

## Classification of diseases having five types:

पञ्च गुल्मा इति वातपित्तकफसन्निपातशोणितजाः, पञ्च प्लीहदोषा इति गुल्मैर्व्याख्याताः, पञ्च कासा इति वातपित्तकफक्षतक्षयजाः, पञ्च श्वासा इति महोर्ध्वच्छिन्नतमकक्षुद्राः, पञ्च हिक्का इति महती गम्भीरा व्यपेता क्षुद्राऽन्नजा च, पञ्च तृष्णा इति वातपित्तामक्षयोपसर्गात्मिकाः, पञ्च छर्दय इति द्विष्टार्थसंयोगजा वातपित्तकफसन्निपातोद्रेकोत्थाश्च, पञ्च भक्तस्यानशनस्थानानीति वातपित्तकफसन्निपातद्वेषाः, पञ्च शिरोरोगा इति पूर्वोद्देशमभिसमस्य वातपित्तकफसन्निपातक्रिमिजाः, पञ्च हृद्रोगा इति शिरोरोगैर्व्याख्याताः, पञ्च पाण्डुरोगा इति वातपित्तकफसन्निपातमृद्भक्षणजाः, पञ्चोन्मादा इति वातपित्तकफसन्निपातागन्तुनिमिताः (४)

10. Five types of Gulmas (abdominal tumor) – Vatika, Paittika, Shlaismika, Sannipatika and Raktaja (due to blood)
11. Five types of Pleeha – Splenic disorders (as above)
12. Five types of Kasa (coughing) - Vatika, Paittika, Shlaismika, Kshataja (due to ulceration / injury) and Kshayaja (due to tissue wasting, as in tuberculosis).
13. Five types of Shvasa (dyspnoea) – Maha Shvasa, Urdhva Shvasa, Chinna Shvasa, Tamaka Shvasa and Kshudra Svasa
14. Five types of Hikkas (hiccup) – Maha Hikka, Gambhira Hikka, Vyapeta Hikka (intermittent), Kshudra Hikka and Annaja Hikka (due to food)
15. Five types of Trsna (Thirst) - Vatika, Paittika, Amaja (due to improper digestion), Kshayaja (due to tissue depletion) and Upasargatmika (as a secondary development, due to another disease)
16. Five types of Chardi (Vomiting) - Dvishtartha Samyogaja (that which is caused by coming in contact with obnoxious articles), Vatika, Paittika, Slaismika and Sannipatika
17. Five types of Aruchi (Anorexia) - Vatika, Paittika, Shlaismika, Sannipatika and Dveshaja (due to repugnance)
18. Five types of Shiro roga (head disorder) - Vatika, Pittika, Shlaismika, Sannipatika and Krimija (due to infection)
19. Five types of Hrdroga (heart diseases) (as above) – Vatika, Pittika, Shlaismika, Sannipatika and Krimija (due to infection)
20. Five types of Pandu (anemia) - Vatika, Paittika, Shlaismika, Sannipatika and Mrit bhaksanaja (due to eating mud)
21. Five types of Uamada (insanity) - Vatika, Paittika, Shlaismika, Sannipatika and Agantuja (due to exogenous causes)

## Classification of diseases having four types:

चत्वारोऽपस्मारा इति वातपित्तकफसन्निपातनिमिताः, चत्वारोऽक्षिरोगाश्चत्वारः कर्णरोगाश्चत्वारः प्रतिश्यायाश्चत्वारो मुखरोगाश्चत्वारो ग्रहणीदोषाश्चत्वारो मदाश्चत्वारो मूर्च्छाया इत्यपस्मारैर्व्याख्याताः, चत्वारः शोषा इति साहससन्धारणक्षयविषमाशनजाः, चत्वारि

क्लैब्यानीति बीजोपघातादुद्धवजभङ्गाज्जरायाः शुक्रक्षयाच्च (५)

22. Four types of Apasmara (epilepsy) - Vatika, Paittika, Shlaishmika and Sannipatika
23. Four types of Eye diseases, same as above
24. Four types of Ear diseases, same as above
25. Four types of Pratisyayas (coryza), same as above
26. Four types of Grahani (malabsorption syndrome / IBS) – same as above
27. Four types of Mada (intoxication), same as above
28. Four types of Muka Roga (diseases of oral cavity) – same as above
29. Four types of Murcha (fainting / syncope) – same as above
30. Four types of Shosha (emaciation) - due to overstrain, suppression of natural urges, tissue wasting and irregular dieting.
31. Four types of Klaibya (impotency) – bejeopaghataja (due to the affliction sperm /ovum), dhvajabhanagaja (due to erectile dysfunction), Jaraja (due to old age) and Sukra kshayaja (due to diminution of semen)

**Classification of diseases having three types:**

त्रयः शोथा इति वातपित्तश्लेष्मनिमित्ताः, त्रीणि किलासानीति रक्तताम्रशुक्लानि, त्रिविधं लोहितपित्तमिति ऊर्ध्वभागमधोभागमुभयभागं च (६)

32. Three types of Shothas (oedema) - Vatika, Paittika, Slaismika .
33. Three types of Kilasas (an obstinate skin diseases) – leucoderma, coppery and white colored
34. Three types of Raktapittas (a disease characterized by bleeding from various parts of the body) - Urdhvabhaga (affecting the upper channel), Adhobhaga (affecting the lower channel) and Ubhayabhaga (affecting both upper and lower channels).

**Classification of diseases having two types:**

द्वौ ज्वराविति उष्णाभिप्रायः शीतसमुत्थश्च शीताभिप्रायश्चोष्णसमुत्थः, द्वौ व्रणाविति निजश्चागन्तुजश्च, द्वावायामाविति बाह्यश्चाभ्यन्तरश्च, द्वे गृध्रस्याविति वाताद्वातकफाच्च, द्वे कामले इति कोष्ठाश्रया शाखाश्रया च, द्विविधमाममिति अलसको विसूचिका च, द्विविधं वातरक्तमिति गम्भीरमुत्तानं च, द्विविधान्यर्शांसीति शुष्काण्यार्द्राणि च (७)

35. Two types of Jvara (fever)
**(1) Ushnabhipraya – Arising out of cold where the patient is desirous of hot substance,**
**(2) Sheeta Samuttha – arising out of heat where the patient is desirous of cold substances.**
36. Two types of Vranas (ulcer) Nija – Endogenous and Agantuja – exogenous.
37. Two types of Ayamas (body bending) – Bahirayama – Opisthotonus and Antarayama – emprosthotonos.
38. Two types of Gridhrasi (sciatica) - Vatika and Vata-Shlaismika
39. Two types of Kamala (Jaundice) - Kostashraya (Hepatic and Prehepatic) and Shakhasraya (Obstructive)
40. Two types of Ama (disorders due to improper digestion and metabolism) - Alasaka and Visuchika
41. Two types of Vatarakta (Gout) – Gambhira (deep) and utthana (superficial)
42. Two types of Arshas (piles) – Shushka (non-bleeding) and Ardra (bleeding)

**Diseases having only one type:**

एक ऊरुस्तम्भ इत्यामत्रिदोषसमुत्थः, एकः सन्न्यास इति त्रिदोषात्मको मनःशरीराधिष्ठानः, एको महागद इति अतत्त्वाभिनिवेशः (८)

43. One type of Urustamabha - caused by - Ama-Tridoshaja
44. One types of Sanyasa (Coma) – Sannipatika
45. One Mahagada (Psychic perversion) due to mental and moral perversion

**Classification of diseases having twenty types:**

एक ऊरुस्तम्भ इत्यामत्रिदोषसमुत्थः, एकः सन्न्यास इति त्रिदोषात्मको मनःशरीराधिष्ठानः, एको महागद इति अतत्त्वाभिनिवेशः (८)
विंशतिः क्रिमिजातय इति यूका पिपीलिकाश्चेति द्विविधा बहिर्मलजाः, केशादा लोमादा लोमद्वीपाः सौरसा औदुम्बरा जन्तुमातरश्चेति षट्
शोणितजाः, अन्त्रादा उदरावेष्टा हृदयादाश्चुरवो दर्भपुष्पाः सौगन्धिका महागुदाश्चेति सप्त कफजाः, ककेरुका मकेरुका लेलिहाः सशूलकाः
सौसुरादाश्चेति पञ्च पुरीषजा; विंशतिः प्रमेहा इत्युदकमेहश्चेक्षुबालिकारसमेहश्च सान्द्रमेहश्च सान्द्रप्रसादमेहश्च शुक्लमेहश्च शुक्रमेहश्च
शीतमेहश्च शनैर्मेहश्च सिकतामेहश्च लालामेहश्चेति दश श्लेष्मनिमित्ताः, क्षारमेहश्च कालमेहश्च नीलमेहश्च लोहितमेहश्च मञ्जिष्ठामेहश्च
हरिद्रामेहश्चेति षट् पित्तनिमित्ताः, वसामेहश्च मज्जामेहश्च हस्तिमेहश्च मधुमेहश्चेति चत्वारो वातनिमित्ताः, इति विंशतिः प्रमेहाः;
विंशतिर्योनिव्यापद इति वातिकी पैत्तिकी श्लेष्मिकी सान्निपातिकी चेति चतस्रो दोषजाः, दोषदूष्यसंसर्गप्रकृतिनिर्देशैरवशिष्टाः षोडश
निर्दिश्यन्ते, तद्यथा- रक्तयोनिश्चारजस्का चाचरणा चातिचरणा च प्राक्चरणा चोपप्लुता च परिप्लुता चोदावर्तिनी च कर्णिनी च पुत्रघ्नी
चान्तर्मुखी च सूचीमुखी च शुष्का च वामिनी च षण्ढयोनिश्च महायोनिश्चेति विंशतिर्योनिव्यापदो भवन्ति (९)

**46. Twenty Krimis (germs including parasites):**

Yuka and Pipilika both reside outside the body in the excreta,
6 - Due to blood vitiation – Keshada, Lomada, Saurasa, Audumbara and Jantumatr
7 – Due to Kapha vitiation – Antra, Udaravesta, Hrdayada, Curu, Darbhapuspa, saugandhika and Mahaguda
5 – Pureeshaja – inhabit in feces – Kakeruka, Makeruka, Leliha, Sasulaka, and Sausurada

**47. Twenty Prameha (a kind of urinary disorder):**

10 types due to Kapha imbalance – Udakameha, Iksudalikarasameha, sandrameha, sandraprasadameha, Suklameha, Sukrameha, Sutameha, Sanairmeha, Sikatameha and Lalameha
6 types due to Pitta imbalance – Ksharameha, Kalameha, Nilameha Lohitameha, Manjisthameha and Haridrameha
4 types due to Vata imbalance – Vasameha, Majjameha, Hastimeha and Madhumeha.

**48. Twenty Yoniroga** - (diseases of the female genital tract), Vatika, Paittika, Slaismika and Sannipatika, Raktayoni (menorrhagia), Arajaska (Amenorrhea), Acharana (colpitis mycotica), Aticharana (chronic vaginitis), Prakcharana (deflorative vaginitis), Upapluta (secondary dysmenorrhea), Paripluta (acute vaginitis), Udavartini (primary dysmenorrhea), Karnini (endo-cervicitis), Putraghni (abortive tendency), Antarmukhi (inversion of uterus), Suchimukhi (pin hole os), Shushka (Colo-xerosis), Vamini (Profluvium seminis), Sandhyaoni (undeveloped female sex organs) and Mahayoni (Prolapse of the uterus).

केवलश्चायमुद्देशो यथोद्देशमभिनिर्दिष्टो भवति||४||

The above mentioned are the forty-eight diseases described in brief. Details thereof will be enumerated subsequently. [4]

**Simile regarding the role of doshas in etiopathogenesis of diseases:**

सर्व एव निजा विकारा नान्यत्र वातपित्तकफेभ्यो निर्वर्तन्ते, यथाहि- शकुनिः सर्वं दिवसमपि परिपतन् स्वां छायां नातिवर्तते, तथा
स्वधातुवैषम्यनिमित्ताः सर्वे विकारा वातपित्तकफान्नातिवर्तन्ते|
वातपित्तश्लेष्मणां पुनः स्थानसंस्थानप्रकृतिविशेषानभिसमीक्ष्य तदात्मकानपि च सर्वविकारां स्तानेवोपदिशन्ति बुद्धिमन्तः||५||

All the endogenous diseases occur invariably due to the vitiation of Vata, Pitta and Kapha. The bird cannot transgress its own shadow even though flying throughout the day. Similarly no endogenous diseases caused by the disturbance of equilibrium of Dhatus can occur without the vitiation of Vata, Pitta and Kapha. So, considering the location, signs, symptoms and causes of vitiation of Vata, Pitta and Kapha, all the diseases caused by them are diagnosed on the basis of the vitiation of respective Doshas. [5]

**Difference in the exogenous and endogenous diseases:**

भवतश्चात्र-
स्वधातुवैषम्यनिमित्तजा ये विकारसङ्घा बहवः शरीरे।
न ते पृथक् पित्तकफानिलेभ्य आगन्तवस्त्वेव ततो विशिष्टाः॥६॥

Thus, it is said:
All the bodily diseases arising due to disturbance of the equilibrium of Dhatus are ultimately caused by nothing but the imbalance of Pitta, Kapha and or Vata. It is only the exogenous diseases which are caused otherwise. [6]

**Coexistence of exogenous and endogenous diseases:**

आगन्तुरन्वेति निजं विकारं निजस्तथाऽऽगन्तुमपि प्रवृद्धः।
तत्रानुबन्धं प्रकृतिं च सम्यग् ज्ञात्वा ततः कर्म समारभेत॥७॥

**Coexistence of exogenous and endogenous diseases:**

The endogenous diseases are at times followed by the exogenous ones and even the exogenous ones are followed by the endogenous ones of the most vehement type. One should accordingly start the treatment paying due regard to the secondary development (anubandha) and the primary nature of the disease [7].

**Summary:**

तत्र श्लोकौ-
विंशकाश्चैककाश्चैव त्रिकाश्चोक्तास्त्रयस्त्रयः।
द्विकाश्चाष्टौ, चतुष्काश्च दश, द्वादश पञ्चकाः॥८॥
चत्वारश्चाष्टका वर्गाः, षट्कौ द्वौ, सप्तकास्त्रयः।
अष्टोदरीये रोगाणां रोगाध्याये प्रकाशिताः॥९॥

In the chapter Ashtodareeya Adhyaya, three diseases in each having twenty varieties, one variety an three varieties, eight diseases having two varieties, ten diseases having four varieties, twelve diseases having five varieties, four diseases having eight varieties, two diseases having six varieties and three diseases having seven varieties are described. [8-9]

इत्यग्निवेशकृते तन्त्रे चरकप्रतिसंस्कृते श्लोकस्थानेऽष्टोदरीयो नामोनविंशोऽध्यायः॥१९॥
Thus ends this chapter, written by Master Agnivesha and redacted by Master Charaka. [19]

# 20

# Sutrasthana Chapter 20 Maharogam

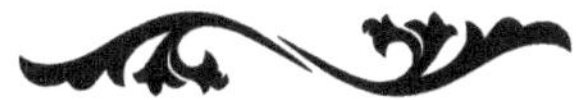

**Maharoga Adhyaya**
**Qualities, Diseases, Treatment of Vata, Pitta and Kapha:**
अथातो महारोगाध्यायं व्याख्यास्यामः॥१॥
इति ह स्माह भगवानात्रेयः॥२॥

The 20th Chapter of Charaka Samhita Sutrasthana is called Maharoga Adhyaya. This is one of the most important chapters. It enlists diseases caused by individual Tridosha – Vata, Pitta and Kapha, qualities of Tridosha, how they cause disease, patho-physiology and their line of treatment

**General classifications of diseases:**
चत्वारो रोगा भवन्ति- आगन्तुवातपित्तश्लेष्मनिमित्ताः; तेषां चतुर्णामपि रोगाणां रोगत्वमेकविधं भवति,
रुक्सामान्यात्; द्विविधा पुनः प्रकृतिरेषाम्, आगन्तुनिजविभागात्; द्विविधं चैषामधिष्ठानं,
मनःशरीरविशेषात्; विकाराः पुनरपरिसङ्ख्येयाः, प्रकृत्यधिष्ठानलिङ्गायतनविकल्पविशेषापरिसङ्ख्येयत्वात्॥३॥

**General classifications of diseases:**
There are four types of diseases viz.
Agantuja – due to exogenous causes such as injury, poison etc.,
Vatika – Vata imbalance disorders,
Paittika – Pitta imbalance disorders and
Shlaishmika – Kapha imbalance disorders.

Pain being common to all, diseases are finally of one type (ruk samanyaat).
Diseases are again of two types depending on their nature,
Agantuja – that is exogenous
Nija – endogenous.

They are again of two types
Shareera Adhishtana – somatic
Mano Adhishtana – psychic-depending on the sites of their manifestation viz. body and mind.

Diseases are in fact innumerable in as much as the immediate causes, (like improper diet and regimen) permutation and combination of various factors of Doshas are innumerable (Aparisankhyeya). [3]

**General causative factors:**

मुखानि   तु   खल्वागन्तोर्नखदशनपतनाभिचाराभिशापाभिषङ्गाभिघातव्यध-   बन्धनवेष्टनपीडनरज्जुदहनशस्त्राशनिभूतोपसर्गादीनि,
निजस्य तु मुखं वातपित्तश्लेष्मणां वैषम्यम्||४||

**General causative factors:**

The Agantuja Roga – exogenous diseases are caused by:

- Nakha – injury caused by nails / scratch,
- Dashana – injury caused by teeth / bite,
- Patana – fall,
- Abhichara – spell,
- Shaapa – curse,
- Abhishanga – psychic afflictions including demoniac seizure,
- Abhighata – injury,
- Vyadha – piercing,
- Bandhana – bandage,
- Veshtana – rapping,
- Peedana – application of pressure,
- Rajju – binding by rope,
- Dahana – fire,
- Shastra – weapon,
- Ashani – thunderbolt,
- Bhuta – demoniac seizure,
- Upasarga – natural calamities etc.

The Nija Rogas – endogenous diseases are caused by the imbalance of Tridosha – Vata, Pitta and Kapha. [4]
**Three basic causative features all diseases:**

द्वयोस्तु खल्वागन्तुनिजयोः प्रेरणमसात्म्येन्द्रियार्थसंयोगः, प्रज्ञापराधः, परिणामश्चेति||५||

**Three basic causative features all diseases:**

The below mentioned three constitute the common causative factors for both the exogenous and endogenous types of diseases :

**Asatmya Indriya Artha Samyoga** – Unwholesome contacts between the sense organs and their objects,
**Prajnaparadha** – intellectual blasphemy, acting against one's conscience
**Parinama** – Effects of time [5]

सर्वेऽपि तु खल्वेतेऽभिप्रवृद्धाश्चत्वारो रोगाः परस्परमनुबध्नन्ति, न चान्योन्येन सह सन्देहमापद्यन्ते ||६||

All these four types of diseases when aggravated do share the symptoms of each other. Even then, the distinctive features of each one of them are too clearly manifested avoiding any confusion. [6]

**Role of Doshas in the pathogenesis of exogenous and endogenous diseases:**

आगन्तुर्हि व्यथापूर्वं समुत्पन्नो जघन्यं वातपित्तश्लेष्मणां वैषम्यमापादयति; निजे तु वातपित्तश्लेष्माणः पूर्वं वैषम्यमापद्यन्ते जघन्यं व्यथामभिनिर्वर्तयन्ति||७||

**Role of Doshas in the pathogenesis of exogenous and endogenous diseases:**

The exogenous diseases (Agantu Roga) begin with pain and then they bring about the disturbance in the Tridosha balance. The endogenous diseases begin with the disturbance in the Tridosha balance, and then result in pain. [7] So, in both Njia and Agantu diseases, ultimately Tridosha imbalance is noted.

**Physiological sites of Doshas in the body:**

**Place of Vata Dosha :**

तेषां त्रयाणामपि दोषाणां शरीरे स्थानविभाग उपदेक्ष्यते; तद्यथा- बस्तिः पुरीषाधानं कटिः सक्थिनी पादावस्थीनि पक्वाशयश्च वातस्थानानि, तत्रापि पक्वाशयो विशेषेण वातस्थानं;

Basti – Urinary bladder, urinary system
Pureeshaadhaana – rectum,
Sakthi – waist,
Padau – thighs, legs,
Asthi – bones and
Pakvashaya – colon are the sites of Vata
Among them, Pakvashaya (colon) is the most important site.

**Place of Pitta Dosha :**

स्वेदो रसो लसीका रुधिरमामाशयश्च पित्तस्थानानि, तत्राप्यामाशयो विशेषेण पित्तस्थानम्;

**Place of Pitta Dosha :**

The important sites of location of these three Doshas are as below:
Svedo – Sweat,
Rasa – Rasa dhatu – end product of food digestion, containing all nutrients
Lasika – Lymph,
Rudhira – blood,
Amashaya – small intestine (lower part of Amashaya) are the sites of pitta;
Among them, small intestine (lower part of Amashaya) is the most important site of Pitta Dosha.

**Place of Kapha Dosha :**

उरः शिरो ग्रीवा पर्वाण्यामाशयो मेदश्च श्लेष्मस्थानानि, तत्राप्युरो विशेषेण श्लेष्मस्थानम्||८||

Ura – Chest,
Shira – head,
Greeva – neck,
Parva – joint,
Amashaya – stomach (upper part of Amashaya) and

Meda – fat are the sites of Shleshma (Kapha).
Among them, chest is the most important site of Kapha Dosha. [8]

**General functions of balanced Doshas:**

सर्वशरीरचरास्तु वातपित्तश्लेष्माणः सर्वस्मिञ्छरीरे कुपिताकुपिताः शुभाशुभानि कुर्वन्ति- प्रकृतिभूताः शुभान्युपचयबलवर्णप्रसादादीनि, अशुभानि पुनर्विकृतिमापन्ना विकारसञ्ज्ञकानि||९||

All the three Doshas are present in all parts of the body. These Doshas, in normal balanced condition, cause good health and in imbalanced condition, they cause illness.
When they are balanced, they cause
Upachaya – body nourishment
Bala – improvement of strength and immunity
Varna Prasada – improvement of skin health and complexion [9]

**Diseases caused by Tridosha Imbalance:**

Endogenous diseases (Nija Roga) are again of two types viz,
Samanyaja Vyadhi – diseases caused by Vata, Pitta and Kapha in different combinations and
Nanatmaja Vyadhi – specific diseases caused by individual Doshas – Vata, Pitta and Kapha.

**Samanyaja Vyadhi –** Diseases of the combined Doshas are explained in the preceding chapter and diseases caused by individual imbalanced Doshas are being explained here.

**Nanatmaja Vyadhi :**

तत्र विकाराः सामान्यजा, नानात्मजाश्च|
तत्र सामान्यजाः पूर्वमष्टोदरीये व्याख्याताः, नानात्मजांस्त्विहाध्यायेऽनुव्याख्यास्यामः|
तद्यथा- अशीतिर्वातविकाराः, चत्वारिंशत् पित्तविकाराः, विंशतिः श्लेष्मविकाराः||१०||

**Diseases caused by individual Doshas :**

Vata when imbalanced alone, causes 80 types of disorders
Pitta when imbalanced alone, causes 40 types of disorders
Kapha, when imbalanced alone, causes 20 types of disorders. [10]

**Eighty diseases caused by Vata alone – Vataja Nanatmaja Vyadhi:**

तत्रादौ वातविकाराननुव्याख्यास्यामः|
तद्यथा- नखभेदश्च, विपादिका च, पादशूलं च, पादभ्रंशश्च, पादसुप्तता च, वातखुड्डता च, गुल्फग्रहश्च, पिण्डिकोद्वेष्टनं च, गृध्रसी च, जानुभेदश्च, जानुविश्लेषश्च, ऊरुस्तम्भश्च, ऊरुसादश्च, पाङ्गुल्यं च, गुदभ्रंशश्च, गुदार्तिश्च, वृषणाक्षेपश्च, शेफस्तम्भश्च, वङ्क्षणानाहश्च, श्रोणिभेदश्च, विड्भेदश्च, उदावर्तश्च, खञ्जत्वं च, कुब्जत्वं च, वामनत्वं च, त्रिकग्रहश्च, पृष्ठग्रहश्च, पार्श्वावमर्दश्च, उदरावेष्टश्च, हृन्मोहश्च, हृद्द्रवश्च, वक्षौद्घर्षश्च, वक्षौपरोधश्च, वक्षस्तोदश्च, बाहुशोषश्च, ग्रीवास्तम्भश्च, मन्यास्तम्भश्च, कण्ठोद्ध्वंसश्च, हनुभेदश्च, ओष्ठभेदश्च, अक्षिभेदश्च, दन्तभेदश्च, दन्तशैथिल्यं च, मूकत्वं च, वाक्सङ्गश्च, कषायास्यता च, मुखशोषश्च, अरसज्ञता च, घ्राणनाशश्च, कर्णशूलं च, अशब्दश्रवणं च, उच्चैःश्रुतिश्च, बाधिर्यं च, वर्त्मस्तम्भश्च, वर्त्मसङ्कोचश्च, तिमिरं च, अक्षिशूलं च, अक्षिव्युदासश्च, भ्रूव्युदासश्च, शङ्खभेदश्च, ललाटभेदश्च, शिरोरुक् च, केशभूमिस्फुटनं च, अर्दितं च, एकाङ्गरोगश्च, सर्वाङ्गरोगश्च, पक्षवधश्च, आक्षेपकश्च, दण्डकश्च, तमश्च , भ्रमश्च, वेपथुश्च, जृम्भा च, हिक्का च, विषादश्च, अतिप्रलापश्च, रौक्ष्यं च, पारुष्यं च, श्यावारुणावभासता

च, अस्वप्नश्च, अनवस्थितचित्तत्वं च; इत्यशीतिर्वातविकारा वातविकाराणामपरिसङ्ख्येयानामाविष्कृततमा व्याख्याताः ||११||

**Eighty diseases caused by Vata alone – Vataja Nanatmaja Vyadhi: |**

Though Vata imbalance diseases are innumerable, the following eighty diseases are the most commonly manifested ones:

1. Nakhabheda (cracking of nails)
2. Vipadika (cracking of feet)
3. Pada shoola (pain in foot)
4. Pada Bhramsha (foot Drop)
5. Pada Suptata (numbness of foot)
6. Vata khuddata (club foot)
7. Gulpha Graha (stiff ankle)
8. Pindikodveshtana (cramps in calf muscle)
9. Gridhrasi (sciatica)
10. Janu Bheda (Genu varum)- Bow leggedness, bandiness
11. Januvishlesha (Genu valgum) – Knock Knee
12. Urustambha (stiffness of thigh)
13. Urusada (pain in the thigh)
14. Pangulya (paraplegia)
15. Guda Bhramsa (prolapsed rectum)
16. Gudarti (Tenasmus)
17. Vrushanakshepa (pain in scrotum)
18. Shepha Stambha (stiffness of penis)
19. Vankshana anaha (tension of groin)
20. Shroni Bheda (pain around the pelvic girdle)
21. Vidheda (diarrhea)
22. Udavarta (bloating)
23. Khanjatva (lameness)
24. Kubjatva (kyphosis)
25. Vamanatava(dwarfism)
26. Trikagraha (stiffness of sacro-iliac joint)
27. Prsistagraha (stiffness of back)
28. Parshva Marda (pain in chest)
29. Udaraveshta (Gripping pain in abdomen)
30. Hrit Moha (brabycardia)
31. Hrit Drava (tachycardia)
32. Vaksha- Udgharsha (rubbing pain in chest)
33. Vaksha- Uparodha (impairment of thoracic movement)
34. Vakshastoda (stabbing pain in chest)
35. Bahu Shosha (atrophy of arm)
36. Greeva Stambha (stiffness of the neck)
37. Manyastambha (torticollis)
38. Kanthoddhvamsa (hoarseness of voice)
39. Hanu Bheda (pain in jaw)
40. Ostha Bheda (pain in lips)
41. Akshi Bheda (pain in eye)
42. Danta Bheda (toothache)

43. Danta Shaithilya (looseness of tooth)
44. Mookatva (aphasia / dumbness)
45. Vak Sanga (stalling speech)
46. Kashaya asyata (astringent taste in mouth)
47. Mukha shosha (dryness of mouth)
48. Arasajnata (ageusia) – loss of taste function
49. Ghrana Nasha (anosmia) – loss of smell function
50. Karna Shoola (ear ache)
51. Ashabda Shravana (tinnitus)
52. Ucchaih Shruti (hard hearing)
53. Badhirya (deafness)
54. Vartma Stambha (Ptosis of eyelid)
55. Vartma Samkocha (entropies)
56. Timira(amaurosis) – a type of vision loss
57. Akshi Shoola (pinching pain in eye)
58. Akshi Vyudasa (Ptosis of eye ball)
59. Bhru Vyudasa (ptosis of eye brow)
60. Shankha Bheda (pain in temporal region)
61. Lalata Bheda (pain in frontal region)
62. Shiro Ruk (headache)
63. Kesha bhumi sphutana (dandruff)
64. Ardita(facial paralysis)
65. Ekanga Roga (monoplegia)
66. Sarvanga Roga (polyplegia)
67. Pakshavaha (hemiplegia)
68. Akshepaka (convulsion)
69. Dandaka (tonic convulsion)
70. Tama (fainting)
71. Bhrama (giddiness, dizziness)
72. Vepathu (tremor)
73. Jrumbha (yawning)
74. Hikka (hiccup)
75. Vishaada(asthenia) – weakness, depression
76. Ati Pralapa (delirium) – excessive irrelevant talk
77. Raukshya (dryness)
78. Parushya (hardness)
79. Shyava Arunaava Bhasata (dusky red appearance)
80. Asvapna (sleeplessness)
81. Anavasthita chittatva (unstable mind). [9-11]


**Qualities of Vata Dosha – how it is exhibited in Vata Nanatmaja diseases :**

सर्वेष्वपि खल्वेतेषु वातविकारेषूक्तेष्वन्येषु चानुक्तेषु वायोरिदमात्मरूपमपरिणामि कर्मणश्च स्वलक्षणं, यदुपलभ्य तदवयवं वा विमुक्तसन्देहा वातविकारमेवाध्यवस्यन्ति कुशलाः; तद्यथा- रौक्ष्यं शैत्यं लाघवं वैशद्यं गतिरमूर्त्तत्वमनवस्थितत्वं चेति वायोरात्मरूपाणि; एवंविधत्वाच्च वायोः कर्मणः स्वलक्षणमिदमस्य भवति तं तं शरीरावयवमाविशतः;

तद्यथा- संसभ्रंसव्याससङ्गभेदसादहर्षतर्षकम्पवर्तचालतोदव्यथाचेष्टादीनि, तथा खरपरुषविशदसुषिरारुणवर्णकषायविरसमुखत्वशोषशूलसुप्तिसङ्कोचनस्तम्भनखञ्जतादीनि च वायोः कर्मणि; तैरन्वितं वातविकारमेवाध्यवस्येत्||१२||

**Qualities of Vata Dosha – how it is exhibited in Vata Nanatmaja diseases :**

In all the pure Vata diseases, enumerated or implied, the inherent natural qualities and actions of Vata are quite obviously manifested wholly or partially and as such it is not difficult for a competent physician to correctly diagnose the Vatika type of diseases;
Raukshya – Rookshata – roughness,
Shaitya – Sheetata – coolness,
Laaghava – Laghu – lightness
Vaishadya – clarity, non-sliminess,
Gati – movement,
Amoortata – shapelessness,
Anavastitatva – instability- these are the inherent qualities of Vata.

Vata Dosha while moving from one part of the body, if abnormal, exhibits symptoms like :
Sramsa – looseness,
Bhramsa – dislocation,
Vyasa – expansion,
Sangha – obstruction,
Bheda – separation,
Saada – depression,
Harsha – excitation,
Tarsha – thirst,
Kampa – trembling,
Varta – circular movement,
Chaala – motion,
Toda – piercing pain,
Vyatha – aching pain,
Cheshta action, etc.
Khara – coarseness,
Parusha – harshness,
Vishada – non-sliminess,
Sushira – porousness,
Aruna Varna – reddishness, (color of sunrise)
Kashaya – Astringent taste
Virasa Mukhatva – tastelessness in the mouth,
Shosha – wasting pain,
Shoola – pain,
Supti – numbness,
Samkocha – contraction,
Sthambhana- rigidity and
Khanjata – lameness, etc. – these are the actions that help a competent physician to diagnose the pure Vatik type diseases.[12]

**General principles of treatment of Vata disorders:**

Madhura, Amla Lavana Snigdha Ushna Upakrama – The vitiated Vata should be treated by drugs having sweet, sour and saline taste and unctuous and hot qualities

Snehana – oleation,
Sveda – fomentation, sweating treatment
Asthapana – decoction enema
Anuvasana – oil enema
Nasyakarma – nasal instillation of drops,
Bhojana – healthy diet,
Abhyanga – massage,
Utsadana – unction,
Parisheka – sprinkling of oil / liquid containing materials having anti-Vata properties.
This is to be done with due regard to the dosage and the season.

**Importance of Basti treatment in Vata disorders :**

तं मधुराम्ललवणस्निग्धोष्णैरुपक्रमैरुपक्रमेत, स्नेहस्वेदास्थापनानुवासननस्तःकर्मभोजनाभ्यङ्गोत्सादनपरिषेकादिभिर्वातहरैर्मात्रां कालं च प्रमाणीकृत्य; तत्रास्थापनानुवासनं तु खलु सर्वत्रोपक्रमेभ्यो वाते प्रधानतमं मन्यन्ते भिषजः, तदद्ध्यादित एव पक्वाशयमनुप्रविश्य केवलं वैकारिकं वातमूलं छिनत्ति; तत्रावजितेऽपि वाते शरीरान्तर्गता वातविकाराः प्रशान्तिमापद्यन्ते, यथा वनस्पतेर्मूले छिन्ने स्कन्धशाखाप्ररोहकुसुमफलपलाशादीनां नियतो विनाशस्तद्वत्||१३|| |

**Importance of Basti treatment in Vata disorders :**

Of all the treatments stated above, the Asthapana (decoction enema) and Anuvasana (oil enema) are the treatment par excellence for the cure of Vatik diseases, because immediately after entering the colon, they strike at the very root of the vitiated Vata and when Vata is overcome in the colon, even the entire vitiated Vata dwelling in other parts of the body is automatically alleviated.

This can be compared and understood in terms of cutting of the root off a tree which results in the automatic fall of the trunk, branches, sprouts, flowers, fruits, leaves, etc. [13]

**Forty specific diseases of Pitta – Pittaja Nanatmaja Vyadhi :**

पित्तविकारांश्चत्वारिंशतमत ऊर्ध्वमनुव्याख्यास्यामः- ओषश्च, प्लोषश्च, दाहश्च, दवथुश्च, धूमकश्च, अम्लकश्च, विदाहश्च, अन्तर्दाहश्च, अंसदाहश्च, ऊष्माधिक्यं च, अतिस्वेदश्च (अङ्गस्वेदश्च), अङ्गगन्धश्च, अङ्गावदरणं च, शोणितक्लेदश्च, मांसक्लेदश्च, त्वग्दाहश्च, (मांसदाहश्च), त्वगवदरणं च, चर्मदलनं च, रक्तकोठश्च, रक्तविस्फोटश्च, रक्तपित्तं च, रक्तमण्डलानि च, हरितत्वं च, हारिद्रत्वं च, नीलिका च, कक्षा(क्ष्या)च, कामला च, तिक्तास्यता च, लोहितगन्धास्यता च, पूतिमुखता च, तृष्णाधिक्यं च, अतृप्तिश्च, आस्यविपाकश्च, गलपाकश्च, अक्षिपाकश्च, गुदपाकश्च, मेढ्रपाकश्च, जीवादानं च, तमःप्रवेशश्च, हरितहारिद्रनेत्रमूत्रवर्चस्त्वं च; इति चत्वारिंशत्पित्तविकाराः पित्तविकाराणामपरिसङ्ख्येयानामाविष्कृततमा व्याख्याताः||१४||

Now we shall explain the forty varieties of diseases due to the vitiation of Pitta. Even though the diseases due to the vitiation of Pitta are innumerable, the following forty varieties are the most commonly manifested.
1. Osha (heating)
2. Plosha (scorching)
3. Daha (burning)
4. Davathu (boiling)
5. Dhoomaka (fuming)
6. Amlaka (acid eructation)
7. Vidaaha (pyrosis) – heartburn
8. Antar daaha (burning sensation inside the body)

9. Amsa daha (burning sensation in shoulder)
10. Ushmaadhikya (excessive temperature)
11. Ati Sveda (excessive sweating)
12. Anga gandha (bad odour of the body)
13. Angaavadarana (cracking pain in the body)
14. Shonita kleda (sloughing of the blood)
15. Mamsa kleda (sloughing of the muscle)
16. Tvak Daaha (burning sensation in the skin)
17. Charma dalana (itching of the skin)
18. Tvagavadarana (cracking of the skin)
19. Rakta kotha (urticaria)
20. Rakta visphota (red vesicle)
21. Rakta Pitta (bleeding tendency)
22. Rakta mandala (red wheals)
23. Haritatva (greenishness)
24. Haaridratva (yellowishness)
25. Neelika (blue moles)
26. Kaksha (herpes)
27. Kaamala (jaundice)
28. Tiktaasyata (bitter taste in month)
29. Lohita Gandhasyata (smell of blood from the mouth)
30. Pooti mukhata (foetid odour of mouth)
31. Trishnaadhikya (excessive thirst)
32. Atrupti (non-satisfaction)
33. Aasya Vipaka (stomatitis)
34. Gala paka (pharyngitis)
35. Akshi paka (conjunctivitis)
36. Guda paka (proctitis)
37. Medhra Paka (inflammation of the penis)
38. Jivadana (haemorrhage)
39. Tamah pravesha (fainting)
40. Harita haridra netra mutra varchas (greenish and yellowish coloration of eyes, urine & feces) [14]

**Patho-physiology of Pitta diseases:**

सर्वेष्वपि खल्वेतेषु पित्तविकारेष्वूक्तेष्वन्येषु चानुक्तेषु पित्तस्येदमात्मरूपमपरिणामि कर्मणश्च स्वलक्षणं, यदुपलभ्य तदवयवं वा विमुक्तसन्देहाः पित्तविकारमेवाध्यवस्यन्ति कुशलाः; तद्यथा- औष्ण्यं तैक्ष्ण्यं द्रवत्वमनतिस्नेहो वर्णश्च शुक्लारुणवर्जो गन्धश्च विस्रो रसौ च कटुकाम्लौ सरत्वं च पित्तस्यात्मरूपाणि; एवंविधत्वाच्च पित्तस्य कर्मणः स्वलक्षणमिदमस्य भवति तं तं शरीरावयवमाविशतः; तद्यथा- दाहौष्ण्यपाकस्वेदक्लेदकोथकण्डूस्रावरागा यथास्वं च गन्धवर्णरसाभिनिर्वर्तनं पित्तस्य कर्माणि; तैरन्वितं पित्तविकारमेवाध्यवस्येत्||१५||

In all the Paittika types of diseases enumerated or implied, the inherent natural qualities and actions of Pitta are quite obviously manifested wholly or partially and as such it is not difficult for a competent physician to correctly diagnose the Paittika type of diseases.

**Qualities of Pitta –**
The inherent natural qualities of Pitta are
Aushnya – Ushna – heat,
Taikshnya – Teekshna – sharpness,
Dravatva – liquidity,

Anati Sneha – slight unctuousness, mild oiliness,
all colors except white and red,
Visra Gandha – fishy smell,
Katu, Amla – acrid and sour tastes
Saratva – fluidity.

**Pitta imbalance symptoms -**
Daaha – burning sensation,
Aushnya – ushna – heat,
Paaka – suppuration,
Sveda – perspiration,
Kleda – sloughing,
Kotha – putrefaction,
Kandu – itching,
Srava – discharge,
Raaga – redness,
and exhibition of its inherent smell, color and taste.

**General principles of treatment for Pitta diseases:**

तं मधुरतिक्तकषायशीतैरुपक्रमैरुपक्रमेत स्नेहविरेकप्रदेहपरिषेकाभ्यङ्गादिभिः पित्तहरैर्मात्रां कालं च प्रमाणीकृत्य; विरेचनं तु सर्वोपक्रमेभ्यः पित्ते प्रधानतमं मन्यन्ते भिषजः; तद्ध्यादित एवामाशयमनुप्रविश्य केवलं वैकारिकं पित्तमूलमपकर्षति, तत्रावजिते पित्तेऽपि शरीरान्तर्गताः पित्तविकाराः प्रशान्तिमापद्यन्ते, यथाऽग्नौ व्यपोढे केवलमग्निगृहं शीतीभवति तद्वत्||१६||

**General principles of treatment for Pitta diseases:**

Madhura, Tikta Kashaya – Pitta is treated with herbs having sweet, bitter and astringent tastes
Sheeta – cooling qualities and
Snehana – oleation
Virechana – purgation,
Pradeha – unction,
Parisheka – effusion,
Abhyanga – massage, etc. procedures done with herbs having anti Pitta qualities.
This is of course to be done with due regard to the dosage and season.

**Importance of Virechana in Pitta imbalance :**

Of all the devices stated above, the purgation is the treatment par excellence for curing the Paittika diseases because, immediately after it is administered, it eliminates the vitiated Pitta from its very root from the level of intestines. When it is overcome in the Amasaya (small intestine), it alleviates the entire vitiated Pitta dwelling in other parts of the body. This can be likened to a hot chamber being cooled by removing the fire from inside it. [16]

**Twenty types of kaphaja diseases – Kaphaja Nanatmaja Vikara:**

श्लेष्मविकारांश्च विंशतिमत ऊर्ध्वं व्याख्यास्यामः; तद्यथा- तृप्तिश्च, तन्द्रा च, निद्राधिक्यं च, स्तैमित्यं च, गुरुगात्रता च, आलस्यं च, मुखमाधुर्य च, मुखस्रावश्च, श्लेष्मोद्गिरणं च, मलस्याधिक्यं च, बलासकश्च, अपक्तिश्च, हृदयोपलेपश्च, कण्ठोपलेपश्च, धमनीप्रति(वि)चयश्च, गलगण्डश्च, अतिस्थौल्यं च, शीताग्निता च, उद्दर्दश्च, श्वेतावभासता च, श्वेतमूत्रनेत्रवर्चस्त्वं च; इति विंशतिः

श्लेष्मविकाराः श्लेष्मविकाराणामपरिसङ्ख्येयानामाविष्कृततमा व्याख्याता भवन्ति||१७||

Now we shall explain the twenty varieties of diseases due to the vitiation of Kapha. Even though, the diseases due to the vitiation of Kapha are innumerable; the following are the twenty varieties which are most commonly manifested.

1. Trupti (anorexia nervosa)
2. Tandra (drowsiness)
3. Nidraadhikya (excessive sleep)
4. Staimitya (timidness)
5. Guru Gatrata (heaviness of the body)
6. Alasya (laziness)
7. Mukha Maadhurya (sweet taste in mouth)
8. Mukha Srava (salivation)
9. Shleshmodgirana (mucus expectoration)
10. Malaadhikya (excessive excretion of excreta)
11. Balasaka (loss of strength)
12. Apakti (indigestion)
13. Hrudayopalepa (feeling as if heart is wrapped up with moisture)
14. Kantopalepa (phlegm adhered to throat)
15. Dhamani Pratichaya (hardening of vessels)
16. Galaganda (goiter)
17. Ati Sthaulya (obesity)
18. Sheetaagnita (suppression of digestive powder)
19. Udarda (urticaria)
20. Shvetaavabhasata (pallor), Shveta Mutra Netra Varchastva (whiteness of urine, eye and faces) [17]

## Pathophysiology of kaphaja diseases:

सर्वेष्वपि खल्वेतेषु श्लेष्मविकारेषूक्तेष्वन्येषु चानुक्तेषु श्लेष्मण इदमात्मरूपमपरिणामि कर्मणश्च स्वलक्षणं यदुपलभ्य तदवयवं वा विमुक्तसन्देहाः श्लेष्मविकारमेवाध्यवस्यन्ति कुशलाः; तद्यथा- स्नेहशैत्यशौक्ल्यगौरवमाधुर्यस्थैर्यपैच्छिल्यमात्स्न्र्यानि श्लेष्मण आत्मरूपाणि; एवंविधत्वाच्च श्लेष्मणः कर्मणः स्वलक्षणमिदमस्य भवति तं तं शरीरावयवमाविशतः; तद्यथा- श्वैत्यशैत्यकण्डूस्थैर्यगौरवस्नेहसुप्तिक्लेदोपदेहबन्धमाधुर्यचिरकारित्वानि श्लेष्मणः कर्माणि; तैरन्वितं श्लेष्मविकारमेवाध्यवस्येत्||१८||

In all the Shlaishmika (Kaphaja) type of diseases enumerated or implied, the inherent natural qualities and actions of Kapha are quite obviously manifested fully or partly and as such it is not difficult for a competent physician to correctly diagnose the shlaishmika type of diseases.

## Qualities of Kapha :

तद्यथा- स्नेह शैत्य शौक्ल्य गौरव माधुर्य स्थैर्य पैच्छिल्य मात्स्न्र्यानि श्लेष्मण आत्मरूपाणि;

Sneha - unctuousness
Shaitya - coldness
Shauklya - Shukla - whiteness
Gaurava - heaviness
Madhurya - sweetness
Sthairya - stability
Paichchilya - stickiness
Martsnya - smoothness

## Kapha imbalance symptoms

Kapha brings about following attributes to the body
Shvaitya – Shveta – whiteness
Shaitya – Sheeta – coolness
Kandu – itching
Sthairya – steadiness, stability
Gaurava – heaviness,
Sneha – unctuousness, oiliness,
Supti – numbness,
Kleda – moistness, stickiness,
Upadeha – sliminess, as if being anointed with oil,
Bandha – binding, obstruction
Madhurya – sweetness,
Chirakaritva – slowness, delay in manifestation- these are the actions that help a competent physician to diagnose diseases caused by kapha.[18]

## General principle of treatment for Kaphaja diseases:

तं कटुकतिक्तकषायतीक्ष्णोष्णरूक्षैरुपक्रमैरुपक्रमेत स्वेदवमनशिरोविरेचनव्यायामादिभिः श्लेष्महरैर्मात्रां कालं च प्रमाणीकृत्य; वमनं तु सर्वोपक्रमेभ्यः श्लेष्मणि प्रधानतमं मन्यन्ते भिषजः, तद्ध्यादित एवामाशयमनुप्रविश्योरोगतं केवलं वैकारिकं श्लेष्ममूलमूर्ध्वमुत्क्षिपति, तत्रावजिते श्लेष्मण्यपि शरीरान्तर्गताः श्लेष्मविकाराः प्रशान्तिमापद्यन्ते, यथा भिन्ने केदारसेतौ शालियवषष्टिकादीन्यनभिष्यन्द्यमानान्यम्भसा प्रशोषमापद्यन्ते तद्वदिति॥१९॥
They (diseases due to vitiated Kapha) should be treated with
Katu Tikta Kashaya – herbs having pungent, bitter, astringent taste,
Teekshna Ushna Rooksha – treatments and medicines having sharp, hot and dryness qualities
Sveda – fomentation, sweating
Vamana – emesis, vomiting therapy,
Shiro Virechana – elimination of Doshas from the head by Nasya procedure,
Vyayama – exercise etc., which should all contain materials having Anti- Slaismika properties.

## Importance of Vamana in Kapha imbalance :

This is of course to be done with due regard to the dosage and season. Of all the devices stated above, emetic therapy is the treatment par excellence for the cure of diseases due to Kapha because immediately after entering the Amashaya – stomach, it strikes at the very root cause of the vitiation of Kapha and when it is overcome in the stomach, even the entire vitiated Kapha dwelling in other parts of the body is automatically alleviated. This can be compared to the withering away of paddy, barley, etc. for want of a barrier of the cornfield (full of water) being broken. [19]

## Importance of diagnosis in treatment:

भवन्ति चात्र-
रोगमादौ परीक्षेत ततोऽनन्तरमौषधम्।
ततः कर्म भिषक् पश्चाज्ज्ञानपूर्वं समाचरेत्॥२०॥
यस्तु रोगमविज्ञाय कर्माण्यारभते भिषक्।

अप्यौषधविधानज्ञस्तस्य सिद्धिर्यदृच्छया||२१||
यस्तु रोगविशेषज्ञः सर्वभैषज्यकोविदः|
देशकालप्रमाणज्ञस्तस्य सिद्धिरसंशयम्||२२||

## Importance of diagnosis in treatment:

Thus, it is said: A physician should first of all diagnose the disease and then he should select proper medicine. Thereafter, he should administer the therapy applying the knowledge of the science of medicine he had already gained.

A physician who initiates treatment without proper diagnosis of the diseases can accomplish the desired object only by chance (he cannot be sure of his success); The fact that he is well- acquainted with the knowledge of application of medicine does not necessarily guarantee his success. On the other hand, the physician who is well-versed in diagnosing diseases, who is proficient in the administration of medicines and who knows about the dosage of the therapy that varies from place to place and season to season, is sure to accomplish the desired objective. [20-22]

## To sum up:

तत्र श्लोकाः-
सङ्ग्रहः प्रकृतिर्देशो विकारमुखमीरणम् |
असन्देहोऽनुबन्धश्च रोगाणां सम्प्रकाशितः||२३||
दोषस्थानानि रोगाणां गणा नानात्मजाश्च ये|
रूपं पृथक् च दोषाणां कर्म चापरिणामि यत्||२४||
पृथक्त्वेन च दोषाणां निर्दिष्टाः समुपक्रमाः|
सम्यङ्महति रोगाणामध्याये तत्त्वदर्शिना||२५||

In this chapter – Maha Roga Adhyaya, the enlightened sage has fully dealt with the following subjects: classification, nature, sites of manifestation, specific and general causative factors, interchangeability and specific identity of diseases, sites of Doshas, enumeration of specific diseases due to Doshas, invariable signs and actions of Doshas separately along with their treatment. [23-25]

इत्यग्निवेशकृते तन्त्रे चरकप्रतिसंस्कृते श्लोकस्थाने महारोगाध्यायो नाम विंशोऽध्यायः||२०||
समाप्तो रोगचतुष्कः||५||
Thus ends the twentieth chapter of Charaka Samhita Sutrasthana, of Agnivesa's work as redacted by Charaka.[20]
This ends Roga Chatushka.

# 21

# Sutrasthana Chapter 21 Ashtau Ninditeeyam

**Ashtau Ninditeeya Adhyaya - Weight Loss, Weight Gain Treatment, Sleep**

अथातोऽष्टौनिन्दितीयमध्यायंव्याख्यास्यामः||१||

इतिहस्माहभगवानात्रेयः||२||

The twenty first chapter is one of the most important chapters of Charaka Samhita Sutrasthana. It explains the process of obesity, its treatment, methods of gaining weight, importance of sleep and more. It is called as Ashtau Ninditeeya Adhyaya. Ashta means eight. Nindita means undesirable. It deals with eight types of undesirable body constitutions.

**Eight undesirable constitutions:**

इहखलुशरीरमधिकृत्याष्टौपुरुषानिन्दिताभवन्ति; तद्यथा-अतिदीर्घश्च, अतिह्रस्वश्च, अतिलोमाच, अलोमाच, अतिकृष्णश्च, अतिगौरश्च, अतिस्थूलश्च, अतिकृशश्चेति||३||

Following are the eight types of undesirable physical constitution.
Ati Deergha – too tall,
Ati Hrasva – too short,
Ati Loma – too hairy,
Aloma – hairless,
Ati Krishna – too black,
Ati Gaura – too white,
Ati Sthoola – too corpulent,
Ati Krisha – too emaciated. [3]

(The word undesirable should only be understood from the health perspective. The term undesirable in present context means, extra healthcare efforts are required to maintain good health of the above individuals. Very tall person is correlated to gigantism, a very short person means dwarfism. In a normal colored family, if someone is born with abnormally excess white or black skin color, then they are grouped under ati krishna and ati gaura. This does not apply to tall or short or white or black skin-colored persons in general).

**Eight difficulties of being very obese:**

तत्रातिस्थूलकृशयोर्भूय एवापरे निन्दितविशेषा भवन्ति|

अतिस्थूलस्य तावदायुषो ह्रासो जवोपरोधः कृच्छ्रव्यवायता दौर्बल्यं दौर्गन्ध्यं स्वेदाबाधः क्षुदतिमात्रं पिपासातियोगश्चेति भवन्त्यष्टौ दोषाः|

**Eight difficulties of being very obese:**

Highly obese people have following health issues.
Ayusho Hrasa – Deficient in longevity, short life term (short lifespan),
Javoparodha – slow in movement
Krichra Vyavayata – Difficulty in intercourse
Daurbalya – weakness
Daurgandhya – bad / foul body odor
Svedaabadha – excess sweating
Kshudha atimatram – excessive hunger
Pipasa Atiyoga – excessive thirst.

**Causes for obesity:**

तदतिस्थौल्यमतिसम्पूरणाद्गुरुमधुरशीतस्निग्धोपयोगादव्यायामादव्यवायादिदिवास्वप्नाद्धर्षनित्यत्वाद-
चिन्तनाद्बीजस्वभावाच्चोपजायते|
**Causes for obesity:**

Ati Sampooranat – excess intake of food;
Guru Madhura Ahara – heavy to digest foods, sweet foods,
Sheeta Snigdha Ahara – cooling foods and unctuous (oily) food,
Avyayamaat – lack of physical exercise,
Avyavaayaat – abstinence from sexual intercourse,
Divasvapnaat – due to day sleeping,
Harsha Nityatvaat – uninterrupted cheerfulness, happy all the time,
Achintana – lack of mental exercise, lack of thinking
Beeja Svabhaavaat – heredity.

**Reasoning for symptoms in obesity:**

तस्य ह्यतिमात्रमेदस्विनो मेद एवोपचीयते न तथेतरे धातवः, तस्मादस्यायुषो ह्रासः; शैथिल्यात् सौकुमार्याद्गुरुत्वाच्च मेदसो जवोपरोधः ,
शुक्राबहुत्वान्मेदसाऽऽवृतमार्गत्वाच्च कृच्छ्रव्यवायता, दौर्बल्यमसमत्वाद्धातूनां, दौर्गन्ध्यं मेदोदोषान्मेदसः स्वभावात् स्वेदनत्वाच्च, मेदसः
श्लेष्मसंसर्गादिवष्यन्दित्वाद्बहुत्वाद्गुरुत्वाद्व्यायामासहत्वाच्च स्वेदाबाधः, तीक्ष्णाग्नित्वात् प्रभूतकोष्ठवायुत्वाच्च क्षुदतिमात्रं
पिपासातियोगश्चेति||४||
**Reasoning for symptoms in obesity:**

In obese people, only Medo Dhatu (fat tissue) gets nourishment. Hence, other body tissues are deprived of nourishment. Hence, longevity is affected. The bodily movement is impaired due to the looseness, tenderness and heaviness of fats. Due to deprived Shukra Dhatu (reproductive system), there will be difficulty in intercourse. It is also caused by less quantity of semen and obstruction of related channels.
Bad smell is caused by the inherent defect and nature of the fat tissue and also due to excessive sweating;
As the fat is associated with Kapha and its fluidity, bulkiness and heaviness, the person cannot withstand physical exercise and it brings about excessive sweating; Because of the sharp digestive power and the presence of excess Vata Dosha in the digestive tract, there is excessive hunger and thirst. [4]

**Pathophysiology of obesity:**

भवन्ति चात्र-
मेदसाऽऽवृतमार्गत्वाद्वायुः कोष्ठे विशेषतः|
चरन् सन्धुक्षयत्यग्निमाहारं शोषयत्यपि||५||
तस्मात् स शीघ्रं जरयत्याहारं चातिकाङ्क्षति|
विकारांश्चाश्नुते घोरान् कांश्चित्कालव्यतिक्रमात्||६||
एतावुपद्रवकरौ विशेषादग्निमारुतौ|
एतौ हि दहतः स्थूलं वनदावो वनं यथा||७||
मेदस्यतीव संवृद्धे सहसैवानिलादयः|
विकारान् दारुणान् कृत्वा नाशयन्त्याशु जीवितम्||८||
मेदोमांसातिवृद्धत्वाच्चलस्फिगुदरस्तनः|
अयथोपचयोत्साहो नरोऽतिस्थूल उच्यते||९||
इति मेदस्विनो दोषा हेतवो रूपमेव च|
निर्दिष्टं वक्ष्यते वाच्यमतिकार्श्ये त्वतः परम्||१०||

**Pathophysiology of obesity:**

In obesity, Medo Dhatu obstructs the channels related to digestive system (Koshta). This results in obstruction of Vata Dosha in the digestive system. It increases Agni (digestive fire, like wind increases fire) and dries up food in the stomach and intestines. Hence, digestion of food speeds up hunger. So the patient digests food quickly and becomes a voracious eater. If he does not get food on time, he becomes prone to serious disorders. The Agni (digestive fire), influenced by Pitta and Vata Dosha get vitiated. They burn the food as the forest fire burns the forest. Consequently, there is more craving for food and the person eats repeatedly. Hence the body weight increases. Due to a disproportionate increase of fat, diseases of very serious types are caused, all of a sudden, by Vata, etc. This may lead to instantaneous death. Owing to an excessive increase of fat and muscle tissue, the buttock, abdomen and breast become pendulous and his strength is rendered disproportionate with his physical growth. Thus, the defects of the corpulent persons, their causes, signs and symptoms have been explained. [5-10]

**Causes for emaciation – lean person:**
      ... वक्ष्यते वाच्यमतिकार्श्ये त्वतः परम्||१०||
सेवा रूक्षान्नपानानां लङ्घनं प्रमिताशनम्|
क्रियातियोगः शोकश्च वेगनिद्राविनिग्रहः||११||
रूक्षस्योद्वर्तनं स्नानस्याभ्यासः प्रकृतिर्जरा|
विकारानुशयः क्रोधः कुर्वन्त्यतिकृशं नरम्||१२||

**Causes for emaciation – lean person:**

Rooksha Annapana – consumption of food and drinks that are dry in nature
Langhana – fasting for long periods of time
Pramitashana – taking very less quantities of food
Kriya Atiyoga – excessive Panchakarma therapies,
Shoka – grief,
Vega Nidra Vinigraha – suppression of the natural urges including sleep,
Rookshasya Udvartana – performing powder massage on a naturally dry person
Snana – repeated baths,
Prakruti – heredity,
Jara – old age,

Vikara Anushaya – continued illness
Krodha – anger

**Features of very lean person:**

व्यायाममतिसौहित्यं क्षुत्पिपासामयौषधम् [१] |
कृशो न सहते तद्वदतिशीतोष्णमैथुनम्||१३||
प्लीहा कासः क्षयः श्वासो गुल्मोऽर्शास्युदराणि च|
कृशं प्रायोऽभिधावन्ति रोगाश्च ग्रहणीगताः||१४||

**Features of very lean person:**

Vyayama Asauhitya – cannot stand physical exercise,
Kshut, Pipasa Amaya, Aushadham – cannot stand the intake of food in large quantities, hunger, thirst, diseases and drugs.
Na Sahate Ati Sheeta Ushna Maithuna – cannot stand excessive cold, heat and sexual acts.
Such emaciated persons are prone to
Pleeha – splenic diseases,
Kasa – cough, cold
Kshaya – muscle wasting,
Shwasa – dyspnoea, asthma
Gulma – abdominal tumour,
Arsha – piles, and diseases of the duodenum and small intestine.

**Features of lean person:**

शुष्कस्फिगुदरग्रीवो धमनीजालसन्ततः|
त्वगस्थिशेषोऽतिकृशः स्थूलपर्वा नरो मतः||१५||

Their buttocks, abdomen and neck are emaciated, veins are prominent underneath skin;
The joints are prominently seen and the man appears to have bone and skin only. [10-15]

**Comparative disadvantage of corpulence and emaciation:**

सततं व्याधितावेतावतिस्थूलकृशौ नरौ|
सततं चोपचर्यौ हि कर्शनैर्बृंहणैरपि||१६||
स्थौल्यकार्श्ये वरं कार्श्यं समोपकरणौ हि तौ|
यद्युभौ व्याधिरागच्छेत् स्थूलमेवातिपीडयेत्||१७||

Comparative disadvantage of corpulence and emaciation:

Both the types – i.e., patients who are too obese or lean suffer from diseases all the time. They are to be treated by slimming and nourishing therapies respectively. Of the two, leanness is less harmful than obesity, though both of them are equally in need of treatment. When subjected to diseases, the volume of suffering in case of obese persons is far greater than in emaciated ones. [16-17]

**Features of a good physical health :**

सममांसप्रमाणस्तु समसंहननो नरः|
दृढेन्द्रियो विकाराणां न बलेनाभिभूयते||१८||
क्षुत्पिपासातपसहः शीतव्यायामसंसहः|
समपक्ता समजरः सममांसचयो मतः||१९||

## Features of a good physical health :

Sama Mamsa pramana – proportionate musculature
Sama Samhana – compactness of the body
Druda indriya – strong sensory and motor organs
Cannot be overcome by the onslaught of diseases
Kshut Pipasa Atapa Saha – Ability to stand hunger, thirst, the heat of the sun,
Sheeta Vyayama Samsaha – Ability to stand cold and physical exercises.
Samapakta, Samajara – Ability to digest and assimilate food easily,
Sama Mamsa Upachaya – good muscular body / good nourishment of muscles. [18-19]

## Principles of treatment for obese and emaciated persons:

गुरु चातर्पणं चेष्टं स्थूलानां कर्शनं प्रति|
कृशानां बृंहणार्थं च लघु सन्तर्पणं च यत्||२०||

Heavy-to-digest and non-nourishing diet is prescribed to treat obesity.
Light and nourishing diet is prescribed for lean persons. [20]

## Management of obesity:

वातघ्नान्यन्नपानानि श्लेष्ममेदोहराणि च|
रूक्षोष्णा बस्तयस्तीक्ष्णा रूक्षाण्युद्वर्तनानि च||२१||
गुडूचीभद्रमुस्तानां प्रयोगस्त्रैफलस्तथा|
तक्रारिष्टप्रयोगश्च प्रयोगो माक्षिकस्य च||२२||
विडङ्गं नागरं क्षारः कालललोहरजो मधु|
यवामलकचूर्णं च प्रयोगः श्रेष्ठ उच्यते||२३||
बिल्वादिपञ्चमूलस्य प्रयोगः क्षौद्रसंयुतः|
शिलाजतुप्रयोगश्च साग्निमन्थरसः परः||२४||
प्रशातिका प्रियङ्गुश्च श्यामाका यवका यवाः|
जूर्णाह्वाः कोद्रवा मुद्गाः कुलत्थाश्चक्रमुद्गकाः ||२५||
आढकीनां च बीजानि पटोलामलकैः सह|
भोजनार्थं प्रयोज्यानि पानं चानु मधूदकम्||२६||
अरिष्टांश्चानुपानार्थं मेदोमांसकफापहान्|
अतिस्थौल्यविनाशाय संविभज्य प्रयोजयेत्||२७||
प्रजागरं व्यवायं च व्यायामं चिन्तनानि च|
स्थौल्यमिच्छन् परित्यक्तुं क्रमेणाभिप्रवर्धयेत्||२८||

## Management of obesity:

For reducing over corpulence, the following prescriptions are suitable:

1. Diets and drinks that alleviate Vata and Kapha Dosha and which can reduce fat.

2. Rooksha, Ushna Teekshna Basti – Enema prepared with drugs that are non-unctuous, hot and sharp.

3. Rooksha Udvartana – powder massage with herbs having dry quality

4. Intake of Guduchi (Tinospora cordifolia), Musta (Cyperus rotundus), Triphala i.e. Haritaki (Terminalia chebula Linn.), Bibhitaki (Terminalia belerica Roxb.) and Amalaka (Emblica officinalis Gaertn.))

5. Administration of Takrarista – buttermilk, fermented with spices

6. Administration of honey

7. Intake of Vidanga (Embelia ribes Burm f.), Nagara (ginger), Yavaksara (Kshara prepared from Barley), Loha Bhasma with honey and powder of Yava – barley and Amla.

8. Administration of honey along with decoction of Bilvadi panchamula (roots of Bael, Oroxylum indicum, Gmelina arborea, Stereospermum suaveolens and Clerodendrum phlomidis)

9. Administration of Silajatu (asphaltum / mineral pitch)

10. Administration of the juice of Agnimantha (Clerodendrum phlomidis Linn. f.)

11. Intake of Prashatika (Setaria italica Beauv.), Priyangu (Callicara macrophylla), Syamaka (Echinochloa frumentacea Linn.), Yavaka (small variety of barley), Yava – Barley, Jurnahva (Sorghum vulgare Pers.), Kodrava (Paspalum scrobiculatum Linn.), Mudga (green gram), Kulattha (horse gram), Chakramudgaka (?), seeds of Adhaki (Cajanus cajan Millsp.) along with Patola (Trichosanthes cucumerina Linn.) and Amalaki (Indian gooseberry) as food,

12. Madhudhaka – combination of honey and water.

13. Alcoholic preparations that help to reduce fat, muscle and Kapha may be used as after-food-drinks.

The above are to be prescribed in proper dosage for the reduction of obesity. One desirous of reducing obesity should indulge more and more in having less sleep, sexual act, physical and mental exercises. [21-78]

**The management of leanness:**

स्वप्नो हर्षः सुखा शय्या मनसो निर्वृतिः शमः।
चिन्ताव्यवायव्यायामविरामः प्रियदर्शनम्॥२९॥
नवान्नानि नवं मद्यं ग्राम्यानूपौदका रसाः।
संस्कृतानि च मांसानि दधि सर्पिः पयांसि च॥३०॥
इक्षवः शालयो माषा गोधूमा गुडवैकृतम्।
बस्तयः स्निग्धमधुरास्तैलाभ्यङ्गश्च सर्वदा॥३१॥
स्निग्धमुद्वर्तनं स्नानं गन्धमाल्यनिषेवणम्।
शुक्लं वासो यथाकालं दोषाणामवसेचनम्॥३२॥
रसायनानां वृष्याणां योगानामुपसेवनम्।
हत्वाऽतिकार्श्यमाधत्ते नृणामुपचयं परम्॥३३॥
अचिन्तनाच्च कार्याणां ध्रुवं सन्तर्पणेन च।
स्वप्नप्रसङ्गाच्च नरो वराह इव पुष्यति॥३४॥

**The management of leanness:**

Swapna – Sleep,

Harsha – joy,

Sukha Shayya – comfortable bed,

Manasonivrutti, shama – contentment, tranquility of mind,

Abstinence from anxiety, sexual act and physical exercise,

Priya Darshana – pleasant sights and people,

Nava Anna – Intake of freshly harvested rice,

Nava Madya – fresh wine,

Gramya, Anupa and Audaka Mamsarasa – Meat soup of domestic, marshy and aquatic animals,

Well prepared meat, curd, ghee, milk, sugar cane, rice, Masha (black gram), wheat, sugar candy preparations,

Snigdha Madhura Basti – enema consisting of oily and sweet drugs,

Taila Abhyanga – regular oil massage,

unctuous unction bath, use of scents and garlands, use of white apparel, elimination of Doshas in time and administration of rejuvenating and aphrodisiac drugs

All the above said measures remove emaciation and bring out nourishment in the body. Freedom from anxiety about any work, intake of nourishing diet and adequate sleep makes the person fatty - like a boar. [29-34]

**Physiology of Sleep:**

यदा तु मनसि क्लान्ते कर्मात्मानः क्लमान्विताः |
विषयेभ्यो निवर्तन्ते तदा स्वपिति मानवः||३५||

**Physiology of Sleep:**

When the mind including sensory and motor organs is exhausted and they dissociate themselves from their objects, then the individual sleeps. [25]

**Effect of Sleep:**

निद्रायत्तं सुखं दुःखं पुष्टिः कार्श्यं बलाबलम्|
वृषता क्लीबता ज्ञानमज्ञानं जीवितं न च||३६||
अकालेऽतिप्रसङ्गाच्च न च निद्रा निषेविता|
सुखायुषी पराकुर्यात्का लरात्रिरिवापरा||३७||
सैव युक्ता पुनर्युङ्क्ते निद्रा देहं सुखायुषा|
पुरुषं योगिनं सिद्ध्या सत्या बुद्धिरिवागता||३८||

**Effect of Sleep:**

Happiness, misery, nourishment, emaciation, strength, weakness, virility, sterility, knowledge, ignorance, life and death – all these occur depending on the proper or improper sleep. Like the night of destruction, untimely and excessive sleep and prolonged vigil (waking up at night), take away both happiness and longevity. The same sleep, if properly enjoyed, brings about happiness and longevity in human beings as the real knowledge brings about Siddhi (spiritual power) in a Yogin.

**Indications of day sleep:**

गीताध्ययनमद्यस्त्रीकर्मभाराध्वकर्शिताः|
अजीर्णिनः क्षताः क्षीणा वृद्धा बालास्तथाऽबलाः||३९||
तृष्णातीसारशूलार्ताः श्वासिनो हिक्किनः कृशाः|
पतिताभिहतोन्मत्ताः क्लान्ता यानप्रजागरैः||४०||
क्रोधशोकभयक्लान्ता दिवास्वप्नोचिताश्च ये|
सर्व एते दिवास्वप्नं सेवेरन् सार्वकालिकम्||४१||
धातुसाम्यं तथा ह्येषां बलं चाप्युपजायते|
श्लेष्मा पुष्णाति चाङ्गानि स्थैर्यं भवति चायुषः||४२||
ग्रीष्मे त्वादानरूक्षाणां वर्धमाने च मारुते|

रात्रीणां चातिसङ्क्षेपादिदिवास्वप्नः प्रशस्यते||४३||

## Indications of day sleep:

Sleeping during the day time in all seasons is prescribed for those who are exhausted by singing, study, alcoholic drinks, sexual acts, Panchakarma therapy, carrying heavy weight, walking long distance; those suffering from indigestion, injuries, muscle wasting, thirst, diarrhea, colic pain, dyspnea (as in Asthma), hiccup, leanness, insanity, those who are too old, too young, weak and emaciated; those injured by fall and assault, those exhausted by journey by a vehicle, vigil, anger, grief and fear, and those who are accustomed to day sleep.

By this the equilibrium of Dhatus and strength are maintained and the Kapha nourishes the organs and ensures longevity.In summer, nights become shorter and Vata gets aggravated in the body due to the absorption of fluid (Adana). Therefore, during this season, sleep during day time is prescribed for all. [39-43]

## Contra-indications of day sleep:

ग्रीष्मवर्ज्येषु कालेषु दिवास्वप्नात् प्रकुप्यतः|
श्लेष्मपित्ते दिवास्वप्नस्तस्मातेषु न शस्यते||४४||
मेदस्विनः स्नेहनित्याः श्लेष्मलाः श्लेष्मरोगिणः|
दूषीविषार्ताश्च दिवा न शयीरन् कदाचन||४५||
हलीमकः शिरःशूलं स्तैमित्यं गुरुगात्रता|
अङ्गमर्दोऽग्निनाशश्च प्रलेपो हृदयस्य च||४६||
शोफारोचकहृल्लासपीनसार्धावभेदकाः|
कोठारुःपिडकाः कण्डूस्तन्द्रा कासो गलामयाः||४७||
स्मृतिबुद्धिप्रमोहश्च संरोधः स्रोतसां ज्वरः|
इन्द्रियाणामसामर्थ्यं विषवेगप्रवर्त(र्ध)नम्||४८||
भवेन्नृणां दिवास्वप्नस्याहितस्य निषेवणात्|
तस्मादिधताहितं स्वप्नं बुद्ध्वा स्वप्यात् सुखं बुधः||४९||

## Contra-indications of day sleep:

Sleeping during day time in the seasons other than summer is not advisable as it causes vitiation of Kapha and Pitta. Obese persons, those who are addicted to taking oily foods, those with Kapha body type, those suffering from diseases due to the vitiation of Kapha and those suffering from Dooshivisha (artificial poisoning) should never sleep during day time. If one violates the prescription regarding sleep during the day time, he would subject himself to

Halimaka (serious type of jaundice),
Shirashoola – headache,
Agninasha – loss of digestion strength,
Pralepo Hrudayasya – coating of heart region, feeling of heaviness,
Shopha – oedema,
Aruchi - Anorexia
Hrullasa – nausea,
Peenasa – rhinitis,
Ardhavabhedhaka – hemicrania, migraine,

Kotha, Pidaka, Kandu – urticaria, eruption, abscess, pruritus,
Tandra – drowsiness,
Kasa – cough,
Galaamaya – diseases of the throat, impairment of the memory and intelligence, obstruction of the channels of the body, fever, weakness of sensory and motor organs and enhancement of the toxic effects of artificial poisons (Gara Visha).

So, one should keep in view the merits and demerits of sleep in various seasons and situations. By doing so, proper sleep would bring happiness to that person. [44-49]

**Effect of waking up till late night :**

रात्रौ जागरणं रूक्षं स्निग्धं प्रस्वपनं दिवा|
अरूक्षमनभिष्यन्दि त्वासीनप्रचलायितम्||५०||

**Effect of waking up till late night :**

Vigil during night causes roughness in the body; sleep during day time causes increased oiliness.
'Sleeping in sitting posture' neither cause roughness nor unctuousness. [50]

**The role of sleep-in obesity:**
देहवृत्तौ यथाऽऽहारस्तथा स्वप्नः सुखो मतः|
स्वप्नाहारसमुत्थे च स्थौल्यकार्श्ये विशेषतः||५१||

**The role of sleep-in obesity:**

Like proper diet, proper sleep is also essential for the maintenance of the body. Obesity and emaciation are specially conditioned by proper or improper sleep and diet. [51]

**Methods to induce good sleep:**

अभ्यङ्गोत्सादनं स्नानं ग्राम्यानूपौदका रसाः|
शाल्यन्नं सदधि क्षीरं स्नेहो मद्यं मनःसुखम्||५२||
मनसोऽनुगुणा गन्धाः शब्दाः संवाहनानि च|
चक्षुषोस्तर्पणं लेपः शिरसो वदनस्य च||५३||
स्वास्तीर्णं शयनं वेश्म सुखं कालस्तथोचितः|
आनयन्त्यचिरान्निद्रां प्रनष्टा या निमित्ततः||५४||

**Methods to induce good sleep:**

Abhyanga – massage,
Utsadana – body massage,
bath, intake of soup of domestic, marshy and aquatic animals, rice with curd, milk, unctuous substance and alcohol, psychic pleasure, smell of scents and hearing of sounds of one's own taste, Samvahana (rubbing the body by hand), application of soothing ointment to the eyes, head and face, comfortable bed and home and proper time. [52-54]

**Causes of Insomnia:**

कायस्य शिरसश्चैव विरेकश्छर्दनं भयम्|
चिन्ता क्रोधस्तथा धूमो व्यायामो रक्तमोक्षणम्||७५||
उपवासोऽसुखा शय्या सत्त्वौदार्य तमोजयः|
निद्राप्रसङ्गमहितं वारयन्ति समुत्थितम्||७६||
एत एव च विज्ञेया निद्रानाशस्य हेतवः|
कार्यं कालो विकारश्च प्रकृतिर्वायुरेव च||७७||

## Causes of Insomnia:

Elimination of Doshas from the body and head through Panchakarma therapies,
Fear, anxiety, anger, herbal smoke, physical exercise, bloodletting (Rakta Mokshana), fasting, uncomfortable bed, predominance of Satva and suppression of Tamas help in overcoming excess sleep.
The above-mentioned factors along with overwork, old age, diseases - especially those caused due to the vitiation of Vata like colic pain, etc. are known to cause sleeplessness even in normal individuals. Some have less sleep by nature. [55-57]

## Classification of sleep:

तमोभवा श्लेष्मसमुद्भवा च मनःशरीरश्रमसम्भवा च|
आगन्तुकी व्याध्यनुवर्तिनी च रात्रिस्वभावप्रभवा च निद्रा||७८||

## Types of sleep
1.Tamo Bhava – Caused by excess of Tamas quality;
2. Shleshma Samudbhava – Caused by (vitiated) Kapha;
3. Mana Shrama Sambhava – Caused by mental exertion;
4. Shareera shrama sambhava – Caused by physical exhaustion;
5. Agantuka – caused by external causes such as injury,
6. Vyadhi anuvartini – Caused as a complication of other diseases like Samnipata Jvara, etc.; and
7. Ratri Svabhavaja – Caused by the very nature of the night (physiological sleep). [58]

## Good and bad sleep:
रात्रिस्वभावप्रभवा मता या तां भूतधात्रीं प्रवदन्ति तज्ज्ञाः|
तमोभवामाहुरघस्य मूलं शेषाः पुनर्व्याधिषु निर्दिशन्ति||७९||

The sleep caused by the nature of the night is the sleep par excellence. This is known as "Bhutadhatri" (that which nurses all the living beings). The one caused by Tamas is the root cause of all sinful acts. The remaining types are to be treated as diseases. [59]

## To sum up:
तत्र श्लोकाः-
निन्दिताः पुरुषास्तेषां यौ विशेषेण निन्दितौ|
निन्दिते कारणं दोषास्तयोर्निन्दितभेषजम्||६०||
येभ्यो यदा हिता निद्रा येभ्यश्चाप्यहिता यदा|
अतिनिद्रायानिद्राय भेषजं यद्भवा च सा||६१||
या या यथाप्रभावा च निद्रा तत् सर्वमत्रिजः|
अष्टौनिन्दितसङ्ख्याते व्याजहार पुनर्वसुः||६२||

Lord Punarvasu on the chapter on "Eight types of Undesirable Constitutions" has explained the following.

1. Enumeration of undesirable constitutions;
2. The two most undesirable types of persons;
3. Cause of undesirability;
4. Demerits of undesirable persons;
5. Their treatment;
6. Indications and contra-indications of sleep depending upon the nature of the individual and time;
7. Treatment of excessive sleep and sleeplessness;
8. Factors responsible for causation of sleep
9. Types and effects of sleep [60-62]

इत्यग्निवेशकृते तन्त्रे चरकप्रतिसंस्कृते श्लोकस्थानेऽष्टौनिन्दितीयो नामैकविंशतितमोऽध्यायः||२१||

Thus, ends the twenty-first chapter on "Eight types of Undesirable Constitutions" of the Sutra section of Agnivesha's work as redacted by Charaka.

# 22

# Sutrasthana Chapter Langhana Brumhaneeyam

**Langhana Brimhaneeya Adhyaya - Six Basic Ayurvedic Therapies – Shat Upakrama**

अथातो लङ्घनबृंहणीयमध्यायं व्याख्यास्यामः ||१||

इति ह स्माह भगवानात्रेयः||२||

**Langhana** – De-nourishing, or deprivation therapy and Brimhana – nourishing therapy – these two types, along with four others, form the basis of Ayurvedic therapies. This is not only applicable to weight loss or weight gain treatments but is also applicable to a plethora of diseases in Ayurveda. This concept is very impressively explained in Langhana Brimhaneeya Adhyaya, 22nd chapter of Charaka Samhita Sutrasthana.

**Six main therapies of Ayurveda:**

तपःस्वाध्यायनिरतानात्रेयः शिष्यसत्तमान्|

षडग्निवेशप्रमुखानुक्तवान् परिचोदयन्||३||

लङ्घनं बृंहणं काले रूक्षणं स्नेहनं तथा|

स्वेदनं स्तम्भनं चैव जानीते यः स वै भिषक्||४||

तमुक्तवन्तमात्रेयमग्निवेश उवाच ह||५||

भगवँल्लङ्घनं किंस्विल्लङ्घनीयाश्च कीदृशाः|

बृंहणं बृंहणीयाश्च रूक्षणीयाश्च रूक्षणम्||६||

के स्नेहाः स्नेहनीयाश्च स्वेदाः स्वेद्याश्च के मताः|

स्तम्भनं स्तम्भनीयाश्च वक्तुमर्हसि तद्गुरो!||७||

लङ्घनप्रभृतीनां च षण्णामेषां समासतः|

कृताकृतातिवृतानां लक्षणं वक्तुमर्हसि||८||

**Six main therapies of Ayurveda :**

With a view to initiating discussion, Lord Atreya spoke to his six illustrious disciples headed by Agnivesa (the other five are – Bhela, Harita, Ksharaparni, Jatukarna and Parashara)., who are engaged in penance and studies.

The Vaidya (doctor) is the one, who knows about

Langhana – deprivation treatment

Brumhana – nourishing therapy,

Rookshana – Drying treatment

Snehana – oiling / oleating therapy

Svedana – sweating treatment

Stambhana – blocking/ stopping treatment, astringent therapy.

**Questions related to six main therapies**

Agnivesha asks the below mentioned questions to Master Atreya -

What is Langhana?

Who are eligible for Langhana therapy?

What is Brimhana?

Who are eligible for Brimhana therapy?

What is Rookshana?

Who are eligible for Rookshana therapy?

What is Snehana?

Who are eligible for Snehana therapy?

What is Swedana?

Who are eligible for Swedana therapy?

What is Stambhana?

Who are eligible for Stambhana therapy?

"Hey Great teacher, kindly explain in detail about these therapies and also tell us breifly about the signs of proper, less and excessive administration of these six therapies."

**Reply by Master Atreya**

**Definition of Langhana, Brimhana etc.:**

तदग्निवेशस्य वचो निशम्य गुरुरब्रवीत्।
यत् किञ्चिल्लाघवकरं देहे तल्लङ्घनं स्मृतम्||९||
बृहत्वं यच्छरीरस्य जनयेत्तच्च बृंहणम्।
रौक्ष्यं खरत्वं वैशद्यं यत् कुर्यात्तदिध रूक्षणम्||१०||
स्नेहनं स्नेहविष्यन्दमार्दवक्लेदकारकम् [ १ ] ।
स्तम्भगौरवशीतघ्नं स्वेदनं स्वेदकारकम्||११||
स्तम्भनं स्तम्भयति यद्गतिमन्तं चलं ध्रुवम्।
लघूष्णतीक्ष्णविशदं रूक्षं सूक्ष्मं खरं सरम्||१२||
कठिनं चैव यद्द्रव्यं प्रायस्तल्लङ्घनं स्मृतम्।
गुरु शीतं मृदु स्निग्धं बहलं स्थूलपिच्छिलम्||१३||
प्रायो मन्दं स्थिरं श्लक्ष्णं द्रव्यं बृंहणमुच्यते।
रूक्षं लघु खरं तीक्ष्णमुष्णं स्थिरमपिच्छिलम्||१४||
प्रायशः कठिनं चैव यद्द्रव्यं तदिध रूक्षणम्।
द्रवं सूक्ष्मं सरं स्निग्धं पिच्छिलं गुरु शीतलम्।
प्रायो मन्दं मृदु च यद्द्रव्यं तत्स्नेहनं मतम्||१५||
उष्णं तीक्ष्णं सरं स्निग्धं रूक्षं सूक्ष्मं द्रवं स्थिरम्।
द्रव्यं गुरु च यत् प्रायस्तदिध स्वेदनमुच्यते||१६||
शीतं मन्दं मृदु श्लक्ष्णं रूक्षं सूक्ष्मं द्रवं स्थिरम्।
यद्द्रव्यं लघु चोद्दिष्टं प्रायस्तत् स्तम्भनं स्मृतम्||१७||

**Langhana** – This word is derived from Laghu (lightness). Whatever the procedures or medicines that bring about lightness in the body are called Langhana. – Deprivation treatment.

**Brimhana** – Brimhana is derived from brihat (big). Whatever causes improvement in body size / weight or causes nourishment of the body, is called Brimhana – nourishing treatment.

**Rookshana** - Rooksha means dry. Treatment that causes / increases Raukshya (dryness), Kharatva (roughness) and Vaishadya (clarity, non- sliminess) is called Rookshana – drying treatment.

**Snehana** – Whatever causes unctuousness / oiliness (Sneha), fluidity (Vishyanda), softness (Mardava) and moistness (Kleda) is Snehana or Oleating therapy;

**Swedana** – whatever cures stiffness (Stambha), heaviness (Gaurava) and coldness (Sheeta) is 'Swedana' or sweating therapy

**Sthambhana** - The therapy that prevents mobility and flow of bodily substances and fluids is known as 'Stambhana' or astringent therapy.

## Qualities of each of the above said therapies:

### Characteristic Features of Drugs used in these therapies:

1. Langhana or Lightening Therapy – Light (Laghu), hot (Ushna), sharp (Teekshna), non-slimy (Vishada), dry (rooksha), minute (sookshma), rough (khara), mobility (Sara) and hardness (Katina)

2. **Brimhana** or Nourishing Therapy – Heavy (Guru), cold (Sheeta), soft (Mrudu), unctuous (Snigdha), thick (Sthoola), bulky (bahala), sticky (Picchila), sluggish (Manda), stable (sthira), and smooth (Shlakshna).

3. **Rookshana** or Drying Therapy – Dry (rooksha), light (laghu), rough (Khara), sharp (teekshna), hot (ushna), stable (sthira), non-non sticky (Apicchila) and hard (Katina).

4. **Snehana** or Oleation Therapy – Liquid (Drava), minute (Sookshma), fluid (Sara), oily (snigdha), slimy (picchila), heavy (Guru), cold (Sheeta), sluggish (manda) and soft (mridu).

5. **Swedana** or Fomentation Therapy – Hot (ushna), Sharp (teekshna), fluid (sara), oily (snigdha) / rough (dry), subtle (minute), liquid (drava), stable (sthira), and heavy (guru).

6. **Stambhana** or Astringent Therapy - Cold (sheeta), sluggish (manda), soft (mrudu), smooth (shlakshna), rough (rooksha), subtle (sookshma), liquid (drava), stable (sthira) and light (laghu).

## 10 Types of Langhana Therapy (depriving / de-nourishing therapy):

चतुष्प्रकारा संशुद्धिः पिपासा मारुतातपौ|
पाचनान्युपवासश्च व्यायामश्चेति लङ्घनम्||१८||

The four types of Panchakarma purifying therapies – Vamana (emesis), Virechana (purgation), Niruha basti (decoction enema) and Nasya (nasal instillation)

Pipasa – controlling thirst

Maruta – exposure to wind

Atapa – exposure to sun

Pachana – administration of digestive foods and medicine

Upavasa – fasting

Vyayama – physical exercise

All the above said constitute Langhana Therapy. [18]

## Indication for ten types of Langhana therapies:

### 1-4 Indication for four types of Panchakarma procedures:

प्रभूतश्लेष्मपित्तास्रमलाः संसृष्टमारुताः|
बृहच्छरीरा बलिनो लङ्घनीया विशुद्धिभिः||१९||

4 Panchakarma therapies as deprivation treatment is useful in

**Prabhuta Shleshma, Pitta Asra** – person having Kapha Pitta imbalance and blood vitiation

**Prabhuta mala** – in person with excess toxicity / waste products in the body,

**Samsrushta Maruta** - in person where Vata is obstructed

**Brihat shareera** – those having good physical built / obesity
**Balina** – strong person

## 5. Indication for Pachana (digestive) treatment :

येषां मध्यबला रोगाः कफपित्तसमुत्थिताः|
वम्यतीसारहृद्रोगविसूच्यलसकज्वराः||२०||
विबन्धगौरवोद्गारहृल्लासारोचकादयः|
पाचनैस्तान् भिषक् प्राज्ञः प्रायेणादावुपाचरेत्||२१||

**Madhya bala roga** – in diseases with moderate strength of the below mentioned types, a wise physician shall first administer pachana treatments –
**Kapha Pitta Samutha** – diseases with Kapha and Pitta imbalance, vomiting (Chardi), diarrhoea (Atisara), heart diseases (Hrit Roga), cholera (visuchika), severe kind of digestive disorder (Alasaka), fever (Jwara), constipation (vibandha), heaviness of the body (gaurava), eructation (udgara), nausea (hrullasa) and anorexia (aruchi).

## 6, 7 – Indication for control of thirst and fasting :

एत एव यथोद्दिष्टा येषामल्पबला गदाः|
पिपासानिग्रहैस्तेषामुपवासैश्च ताञ्जयेत्||२२||

If the same diseases mentioned above are of mild nature, they are to be treated by the control of thirst and hunger (fasting).

## 8-10 – Indication for exercise, sun and wind exposure:

रोगाञ्जयेन्मध्यबलान् व्यायामातपमारुतैः|
बलिनां किं पुनर्येषां रोगाणामवरं बलम्||२३||

If strong individuals suffer from diseases of moderate nature, such diseases can be cured by Physical exercise and Exposure to Sun and Wind. It goes without saying that diseases of mild nature of these individuals can also be cured by the same devices.

## Indication for Langhana therapy even for Vata disorders:

त्वग्दोषिणां प्रमीढानां स्निग्धाभिष्यन्दिबृंहिणाम्|
शिशिरे लङ्घनं शस्तमपि वातविकारिणाम्||२४|

As we have seen above, Langhana is more suited for Kapha-Pitta imbalance disorders. However, it is suited in Vata disorders also,
Tvak Dosha – skin diseases
Prameha – urinary tract disorders
Snigdha, Abhishyanda - those having excess oiliness, fluidity
Brumhina – excessively nourished body
Shishire – during the winter [19-24]

## Brimhana (nourishing therapy):

**Non veg foods that have nourishing qualities:**

अदिग्धविद्धमक्लिष्टं वयस्थं सात्म्यचारिणाम्|
मृगमत्स्यविहङ्गानां मांसं बृंहणमुच्यते||२५||

Fresh meat of young animals, fishes and birds moving in their natural surroundings and killed by non-poisonous devices like arrows, etc. is nourishing.

**Indication for Brimhana (nourishing therapy) :**

क्षीणाः क्षताः कृशा वृद्धा दुर्बला नित्यमध्वगाः|
स्त्रीमद्यनित्या ग्रीष्मे च बृंहणीया नराः स्मृताः||२६||
शोषार्शोग्रहणीदोषैर्व्याधिभिः कर्शिताश्च ये|
तेषां क्रव्यादमांसानां बृंहणा लघवो रसाः||२७||

Ksheena – debilitated, having muscle wasting
Kshata – injured
Krusha – emaciated patients
Vruddah – elderly patients
Durbala – weak
Nityam adhwaga – who walk excessively on a daily basis
Stree nitya – who indulge in sexual activity on daily basis
Madya nitya – who take alcohol daily
Greeshme – for all persons, during summer
Patients who are debilitated by
Shosha – wasting
Arsha – haemorrhoids
Grahani – malabsorption disorder / IBS

For patients emaciated due to above disorders, soup of meat eating birds and animals, which are light by nature is ideal. This helps in bringing about nourishment.

**Other methods of Brimhana :**

स्नानमुत्सादनं स्वप्नो मधुराः स्नेहबस्तयः|
शर्कराक्षीरसर्पींषि सर्वेषां विद्धि बृंहणम्||२८||

Snana – Bath,
Utsadana – unction, massage
Svapna – sleep,
Madhura Sneha Basti – oil enema prepared with sweet substances,
Sharkara – sugar candy
Ksheera – milk
Sarpi – ghee

These are universal diet for Brimhana. [25-28]

**Definition of Rookshana (drying therapy):**

कटुतिक्तकषायाणां सेवनं स्त्रीष्वसंयमः|
खलिपिण्याकतक्राणां मध्वादीनां च रूक्षणम्||२९||

Intake of pungent, bitter and astringent substances, sexual indulgence, and oil cake made of mustard and sesame, honey, etc. constitute drying therapy.

**Indication for Rookshana :**

अभिष्यण्णा महादोषा मर्मस्था व्याधयश्च ये|
ऊरुस्तम्भप्रभृतयो रूक्षणीया निदर्शिताः||३०||
स्नेहाः स्नेहयितव्याश्च स्वेदाः स्वेद्याश्च ये नराः|
स्नेहाध्याये मयोक्तास्ते स्वेदाख्ये च सविस्तरम्||३१||

Patients suffering from diseases characterised by the obstruction of bodily channels, domination of the aggravated Dosha in excess and manifested in vital organs of the body like 'spasticity of thighs' (Urustambha), gout, should be treated by "Drying Therapy".

**Snehana and Swedana** - The oleation (Snehana) and sweating treatment (Swedana), along with the indication and methods are already explained in separate chapters [29-31]

**Definition and Indication of Stambhana – astringent / blocking therapy:**

द्रवं तन्वसरं यावच्छीतीकरणमौषधम्|
स्वादु तिक्तं कषायं च स्तम्भनं सर्वमेव तत्||३२||
पित्तक्षाराग्निदग्धा ये वम्यतीसारपीडिताः|
विषस्वेदातियोगार्ताः स्तम्भनीया निदर्शिताः||३३||

**Definition and Indication of Stambhana – astringent / blocking therapy:**

The drugs constituting Astringent therapy are characterized by liquidity, thinness, consistency, coldness, sweetness, bitterness and astringency. Patients afflicted with Pitta, Alkalies (Kshara) and fire, and those suffering from vomiting, diarrhea, poisoning, excessive administration of sweating therapy are fit to be treated by "Astringent Therapy". [32-33]

**Signs and symptoms of successful Langhana therapy:**

वातमूत्रपुरीषाणां विसर्गे गात्रलाघवे|
हृदयोद्गारकण्ठास्यशुद्धौ तन्द्राक्लमे गते||३४||
स्वेदे जाते रुचौ चैव क्षुत्पिपासासहोदये|
कृतं लङ्घनमादेश्यं निर्व्यथे चान्तरात्मनि||३५||

**Signs and symptoms of successful Langhana therapy:**

Vata Mutra Pureesha Visarga – Proper excretion of flatus, urine and feces,

Laghava – lightness of the body,
Hrudaya Shuddhi – feeling of purity in heart,
Udgara shuddhi – feeling purity in eructation,
Kanta Shuddhi – feeling purity in throat,
lack of Tandra (drowsiness) and Klama (excretion),
appearance of sweat and appreciation of taste for food,
hunger and thirst and contentment. These symptoms indicate proper administration of "Langhana therapy"

**Adverse effects of excess Langhana treatment:**

पर्वभेदोऽङ्गमर्दश्च कासः शोषो मुखस्य च|
क्षुत्प्रणाशोऽरुचिस्तृष्णा दौर्बल्यं श्रोत्रनेत्रयोः||३६||
मनसः सम्भ्रमोऽभीक्ष्णमूर्ध्ववातस्तमो हृदि|
देहाग्निबलनाशश्च लङ्घनेऽतिकृते भवेत्||३७||

**Adverse effects of excess Langhana treatment:**

Parva bheda – Cracking of the skin, crackling sound in small joints
Angamarda – Malaise, body ache,
Kasa – cough,
Mukha Shosha – dryness of mouth,
Kshut pranasa – loss of appetite,
Aruchi – anorexia,
Trishna – thirst,
Weakness of the ears and eyes (impairment of the power of hearing and sight),
Sambhrama – loss of memory, dizziness,
frequent upward movement of Vayu,
Tamo hrudi – bradycardia, lowered functioning of heart,
emaciation of body, loss of the power of digestion and body strength
These are the signs and symptoms of excessive administration of "Langhana Therapy " [34-37]

**Symptoms of normal and excessive nourishing therapy :**

बलं पुष्ट्युपलम्भश्च कार्श्यदोषविवर्जनम्|
लक्षणं बृंहिते स्थौल्यमति चात्यर्थबृंहिते||३८||
कृतातिकृतलिङ्गं यल्लङ्घिते तद्धि रूक्षिते |३९|

**Symptoms of normal and excessive nourishing therapy :**
Strength, body bulk, disappearance of the defects of emaciation- these are the symptoms of proper administration of "Nourishing Therapy. Obesity is the result of the excessive administration of "Nourishing Therapy", The signs and symptoms of proper and excessive administration of Rookshana (Drying therapy) are the same as those of Langhana treatment [38]

**Signs and symptoms of proper and improper Stambhana (astringent therapy):**

स्तम्भितः स्यादबले लब्धे यथोक्तैश्चामयैर्जितैः||३९||
श्यावता स्तब्धगात्रत्वमुद्वेगो हनुसङ्ग्रहः|

हृद्वर्चोनिग्रहश्च स्यादतिस्तम्भितलक्षणम्||४०||

By the proper administration of Astringent treatment, the patient gains strength and the indicated diseases subside. The signs and symptoms of the excessive Stambhana are
Shyavata – blackish appearance,
Stabda gatrata – stiffness of the body,
Udvega – upward movement of Vata,
Hanu Sangraha – rigidity of Jaw,
Hrudaya nigraha – bradycardia and
Varcha nigraha – constipation [39-40].

**Features of effective administration of six types of therapies:**

लक्षणं चाकृतानां स्यात् षण्णामेषां समासतः|
तदौषधानां धातूनामशमो वृद्धिरेव च||४१||
इति षट् सर्वरोगाणां प्रोक्ताः सम्यगुपक्रमाः|
साध्यानां साधने सिद्धा मात्राकालानुरोधिनः||४२||

**Features of effective administration of six types of therapies:**
Signs and symptoms of non-utilization of all the six therapies in brief are the non-alleviation, rather aggravation of diseases for which these therapies have been administered. These are the six therapies which if administered properly with due regard to the dosage and the season can cure all the curable diseases. [41-42]

**Place of six types of the therapies among the measures of treatment:**

भवति चात्र-
दोषाणां बहुसंसर्गात् सङ्कीर्यन्ते ह्युपक्रमाः|
षट्त्वं तु नातिवर्तन्ते त्रित्वं वातादयो यथा||४३||

**Place of six types of the therapies among the measures of treatment:**

Depending upon the permutation and combination of diseases, these therapies are often required to be complied with one another (for example, sometimes Langhana and sweating therapies, some rimes nourishing and sweating therapies are required to be administered jointly). But in spite of this, the number of these therapies is six only as the number of Doshas is only three. [43]

तत्र श्लोकाः:-
इत्यस्मिँल्लङ्घनाध्याये व्याख्याताः षड्पक्रमाः|
यथाप्रश्नं भगवता चिकित्सा यैः प्रवर्तते||४४||
Thus, the six therapies which serve as the basis of treatment have been explained by Lord Atreya in this chapter.
इत्यग्निवेशकृते तन्त्रे चरकप्रतिसंस्कृते श्लोकस्थाने लङ्घनबृंहणीयो नाम द्वाविंशोऽध्यायः||२२||
This ends the 22nd chapter - Langhana Brimhaniya Adhyaya, written by Acharya Agnivesha and redacted by Acharya Charaka.

# 23

# Sutrasthana Chapter 23
# Santarpaneeyam

**Santarpaneeya Adhyaya**
**Treatment for Diseases of Over and Under Nourishment :**

अथातः सन्तर्पणीयमध्यायं व्याख्यास्यामः||१||

इति ह स्माह भगवानात्रेयः||२||

Ayurveda emphasises that over nourishment and under nourishment are the two major causes of many diseases. Based on this principle, many diseases can be categorized into these two divisions. This concept and detailed treatment and remedies are explained in chapter Santarpaneeya Adhyaya – "the Nourishment Regimen". As a learner of Ayurveda, please concentrate on the herbs that are listed in this chapter which are used to treat over or under nourishment.

**Disadvantages of taking excessive nourishing diet:**

सन्तर्पयति यः स्निग्धैर्मधुरैर्गुरुपिच्छिलैः|
नवान्नैर्नवमद्यैश्च मांसैश्चानूपवारिजैः||३||
गोरसैर्गौडिकैश्चान्नैः पैष्टिकैश्चातिमात्रशः|
चेष्टाद्वेषी दिवास्वप्नशय्यासनसुखे रतः||४||
रोगास्तस्योपजायन्ते सन्तर्पणनिमित्तजाः|
प्रमेहपिडकाकोठकण्डूपाण्ड्वामयज्वराः||५||
कुष्ठान्यामप्रदोषाश्च मूत्रकृच्छ्रमरोचकः|
तन्द्रा क्लैब्यमतिस्थौल्यमालस्यं गुरुगात्रता||६||
इन्द्रियस्रोतसां लेपो बुद्धेर्मोहः प्रमीलकः|
शोफाश्चैवंविधाश्चान्ये शीघ्रमप्रतिकुर्वतः||७||

**Disadvantages of taking excessive nourishing diet:**

One who over indulges in nourishing himself with
Snigdha, Madhura Guru Picchila Ahara – food with oily, sweet, heaviness and stickiness qualities,
Nava anna – newly harvested rice and grains
Nava Madya – newly made wine,
Anupa Mamsa, Varija Mamsa – meat of marshy and aquatic animals,
Gorasa, Gaudika, Paishtika – cow's milk and its preparations and food preparations made of jaggery and pastry
Cheshtadveshi – who is averse to physical activities,

Divaswapna – indulges in sleep during daytime.

Shayyasukhe rata – indulging in sleeping and resting all the time,

Such a person often suffers from diseases like

Prameha – urinary disorders including diabetes,

Pidaka - carbuncles,

Kota – urticaria,

Kandu – itching,

Pandu - anaemia,

Jwara – fever,

Kushta – skin diseases,

diseases due to Ama,

Mutrkrichra – dysuria,

Arochaka - anorexia,

Tandra – drowsiness,

Klaibya – sterility, infertility,

Atisthoulya – excessive obesity,

Alasya – laziness,

Gurutva – heaviness of the body,

adhesion of the channels in sensory organs,

Moha – delusion,

Pramilaka – wandering,

Shopha – oedema and such other diseases.

Unless the effects of a nourishing regimen are neutralised by suitable antidotes, these diseases are bound to occur. [3-7]


**Management of the diseases caused by over nourishment:**

शस्त्रमुल्लेखनं तत्र विरेको रक्तमोक्षणम्।
व्यायामश्चोपवासश्च धूमाश्च स्वेदनानि च॥८॥
सक्षौद्रश्चाभयाप्राशः प्रायो रूक्षान्नसेवनम्।
चूर्णप्रदेहा ये चोक्ताः कण्डूकोठविनाशनाः॥९॥
त्रिफलारग्वधं पाठां सप्तपर्णं सवत्सकम्।
मुस्तं समदनं निम्बं जलेनोत्क्वथितं पिबेत्॥१०॥
तेन मेहादयो यान्ति नाशमभ्यस्यतो ध्रुवम्।
मात्राकालप्रयुक्तेन सन्तर्पणसमुत्थिताः॥११॥
मुस्तमारग्वधः पाठा त्रिफला देवदारु च।
श्वदंष्ट्रा खदिरो निम्बो हरिद्रे त्वक्च वत्सकात्॥१२॥
रसमेषां यथादोषं प्रातः प्रातः पिबन्नरः।
सन्तर्पणकृतैः सर्वव्याधिभिः सम्प्रमुच्यते॥१३॥
एभिश्चोद्वर्तनोद्धर्षस्नानयोगोपयोजितैः।
त्वग्दोषाः प्रशमं यान्ति तथा स्नेहोपसंहितैः॥१४॥
कुष्ठं गोमेदको हिङ्गु क्रौञ्चास्थि त्र्यूषणं वचा।
वृषकैले श्वदंष्ट्रा च खराह्वा चाश्मभेदकः॥१५॥
तक्रेण दधिमण्डेन बदराम्लरसेन वा।
मूत्रकृच्छ्रं प्रमेहं च पीतमेतद्व्यपोहति॥१६॥
तक्राभयाप्रयोगैश्च त्रिफलायास्तथैव च।

अरिष्टानां प्रयोगैश्च यान्ति मेहादयः शमम्||१७||
त्र्यूषणं त्रिफला क्षौद्रं क्रिमिघ्नमजमोदकः|
मन्थोऽयं सक्तवस्तैलं हितो लोहोदकाप्लुतः||१८||
व्योषं विडङ्गं शिग्रूणि त्रिफलां कटुरोहिणीम्|
बृहत्यौ द्वे हरिद्रे द्वे पाठामतिविषां स्थिराम्||१९||
हिङ्गु केबुकमूलानि यवानीधान्यचित्रकान्|
सौवर्चलमजाजीं च हपुषां चेति चूर्णयेत्||२०||
चूर्णतैलघृतक्षौद्रभागाः स्युर्मानतः समाः|
सक्तूनां षोडशगुणो भागः सन्तर्पणं पिबेत्||२१||
प्रयोगादस्य शाम्यन्ति रोगाः सन्तर्पणोत्थिताः|
प्रमेहा मूढवाताश्च कुष्ठान्यर्शांसि कामलाः||२२||
प्लीहा पाण्ड्वामयः शोफो मूत्रकृच्छ्रमरोचकः|
हृद्रोगो राजयक्ष्मा च कासः श्वासो गलग्रहः||२३||
क्रिमयो ग्रहणीदोषाः श्वैत्र्यं स्थौल्यमतीव च।
नराणां दीप्यते चाग्निः स्मृतिर्बुद्धिश्च वर्धते||२४||

**Management of the diseases caused by over nourishment:**

Ullekhana – Vamana – Emesis therapy,

Virechana – purgation therapy,

Raktamokshana – blood-letting,

Vyayama – physical exercise,

Upavasa – fasting,

Dhumapana – herbal smoking,

Swedana – fomentation / sweating treatment,

intake of Abhayaprasha, Agastya Haritaki etc. with honey,

Rooksha anna sevana – intake of rough and dry food,

Churna Pradeha – application of powders and ointments that are mentioned (in the Aragvdheeya chapter of Sutrasthana) for the cure of pruritus and urticaria,

Water decoction made of Triphala, Aragvadha (Cassia fistula), Patha (Cissampelos pareira Linn), Saptaparna (Alstonia scholaris Br), Vatsaka (Holarrhena antidysenterica Wall.), Musta (Cyperus rotundus), Madana (Randia dumetorum Lam), and nimba – neem.

One can be cured of all the above listed diseases if he takes the Kashaya (water decoction) of the below mentioned herbs every morning :

Musta (Cyperus rotundus), Aragvadha (Cassia fistula Linn), Patha (Cissampelos pareira Linn), Triphala, Devadaru (Cedrus deodara), Shvadamstra (Tribulus terrestris Linn), Khadira (Acacia catechu), Nimba – Neem, Haridra (turmeric), Daru Haridra – Tree Turmeric (stem) – (Berberis aristata) and the skin of Vatsaka (Holarrhena antidysenterica Wall.).

The above mentioned drugs are mixed with oily substances and applied as unction with or without massage or as bath. These measures would help to cure skin diseases.

**Medicine for dysuria, urinary disorder and diabetes:**

Kustha (Saussurea lappa C.B Clarke), Gomedaka (Onyx), Hingu – Asafetida (Ferula narthex Boiss), bone of Krauilca (Demoiselle crane), Shunthi (ginger), Pippali (Long pepper fruit), Maricha (Black pepper fruit), Vacha (Acorus calamus Linn.), Vasa (Adhatoda vasica Nees), Ela (cardamom), Gokshura (Tribulus terrestris Linn), Kharahva

(Trachyspermum roxburghianum), Ashmabheda (Bergenia ligulata Eng;).

These drugs mixed with buttermilk, whey and the juice of sour type of Badara – Zizyphus jujuba when taken, are useful in dysuria and urinary disorders including diabetes mellitus.

By the administration of Haritaki (Terminalia chebula Linn), with buttermilk, Triphala and Arishtas (different types of alcoholic preparation) are useful in urinary disorders, diabetes mellitus and such other diseases.

Mantha (thin gruel) prepared with Trikatu (pepper, long pepper and ginger), Triphala, honey, Vidanga (Embelia ribes Burm f.) Ajamoda – Ajowan (fruit) – Trachyspermum roxburghianum, roasted corn flour, oil and the decoction of Agaru (Aquilaria agallocha Roxb.) help to cure diseases due to over nourishment.

Trikatu (pepper, long pepper and ginger), Vidanga (Embelia ribes Rurm.f.), varieties of Shigru (Moringa oleifera Lam), Triphala, Katurohini – Picrorhiza kurroa, Brihati – Solanum indicum, Kantakari – Solanum xanthocarpum, Haridra (turmeric), Daru Haridra – Tree Turmeric (stem), two varieties of Patha (Cissampelos pareira Linn), Ativisha (Aconitum heterophyllum wall), Shalaparni (Desmodium, gangeticum DC), Hingu – Asafetida (Ferula narthex Boiss), root of Kebuka, Yavani (Trachysperumum ammi Sprague), Dhanyaka (Coriander), Chitraka – Leadwort – Plumbago zeylanica, sochal salt, Ajaji (Cuminum cyminum Linn), and Hapusha (Juniperus communis Linn).

The recipe prepared with the powder of these drugs along with equal quantity of each of the oil, ghee and honey added with sixteen times of roasted corn flour and water is useful in the treatment of urinary disorders including diabetes mellitus, Mudhavata (claudicating caused by Vata), skin diseases including leprosy, piles, jaundice, diseases of spleen, anemia, edema, anorexia, heart disease, tuberculosis, cough, dyspnoea, spasmodic obstruction of the throat, parasitic infestation, sprue, leukoderma and over corpulence caused by enhances memory and intellect.

**Exercise and diet for losing weight:**

व्यायामनित्यो जीर्णाशी यवगोधूमभोजनः|
सन्तर्पणकृतैर्दोषैः स्थौल्यं मुक्त्वा विमुच्यते||२५||
उक्तं सन्तर्पणोत्थानामपतर्पणमौषधम्|२६|

**Exercise and diet for losing weight:**
Individuals desirous of reducing obesity should take to daily exercise, intake of food like barley and wheat only after the digestion of the previous meal. Thus, the emaciating therapies (Apatarpana) for the cure of diseases caused by over-nourishment (Santarpana) have been described. [9-25]

**Diseases caused by nutritional deficiency – Apatarpana Janya Vikara:**

वक्ष्यन्ते सौषधाश्चोर्ध्वमपतर्पणजा गदाः||२६||
देहाग्निबलवर्णौजःशुक्रमांसपरिक्षयः|
ज्वरः कासानुबन्धश्च पार्श्वशूलमरोचकः||२७||
श्रोत्रदौर्बल्यमुन्मादः प्रलापो हृदयव्यथा|
विण्मूत्रसङ्ग्रहः शूलं जङ्घोरुत्रिकसंश्रयम्||२८||
पर्वास्थिसन्धिभेदश्च ये चान्ये वातजा गदाः|
ऊर्ध्ववातादयः सर्वे जायन्ते तेऽपतर्पणात्||२९||
तेषां सन्तर्पणं तज्ज्ञैः पुनराख्यातमौषधम्|

यत्तदात्वे समर्थं स्यादभ्यासे वा तदिष्यते ||३०||

**Diseases caused by nutritional deficiency – Apatarpana Janya Vikara:**

Diseases caused by the improper use of emaciating regimen along with their treatment are as follows:

- Deha kshaya – Emaciation of the body
- reduction in the power of digestion, strength, complexion, Ojas, Semen and muscle tissue
- continuous fever and cough, pain in chest, anorexia, weakness in the power of hearing sounds, insanity, pain in cardiac region, obstruction to the passage of stool and urine, pain in calf, thigh and lumbar regions.
- Cracking pain in fingers, bones and joints and such diseases due to the vitiation of Vata like Urdhvavata (upward movement of Vayu) etc.
- For their treatment, therapies resulting in long term nourishment should be administered. [26-30]

**Management of the patients suffering from nutritional deficiency:**

सद्यःक्षीणो हि सद्यो वै तर्पणेनोपचीयते|
नर्ते सन्तर्पणाभ्यासाच्चिरक्षीणस्तु पुष्यति||३१||
देहाग्निदोषभैषज्यमात्राकालानुवर्तिना|
कार्यमत्वरमाणेन भेषजं चिरदुर्बले||३२||
हिता मांसरसास्तस्मै पयांसि च घृतानि च|
स्नानानि बस्तयोऽभ्यङ्गास्तर्पणास्तर्पणाश्च ये||३३||
ज्वरकासप्रसक्तानां कृशानां मूत्रकृच्छ्रणाम्|
तृष्यतामूर्ध्ववातानां वक्ष्यन्ते तर्पणा हिताः||३४||
शर्करापिप्पलीतैलघृतक्षौद्रैः समांशकैः|
सक्तुद्विगुणितो वृष्यस्तेषां मन्थः प्रशस्यते||३५||
सक्तवो मदिरा क्षौद्रं शर्करा चेति तर्पणम्|
पिबेन्मारुतविण्मूत्रकफपित्तानुलोमनम्||३६||
फाणितं सक्तवः सर्पिर्दधिमण्डोऽम्लकाञ्जिकम्|
तर्पणं मूत्रकृच्छ्रघ्नमुदावर्तहरं पिबेत्||३७||

**Management of the patients suffering from nutritional deficiency:**

One suffering from emaciation can soon be cured by the administration of refreshing regimen but one suffering from chronic type of emaciation would require slow and long-acting nourishment therapy. In cases of patients having chronic types of emaciation, the nourishing therapy (Santarpana) should be administered slowly –
Mamsarasa – meat-soup,
Paya, Ghrita – milk and ghee of different animals,
different types of baths, enema, massage and nourishing drinks are useful.

For those patients suffering from continuous fever, cough, emaciation, dysuria, thirst and upward movement of Vata, the following type of nourishing drink is useful:
**Aphrodisiac gruel:** Mantha (thin gruel) prepared of sugar candy, Pippali (Long pepper fruit), Oil, Ghee, honey – all in equal quantity added with double the quantity of roasted corn flour is aphrodisiac and useful for such conditions.

These patients may be given drinks prepared of roasted corn flour, Alcohol, Honey and sugar which help in elimination of feces, urine, Vayu, Kapha and Pitta. The nourishing drink prepared of Phanita (a preparation of sugar candy), roasted corn flour, ghee, whey, sour gruel which cures dysuria and Udavarta should be given.

## Recipe for alcoholism:

मन्थः खर्जूरमृद्वीकावृक्षाम्लाम्लीकदाडिमैः|
परूषकैः सामलकैर्युक्तो मद्यविकारनुत्||३८||

Mantha (thin gruel) prepared of Date-palm, dry grapes, Vrikshamala (Garcinia indica Chois), Amlika (Tamarindus indica Linn), Dadima – Pomegranate – Punica granatum Linn, Parushaka (Grewia asiatica Linn), and Amalaki (Emblica officinalis Gaertn), are useful for curing alcoholism. [31-38]

## Recipe of nutrition therapy:

स्वादुरम्लो जलकृतः सस्नेहो रूक्ष एव वा|
सद्यः सन्तर्पणो मन्थः स्थैर्यवर्णबलप्रदः||३९||

Mantha (gruel) prepared of water by adding sweet or sour things like Dadima – Pomegranate, with or without oily substance refreshes immediately, and promotes steadiness, complexion and strength.[39]

To sum up:-
तत्र श्लोकः-
सन्तर्पणोत्था ये रोगा रोगा ये चापतर्पणात्|
सन्तर्पणीये तेऽध्याये सौषधाः परिकीर्तिताः||४०||
Diseases due to over refreshing and emaciating regime along with their management are described in the chapter on "Refreshing Regimen" [40]

इत्यग्निवेशकृते तन्त्रे चरकप्रतिसंस्कृते श्लोकस्थाने सन्तर्पणीयो नाम त्रयोविंशोऽध्यायः||२३||
Thus, ends the twenty-third chapter Santarpaneeya Adhyaya of the Sutra of Agnivesa's work as redacted by Charaka.[23]

# 24

# Sutrasthana Chapter 24 Vidhi Shoniteeyam

**Vidhishoniteeya Adhyaya**

**Blood Formation, Causes of Impurity, Diseases, Treatment :**

अथातो विधिशोणितीयमध्यायं व्याख्यास्यामः ||१||

इति ह स्माह भगवानात्रेयः||२||

Blood is explained as the reason for life, strength and immunity in Ayurveda. How is it produced? What are its functions? What causes blood impurity? What are diseases that result? How to treat this? These aspects are explained in detail in the 24th chapter of Charaka Samhita Sutrasthana – Vidhi Shoniteeya Adhyaya (Shonita and rakta means blood).

**Factors responsible for normal Haemopoiesis (Blood production):**

विधिना शोणितं जातं शुद्धं भवति देहिनाम्|

देशकालौकसात्म्यानां विधिर्यः सम्प्रकाशितः||३||

By the administration of proper regimen, with due regard to the place, time and habit as described in the sixth chapter of this section, pure blood is formed in human beings.[3]

**Function of normal Blood:**

तद्विशुद्धं हि रुधिरं बलवर्णसुखायुषा|

युनक्ति प्राणिनं प्राणः शोणितं ह्यनुवर्तते||४||

Living creatures are endowed with the below mentioned virtues due to pure blood in the body –

- Bala- strength and immunity,
- Varna- skin complexion,
- Sukha – happiness, comfort and
- Ayusha – longevity

Blood plays a vital role in the sustenance of Vital force of life [4]

**Causes for blood impurity:**

प्रदुष्टबहुतीक्ष्णोष्णैर्मद्यैरन्यैश्च तद्विधैः|

तथाऽतिलवणक्षारैरम्लैः कटुभिरेव च||५||

कुलत्थमाषनिष्पावतिलतैलनिषेवणैः|

पिण्डालुमूलकादीनां हरितानां च सर्वशः||६||

जलजानूपबैलानां प्रसहानां च सेवनात्|
दध्यम्लमस्तुसुक्तानां सुरासौवीरकस्य च||७||

**Food that cause blood impurity:**

a. Unwholesome, hot and sharp (teekshna) wine and food in large quantity (bahala)

b. Ati Lavana Amla Kshara Katu – Excessive saline, sour, alkaline, acidic and pungent food

c. Kulattha (horse gram), Masha (black gram), Nishpava (flat bean) and sesame oil

d. Pindalu (Dioscorea alata Linn (Water yam) / Moonseed plant / Tamilnadia uliginosa), radish, and all green eatables

e. Meat of aquatic (Jalaja), marshy (Anupa) and Prasaha (living beings which catch food by teeth, tear and eat) types of animal and Bileshaya (animals living in holes).

f. Curd, sour whey (Amla mastu), vinegar (Saktu), wine (Sura) and Sauviraka type of liquor.

g. Rotten (Upaklinna), putrefied food articles (Pooti) and those having bad food combinations.

h. Any other type of food in excessive quantity

**Activities that cause impure blood:**

विरुद्धानामुपक्लिन्नपूतीनां भक्षणेन च|
भुक्त्वा दिवा प्रस्वपतां द्रवस्निग्धगुरूणि च||८||
अत्यादानं तथा क्रोधं भजतां चातपानलौ|
छर्दिवेगप्रतीघातात् काले चानवसेचनात्||९||
श्रमाभिघातसन्तापैरजीर्णाध्यशनैस्तथा|
शरत्कालस्वभावाच्च शोणितं सम्प्रदुष्यति||१०||

a. Sleeping during day time after taking liquid, oily and heavy food.

b. Excessive anger, excessive exposure to the sun and fire.

c. Suppression of the urge for vomiting.

d. Not conducting blood-letting therapy (in the autumn – Sharat Ritu).

e. Exertion, external injury, heat, taking food before the previous meal is digested.

f. By the very nature of the autumn season – Sharat Rutu [5-10].

**Diseases caused by vitiated blood :**

ततः शोणितजा रोगाः प्रजायन्ते पृथग्विधाः|
मुखपाकोऽक्षिरागश्च पूतिघ्राणास्यगन्धिता||११||
गुल्मोपकुशवीसर्परक्तपित्तप्रमीलकाः|
विद्रधी रक्तमेहश्च प्रदरो वातशोणितम्||१२||
वैवर्ण्यमग्निसादश्च पिपासा गुरुगात्रता|
सन्तापश्चातिदौर्बल्यमरुचिः शिरसश्च रुक्||१३||
विदाहश्चान्नपानस्य तिक्ताम्लोद्गिरणं क्लमः|
क्रोधप्रचुरता बुद्धेः सम्मोहो लवणास्यता||१४||
स्वेदः शरीरदौर्गन्ध्यं मदः कम्पः स्वरक्षयः|
तन्द्रानिद्रातियोगश्च तमसश्चातिदर्शनम्||१५||
कण्ड्वरुःकोठपिडकाकुष्ठचर्मदलादयः|
विकाराः सर्व एवैते विज्ञेयाः शोणिताश्रयाः||१६||

**Diseases caused by vitiated blood :**

The following diseases occur due to the vitiation of blood:

Mukhapaka – Stomatitis,

Akshiraga – conjunctivitis,

Pooti ghrana – rhinitis,

Asya Gandhita – foul odour from mouth,

Gulma - abdominal tumor,

Upakusha – type of mouth diseases,

Visarpa - a skin diseases characterized by an acute spread,

Raktapitta - a disease characterized by bleeding from different parts of the body,

Prameelaka - drowsiness,

Vidradhi – abscess,

Raktameha – hematuria, blood in urine,

Pradara – menorrhagia,

Vata Shonita – gout,

Vaivarnya – Palor,

Agnisada – Suppression of the power of digestion,

Pipasa - thirst,

Guru Gatrata – heaviness of the body,

Santapa – burning sensation,

Ati daurbalya – excessive weakness,

Aruchi - anorexia,

Shiro Ruk – headache,

Vidaha – internal burning sensation

Tikta Amla Udgirana – bitter & sour eructation specially of the diet and drink that are not properly digested,

Klama – tiredness,

Krodha – excessive anger,

Sammoha – bewilderment,

Lavanasyata – saline taste in mouth,

Sveda – excessive sweating,

foul smell of the body,

Mada – intoxication, shivering,

Svara Kshaya – aphonia,

Tandra – drowsiness, excessive sleep,

Tamo Darshana – frequent attack of fainting,

pruritis (Kandu), eruption (Kota), urticaria, pimples, skin diseases, Charmadala - skaling, etc.

**Differential diagnosis criteria for disorders due to blood vitiation:**

शीतोष्णस्निग्धरूक्षाद्यैरुपक्रान्ताश्च ये गदाः|
सम्यक् साध्या न सिध्यन्ति रक्तजांस्तान् विभावयेत्||१७||

If any curable disease does not get cured by cold, hot, unctuous (oily), drying and such other therapies, they are to be taken as diseases due to the vitiation of blood.

**Principles of treatment for the diseases of blood:**

कुर्याच्छोणितरोगेषु रक्तपित्तहरीं क्रियाम्|
विरेकमुपवासं च स्रावणं शोणितस्य च||१८||

Therapies like purgation, fasting and blood-letting indicated for the treatment of Raktapitta (a disease characterized by bleeding from different parts of the body) are also useful for curing diseases due to the vitiation of blood.

**Caution for blood- letting:**

बलदोषप्रमाणाद्वा विशुद्ध्या रुधिरस्य वा|
रुधिरं स्रावयेज्जन्तोराशयं प्रसमीक्ष्य वा||१९||

Bloodletting is to be done, with due regard to

Bala – the strength of the patient (both physical and mental)

Dosha Pramana – the quantity of vitiation of dosha (morbidity of blood and its contamination by doshas) nature as well as seriousness of the disease.

Vishudhya va rudhirasya – until the blood is entirely purified of its doshas / morbidity.

Jantoh ashayam prasamikshya – taking into consideration the site / seat of blood [19]

**Changes in blood due to vitiation of different Doshas:**

अरुणाभं भवेद्वातादिवशदं फेनिलं तनु|
पित्तात् पीतासितं रक्तं स्त्यायत्यौष्ण्याच्चिरेण च||२०||
ईषत्पाण्डु कफाद्दुष्टं पिच्छिलं तन्तुमद्घनम्|
संसृष्टलिङ्गं संसर्गात्त्रिलिङ्गं सान्निपातिकम्||२१||

**Changes in blood due to vitiation of different Doshas:**

- Rakta (blood), vitiated by Vata becomes reddish (Arunabha), non-slimy (Vishada), foamy (Phenila) and thin (Tanu).
- Shonita (blood) vitiated by Pitta is yellow (Peeta) and black (Asita), and it takes a longer time to coagulate because of the inherent heat (of Pitta).
- Blood vitiated by Kapha is slightly Pale (Pandu) in color, slimy (Picchila), sticky and thick (ghana).
- Blood due to vitiation by more than one Dosha shares the characteristics of the respective symptoms of all the vitiated Doshas. [21-22]

**Features of pure blood:**

तपनीयेन्द्रगोपाभं पद्मालक्तकसन्निभम्|
गुञ्जाफलसवर्णं च विशुद्धं विद्धि शोणितम्||२२||

- Tapaneeya – Pure blood can be likened to gold, purified by fire
- Indragopaabha – The color can be compared with firefly
- Padmalaktaka – like red lotus, lac.
  Like fruit of Gunja (Abrus precatorius Linn) in color (depending upon the individual constitution).[22]

**Dietetic management after bloodletting therapy:**

नात्युष्णशीतं लघु दीपनीयं रक्तेऽपनीते हितमन्नपानम्|
तदा शरीरं ह्यनवस्थितासृग्ग्निर्विशेषेण च रक्षितव्यः||२३||

After bloodletting, intake of food and drink which are neither very hot nor very cold, that are light and stimulants of digestion are recommended. At this stage, because of the instability of the body, the power of digestion and metabolism is specially required to be maintained. [23]

**Features of men having normal blood:**

प्रसन्नवर्णेन्द्रियमिन्द्रियार्थानिच्छन्तमव्याहतपक्तृवेगम्|
सुखान्वितं तु(पु)ष्टिबलोपपन्नं विशुद्धरक्तं पुरुषं वदन्ति||२४||

The signs and symptoms of persons endowed with pure blood are
Prasanna Varna – clarity in complexion,
Prasanna Indriya – Indriya artha – normal functioning of sense organs and perception of objects,
unobstructed digestion and motion, happiness, contentment (nourishment) and strength. [24]

**Description of Mada, Murcha, Sanyasa :**

**Causes and pathology of cerebro-vascular accidents and cerebral symptoms:**

यदा तु रक्तवाहीनि रससञ्ज्ञावहानि च|
पृथक् पृथक् समस्ता वा स्रोतांसि कुपिता मलाः||२५||
मलिनाहारशीलस्य रजोमोहावृतात्मनः|
प्रतिहत्यावतिष्ठन्ते जायन्ते व्याधयस्तदा||२६||
मदमूर्च्छायसन्न्यासास्तेषां विद्याद्विचक्षणः|
यथोत्तरं बलाधिक्यं हेतुलिङ्गोपशान्तिषु||२७||
दुर्बलं चेतसः स्थानं यदा वायुः प्रपद्यते|
मनो विक्षोभयञ्जन्तोः सञ्ज्ञां सम्मोहयेत्तदा||२८||
पित्तमेवं कफश्चैवं मनो विक्षोभयन्नृणाम्|
सञ्ज्ञां नयत्याकुलतां विशेषश्चात्र वक्ष्यते||२९||

**Causes and pathology of cerebro-vascular accidents and cerebral symptoms:**

When someone indulges in habitual intake of unwholesome diet and when their mind is covered with Rajas and Tamas, the Doshas get jointly and severely vitiated. Then they obstruct the three channels mentioned below –
1. Blood channel – Ratktavaha srotas
2. Rasa Dhatu Vaha srotas (the channels that carry nutrients)
3. Nerve channels – Sanjna Vaha Srotas.
This results in manifestation of three diseases like –

- Mada – intoxication
- Murcha – unconsciousness, fainting
- Sanyasa – Coma, syncope.
  From the view of etiology, symptomatology and cure, syncope (Sanyasa) is more serious than fainting (Murcha) and Fainting (Murcha) is more serious than intoxication (Mada).

**Pathogenesis of Mada disease** - When the Vata attacks the site of mind which has become weak, it disturbs the mind (Mano Vikshobha) and brings about unconsciousness. Similarly Pitta and Kapha also disturb the mind, resulting in the unconsciousness of the individual. The special features of these conditions are described here. [25-29]

**Signs and symptoms of Mada Roga (intoxication):**

सक्तानल्पद्रुताभाषं चलस्खलितचेष्टितम् |
विद्याद्वातमदाविष्टं रूक्षश्यावारुणाकृतिम्||३०||
सक्रोधपरुषाभाषं सम्प्रहारकलिप्रियम्|
विद्यात् पित्तमदाविष्टं रक्तपीतासिताकृतिम्||३१||
स्वल्पासम्बद्धवचनं तन्द्रालस्यसमन्वितम्|
विद्यात् कफमदाविष्टं पाण्डुं प्रध्यानतत्परम्||३२||
सर्वाण्येतानि रूपाणि सन्निपातकृते मदे|३३|

**Signs and symptoms of Mada Roga (intoxication):**

**Signs and symptoms of Vatic (Vata) type of Mada** – making incoherent, excessive and fast speeches, instability and non-coordination in action, dryness, blackish (shyava) and redness (Arunata) in complexion;
**Signs and symptoms of Paittika type of Mada** – anger and harsh speeches, tempted to assaults and quarrels, and redness, yellowness and blackness in complexion.
**Signs and Symptoms of Shlaishmika (Kapha) type of Mada** - feeble incoherent speeches, drowsiness, laziness, paleness and wandering.
**Signs and symptoms of Sannipatika type of Mada (due to all three Doshas combined)** - shares all the above mentioned signs and symptoms. [30-32]

**Treatment of Mada Roga:**

जायते शाम्यति क्षिप्रं मदो मद्यमदाकृतिः||३३||

This intoxication (Mada) which can be likened to the one caused by alcoholic drinks is manifested and cured immediately. The treatment line is similar to that of alcoholism. [33]

**Mada and Dosha:**

यश्च मद्यकृतः प्रोक्तो विषजो रौधिरश्च यः|
सर्व एते मदा नर्ते वातपित्तकफत्रयात्||३४||

Mada of all types produced either by alcoholic drinks or by the intake of poison or by the vitiation of blood are, on an ultimate analysis, caused by nothing but the vitiation of Vata, Pitta and or Kapha. So, all varieties of intoxication are of four types viz, Vatika Paittika, Slaishmika and Sannipatika). [34]

**Signs and symptoms of Murcha (fainting / unconsciousness):**

नीलं वा यदि वा कृष्णमाकाशमथवाऽरुणम्|
पश्यंस्तमः प्रविशति शीघ्रं च प्रतिबुध्यते ||३५||
वेपथुश्चाङ्गमर्दश्च प्रपीडा हृदयस्य च|
कार्श्यं श्यावारुणा च्छायामूर्च्छायै वातसम्भवे||३६||
रक्तं हरितवर्णं वा वियत् पीतमथापि वा|
पश्यंस्तमः प्रविशति सस्वेदः प्रतिबुध्यते||३७||
सपिपासः ससन्तापो रक्तपीताकुलेक्षणः|
सम्भिन्नवर्चाः पीताभो मूर्च्छायै पित्तसम्भवे||३८||
मेघसङ्काशमाकाशमावृतं वा तमोघनैः|

पश्यंस्तमः प्रविशति चिराच्च प्रतिबुध्यते||३९||
गुरुभिः प्रावृतैरङ्गैर्यथैवार्द्रेण चर्मणा|
सप्रसेकः सहल्लासो मूर्च्छाये कफसम्भवे||४०||
सर्वाकृतिः सन्निपातादपस्मार इवागतः|
स जन्तुं पातयत्याशु विना बीभत्सचेष्टितैः||४१||

## Signs and symptoms of Murcha (fainting / unconsciousness):

To an individual suffering from Vatika type of Moorcha – the sky appears as blue, black or red. Thereafter he becomes unconscious but soon he recovers: there is trembling (Vepathu), malaise (Angamarda), cardiac pain, emaciation (Karshya) and blackish brown or red complexion (Shyava Arunata).

To an individual suffering from Pattika type of Murcha, – the sky appears as red, green or yellow. Thereafter he becomes unconscious and recovers with sweating; there is a feeling of thirst and heat, there is redness and yellowness in eyes, diarrhea and yellow complexion.

To an individual suffering from Shlaismika (Kapha) type of fainting, the sky appears as if raining or as if covered by dark cloud (or darkness and cold); Thereafter he becomes unconscious: he recovers after a long time; he feels as if his body is covered with a heavy blanket, like a wet hide; he gets salivation and nausea.
In case of Sannipatika type of Moorcha (Vata, Pitta and Kapha combined) –all the above signs and symptoms are manifested and the individual is laid down like a patient suffering from epilepsy (apasmara); but unlike epilepsy there is no awkward behavior such as biting teeth, throwing out limbs etc.[35-41]

## Differential diagnosis and treatment of Sanyasa (Coma):

दोषेषु मदमूर्च्छायाः कृतवेगेषु देहिनाम्|
स्वयमेवोपशाम्यन्ति सन्न्यासो नौषधैर्विना||४२||

As regards Mada and Murcha, they are cured automatically soon after the manifestation of attack by the aggravated Doshas. The syncope (Sanyasa), however, does not subside without the administration of proper medicines.

## Importance of emergency treatment in Sanyasa :

वाग्देहमनसां चेष्टामाक्षिप्यातिबला मलाः|
सन्न्यस्यन्त्यबलं जन्तुं प्राणायतनसंश्रिताः||४३||
स ना सन्न्याससन्न्यस्तः काष्ठीभूतो मृतोपमः|
प्राणैर्वियुज्यते शीघ्रं मुक्त्वा सद्यःफलाः क्रियाः||४४||
दुर्गेऽम्भसि यथा मज्जद्भाजनं त्वरया बुधः|

## Importance of emergency treatment in Sanyasa :

The aggravated Doshas weaken the individual and bring about loss of functions of mind, body and speech in him. Due to Sanyasa, there is absolute loss of consciousness. He lies down as a piece of wood or corpse. As a wise person takes out a pitcher sinking in very deep water much before it touches the bottom, in Sanyasa, if proper therapy having immediate action is not administered, it may lead to death.

## Treatment methods to bring back consciousness in Sanyasa :

गृह्णीयात्तमप्राप्तं तथा सन्न्यासपीडितम्‌||४५||
अञ्जनान्यवपीडाश्च धूमाः प्रधमनानि च|
सूचीभिस्तोदनं शस्तं दाहः पीडा नखान्तरे||४६||
लुञ्चनं केशलोम्नां च दन्तैर्दशनमेव च|
आत्मगुप्तावघर्षश्च हितं तस्यावबोधने||४७||
सम्मूर्च्छितानि तीक्ष्णानि मद्यानि विविधानि च|
प्रभूतकटुयुक्तानि तस्यास्ये गालयेन्मुहुः||४८||
मातुलुङ्गरसं तद्वन्महौषधसमायुतम्‌|
तद्वत्सौवर्चलं दद्याद्युक्तं मद्याम्लकाञ्जिकैः||४९||
हिङ्गूषणसमायुक्तं यावत्‌ सञ्ज्ञाप्रबोधनम्‌|
प्रबुद्धसञ्ज्ञमन्नैश्च लघुभिस्तमुपाचरेत्‌||५०||
विस्मापनैः स्मारणैश्च प्रियश्रुतिभिरेव च|
पटुभिर्गीतवादित्रशब्दैश्चित्रैश्च दर्शनैः||५१||
संसनोल्लेखनैर्धूमैरञ्जनैः कवलग्रहैः|
शोणितस्यावसेकैश्च व्यायामोद्घर्षणैस्तथा||५२||
प्रबुद्धसञ्ज्ञं मतिमाननुबन्धमुपक्रमेत्‌|
तस्य संरक्षितव्यं हि मनः प्रलयहेतुतः||५३||

- Anjana – Application of collyrium
- Avapeeda Nasya – nasal drops by juice extracts of herbs
- Dhooma – smoke
- Pradhamana nasya – snuff
- Soochi Todana – pricking with needle
- heating causing pain in the nail bed, plucking the hair from the head and body
- biting with teeth and rubbing the body with Atmagupta ( Mucuna prurita Hook).
  These are helpful in bringing about consciousness.

Various types of strong alcoholic drinks mixed together with other drugs of pungent taste should be carefully put in his mouth frequently. The physician should further administer the juice of Matulunga (Lemon variety – Citrus decumana / Citrus limon), Mahausadha (ginger), Asafetida and Black pepper until the patient regains consciousness.

After the patient regains consciousness, he should be given light diet. Thereafter, his consciousness should be maintained by various psychological and physical devices and his mind should be diverted from the etiological factors of unconsciousness. He should be made to remember some surprising events (Vismapana, Smarana), hear pleasing fine songs and music. He should be administered with Panchakarma procedures – purgation, emesis, smoke, collyrium, gargle, blood-letting physical exercise and rough massage (Udgarshana). [45-53]

**Management of Mada and Murcha :**

स्नेहस्वेदोपपन्नानां यथादोषं यथाबलम्‌|
पञ्च कर्माणि कुर्वीत मूर्च्छायेषु मदेषु च||५४||
अष्टाविंशत्यौषधस्य तथा तिक्तस्य सर्पिषः|
प्रयोगः शस्यते तद्वन्महतः षट्पलस्य वा||५५||
त्रिफलायाः प्रयोगो वा सघृतक्षौद्रशर्करः|
शिलाजतुप्रयोगो वा प्रयोगः पयसोऽपि वा||५६||

पिप्पलीनां प्रयोगो वा पयसा चित्रकस्य वा|
रसायनानां कौम्भस्य सर्पिषो वा प्रशस्यते||५७||
रक्तावसेकाच्छास्त्राणां सतां सत्त्ववतामपि|
सेवनान्मदमूर्च्छायाः प्रशाम्यन्ति शरीरिणाम्||५८||

**Management of Mada and Murcha :**

In the case of intoxication and fainting, the patient should be administered the Panchakarma therapies after oleation and fomentation with due regard to the strength and the vitiation of the Doshas of the individual.

Besides the Kalyanaka Ghrita (herbal ghee containing twenty eight drugs), Mahatiktaka Ghrita and Satpala Ghrita (reference: Charaka Chikitsa 7th chapter) may be given. Triphala along with ghee, honey and sugar, Shilajatu (mineral pitch), milk, pippali (Piper longum Linn), Chitraka (Lead word – Plumbago zeylanica) with milk, Kaumbha Sarpi – ten year old ghee and such other elixirs (Rasayana) may also be administered. Raktamokshana (Bloodletting). Study of religious books and devotion to spiritually enlightened good persons also cure intoxication and fainting. [54-58]

**To sum up:**

तत्र श्लोकौ-
विशुद्धं चाविशुद्धं च शोणितं तस्य हेतवः|
रक्तप्रदोषजा रोगास्तेषु रोगेषु चौषधम्||५९||
मदमूर्च्छायसन्न्यासहेतुलक्षणभेषजम्|
विधिशोणितकेऽध्याये सर्वमेतत् प्रकाशितम्||६०||

Causes and signs of pure and impure blood, disease due to impurity in blood, their treatment, etiology, signs, symptoms and treatment of intoxication, fainting and syncope - all these are explained in the chapter on Vidhi Shoniteeya Adhyaya [59-60]

इत्यग्निवेशकृते तन्त्रे चरकप्रतिसंस्कृते श्लोकस्थाने विधिशोणितीयो नाम चतुर्विंशोऽध्यायः||२४||
समाप्तो योजनाचतुष्कः||६||
Thus ends the twenty fourth chapter on Blood Tissue of the Sutra section of Agnivesha's work as redacted by Charaka.[24]
This ends Yogana Chatushka.

# 25

# Sutrasthana Chapter 25 Yajja Purusheeyam Adhyayam

**Yajja Purusheeya Adhyaya**
**Best and Worst Things for Health and Disease**
The 25th chapter of Sutrasthana of Charaka Samhita is structured in a form of group discussion. This chapter enlists the best among the food types, like which type of fish is the best, which type of fruit is the best etc. The chapter is called Yajja Purusheeya Adhyaya – origin of Living Being and Diseases.

अथातो यज्जःपुरुषीयमध्यायं व्याख्यास्यामः||१||

इति ह स्माह भगवानात्रेयः||२||

**A seminar of olden times:**

पुरा प्रत्यक्षधर्माणं भगवन्तं पुनर्वसुम्|
समेतानां महर्षीणां प्रादुरासीदियं कथा ||३||
आत्मेन्द्रियमनोर्थानां योऽयं पुरुषसञ्ज्ञकः|
राशिरस्यामयानां च प्रागुत्पत्तिविनिश्चये||४||

**A seminar of olden times:**
Once upon a time sages assembled together before Lord Punarvasu who had the direct realisation of the virtuous qualities, for a discussion on the determination of the origin of man – an aggregate of soul, senses, mind and objects and his diseases. [3-4]

**Kashiraja's doubt:**

तदन्तरं काशिपतिर्वामको वाक्यमर्थवित्|
व्याजहारर्षिसमितिमुपसृत्याभिवाद्य च||५||
किन्नु भोः पुरुषो यज्जस्तज्जास्तस्यामयाः स्मृताः|
न वेत्युक्ते नरेन्द्रेण प्रोवाचर्षीन् पुनर्वसुः||६||
सर्व एवामितज्ञानविज्ञानच्छिन्नसंशयाः|
भवन्तश्छेतुमर्हन्ति काशिराजस्य संशयम्||७||

**Kashiraja's doubt:**

Vamaka, the king of Kashi, who was well versed in the science of medicine approached the assembly of sages with respect and asked the following question:
Do the diseases also originate from the same source as that of man or not?
At this, Lord Punarvasu directed the sages as follows:

"You are all enlightened, with your doubts fully cleared by virtue of your unlimited knowledge and skill. You are capable of clarifying unlimited knowledge and skill. You are capable of clarifying the point raised by the king of kashi". [5-7]

**Parikshi Maudgalya – Atma is the cause:**

पारीक्षिस्तत्परीक्ष्याग्रे मौद्गल्यो वाक्यमब्रवीत्|
आत्मजः पुरुषो रोगाश्चात्मजाः कारणं हि सः||८||
स चिनोत्युपभुङ्क्ते च कर्म कर्मफलानि च|
नह्यृते चेतनाधातोः प्रवृत्तिः सुखदुःखयोः||९||

**Parikshi Maudgalya – Atma is the cause:**

Parikshi, a descendant of Mudgala, after due examination, said,
"The living being originates from the soul and so also the disease. It is the soul which is the root cause of living beings and their diseases. The soul alone collects and enjoys the actions (Karma) and their results (Karma Phala) respectively.

Happiness (that is freedom from diseases) and miseries (that is affliction with diseases) can never occur without the soul. [8-9]

**Sharaloma – Satva (mind) is the cause:**

शरलोमा तु नेत्याह न ह्यात्माऽऽत्मानमात्मना|
योजयेद्व्याधिभिर्दुःखैर्दुःखद्वेषी कदाचन||१०||
रजस्तमोभ्यां तु मनः परीतं सत्त्वसञ्ज्ञकम्|
शरीरस्य समुत्पत्तौ विकाराणां च कारणम्||११||

**Sharaloma – Satva (mind) is the cause:**

Sharaloma, expressed that the soul which is by nature averse to all miseries cannot by itself be responsible for bringing about diseases or other miseries. It is the mind (Satva) covered with Rajas and Tamas which causes the body (of the living being) as well as its diseases.

**Vayorvida – Rasa Dhatu (nutritious fluid) is the cause:**

वार्योविदस्तु नेत्याह न ह्येकं कारणं मनः |
नर्ते शरीराच्छारीररोगा न मनसः स्थितिः||१२||
रसजानि तु भूतानि व्याधयश्च पृथग्विधाः|
आपो हि रसवत्यस्ताः स्मृता निर्वृतिहेतवः||१३||

**Vayorvida – Rasa Dhatu (nutritious fluid) is the cause:**

Varyovida did not agree with Sharaloma and said, "the mind alone cannot be the cause. Neither the physical diseases nor mind itself can exist without the body. Living beings and their various diseases are in fact caused by the Rasa (product of nutrition after digestion). As water abounds in Rasa Dhatu, it is the ultimate cause of living beings as well as their diseases". [10-13]

**Hiranyaksha – Six Dhatu School (Atma + five basic principles):**

हिरण्याक्षस्तु नेत्याह न ह्यात्मा रसजः स्मृतः|
नातीन्द्रियं मनः सन्ति रोगाः शब्दादिजास्तथा||१४||
षड्धातुजस्तु पुरुषो रोगाः षड्धातुजास्तथा|
राशिः षड्धातुजो ह्येष साङ्ख्यैराद्यैः प्रकीर्तितः ||१५||

**Hiranyaksha – Six Dhatu School (Atma + five basic principles):**

Hiranyaksha was not in favor of accepting Rasa (product of nutrition after digestion) as the origin of the soul. He was of the view that neither Atma (soul) nor the mind is perceptible, none of them can be said to originate from Rasa Dhatu. Similarly all diseases cannot originate from Rasa. There are diseases which are caused by unfavorable sounds etc. So Hiranyaksha concluded that 'the living beings as well as their diseases originate from six Dhatus'. According to the Samkhya system of philosophy, the six Dhatus consist of Atman (Soul) and five fundamental principles (Prithvi – Solid, Ap – water, Tejas – fire, Vayu – air and Akasha – ether).[14-15]

**Kaushika – 'Father – Mother' School:**

तथा ब्रुवाणं कुशिकमाह तन्नेति कौशिकः|
कस्मान्मातापितृभ्यां हि विना षड्धातुजो भवेत्||१६||
पुरुषः पुरुषाद्गौर्गौरश्वादश्वः प्रजायते|
पित्र्या मेहादयश्चोक्ता रोगास्तावत्र कारणम्||१७||

**Kaushika – Father – Mother School:**

Kaushika did not agree with the above view of Hiranyaksha. How the living beings could be born simply out of six Dhatus without reference to their parents. A human being is born from another human being; a cow out of a cow; a horse out of a horse. It is a well known fact that diseases like Prameha (urinary disorders), Kushta (Skin diseases) and piles are hereditary in nature. Thus, according to Kaushika, the parents represent the root cause of living beings as well as diseases. [16-17]

**Bhadrakapya – Karma:**

भद्रकाप्यस्तु नेत्याह नह्यन्धोऽन्धात् प्रजायते|
मातापित्रोरपि च ते प्रागुत्पत्तिर्न युज्यते||१८||
कर्मजस्तु मतो जन्तुः कर्मजास्तस्य चामयाः|
नह्यृते कर्मणो जन्म रोगाणां पुरुषस्य वा||१९||

**Bhadrakapya – Karma:**

Disagreeing with the above view, Bhadrakapya said, "It is not that the progeny of blind parents is invariably blind. Moreover, if Kaushika's view regarding parental origination of living beings and diseases is accepted, how could the parents themselves be born at the primordial stage? So the living beings as well as their diseases originate from Karma (the past action). For, neither living beings nor diseases can be born without Karma. [18-19]

**Bharadwaja – Swabhava (Nature):**

भरद्वाजस्तु नेत्याह कर्ता पूर्वं हि कर्मणः|
दृष्टं न चाकृतं कर्म यस्य स्यात् पुरुषः फलम्||२०||
भावहेतुः स्वभावस्तु व्याधीनां पुरुषस्य च|
खरद्रवचलोष्णत्वं तेजोन्तानां यथैव हि||२१||

## Bharadwaja – Swabhava (Nature):

Bharadvaja rejected the arguments put forth by Bhadrakapya and said "The Karma always presupposes the existence of an agent. There is no evidence to show that an action, even if not performed, can result in the form of creation of a living being". So Bharadvaja concluded, Svabhava (nature) is the root cause of the existence of living beings as well as diseases. For example, it is by nature that Prithvi, Ap, Tajas and Vayu have roughness, Liquidity, heat and mobility respectively. [20-21]

## Kankayana – Prajapati:

काङ्कायनस्तु नेत्याह न ह्यारम्भफलं भवेत्|
भवेत् स्वभावाद्भावानामसिद्धिः सिद्धिरेव वा||२२||
स्रष्टा त्वमितसङ्कल्पो ब्रह्मापत्यं प्रजापतिः|
चेतनाचेतनस्यास्य जगतः सुखदुःखयोः||२३||

Disagreeing with Bharadvaja, Kankayana said that if Svabhava (nature) is taken to be the root cause of living beings it would mean that individual efforts (e.g., performance of rituals, cultivation, study etc.) are altogether useless. Accomplishment or otherwise of an object, would then depend not on individual action but on Svabhava (nature) itself. So he concluded that Prajapati, the son of Brahma with his infinite creative powers will represent the origin of the happiness and misery of the world-sentient as well as insentient.

## Bhikshu Atreya – Kala (time):

तन्नेति भिक्षुरात्रेयो न ह्यपत्यं प्रजापतिः|
प्रजाहितैषी सततं दुःखैर्युञ्ज्यादसाधुवत्||२४||
कालजस्त्वेव पुरुषः कालजास्तस्य चामयाः|
जगत् कालवशं सर्वं कालः सर्वत्र कारणम्||२५||

## Bhikshu Atreya – Kala (time):

Refuting the above view Bhikshu Atreya said that, interested in the well being of the entire creation as he is, Prajapati cannot afford to bring about miseries for his subjects like any other cruel human being. So Bhiksu Atreya concluded that living beings as well as their diseases are caused by Kala (time) the whole universe is conditioned by Kala and Kala is the causative factor for all. [22-25]

## Punarvasu Atreya's conclusion:

तथर्षीणां विवदतामुवाचेदं पुनर्वसुः|
मैवं वोचत तत्त्वं हि दुष्प्रापं पक्षसंश्रयात्||२६||
वादान् सप्रतिवादान् हि वदन्तो निश्चितानिव|

पक्षान्तं नैव गच्छन्ति तिलपीडकवद्गतौ||२७||
मुक्त्वैवं वादसङ्घट्टमध्यात्ममनुचिन्त्यताम्|
नाविधूते तमःस्कन्धे ज्ञेये ज्ञानं प्रवर्तते||२८||
येषामेव हि भावानां सम्पत् सञ्जनयेन्नरम्|
तेषामेव विपद्व्याधीन्निविधान्समुदीरयेत्||२९||

**Punarvasu Atreya's conclusion:**

During the course of this controversial discussion of sages, Lord Punarvasu observed, "Please do not enter into such a controversy: it is difficult to arrive at the truth by taking sides with its partial aspects. Those who consider the varying controversial aspects of the truth as established facts, go on moving around without reaching the goal like a person sitting on the oil press (who goes around moving all along without a pause). So you should get rid of the riddle of Arguments and try to pursue the real truth. One cannot attain real knowledge without shunning one's basics for the partial aspects of the truth.

The very same factors, which, in the state of their wholesome combination, are responsible for the creation of living beings, in the state of their unwholesome combination are responsible for the various diseases. [26-29]

**Enhancing causes:**

अथात्रेयस्य भगवतो वचनमनुनिशम्य पुनरेव वामकः काशिपतिरुवाच भगवन्तमात्रेयं- भगवन्! सम्पन्निमित्तजस्य पुरुषस्य विपन्निमित्तजानां च रोगाणां किमभिवृद्धिकारणमिति||३०||
तमुवाच भगवानात्रेयः- हिताहारोपयोग एक एव पुरुषवृद्धिकरो भवति, अहिताहारोपयोगः पुनर्व्याधिनिमित्तमिति ||३१||
एवंवादिनं भगवन्तमात्रेयमग्निवेश उवाच- कथमिह भगवन्! हिताहितानामाहारजातानां लक्षणमनपवादमभिजानीमहे; हितसमाख्यातानामाहारजातानामहितसमाख्यातानां च मात्राकालक्रियाभूमिदेहदोषपुरुषावस्थान्तरेषु विपरीतकारित्वमुपलभामह इति||३२||

**Enhancing causes:**

After having listened to Lord Punarvasu, Vamaka, the king of Kashi enquired, "Oh! Lord, what are these factors whose wholesome and unwholesome combinations are responsible for the growth of living beings and their diseases. Lord Atreya said, 'Wholesome food is one of the causes for the growth of living beings and unwholesome food for the growth of diseases'.

**Agnivesha** then asked, "How shall we correctly distinguish between wholesome and unwholesome food articles which bring about opposite effects, depending upon the variations in dose, time, and method of preparation, habitat, and constitution of the body, disease and the age of the individual. [30-32] |

**Sama and Vishama diets – Wholesome and unwholesome diet:**

तमुवाच भगवानात्रेयः- यदाहारजातमग्निवेश! समांश्चैव शरीरधातून् प्रकृतौ स्थापयति विषमांश्च समीकरोतीत्येतदिद्धतं विद्धि, विपरीतं त्वहितमिति; इत्येतदिद्धताहितलक्षणमनपवादं भवति||३३||
एवंवादिनं च भगवन्तमात्रेयमग्निवेश उवाच- भगवन्! न त्वेतदेवमुपदिष्टं भूयिष्ठकल्पाः सर्वभिषजो विज्ञास्यन्ति||३४||

**Sama and Vishama diets – Wholesome and unwholesome diet:**

Lord Punarvasu replied, "The food articles which maintain the equilibrium of Dhatus (Tridosha in balance, body tissues and waste products) and help in eliminating the disturbance of their equilibrium are to be regarded as wholesome, otherwise they are unwholesome".

Agnivesha asked again, "This type of general definition will not be comprehensible for all kinds of physicians". [33-34]

**Multiplicity of dietetic factors:**

तमुवाच भगवानात्रेयः- येषां हि विदितमाहारतत्त्वमग्निवेश! गुणतो द्रव्यतः कर्मतः सर्वावयवशश्च मात्रादयो भावाः, त एतदेवमुपदिष्टं विज्ञातुमुत्सहन्ते|
यथा तु खल्वेतदुपदिष्टं भूयिष्ठकल्पाः सर्वभिषजो विज्ञास्यन्ति, तथैतदुपदेक्ष्यामो मात्रादीन् भावाननुदाहरन्तः; तेषां हि बहुविधविकल्पा भवन्ति|
आहारविधिविशेषांस्तु खलु लक्षणतश्चावयवतश्चानुव्याख्यास्यामः||३५||

**Multiplicity of dietetic factors:**

Lord Punarvasu replied, "Those physicians who are well versed with the food articles, (dravya) their properties, action, dosage etc. in all respects will find no difficulty in ascertaining the wholesomeness or otherwise of a given food article.

With a view of guarding the physicians of all categories, we shall explain the various specifications of food articles. It is however not possible to enumerate the dosage etc. of these food articles as their variations are too many to be specified. As to the dietetic variations, they will be explained in general and specific terms. [35]

**Origin of Ahara – Food, types:**

तद्यथा- आहारत्वमाहारस्यैकविधमर्थाभेदात्; स पुनर्द्विर्योनिः, स्थावरजङ्गमात्मकत्वात्; द्विविधप्रभावः, हिताहितोदर्कविशेषात्; चतुर्विधोपयोगः, पानाशनभक्ष्यलेह्योपयोगात्; षडास्वादः, रसभेदतः षड्विधत्वात्;
आहारत्वमाहारस्यैकविधमर्थाभेदात्;

Defined in general terms, food is the one which can be consumed by living beings. By this virtue, food is only of one type.

स पुनर्द्विर्योनिः, स्थावरजङ्गमात्मकत्वात्;

If we consider source, there are two types of food :
Sthavara – vegetable products, the source which stays at only one place without movement
Jangama – animal products, the source which moves.

द्विविधप्रभावः, हिताहितोदर्कविशेषात्;

From the point of view of specific action, food articles can again be classified into two viz,
Hita – with ultimate wholesome effect and
Ahita – food that causes unwholesome effect

चतुर्विधोपयोगः, पानाशनभक्ष्यलेह्योपयोगात्;

Because of the mode of consumption, food is of four types.

Paana – drinks,
Ashana – eatables,
Bhakshya – chewables and
Lehya – lickables (linctus).

षडास्वादः, रसभेदतः षड्विधत्वात्;

Based on taste, food is of six types – i.e.

- Sweet,
- Salt,
- Sour,
- Pungent,
- Bitter and
- Astringent

**Based on qualities, food is of twenty types:**

विंशतिगुणः, गुरुलघुशीतोष्णस्निग्धरूक्षमन्दतीक्ष्णस्थिरसरमृदुकठिन- विशदपिच्छिलश्लक्ष्णखरसूक्ष्मस्थूलसान्द्रद्रवानुगमात्; अपरिसङ्ख्येयविकल्पः, द्रव्यसंयोगकरणबाहुल्यात्॥३६॥

**Based on qualities, food is of twenty types:**

Guru (heaviness) X Laghu (lightness)
Sheeta (cold) X Ushna (hot)
Snigdha (unctuousness, oiliness) X Rooksha (dryness)
Manda (dullness) X Teekshna (sharpness)
Sthira (stability) X Sara (mobility)
Mridu (softness) X Kathina (hardness)
Vishada (non-sliminess, clarity) X Picchila (sliminess, Stickiness)
Shlakshna (smoothness) X Khara (roughness)
Sookshma (minute, subtleness) X Sthoola (grossness, bulk)
Sandra (solidity) X Drava (liquidity).
Depending upon the combination of different food articles, the food types are innumerable. [36]

तस्य खलु ये ये विकारावयवा भूयिष्ठमुपयुज्यन्ते, भूयिष्ठकल्पानां च मनुष्याणां प्रकृत्यैव हिततमाश्चाहिततमाश्च, तांस्तान् यथावदुपदेक्ष्यामः॥३७॥

**Let us learn in detail about examples of wholesome and unwholesome articles [37]**

**Best foods :**

तद्यथा- लोहितशालयः शूकधान्यानां पथ्यतमत्वे श्रेष्ठतमा भवन्ति, मुद्गाः शमीधान्यानाम्, आन्तरिक्षमुदकानां, सैन्धवं लवणानां, जीवन्तीशाकं शाकानाम्, ऐणेयं मृगमांसानां, लावः पक्षिणां, गोधा बिलेशयानां, रोहितो मत्स्यानां, गव्यं सर्पिः सर्पिषां, गोक्षीरं क्षीराणां, तिलतैलं स्थावरजातानां स्नेहानां, वराहवसा आनूपमृगवसानां, चुलुकीवसा मत्स्यवसानां, पाकहंसवसा जलचरविहङ्गवसानां, कुक्कुटवसा विष्किरशकुनिवसानां, अजमेदः शाखादमेदसां, शृङ्गवेरं कन्दानां, मृद्वीका फलानां, शर्करेक्षुविकाराणाम्, इति प्रकृत्यैव हिततमानामाहारविकाराणां प्राधान्यतो द्रव्याणि व्याख्यातानि भवन्ति॥३८॥

## Best foods:

लोहितशालयः शूकधान्यानां – Red type of rice is the best among Paddy having bristles

मुद्गाःशमीधान्यानाम् – Among pulses, Green gram is the best

आन्तरिक्षमुदकानां – Among waters, Rain water collected before fall on the ground is the best

सैन्धवं लवणानां – Among salts, Rock salt is the best

जीवन्तीशाकं शाकानाम् –Among pot herbs, Jivanti (Leptadenia reticulate W.and A) is the best

ऐणेयं मृगमांसानां – Among the meat of big animals, Ena (antelope)

लावः पक्षिणां – Among meat of Birds Lava (common quail)

गोधा बिलेशयानां – Among Meat of animals living in holes, Godha (inguana)

रोहितो मत्स्यानां – Among fish, Rohita type of fish

गव्यं सर्पिः सर्पिषां – Among Ghee, Cow ghee

गोक्षीरं क्षीराणां – Among Milk, Cow milk

तिलतैलं स्थावरजातानां स्नेहानां – Among Vegetable fats, <u>Sesame oil</u>

वराहवसा आनूपमृगवसानां – Among the fats of marshy animals, fat of Lard (pig fat)

चुलुकीवसा मत्स्यवसानां – Among the fish fat – Fat of Chuluki (Gangetic dolphin)

पाकहंसवसा जलचरविहङ्गवसानां – Among the fats of aquatic birds – Fat of Pakahamsa (white swan)

कुक्कुटवसा विष्किरशकुनिवसानां – Among the fats of Vishkira (gallinaceous types of birds, with beak) – Fat of hen

अजमेदः शाखादमेदसां – Among the fats of tree branch eating animals – Fat of goat

शृङ्गवेरं कन्दानां – Among the rhizomes – Ginger

मृद्वीका फलानां – Among the fruits – Grapes

शर्करेक्षुविकाराणाम् – Among the preparations / products of sugar cane – Sarkara (Sugar candy) [38]

## Most unwholesome articles:

अहिततमानप्युपदेक्ष्यामः- यवकाः शूकधान्यानामपथ्यतमत्वेन प्रकृष्टतमा भवन्ति, माषाः शमीधान्यानां, वर्षानादेयमुदकानाम्, ऊषरं लवणानां, सर्षपशाकं शाकानां, गोमांसं मृगमांसानां, काणकपोतः पक्षिणां, भेको बिलेशयानां, चिलिचिमो मत्स्यानाम्, आविकं सर्पिः सर्पिषाम्, अविक्षीरं क्षीराणां, कुसुम्भस्नेहः स्थावरस्नेहानां, महिषवसा आनूपमृगवसानां, कुम्भीरवसा मत्स्यवसानां, काकमद्गुवसा जलचरविहङ्गवसानां, चटकवसा विष्किरशकुनिवसानां, हस्तिमेदः शाखादमेदसां, निकुचं फलानाम्, आलुकं कन्दानां, फाणितमिक्षुविकाराणाम्, इति प्रकृत्यैवाहिततमानामाहारविकाराणां प्रकृष्टतमानि द्रव्याणि व्याख्यातानि भवन्ति; (इति) हिताहितावयवो व्याख्यात आहारविकाराणाम्||३९||

## Most unwholesome foods and activities:

यवकाःशूकधान्याना – Among Shuka Dhanya (Paddy having bristles), Yavaka (a variety of Barley) is most unwholesome

माषाःशमीधान्यानां – Among pulses (Shami Dhanya) black gram is most unwholesome

वर्षानादेयमुदकानाम् – Among waters, river water in rainy season is most unwholesome

ऊषरंलवणानां – Among salts, Ushara (salt collected/prepared from saline soil)

सर्षपशाकंशाकानां – Among pot herbs, Mustard is the most unwholesome

गोमांसंमृगमांसानां – Among meet, Beef

काणकपोतःपक्षिणां – Among meat of birds, Kana Kapota (Young dove)

भेकोबिलेशयानां – Among Bileshaya (meat of animals living in the holes) – Frog is the most unwholesome

चिलिचिमोमत्स्यानाम् – Among fish, Chilichima

आविकंसर्पिःसर्पिषाम् – Among ghee, Ghee of sheep milk

अविक्षीरंक्षीराणां – Among milk, Sheep milk

कुसुम्भ स्नेहःस्थावरस्नेहानां – Among the vegetable fat - Oil from Kusumbha (Canthamus tinctorius Linn)

महिषवसा आनूपमृगवसानां – Among the fats of marshy animals – Fat of Buffalo

कुम्भीरवसा मत्स्यवसानां – Among the fats of aquatic animals – Fat of Kumbhira (Crocodile)

काकमद्गुवसा जलचर विहङ्ग वसानां – Fats of aquatic animals – Fat of Kakamadgu (water foul)

चटकवसा विष्किरशकुनिवसानां – Among the fats of gallinaceous types of birds – Fat of Chataka (sparrow)

हस्तिमेदः शाखादमेदसां – Among the fats of tree branch eating animals - Fat of elephant

निकुचं फलानाम् – Among the fruits - Nikucha (Artocarpus lakoocha Roxb)

आलुकं कन्दानां – Among the Rhizomes and roots - Aluka (potato?)

फाणितमिक्षुविकाराणाम् – Among the Preparations of sugar cane - Phanita (treacle)

**Most important drugs, actions, factors:**

अतो भूयः कर्मौषधानां च प्राधान्यतः सानुबन्धानि द्रव्याण्यनुव्याख्यास्यामः|

तद्यथा- अन्नं वृत्तिकराणां श्रेष्ठम्, उदकमाश्वासकराणां (सुरा श्रमहराणां), क्षीरं जीवनीयानां, मांसं बृंहणीयानां, रसस्तर्पणीयानां, लवणमन्नद्रव्यरुचिकराणाम्, अम्लं हृद्यानां, कुक्कुटो बल्यानां, नक्रेतो वृष्याणां, मधु श्लेष्मपित्तप्रशमनानां, सर्पिर्वातपित्तप्रशमनानां, तैलं वातश्लेष्मप्रशमनानां, वमनं श्लेष्महराणां, विरेचनं पित्तहराणां, बस्तिर्वातहराणां, स्वेदो मार्दवकराणां, व्यायामः स्थैर्यकराणां, क्षारः पुंस्त्वोपघातिनां, (तिन्दुकमनन्नद्रव्यरुचिकराणाम्,) आमं कपित्थमकण्ठ्यानाम्, आविकं सर्पिरहृद्यानाम्, अजाक्षीरं शोषघ्नस्तन्यसात्म्यरक्तसाङ्ग्राहिकरक्तपित्तप्रशमनानाम्, अविक्षीरं श्लेष्मपित्तजननानां, महिषीक्षीरं स्वप्नजननानां, मन्दकं दध्यभिष्यन्दकराणां, गवेधुकान्नं कर्शनीयानां, उद्दालकान्नं विरूक्षणीयानां, इक्षुर्मूत्रजननानां, यवाः पुरीषजननानां, जाम्बवं वातजननानां, शष्कुल्यः श्लेष्मपित्तजननानां, कुलत्था अम्लपित्तजननानां, माषाः श्लेष्मपित्तजननानां, मदनफलं वमनास्थापनानुवासनोपयोगिनां, त्रिवृत् सुखविरेचनानां, चतुरङ्गुलो मृदुविरेचनानां, स्नुक्पयस्तीक्ष्णविरेचनानां, प्रत्यक्पुष्पा शिरोविरेचनानां, विडङ्गं क्रिमिघ्नानां, शिरीषो विषघ्नानां, खदिरः कुष्ठघ्नानां, रास्ना वातहराणाम्, आमलकं वयःस्थापनानां, हरीतकी पथ्यानाम्, एरण्डमूलं वृष्यवातहराणां, पिप्पलीमूलं दीपनीयपाचनीयानाहप्रशमनानां, चित्रकमूलं दीपनीयपाचनीयगुदशोथार्शःशूलहराणां, पुष्करमूलं हिक्काश्वासकासपार्श्वशूलहराणां, मुस्तं साङ्ग्राहिकदीपनीयपाचनीयानाम्, उदीच्यं निर्वापणदीपनीयपाचनीयच्छर्द्यतीसारहराणां, कट्वङ्गं साङ्ग्राहिकपाचनीयदीपनीयानां, अनन्ता साङ्ग्राहिकरक्तपित्तप्रशमनानाम्, अमृता साङ्ग्राहिकवातहरदीपनीयश्लेष्मशोणितविबन्धप्रशमनानां, बिल्वं साङ्ग्राहिकदीपनीयवातकफप्रशमनानाम्, अतिविषा दीपनीयपाचनीयसाङ्ग्राहिकसर्वदोषहराणाम्, उत्पलकुमुदपद्मकिञ्जल्कः साङ्ग्राहिकरक्तपित्तप्रशमनानां, दुरालभा पित्तश्लेष्मप्रशमनानां, गन्धप्रियङ्गुः शोणितपित्तातियोगप्रशमनानां, कुटजत्वक् श्लेष्मपित्तरक्तसाङ्ग्राहिकोपशोषणानां, काश्मर्यफल रक्तसाङ्ग्राहिकरक्तपित्तप्रशमनानां, पृश्निपर्णी साङ्ग्राहिकवातहरदीपनीयवृष्याणां, विदारिगन्धा वृष्यसर्वदोषहराणां, बला साङ्ग्राहिकबल्यवातहराणां, गोक्षुरको मूत्रकृच्छ्रानिलहराणां, हिङ्गुनिर्यासश्छेदनीयदीपनीयानुलोमिकवातकफप्रशमनानाम्, अम्लवेतसो भेदनीयदीपनीयानुलोमिकवातश्लेष्महराणां, यावशूकः संसनीयपाचनीयार्श्वघ्नानां, तक्राभ्यासो ग्रहणीदोषशोफार्श्वघृतव्यापत्प्रशमनानां, क्रव्यान्मांसरसाभ्यासो ग्रहणीदोषशोषार्श्वघ्नानां, क्षीरघृताभ्यासो रसायनानां, समघृतसक्तुप्राशाभ्यासो वृष्योदावर्तहराणां, तैलगण्डूषाभ्यासो दन्तबलरुचिकराणां, चन्दनं दुर्गन्धहरदाहनिर्वापणलेपनानां, रास्नागुरुणी शीतापनयनप्रलेपनानां, लामज्जकोशीरं दाहत्वग्दोषस्वेदापनयनप्रलेपनानां, कुष्ठं वातहराभ्यङ्गोपनाहोपयोगिनां, मधुकं चक्षुष्यवृष्यकेश्यकण्ठ्यवर्ण्यविरजनीयरोपणीयानां, वायुः प्राणसञ्ज्ञाप्रदानहेतूनाम्, अग्निरामस्तम्भशीतशूलोद्वेपनप्रशमनानां, जलं स्तम्भनीयानां, मृद्भृष्टलोष्ट्रनिर्वापितमुदक तृष्णाच्छर्द्यतियोगप्रशमनानाम्, अतिमात्राशनमामप्रदोषहेतूनां, यथाग्न्यभ्यवहारोऽग्निसन्धुक्षणानां, यथासात्म्यं चेष्टाभ्यवहारौ सेव्यानां, कालभोजनमारोग्यकराणां, तृप्तिराहारगुणानां, वेगसन्धारणमनारोग्यकराणां, मद्यं सौमनस्यजननानां, मद्याक्षेपो धीधृतिस्मृतिहराणां, गुरुभोजनं दुर्विपाककराणां, एकाशनभोजनं सुखपरिणामकराणां, स्त्रीष्वतिप्रसङ्गः शोषकराणां, शुक्रवेगनिग्रहः षाण्ड्यकराणां, पराघातनमन्नाश्रद्धाजननानाम्, अनशनमायुषो ह्रासकराणां, प्रमिताशनं कर्शनीयानाम्, अजीर्णाध्यशनं ग्रहणीदूषणां, विषमाशनमग्निवैषम्यकराणां, विरुद्धवीर्याशनं निन्दितव्याधिकराणां, प्रशमः पथ्यानां, आयासः सर्वापथ्यानां, मिथ्यायोगो व्याधिकराणां, रजस्वलाभिगमनमलक्ष्मीमुखानां, ब्रह्मचर्यमायुष्याणां, परदाराभिगमनमनायुष्याणां, सङ्कल्पो वृष्याणां, दौर्मनस्यमवृष्याणाम्, अयथाबलमारम्भः प्राणोपरोधिनां, विषादो रोगवर्धनानां, स्नानं श्रमहराणां, हर्षः प्रीणनानां, शोकः शोषणानां, निवृत्तिः पुष्टिकराणां,

पुष्टिःस्वप्नकराणाम्, अतिस्वप्नस्तन्द्राकराणां, सर्वरसाभ्यासो बलकराणाम्, एकरसाभ्यासो दौर्बल्यकराणां, गर्भशल्यमाहार्याणाम्, अजीर्णमुद्धार्याणां, बालो मृदुभेषजीयानां, वृद्धो याप्यानां, गर्भिणी तीक्ष्णौषधव्यवायव्यायामवर्जनीयानां, सौमनस्यं गर्भधारणानां, सन्निपातो दुश्चिकित्स्यानाम्, आमो विषमचिकित्स्यानां, ज्वरो रोगाणां, कुष्ठं दीर्घरोगाणां, राजयक्ष्मा रोगसमूहानां, प्रमेहोऽनुषङ्गिगणां, जलौकसोऽनुशस्त्राणां, बस्तिस्तन्त्राणां, हिमवानौषधिभूमीनां, सोम ओषधीनां, मरुभूमिरारोग्यदेशानाम्, अनूपोहितदेशानां, निर्देशकारित्वमातुरगुणानां, भिषक् चिकित्साङ्गानां, नास्तिकोवर्ज्यानां, लौल्यं क्लेशकराणाम्, अनिर्देशकारित्वमरिष्टानां, अनिर्वेदो वार्तलक्षणानां, वैद्यसमूहो निःसंशयकराणां, योगो वैद्यगुणानां, विज्ञानमौषधीनां, शास्त्रसहितस्तर्कः साधनानां, सम्प्रतिपत्तिः कालज्ञानप्रयोजनानाम्, अव्यवसायः कालातिपत्तिहेतूनां, दृष्टकर्मता निःसंशयकराणाम्, असमर्थता भयकराणां, तद्विद्यसम्भाषा बुद्धिवर्धनानाम्, आचार्यः शास्त्राधिगमहेतूनाम्, आयुर्वेदोऽमृतानां, सद्वचनमनुष्ठेयानां, असद्ग्रहणं सर्वाहितानां, सर्वसन्न्यासः सुखानामिति॥४०॥

**Most important drugs, actions, factors:**

अन्नं वृत्तिकराणां श्रेष्ठम् – Among those which sustain life, food (Anna) is the best.

उदकमाश्वासकराणां – Water is best to generate soothing effect

सुरा श्रमहराणां – Wine is best to Dispel fatigue

क्षीरं जीवनीयानां – Milk is best among enlivening, invigorating substances

मांसं बृंहणीयानां – Meat is best among nourishing food

रसस्तर्पणीयानां – Meat soup (Mamsarasa) is best among refreshing, nourishing food

लवणमन्नद्रव्यरुचिकराणाम् – Salt is best among substances that enhance taste.

अम्लं हृद्यानां – Sour substances are best among cardiac tonics

कुक्कुटो बल्यानां – among foods to improve strength and immunity, Kukkuta – chicken is best.

नक्रेतो वृष्याणां – Among aphrodisiac substances, Nakra Retas – Semen of crocodile is the best.

मधु श्लेष्मपित्तप्रशमनानां – Among substances to balance Kapha and Pitta, Honey is the best.

सर्पिर्वातपित्तप्रशमनानां – Among substances to balance Vata and Pitta, cow ghee is the best.

तैलं वातश्लेष्मप्रशमनानां – Among substances to balance Vata and Kapha, Taila (sesame oil) is the best.

वमनं श्लेष्महराणां – Among Kapha balancing procedures, Vamana (emesis) therapy is the best.

विरेचनं पित्तहराणां – Among Pitta balancing procedures, Virechana is the best

बस्तिर्वातहराणां – Among Vata balancing procedures, Basti – Enema (both Anuvasana and Asthapana) is the best

स्वेदो मार्दवकराणां – Among procedures to bring about softness and tenderness, Swedana – sweating therapy is the best.

व्यायामः स्थैर्यकराणां – Exercise (Vyayama) is the best to bring about body firmness.

क्षारः पुंस्त्वोपघातिनां – Among substances causing impotency, kshara is the best

तिन्दुकमन्नद्रव्यरुचिकराणाम् – Among substances hurting the taste of food, Tinduka (Diospros peregrine Gurke) is the best

आमं कपित्थमकण्ठ्यानाम् – Among those hurting throat and quality of sound, Unripe Kapittha (Feronia Limonia Swingle) is the best

आविकं सर्पिरहृद्यानाम् – Among those damaging heart, Sheep ghee is the best

अजाक्षीरं शोषघ्नस्तन्यसात्म्यरक्तसाङ्ग्राहिकरक्तपित्तप्रशमनानाम् – Among those substances that relieve emaciation, improve breast milk, blood production, absorbant (useful in IBS) and bleeding disorders, goat milk is the best. (Related – goat milk benefits)

अविक्षीरं श्लेष्मपित्तजननानां – Sheep milk is best to Vitiate Kapha and Pitta Dosha

महिषीक्षीरं स्वप्नजननानां – Buffalo milk is best to induce sleep

मन्दकं दध्यभिष्यन्दकराणां – in obstructing the body channels and circulation, half formed curds (Mandaka Dadhi) is best

गवेधुकान्नं कर्शनीयानाम् – Food prepared of Gavedhuka (Triticum aestivum Linn) to cause emaciation

उद्दालकान्नं विरूक्षणीयानाम् – Food prepared with Uddalaka (a variety of black gram) is best to cause drying

इक्षुर्मूत्रजननानां – Sugarcane is best in producing diuretic effect.

यवाः पुरीषजननानां – Barley is best to increase bulk of feces

जाम्बवं वातजननानां – Jambu - (Jamun - Syzygium cumini) is best in aggravating Vata

शष्कुल्यः श्लेष्मपित्तजननानां – Shashkuli type of pastry (Chakkuli in Kannada language) is best in aggravating Pitta and Kapha

कुलत्था अम्लपित्तजननानां – Kulattha (horse gram) is best in causing Amlapitta (acid dyspepsia)

माषाः श्लेष्मपित्तजननानां – Black gram is best in aggravating Kapha and Pitta

मदनफलं वमनास्थापनानुवासनोपयोगिनां – Fruit of Madana ( Randia dumetorum Lam) is best in Vamana (emesis), Asthapana and anuvasana types of enema

त्रिवृत् सुखविरेचनानां – Trivrit (Operculina turpethum R.B) is the best in causing easy purgation

चतुरङ्गुलो मृदुविरेचनानां – Aragvadha (Cassia fistula Linn) is best in causing mild purigation

स्नुक्पयस्तीक्ष्णविरेचननां – Milk of Snuhi (Euphorbia neriifolia Linn) is best in causing strong purgation

प्रत्यक्पुष्पा शिरोविरेचनानां – Apamarga (Achyranthes aspera Linn) is best in eliminating Doshas from the head

विडङ्गं क्रिमिघ्नानां – Vidanga (Embelia ribes Burm .f.) is best in Killing parasites.

शिरीषो विषघ्नानां – Shireesha (Albizia lebbeck Benth) is the best anti poisonous herb.

खदिरः कुष्ठघ्नानां – Khadira (Acacia catechu Wild) is best in curing skin diseases

रास्ना वातहराणाम् – Rasna (Pluchea lanceolata) is best in alleviating vata

आमलकं वयःस्थापनानां – Amalaka (Amla – Emblica officinalis) is best to cause Rasayana (rejuvenation)

हरितकी पथ्यानाम् – Haritaki (Terminalia chebula Linn) is best wholesome fruit

एरण्डमूलं वृष्यवातहराणां – Castor root (Eranda moola) is best in alleviating Vata and is an aphrodisiac

पिप्पलीमूलं दीपनीयपाचनीयानाहप्रशमनानां – Pippalimoola (long pepper root) is best in promoting digestion, carmination and relieving bloating and constipation

चित्रकमूलं दीपनीयपाचनीयगुदशोथार्शःशूलहराणां – Root of Chitraka (Plumbago zeylanica Linn) is best in Promoting digestion, carmination and curing piles and colic pain

पुष्करमूलं हिक्काश्वासकासपार्श्वशूलहराणां – Pushkaramoola (Inula racemosa Hook.f) is best in curing hiccup, asthma, Cough and pain in the chest

मुस्तं साङ्ग्राहिकदीपनीयपाचनीयानाम् – Musta (Cyperus rotunds Linn) is best in causing astringent effect,

उदीच्यं निर्वापणदीपनीयपाचनीयच्छर्द्यतीसारहराणां – Udeechya – Pavonia odorata is best in causing digestion, carmination, anti emetic and anti diarrheal effect.

कट्वङ्गं साङ्ग्राहिकपाचनीयदीपनीयानाम् – Katvanga is best to cause absorption, to improve digestion and carmination.

अनन्ता साङ्ग्राहिकरक्तपित्तप्रशमनानाम् – Ananta (Hemidesmus indicus) is best to cause absorption and in bleeding disorders.

अमृता साङ्ग्राहिकवातहरदीपनीयश्लेष्मशोणितविबन्धप्रशमनानां – Giloy is best to cause astringent effect, promoting digestion, alleviating Vata, Kapha, constipation and Raktapitta (bleeding disorders)

बिल्वं साङ्ग्राहिकदीपनीयवातकफप्रशमनानाम् – Bael is best to cause astringent effect, promoting digestion and alleviating Vata and Kapha.

अतिविषा दीपनीयपाचनीयसाङ्ग्राहिकसर्वदोषहराणाम् – Ativisha (Aconitum heterophyllum) is best in causing astringent effect, promoting digestion, carmination and alleviation of all the Doshas.

उत्पलकुमुदपद्मकिञ्जल्कः साङ्ग्राहिकरक्तपित्तप्रशमनानां – Utpala (Nymphaea alba), Kumuda (a variety of lotus) and Padma (lotus) is best in causing astringent effect, alleviating bleeding disorders.

दुरालभा पित्तश्लेष्मप्रशमनानां – Duralabha (Fagonia cretica) is best in alleviating Kapha and Pitta.

गन्धप्रियङ्गुः शोणितपित्तातियोगप्रशमनानां – Gandha Priyangu (Callicarpa macrophylla) is best in alleviating acute heavy bleeding.

कुटजत्वक् श्लेष्मपित्तरक्तसाङ्ग्राहिकोपशोषणानां – Bark of Kutaja (Holarrhena antidysenterica) is best in balancing Kapha and Pitta, causing astringent effect over blood and to cause drying absorbing effect

काश्मर्यफलं रक्तसाङ्ग्राहिकरक्तपित्तप्रशमनानां – Fruit of Gambhari (Gmelina arborea) is best in causing hemostasis, curing bleeding disorders

पृश्निपर्णी साङ्ग्राहिकवातहरदीपनीयवृष्याणां – Prishniparni – Uraria picta is best in causing astringent and aphrodisiac, digestive effect and alleviating Vata

विदारिगन्धा वृष्यसर्वदोषहराणां – Vidarigandha (Pueraria tuberosa/ Ipomoea digitata) is best as aphrodisiac and to cause Tridosha balance

बला साङ्ग्राहिकबल्यवातहराणां – Bala (Sida cordifolia) is best in causing absorbent effect, improving strength and balancing Vata Dosha.

गोक्षुरको मूत्रकृच्छ्रानिलहराणां – Gokshura (Tribulus terrestris) is best in relieving dysuria

हिङ्गुनिर्यासश्छेदनीय दीपनीयानुलोमिक वातकफप्रशमनानाम् – Asafetida is best in causing excision, promoting digestion, downward movement of wind, and alleviating Vata and Kapha doshas

अम्लवेतसो भेदनीयदीपनीयानुलोमिकवातश्लेष्महराणां – Amlavetasa (Garcinia pedunculata) is best in causing purgation, promoting digestion, downward movement of wind (Anulomna) and balancing Vata and Kapha.

यावशूकः संसनीयपाचनीयार्शोघ्नानां – Ash of Barley (Yavakshara / Yavashuka) is best in causing laxative effect, carmination and curing piles

तक्राभ्यासो ग्रहणीदोषशोफार्शोघृतव्यापत्प्रशमनानां – Regular intake of buttermilk is best in curing Grahani (IBS), Shotha (edema), piles and ghee indigestion

क्रव्यान्मांसरसाभ्यासो ग्रहणीदोषशोषार्शोघ्नानां – habitual use of meat soup of carnivorous animals is best in curing Grahani (IBS), emaciation and piles

क्षीरघृताभ्यासो रसायनानां – habitual use of milk and ghee is best in causing anti aging effect (rasayana)

समघृतसक्तुप्राशाभ्यासो वृष्योदावर्तहराणां – habitual use of mix of equal quantities of ghee and Saktu (roasted corn flour) is best aphrodisiac and Vata balancing.

तैलगण्डूषाभ्यासो दन्तबलरुचिकराणां – sesame oil – oil pulling is best to strengthen teeth and to relieve anorexia

चन्दनं दुर्गन्धहरदाहनिर्वापणलेपनानां – Sandalwood (Chandana) is best in reliving bad odor, burning sensation and best to apply as paste.

रास्नागुरुणी शीतापनयनप्रलेपनानां – Application of Rasna (Pluchea lanceolata) and Agaru (Aquilaria agallocha) is best in removing coldness, on external application.

लामज्जकोशीरं दाहत्वग्दोषस्वेदापनयनप्रलेपनानां – Lamajjaka (Cymbopogon jwarancusa) is best in curing burning sensation, skin diseases and sweating, on external application.

कुष्ठं वातहराभ्यङ्गोपनाहोपयोगिनां – Kushta (Saussurea lappa) is best in causing Vata balance upon usage as massage and poultice.

मधुकं चक्षुष्य वृष्य केश्य कण्ठ्य वर्ण्य विरजनीय रोपणीयानां – Madhuka (Licorice) is best in improving eye health, aphrodisiac effect, improving hair quality, throat/voice quality, skin complexion, imparting colour and wound healing

वायुः प्राणसञ्ज्ञाप्रदानहेतूनाम् – air is best to restore Prana and consciousness

अग्निराम स्तम्भ शीत शूलोद्वेपन प्रशमनानां – fire is best in curing indigestion, stiffness, cold, colic pain and shivering

जलं स्तम्भनीयानां – water is best in causing absorbent / astringent effect

मृद्भृष्ट लोष्ट्र निर्वापितमुदकं तृष्णाच्छद्र्यतियोग प्रशमनानाम् – water from a pot prepared from heated mud, is best in alleviating acute attacks of thirst and vomiting

अतिमात्राशनमामप्रदोषहेतूनां – eating in excess quantities is best in causing excess Ama (Indigestion and impaired metabolism)

यथाग्न्यभ्यवहारोऽग्निसन्धुक्षणानां – Intake of food as per digestion strength, is best to improve digestion power.

यथासात्म्यं चेष्टाभ्यवहारौ सेव्यानां – wholesome diet and regime is best to adopt habits

कालभोजनमारोग्यकराणां – taking food in right time is best to promote health

तृप्तिराहारगुणानां – Trupti (Satiation) is the best quality of food

वेगसन्धारणमनारोग्यकराणां – suppression of urges is the best cause of disease

मद्यं सौमनस्यजननानां – alcohol (Madya) is best in causing soothing mind, exhilaration

मद्याक्षेपो धीधृतिस्मृतिहराणां – alcohol addiction is best to cause loss of intelligence, memory and patience

गुरुभोजनं दुर्विपाककराणाम् – heavy food intake is best to cause indigestion

एकाशनभोजनं सुखपरिणामकराणां – having one meal per day is best to cause digestion and absorption of food

स्त्रीष्वतिप्रसङ्गः शोषकराणां – excessive indulgence in women is best to cause emaciation

शुक्रवेगनिग्रहः षाण्ड्यकराणां – continuous suppression of ejaculation causes impotence

पराघातनमन्नाश्रद्धाजननानाम् – Slaughtering place is the best place to cause aversion for food

अनशनमायुषो ह्रासकराणां – Fasting is best to cause reduction of longevity

प्रमिताशनं कर्शनीयानाम् – Intake of food in reduced quantity is best to cause weight loss

अजीर्णाध्यशनं ग्रहणीदूषणानां – Intake of food before digestion of previous meal is best in causing vitiation of stomach and intestine

विषमाशनमग्निवैषम्यकराणां – Intake of food in irregular timings causes irregularity in digestive power

विरुद्धवीर्याशनं निन्दितव्याधिकराणां – intake of incompatible foods – is best in causing worst of diseases like skin disorders

प्रशमः पथ्यानां – Tranquillity, soothing, calming behaviour is the best healthy regime

आयासः सर्वापथ्यानां – Exertion beyond one's capacity is best Unhealthy regime

मिथ्यायोगो व्याधिकराणां – Mithya Yoga – Improper utilisation of objects and sense organs – like looking at sharp objects, hearing to loud sound etc) is best in causing disease.

रजस्वलाभिगमनमलक्ष्मीमुखानां – sex with a menstruating woman is best inauspicious activity

ब्रह्मचर्यमायुष्याणां – practising celibacy is best to cause longevity

परदाराभिगमनमनायुष्याणां – Adultery is best to reduce longevity

सङ्कल्पो वृष्याणां – Determination is the best aphrodisiac

दौर्मनस्यमवृष्याणाम् – having difference of opinion / different minds is the best un-aphrodisiac

अयथाबलमारम्भःप्राणोपरोधिनां – strenuous efforts beyond one's capacity is best to lose life

विषादो रोगवर्धनानां – Grief/ depression is best to worsen disease

स्नानंश्रमहराणां – Bath is best in removing fatigue

हर्षःप्रीणनानां – Cheerfulness is best to cause Delight

शोकः शोषणानां – Worry is best to cause emaciation, to lose weight

निवृत्तिःपुष्टिकराणां – detachment is best to cause nourishment

पुष्टिःस्वप्नकराणाम् – having nutritious food is best to induce sleep

अतिस्वप्नस्तन्द्राकराणां – Excessive sleep is best in causing drowsiness

सर्वरसाभ्यासोबलकराणाम् – having food with all the tastes is best to promote strength and immunity

एकरसाभ्यासोदौर्बल्यकराणां – having food with only one taste is best to cause debility

गर्भशल्यमाहार्याणाम् – dead foetus is best to be removed immediately

अजीर्णमुद्धार्याणां – indigestion is best to be prevented

बालोमृदुभेषजीयानां – children are best to be administered with mild medicines

वृद्धोद्याप्यानां – aged patients are best to be administered with palliating medicines

गर्भिणी तीक्ष्णौषध व्यवाय व्यायाम वर्जनीयानां -pregnant women are best to avoid strong medicines, sex and exercise

सौमनस्यं गर्भधारणानां – having common minds is best way to achieve conception

सन्निपातो दुश्चिकित्स्यानाम् – Sannipata – involvement of all Doshas is worst condition to treat

आमो विषमचिकित्स्यानां – Ama (altered digestion and metabolism) is best to be considered and treated as Toxicity

ज्वरो रोगाणां – fever is best among diseases

कुष्ठं दीर्घरोगाणां – skin diseases are the longest duration disorders

राजयक्ष्मा रोगसमूहानां – Rajayakshma (tuberculosis / AIDS) is the best disease combination with many diseases

प्रमेहोऽनुषङ्गिगणां – urinary disorders are the best relapsing disorders

जलौकसोऽनुशस्त्राणां – leech is the best accessory surgical devices

बस्तिस्तन्त्राणां – Enema is the best among elimination therapies

हिमवानौषधिभूमीनां – The Himalaya is the best habitat of medicinal plants

सोम ओषधीनां – Soma is the best medicine

मरुभूमिरारोग्यदेशानाम् – Desert is best among healthy places

अनूपोऽहितदेशानाम् – Marshy Land is Unhealthiest place

निर्देशकारित्वमातुरगुणानां – Compliance with the instructions of the physician is the best quality of patient

भिषक् चिकित्साङ्गानां – Physician is the best part of treatment

नास्तिकोवर्ज्यानां – An atheist is best to be rejected treatment

लौल्यं क्लेशकराणाम् – Greed is the most troublesome practice

अनिर्देशकारित्वमरिष्टानां – Disobedience to the instructions of the physician is the worst prognostic sign

अनिर्वेदो वार्तलक्षणानां – Self confidence is the best sign of recovery

वैद्यसमूहो निःसंशयकराणं – An assemblage of physician is best in eradicating doubts (with regard to the line of treatment etc)

योगो वैद्यगुणानां – Sense of propriety is the best quality of physician

विज्ञानमौषधीनां – Knowledge is the best medicine

शास्त्रसहितस्तर्कः साधनानां – Scriptures based logic is best to gain knowledge

सम्प्रतिपत्तिः कालज्ञानप्रयोजनानाम् – Presence of mind is best to understand the situation

अव्यवसायः कालातिपत्तिहेतूनां – Inaction is the best way to waste time

दृष्टकर्मता निःसंशयकराणाम् – Practical experience is best to eradicate doubts

असमर्थता भयकराणां – Incapability is best to cause fear

तद्विद्यसम्भाषा बुद्धिवर्धनानाम् – Clinical seminars, reasoning based discussion is best to improve wisdom and intelligence

आचार्यः शास्त्राधिगमहेतूनाम् – Guru is best tool to understand science

आयुर्वेदोऽमृतानां – Knowledge of Ayurveda (science of life) is the best among nectors

सद्वचनमनुष्ठेयानाम् – Words of noble person is best to be complied with

असद्ग्रहणं सर्वाहितानां – Words of wicked is best to cause harmful result

सर्वसन्न्यासः सुखानामिति – absolute detachment is the best way to achieve happiness [40]


भवन्ति चात्र-
अग्र्याणां शतमुद्दिष्टं यद्दिद्वपञ्चाशदुत्तरम्|
अलमेतद्विकाराणां विघातायोपदिश्यते||४१||


Thus one hundred and fifty two varieties of best drugs and regimen have been explained.
They are sufficient for giving guidance to a physician in connection with the treatment of various diseases. [41]


समानकारिणो येऽर्थास्तेषां श्रेष्ठस्य लक्षणम्|
ज्यायस्त्वं कार्यकर्तृत्वे वरत्वं चाप्युदाहृतम्||४२||
वातपित्तकफानां च यद्यत् प्रशमने हितम्|
प्राधान्यतश्च निर्दिष्टं यद्व्याधिहरमुत्तमम्||४३||
एतन्निशम्य निपुणं चिकित्सां सम्प्रयोजयेत्|

एवं कुर्वन् सदा वैद्यो धर्मकामौ समश्नुते॥४४॥

The best among drugs and regimens having similar actions, the best effects and qualities, have been listed. The drugs and regimen useful for alleviating diseases caused by Vata, Pitta and Kapha and the most useful ones among them have been indicated here. A good physician should know all this before starting the treatment of the various diseases. It is only if he does so, he can enjoy happiness in this world and the world beyond. [42-44]

**Definition of Pathya – wholesome food :**

पथ्यं पथोऽनपेतं यद्यच्चोक्तं मनसः प्रियम्‌।
यच्चाप्रियमपथ्यं च नियतं तन्न लक्षयेत्‌॥४५॥
मात्राकालक्रियाभूमिदेहदोषगुणान्तरम्‌।
प्राप्य तत्तद्धि दृश्यन्ते ते ते भावास्तथा तथा॥४६॥
तस्मात्‌ स्वभावो निर्दिष्टस्तथा मात्रादिराश्रयः।
तदपेक्ष्योभयं कर्म प्रयोज्यं सिद्धिमिच्छता॥४७॥

Pathya – wholesome food is the one, which is –
Patho Anapetha (Patha means path / digestive tract) - which is good for one's digestive system and
Manasaha priyam – which is liked by the person.
Those which adversely affect digestive tract and mind are considered to be Apathya – unwholesome.
But this cannot be accepted as a general rule in absolute terms. The drugs and regimen in fact change their qualities, depending on the –

- Matra – dosage,
- Kala – season,
- Kriya – method of preparation,
- Bhumi – habitat and
- combination with other useful and harmful drugs. [45-47]

**Asava Yoni :**

**Alcoholic preparations:**

तदात्रेयस्य भगवतो वचनमनुनिशम्य पुनरपि भगवन्तमात्रेयमग्निवेश उवाच- यथोद्देशमभिनिर्दिष्टः केवलोऽयमर्थो भगवता श्रुतश्चास्माभिः।
आसवद्रव्याणामिदानीमनपवादं लक्षणमनतिसङ्क्षेपेणोपदिश्यमानं शुश्रूषामह इति॥४८॥
तमुवाच भगवानात्रेयः:- धान्यफलमूलसारपुष्पकाण्डपत्रत्वचो भवन्त्यासवयोनयोऽग्निवेश! सङ्ग्रहेणाष्टौ शर्करानवमीकाः।
तास्वेव द्रव्यसंयोगकरणतोऽपरिसङ्ख्येयासु यथापथ्यतमानामासवानां चतुरशीतिं निबोध।
तद्यथा- सुरासौवीरतुषोदकमैरेयमेदकधान्याम्लाः षड धान्यासवा भवन्ति, मृद्वीकाखर्जूरकाश्मर्यधन्वनराजादनतृणशून्यपरूषकाभयामलकमृगलिण्डिकाजाम्बवकपित्थ-कुवलबदरकर्कन्धुपीलुप्रियालपनसन्यग्रोधाश्वत्थप्लक्षकपीतनोदुम्बराजमोदशृङ्गाटकशाङ्खिनीफलासवाः षड्विंशतिर्भवन्ति, विदारिगन्धाश्वगन्धाकृष्णगन्धाशतावरीश्यामात्रिवृद्दन्तीद्रवन्तीबिल्वोरुबूकचित्रकमूलैरेकादश मूलासवा भवन्ति, शालप्रियकाश्वकर्णचन्दनस्यन्दनखदिरकदरसप्तपर्णार्जुनासनारिमेदतिन्दुककिणिहीशमी-शुक्तिशिंशपाशिरीषवञ्जलधन्वनमधूकैः सारासवा विंशतिर्भवन्ति, पद्मोत्पलनलिकुमुदसौगन्धिककपुण्डरीकशतपत्रमधूकप्रियङ्गुधातकीपुष्पैर्दश पुष्पासवा भवन्ति, इक्षुकाण्डेक्षुवालिकापुण्ड्रकचतुर्थाः काण्डासवा भवन्ति, पटोलताडकपत्रासवौ द्वौ भवतः, तिल्वकलोधैलवालुकक्रमुकचतुर्थास्त्वगासवा भवन्ति, शर्करासव एक एवेति।

एवमेषामासवानां चतुरशीतिः परस्परेणासंसृष्टानामासवद्रव्याणामुपनिर्दिष्टा भवति|
एषामासवानामासुतत्वादासवसञ्ज्ञा|
द्रव्यसंयोगविभागविस्तारस्त्वेषां बहुविधकल्पः संस्कारश्च|
यथास्वं संयोगसंस्कारसंस्कृता ह्यासवाः स्वं कर्म कुर्वन्ति|
संयोगसंस्कारदेशकालमात्रादयश्च भावास्तेषां तेषामासवानां ते ते समुपदिश्यन्ते तत्तत्कार्यमभिसमीक्ष्येति||४९||

Having listened to the above instructions of Lord Atreya, Agnivesha said. "You have answered our questions in entirety and we have followed it. Now we shall like to hear an elaborate and correct description of the ingredients that are used in alcoholic preparations."

Lord Atreya replied, In belief, Asava Yoni – sources of ingredients for alcoholic preparations are eight Viz,
Dhanya – grains (6 preparations)
Phala – fruits, (26 herbs)
Moola – roots, (11 herbs)
Saara – heartwoods, (20)
Pushpa – flowers, (10)
Kanda – branches (4)
Patra – leaves (2)
Twacha – barks; (4)
The ninth one is sugar.

Alcoholic preparations are innumerable depending upon the ingredients, their combinations and the method of preparation; however the most wholesome ones out of them are eighty four in number. They are as follows:-
**1 Six alcoholic preparations made of grains**–- Sura, Sauvira, Tusodaka, Maireya, Medaka and Dhanyamla
    **2. Twenty six alcoholic preparations made of fruits-**
1. Draksa (Vitis vinifera Linn)
2. Kharjura (Phoenix sylvestris Roxb)
3. Kashmarya (Gmelina arborea Linn)
4. Dhanvana (Grewia tiliaefolia Vahl_)
5. Rajadana (Mimusops hexandra Roxb)
6. Ketaka (Pandanus tectorius Soland)
7. Parushaka (Grewia asiatica Linn)
8. Abhaya (Terminalia chebula Linn)
9. Amalaka (Emblica officinalis Gaertn)
10. Mrigelindika (Terminalia bellirica Roxb)
11. Jambu (Syzygium cumini Skeels)
12. Kapittha (Feronia limonia Swingle)
13. Kuvala (Zizyphus jujuba Gaertn)
14. Badara (Zizyphus jujuba Lam)
15Karkandhu (Ziziphus nummularia W.A)
16 Plu (Salvadora persica Linn)
17. Priyala (Buchanania Lanzan Spreng)
18. Panasa (Artocarpus heterophyllus Lam)
19. Nyagrodha (Ficus bengalensis Linn)
20. Asvatha (Ficus religiosa Linn)
21.Plaksa (Ficus locar Buch. Ham.)
22. Kapitana (Albizia lebbeck Benth)

23. Udumara (Ficus racemosa Linn)

24. Ajamoda (Trachyspermum roxburghianum)

25. Srngataka (Trapa bispinosa Roxb)

26. Sankhini (Canscora decussata Roem et. Sch)

### 3. Eleven Alcholic preprations made of roots

1. Salaparni (Desmodium gangeticum DC)

2. Ashvagandha (Withania somnifera Lam)

4. Satavari (Asparagus racemosus Willd)

5. Syama (Operculina turpethum R.B)

6. Trivrt (A variety of Syama)

7. Danti (Baliospermum montanum Muell- Arg)

8. Dravanti (Jatropha glandulifera Roxb)

9. Bilva (Aegle marmelos Corr)

10. Eranda (Ricinus communis Linn)

11. Citraka (Plumbago zeylanica Linn)

### 4. Twenty alcoholic preprations made of heart-wood

1. Sala (Shorea robusta Gaertn.f)

2. Priyaka (Buchanania lanzan spreng)

3. Asvakarna (Dipterocarpus alatus Roxb)

4. Candana (Santalum album Linn)

5. Tinisa (Ougeinia dalbergioides Benth)

6. Khadira (Acacia catechu Willd)

7. Kasara (a variety of Khadira)

8. Saptaparna (Alstonia scholaris R. Br)

9. Arjuna (Terminalia arjuna)

10. Asana (Terminalia tomentosa)

11. Arimeda (a variety of Khadira)

12. Tinduka (Diospyros peregrina Gurke)

13. Kinihi (white variety of Sirisa)

14.Sami (Prosopis spicigera Linn)

15. Badari (Ziziphus jujuba Lam)

16. Simsapa (Dalbergia sissoo Roxb)

17. Sirisa (Albizia lebbeck Benth)

18.Vanjula

19.Dhanvana (Grewia tiliaefolia Vahl)

20. Madhuka (Madhuka indica J.F Gmel)

### 5. Ten alcoholic preparations made of flowers

1. Padma (Nelumbo nucifera Gaertn)

2. Utpala (Nymphaea alba Linn)

3. Nalina (a variety of Padma)

4. Kumuda (a variety of Utpala)

5. Saugandhika

6. Pundarika (Nymphaea lotus Linn)

7. Satapatra (a variety of Kamala)

8. Madhuka (Madhuka indica J.F) Gmel)

9. Priyangu (Calliarpa macrophylla Vahl)

10. Dhataki (Woodfordia fruticosa Kurz)

### 6. Four alcoholic preparations made of branches

1. Iksu (Saccharum officinarum Linn)
2. Kandeksu (Saccharum spontaneum Linn)
3. Iksuvalika (Asteracantha longifolia Ness)
4. Pundraka (a type of sugar cane)

### 7. Two alcoholic preparations made of leaves

1. Patola (Trichosanthes cucumerina Linn)
2. Tadaka (Borassus flabellifer Linn)

### 8. Four alcoholic preparations made of barks

1. Tilvaka (Symplocos racemosa Roxb)
2. Lodhra (a variety of tilvaka)
3. Elavaluka (Prunus cerasus L)
4. Kramuka (Areca catechu Linn)

## 9. One alcoholic preparation made from sugar

The alcoholic preparation made up of sugar is called as Sharkarasava.

### Alcoholic preparations

There is only one variety of alcoholic preparation made of sugar.

When prepared individually from the above mentioned ingredients, they make eighty four varieties of alcoholic preparations. They are known as alcoholic preparation because of the process of fermentation involved. Depending upon the permutation and combination of these ingredients and preparation method, they have in fact innumerable varieties. Actions of these alcoholic preparations are based on the properties of the ingredients and the method of preparation. Keeping in view the effects desired to be produced by a particular alcoholic preparation, combination of ingredients, method, time (duration of fermentation), and place (inside a heap of ashes or grains etc) of the preparation, quantity etc. are prescribed. {48-49}

Again:-

भवति चात्र-

मनःशरीराग्निबलप्रदानामस्वप्नशोकारुचिनाशनानाम्|
संहर्षणानां प्रवरासवानामशीतिरुक्ता चतुरुत्तरैषा||७०||

Thus, it is said:

The eighty-four types of excellent alcoholic preparations have been enumerated. They all strengthen the mind, body and the power of digestion; they help in overcoming sleeplessness, grief and anorexia and are exhilarating.

To sum up:

तत्र श्लोकः-

शरीररोगप्रकृतौ मतानि तत्त्वेन चाहारविनिश्चयं च|
उवाच यज्जःपुरुषादिकेऽस्मिन् मुनिस्तथाऽग्याणि वरासवांश्च||५१||

In this chapter – Yajja Purusheeya Adhyaya, various theories relating to the origin of living beings and diseases, the most wholesome and unwholesome diets and regimen and the most important alcoholic preparations have been described.{51}

इत्यग्निवेशकृते तन्त्रे चरकप्रतिसंस्कृते श्लोकस्थाने यज्जःपुरुषीयो नाम पञ्चविंशोऽध्यायः||२५||
Thus, ends the twenty fifth chapter of the Sutra section of Agnivesa's work as redacted by Charaka.

# 26

# Sutrasthana Chapter 26 Atreya Bhadrakapeeyam

**Atreya Bhadrakapyeeya Adhyaya**

**Ayurvedic Pharmacology**

अथात आत्रेयभद्रकाप्यीयमध्यायं व्याख्यास्यामः||१||

इति ह स्माह भगवानात्रेयः||२||

The 26th Chapter of Charaka Samhita explains Ayurvedic pharmacology in detail, along with incompatible foods, qualities and actions of taste, 5 basic elements. This chapter is called Atreya Bhadrakapyiya Adhyaya.

**A Symposium**

आत्रेयो भद्रकाप्यश्च शाकुन्तेयस्तथैव च|

पूर्णाक्षश्चैव मौद्गल्यो हिरण्याक्षश्च कौशिकः||३||

यः कुमारशिरा नाम भरद्वाजः स चानघः|

श्रीमान् वार्योविदश्चैव राजा मतिमतां वरः||४||

निमिश्च राजा वैदेहो बडिशश्च महामतिः|

काङ्कायनश्च बाह्लीको बाह्लीकभिषजां वरः||५||

एते श्रुतवयोवृद्धा जितात्मानो महर्षयः|

वने चैत्ररथे रम्ये समीयुर्विजिहीर्षवः||६||

तेषां तत्रोपविष्टानामियमर्थवती कथा|

बभूवार्थविदां सम्यग्रसाहारविनिश्चये||७||

**A Symposium**

Once upon a time Atreya, Bhadrakapya, Shakunteya, Purnaksha Maudgalya, Hiranyaksha Kaushika, Kumarashira Bharadvaja, the king Varyovida, Nimi the king of Videha, Kankayana the best among the physicians of Bahlika (Balkh)- all these Ayurveda experts, having self control- assembled in the pleasant woods of Chaitraratha on a pleasant trip. They sat together and then started discussing some of the vital problems relating to correlation between Rasa (taste) and Diet. [3-7]

**Different views of members on the number of taste (Rasa):**

**One type of taste:**

एक एव रस इत्युवाच भद्रकाप्यः, यं पञ्चानामिन्द्रियार्थानामन्यतमं जिह्वावैषयिकं भावमाचक्षते कुशलाः, स पुनरुदकादनन्य इति|

Bhadrakapya opined that there is only one type of taste because taste is perceived by tongue, and it is the object of tongue (sense organ). He said that it is no different than water element (Jala Mahabhuta).

**Two types of tastes:**

द्वौ रसाविति शाकुन्तेयो ब्राह्मणः, छेदनीय उपशमनीयश्चेति||

Shakunteya Brahmana opined that there are two types of tastes:

Chedaneeya – scraping

Upashamaneeya – palliating, calming

## Three types of taste:

त्रयो रसा इति पूर्णाक्षो मौद्गल्यः, छेदनीयोपशमनीयसाधारणा इति|

Purnaksha Maudgalya – 3 types of taste

Chedaneeya – scraping

Upashamaneeya – Nourishing, palliating, calming

Sadharana – in between Chedaneeya and Upashamaneeya

## Four types of taste:

चत्वारो रसा इति हिरण्याक्षः कौशिकः, स्वादुर्हितश्च स्वादुरहितश्चास्वादुर्हितश्चास्वादुरहितश्चेति|

Hiranyaksha Kaushika :

1. Swadu Hita – Palatable and wholesome

2. Swadu Ahita – Palatable but unwholesome

3. Aswadu Hita – Unpalatable, but wholesome

4. Aswadu Ahita – Unpalatable and unwholesome

## Five types of taste:

पञ्च रसा इति कुमारशिरा भरद्वाजः, भौमौदकाग्नेयवायव्यान्तरिक्षाः|

**Kumarashira Bharadwaja – Five types**

1.Parthiva – Originating from earth element

2. Apya – Originating from water element

3. Taijasa – Originating from fire element

4. Vayaviya – Originating from air element

5. Akashiya – Originating from ether / vacuum element

## Six types of taste:

षड्रसा इति वार्योविदो राजर्षिः, गुरुलघुशीतोष्णस्निग्धरूक्षाः|

Royal Sage Varyovida Six types

1. Guru (heavy)

2. Laghu (Light)

3. Sheeta (Cold)

4. Ushna (Hot)

5. Snigdha (Unctuous / oily)

6. Rooksha (Non unctouous)

## Seven types of taste:

सप्त रसा इति निमिर्वैदेहः, मधुराम्ललवणकटुतिक्तकषायक्षाराः|

As per Nimi the king of Videha –

1. Madhura (sweet)

2. Amla (sour)

3. Lavana (Saline)

4. Katu (Pungent)

5. Tikta (Bitter)

6. Kashaya (Astringent)

7. Kshara (Alkaline)

## Eight types of tastes

अष्टौ रसा इति बडिशो धामार्गवः, मधुराम्ललवणकटुतिक्तकषायक्षाराव्यक्ताः|

As per Dhamaragava Badisa :

1. Madhura (sweet)

2. Amla (sour)

3. Lavana (Saline)

4. Katu (Pungent)

5. Tikta (Bitter)

6. Kashaya (Astringent)

7. Kshara (Alkaline)

8. Avyakta (imperceptible)

## Infinite tastes:

अपरिसङ्ख्येया रसा इति काङ्कायनो बाह्लीकभिषक्, आश्रयगुणकर्मसंस्वादविशेषाणामपरिसङ्ख्येयत्वात्||८||

## Infinite tastes:

Kankayana Bahlika opines that tastes are innumerable, because of the innumerability of qualities, actions, that reside in a substance.[8]

## Concluding remarks by Chairperson- Lord Punarvasu:

षडेव रसा इत्युवाच भगवानात्रेयः पुनर्वसुः, मधुराम्ललवणकटुतिक्तकषायाः|

There are only six tastes –

1. Madhura (sweet)

2. Amla (sour)

3. Lavana (Saline)

4. Katu (Pungent)

5. Tikta (Bitter)

6. Kashaya (Astringent)

## Substantiation of six number of tastes:

तेषां षण्णां रसानां योनिरुदकं, छेदनोपशमने द्वे कर्मणी, तयोर्मिश्रीभावात् साधारणत्वं, स्वाद्वस्वादुता भक्तिः, हिताहितौ प्रभावौ, पञ्चमहाभूतविकारास्त्वाश्रयाः प्रकृतिविकृतिविचारदेशकालवशाः, तेष्वाश्रयेषु द्रव्यसञ्ज्ञकेषु गुणा गुरुलघुशीतोष्णस्निग्धरूक्षाद्याः; क्षरणात् क्षारः, नासौ रसः द्रव्यं तदनेकरससमुत्पन्नमनेकरसं कटुकलवणभूयिष्ठमनेकेन्द्रियार्थसमन्वितं करणाभिनिर्वृत्तम्; अव्यक्तीभावस्तु खलु रसानां प्रकृतौ भवत्यनुरसेऽनुरससमन्विते वा द्रव्ये; अपरिसङ्ख्येयत्वं पुनस्तेषामाश्रयादीनां भावानां विशेषापरिसङ्ख्येयत्वान्न युक्तम्, एकैकोऽपि ह्येषामाश्रयादीनां भावानां विशेषानाश्रयते विशेषापरिसङ्ख्येयत्वात्, न च तस्मादन्यत्वमुपपद्यते; परस्परसंसृष्टभूयिष्ठत्वान्न चैषामभिनिर्वृत्तेर्गुणप्रकृतीनामपरिसङ्ख्येयत्वं भवति; तस्मान्न संसृष्टानां रसानां कर्मोपदिशन्ति बुद्धिमन्तः| तच्चैव कारणमपेक्षमाणाः षण्णां रसानां परस्परेणासंसृष्टानां लक्षणपृथक्त्वमुपदेक्ष्यामः||९||

## Substantiation of six number of tastes

The Yoni – source material for the manifestation of all these tastes is water element – Jala Mahabhuta

Chedana – emaciation and Upashamana – nourishment are two types of action of tastes. Hence, they do not taste like themselves. Combination of these two actions leads to the manifestation of tastes having a general action (Sadharana). Swadu (Palatability) or otherwise is the subjective reaction (bhakti); wholesomeness (Hita) or unwholesomeness (Ahita) constitutes the specific action. Hence, four types of taste theory are invalid.

The five basic elements form dravya – substance. Due to different permutations and combinations, due to the effect of time, place, and season on them, the substance exhibits qualities like Guru (heavy), laghu (lightness) etc. Hence six types of tastes based on quality are invalid.

क्षरणात् क्षार: – kṣaraṇāt kṣāraḥ

Because of its corrosive nature, it is known as Kshara / Alkali; Hence, it is a physical effect. Thus kshara cannot be called as taste. This is manifested by the combination of many tastes and it possesses many tastes dominated by pungent and saline ones. Kshara is the object of many senses (for example, it can be seen, it can be touched etc) and it involves a special method of preparation.

Avyakta – imperceptibility of tastes is affected only in Jala Mahabhuta (water element). It happens when the taste is hidden deep in the substance or is exhibited incompletely. Hence, it cannot be said as a type of taste. It is not correct to say that the tastes are innumerable, by just saying that the substances in the world are innumerable. Even in the innumerable substances, the qualities, action and taste of those substances are not innumerable. So we shall now explain the specific characteristics and distinctive features of the six tastes separately. [9]

## Observations regarding the classification of matter:

अग्रे तु तावद्द्रव्यभेदमभिप्रेत्य किञ्चिदभिधास्यामः।

सर्वं द्रव्यं पाञ्चभौतिकमस्मिन्नर्थे; तच्चेतनावदचेतनं च, तस्य गुणाः शब्दादयो गुर्वादयश्च द्रवान्ताः, कर्म पञ्चविधमुक्तं वमनादि॥१०॥

## Observations regarding the classification of matter:

All matter is constituted of five Mahabhutas (five basic elements);
Some of the materials are Chetana (have soul) and others are Achetana (does not have soul)
Qualities of substances are Shabda (sound), Sparsha (touch), Roopa (vision), Rasa (taste) and Gandha (Smell)
also the twenty qualities beginning with heaviness etc 20 qualities
These substances are useful in Vamana etc Panchakarma therapies.[10]

## Physical properties of Pancha Mahabhutas:

तत्र द्रव्याणि गुरुखरकठिनमन्दस्थिरविशदसान्द्रस्थूलगन्धगुणबहुलानि पार्थिवानि, तान्युपचयसङ्घातगौरवस्थैर्यकराणि;
द्रवस्निग्धशीतमन्दमृदुपिच्छिलरसगुणबहुलान्याप्यानि, तान्युपक्लेदस्नेहबन्धविष्यन्दमार्दवप्रह्लादकराणि;
उष्णतीक्ष्णसूक्ष्मलघुरूक्षविशदरूपगुणबहुलान्याग्नेयानि, तानि दाहपाकप्रभाप्रकाशवर्णकराणि;
लघुशीतरूक्षखरविशदसूक्ष्मस्पर्शगुणबहुलानि वायव्यानि, तानि रौक्ष्यग्लानिविचारवैशद्यलाघवकराणि;

## Qualities and function of earth element:

तत्र द्रव्याणि गुरुखरकठिनमन्दस्थिरविशदसान्द्रस्थूलगन्धगुणबहुलानि पार्थिवानि, तान्युपचयसङ्घातगौरवस्थैर्यकराणि;
Substances that have below qualities in abundance are called Parthiva – having earth as the dominant element.
Guru – heavy,
Khara – tough,
Katina – hard,
Manda – dull,
Sthira – stable,
Vishada – non-slimy, clear
Sandra – dense,
Sthoola – bulk, gross and
Gandha – Smell
These Parthiva – earth dominant substances cause
Upachaya – promote plumpness,

Sanghata – compactness, give shape to body and body organs
Gaurava – heaviness
Sthairya – stability.

## Qualities and function of (liquids) materials having water-element dominance – Apya Dravya

द्रवस्निग्ध शीतमन्द मृदुपिच्छिल रसगुणबहुलान्याप्यानि, तान्युपक्लेद स्नेहबन्धविष्यन्द मार्दवप्रह्लादकराणि;

Substances that have below qualities in abundance are called as Apya – having water as dominant element.
Drava – liquid,
Snigdha – unctuous, oily
Sheeta – cold
Manda – dull, slow flowing
Mrudu – soft,
Picchila – slimy, sticky
Rasa – taste
They promote below functions
Upakleda – stickiness,
Sneha – unctuousness, Oiliness
Bandha – compactness,
Vishyanda – moistness,
Mardava – softness and
Prahlada – happiness.

## Qualities and function of materials having fire-element dominance – Agneya Dravya

उष्णतीक्ष्ण सूक्ष्म लघुरूक्ष विशद रूपगुणबहुलान्याग्नेयानि, तानि दाहपाक प्रभा प्रकाशवर्णकराणि;

Substances that have below qualities in abundance are called as Agneya – having fire as dominant element.
Ushna – hot,
Teekshna – sharp,
Sookshma – subtle, minute
Laghu – light,
Rooksha – dryness
Vishada – non-slimy, clarity
Roopa – vision
They promote below functions
Daaha – combustion, burning
Paaka – digestion, metabolism,
Prabha – luster,
Prakasha – radiance
Varna – color.

## Qualities and function of materials having air-element dominance – Vayavya Dravya

लघुशीत रूक्षखर विशद सूक्ष्म स्पर्शगुणबहुलानि वायव्यानि, तानि रौक्ष्यग्लानि विचारवैशद्य लाघवकराणि;

Substances that have below qualities in abundance are called as Vayavya – having air as dominant element.
Laghu – lightness,
Sheeta – cold,
Rooksha – nonuctuous, dry
Khara – rough,
Vishada – Clear, non- slimy,
Sookshma – subtle, minute

Sparsha – touch
They promote
Roukshya – roughness,
Glani – aversion, tiredness
Vichara – movement,
Vaishadya – clarity, non-sliminess and
Laghava – lightness.

## Qualities and function of materials having ether / vacuum – element dominance – Akasheeya Dravya

मृदुलघुसूक्ष्मश्लक्ष्णशब्दगुणबहुलान्याकाशात्मकानि, तानि मार्दवसौषिर्यलाघवकराणि||११||

Substances that have below qualities in abundance are called as Akasheeya – having ether as dominant element.
Mridu – soft,
Laghu – lightness,
Sookshma – smoothness
Shabda – sound
They promote
Mardava – softness,
Soushirya – porosity, emptiness and
Laghava – lightness.[11]

## All the substances in this world can be medicine:

अनेनोपदेशेन नानौषधिभूतं जगति किञ्चिद्द्रव्यमुपलभ्यते तां तां युक्तिमर्थं च तं तमभिप्रेत्य||१२||
With the above explanation, there is no substances in this world, without any medicinal qualities / therapeutic utility.
It is upto the physician to appropriately choose and use the substances as medicine based on
Yukti – planned wisdom and
Artha – knowledge of the exact purpose of the substance. [12]

## How a medicine acts? Pharmaco-dynamics of drugs:

न तु केवलं गुणप्रभावादेव द्रव्याणि कार्मुकाणि भवन्ति; द्रव्याणि हि द्रव्यप्रभावाद्गुणप्रभावाद्द्रव्यगुणप्रभावाच्च तस्मिंस्तस्मिन् काले तत्तदधिकरणमासाद्य तां तां च युक्तिमर्थं च तं तमभिप्रेत्य यत् कुर्वन्ति, तत् कर्म; येन कुर्वन्ति, तद्वीर्यं; यत्र कुर्वन्ति, तदधिकरणं; यदा कुर्वन्ति, स कालः; यथा कुर्वन्ति, स उपायः; यत् साधयन्ति, तत् फलम्||१३||

## How a medicine acts? Pharmaco-dynamics of drugs:

It is not just by the virtue of Guna – qualities, that a substance exhibits action. In fact they act by virtue of their own nature or qualities or both on a proper occasion, in a given location, in appropriate condition and situations; the effect so produced is considered to be their action (Karma);
Yena Kurvanti, tat veeryam – By which a medicine acts, is called as Veerya. The factor responsible for the manifestation of the effect is known as Veerya:

Yatra kurvanti tat adhikaranam – where they act is the Adhisthana / Adhikarana (site of action);
Yada kurvanti, sa kaalaha – when they act is the time,
yathaa kurvanti sa upaayaha – how they act is the Upaya or mode of action;
Yat sadhayati, tat phalam – what they accomplish is the achievement.[13]

## Taste combinations:

भेदश्चैषां त्रिषष्टिविधविकल्पो द्रव्यदेशकालप्रभावाद्भवति, तमुपदेक्ष्यामः||१४||

There are 63 combinations of Rasas (tastes) depending upon the variation of the nature of the substance, location and time, they are being explained here.[14]

**Sixty-three types of Rasa:**
स्वादुरम्लादिभिर्योगं शेषैरम्लादयः पृथक्|
यान्ति पञ्चदशैतानि द्रव्याणि दिवरसानि तु||१५||

**A. By the combination of two Rasas- 15 in number**
1. Sweet and sour
2. Sweet and saline
3. Sweet and pungent
4. Sweet and bitter
5. Sweet and astringent
6. sour and saline
7. sour and pungent
8. sour and bitter
9. sour and astringent
10. saline and pungent
11. saline and bitter
12. saline and astringent
13. pungent and bitter
14. pungent and astringent
15. bitter and astringent

**B. By the combination of three Rasas- 20 in number**
पृथगम्लादियुक्तस्य योगः शेषैः पृथग्भवेत्|
मधुरस्य तथाऽम्लस्य लवणस्य कटोस्तथा||१६||
त्रिरसानि यथासङ्ख्यं द्रव्याण्युक्तानि विंशतिः|१७|

16. Sweet, Sour and Saline
17. Sweet, Sour and Pungent
18. Sweet Sour and bitter
19. Sweet, Sour and Astringent
20. Sweet, saline and Pungent
21. Sweet, Saline and Bitter
22. Sweet, saline and Astringent
23. Sweet, Pungent and bitter
24. Sweet, Pungent and Astringent
25. Sweet, bitter and Astringent
26. Sour, Saline and Pungent
27. Sour, saline and Bitter
28. Sour, Saline and astringent
29. Sour, Pungent and Bitter
30. Sour, Pungent and Astringent
31. Sour, Bitter and Astringent
32. Saline, Pungent and Bitter

33. Saline, Pungent and Astringent
34. Saline, Bitter and Astringent
35. Pungent, Bitter and Astringent

## C. By the combination of four Rasas - 15 in number

वक्ष्यन्ते तु चतुष्केण द्रव्याणि दश पञ्च च||१७||
स्वाद्वम्लौ सहितौ योगं लवणाद्यैः पृथग्गतौ|
योगं शेषैः पृथग्यातश्चतुष्करससङ्ख्यया||१८||
सहितौ स्वादुलवणौ तद्वत् कट्वादिभिः पृथक्|
युक्तौ शेषैः पृथग्योगं यातः स्वादूषणौ तथा||१९||
कट्वाद्यैरम्ललवणौ संयुक्तौ सहितौ पृथक्|
यातः शेषैः पृथग्योगं शेषैरम्लकटू तथा||२०||
युज्यते तु कषायेण सतिक्तौ लवणोषणौ|२१|

36. Sweet, Sour, Saline and Pungent
37. Sweet, Sour, Saline and Bitter
38. Sweet, Sour, Saline and Astringent
39. Sweet, Sour, Pungent and Bitter
40. Sweet, Sour, Pungent and Astringent
41. Sweet, Sour, Bitter and Astringent
42. Sweet, Saline, Pungent and Bitter
43. Sweet, Saline, Bitter and Astringent
44. Sweet, saline, Astringent and Pungent
45. Sweet, Pungent, bitter and Astringent
46. Sour, Saline, Pungent and Bitter
47. Sour, Saline, Bitter and Astringent
48. Sour, Saline, Astringent and Pungent
49. Sour, Pungent, Bitter and Astringent
50. Saline, Pungent, Bitter and Astringent

## D. By the combination of five Rasas- 6 in number

षट् तु पञ्चरसान्याहुरेकैकस्यापवर्जनात्||२१||

51. Sour, Saline, Pungent Bitter and Astringent
52. Sweet, Saline, Pungent, Bitter and Astringent
53. Sweet, Sour, Pungent, Bitter and Astringent
54. Sweet, Sour, Saline, Bitter and Astringent
55. Sweet, Sour, Saline, Pungent and Astringent
56. Sweet, Sour, Saline, Pungent and Bitter

## E. Without any combination - 6 in number

षट् चैवैकरसानि स्युरेकं षड्रसमेव तु|२२|

57. Sweet
58. Sour
59. Saline
60. Pungent

61. Bitter
62. Astringent

**F. By the combination of all the Six Rasas:**
63. Sweet, Sour, Saline, Pungent, Bitter and Astringent. [15-22]

इति त्रिषष्टिर्द्रव्याणां निर्दिष्टा रससङ्ख्यया||२२||
त्रिषष्टिः स्यात्वसङ्ख्येया रसानुरसकल्पनात्|
रसास्तरतमाभ्यां तां सङ्ख्यामतिपतन्ति हि||२३||
संयोगाः सप्तपञ्चाशत् कल्पना तु त्रिषष्टिधा|
रसानां तत्र योग्यत्वात् कल्पिता रसचिन्तकैः||२४||

The number may still go up to the extent of infinity if Anurasa (after tastes or subsidiary tastes) and their relative degrees are taken into account. [23] In view of their therapeutic utility, fifty- seven combinations and sixty-three types of Rasas (tastes) are enunciated. [24]

**General principles of Rasa therapy:**
क्वचिदेको रसः कल्प्यः संयुक्ताश्च रसाः क्वचित्|
दोषौषधादीन् सञ्चिन्त्य भिषजा सिद्धिमिच्छता||२५||
द्रव्याणि द्विरसादीनि संयुक्तांश्च रसान् बुधाः|
रसानेकैकशो वाऽपि कल्पयन्ति गदान् प्रति||२६||

**General principles of Rasa therapy:**
A physician may prescribe drugs having one taste or combination of several tastes, with due regard to the nature of imbalanced Doshas, the resultant manifestation of the disease and specific actions of drugs etc, for the maintenance of health. Similarly for the cure of diseases, drugs having one or more tastes may be prescribed. [25-26]

**Importance of the knowledge of the classification of Rasa and Dosha:**
यः स्याद्रसविकल्पज्ञः स्याच्च दोषविकल्पवित्|
न स मुह्येद्विकाराणां हेतुलिङ्गोपशान्तिषु ||२७||
A physician, well acquainted with the combinations of Rasa (taste) and Doshas, seldom commits blunders in ascertaining the etiology, symptoms and treatment of diseases. [27]

**Identification of Rasa (taste) and Anurasa (after-taste) in a given substance:**
व्यक्तः शुष्कस्य चादौ च रसो द्रव्यस्य लक्ष्यते|
विपर्ययेणानुरसो रसो नास्ति हि सप्तमः||२८||
The taste that is felt at the beginning and end of the time of contact of tongue, by a dry substance, is considered as Rasa. When such a taste is not distinctly perceptible but is inferred only by its actions, it is known as Anurasa (after-taste). It is included in one of the six tastes and there is no separate seventh taste. [28]

**Paradi Guna – special list of qualities:**
परापरत्वे युक्तिश्च सङ्ख्या संयोग एव च|
विभागश्च पृथक्त्वं च परिमाणमथापि च||२९||
संस्कारोऽभ्यास इत्येते गुणा ज्ञेयाः परादयः|
सिद्ध्युपायाश्चिकित्साया लक्षणैस्तान् प्रचक्ष्महे||३०||
देशकालवयोमानपाकवीर्यरसादिषु|
परापरत्वे, युक्तिश्च योजना या तु युज्यते||३१||

सङ्ख्या स्याद्गणितं, योगः सह संयोग उच्यते|
द्रव्याणां द्वन्द्वसर्वैककर्मजोऽनित्य एव च||३२||
विभागस्तु विभक्तिः स्यादि्वयोगो भागशो ग्रहः|
पृथक्त्वं स्यादसंयोगो वैलक्षण्यमनेकता||३३||
परिमाणं पुनर्मानं, संस्कारः करणं मतम्|
भावाभ्यसनमभ्यासः शीलनं सततक्रिया||३४||
इति स्वलक्षणैरुक्ता गुणाः सर्वे परादयः|
चिकित्सा यैरविदितैर्न यथावत् प्रवर्तते||३५||

**Paradi Guna – special list of qualities:**
Apart from the 20 qualities of substances, there are 10 other qualities, known as Paradi Guna (starting from Para).
They are –
Para – superiority
Apara – inferiority
Yukti – planning, propriety (proper application),
Sankhya – number
Samyoga – combination
Vibhaga – division
Pruthaktva – individuality, separation (consisting of non combination, distinctness and plurality),
Parimana – quantification
Samskara – habit, transformation (method of preparation)
Abhyasa – practice, repetition

**Para, Apara (superiority and inferiority)**
देशकाल वयोमान पाकवीर्य रसादिषु | परापरत्वे,

The superiority and inferiority can be appreciated in
Desha – place, parts of body
Kala – season
Vayo – age
Mana – measurements
Paka – digestion
Veerya – potency and
Rasa – taste

**Yukti – planning**
युक्तिश्च योजना या तु युज्यते||३१||
Planning of treatment with one or more components.

**Sankhya – number:**
सङ्ख्या स्याद्गणितं
Sankhya is related with maths, to counting.

**Samyoga – combination :**
योगः सह संयोग उच्यते| द्रव्याणां द्वन्द्वसर्वैककर्मजोऽनित्य एव च||३२||
Samyoga is combining two or more substances.

**Vibhaga – division :**
विभागस्तु विभक्तिः स्यादि्वयोगो भागशो ग्रहः|
Division of a complex thing into many components is Vibhaga.

**Prutaktva :**
पृथक्त्वं स्यादसंयोगो वैलक्षण्यमनेकता||३३||
Prutaktva is individuality, considering each component singularly or differentiation

**Parimana :**
परिमाणं पुनर्मानं
To measure or quantify.

**Samskara :**
संस्कारः करणं मतम्|
Processing, converting, habit, transformation (method of preparation)

**Abhyasa:**
भावाभ्यसनमभ्यासः शीलनं सततक्रिया||३४||
Doing the same thing continuously. Without knowing these Paradi qualities, a physician cannot do well in treatment. [29-35]

**Properties attributed to Rasas really belong to Dravyas:**
गुणा गुणाश्रया नोक्तास्तस्माद्रसगुणान् भिषक्|
विद्याद्द्रव्यगुणान् कर्तुरभिप्रायाः पृथग्विधाः||३६||
A quality, itself cannot hold another quality. So, taste, being a quality, cannot hold other qualities. All the qualities of the taste that were explained are actually the qualities of the substance, which holds that taste.
All the qualities including taste, reside in the substance (Dravya). [36]

अतश्च प्रकृतं बुद्ध्वा देशकालान्तराणि च|
तन्त्रकर्तुरभिप्रायानुपायांश्चार्थमादिशेत्||३७||
In the event of the texts conveying apparently conflicting views, the interpretation should be based on the contextual, local and temporal propriety, the intention of the author and the rules of interpretation (Tantra Yukti). [37]

षड्विभक्तीः प्रवक्ष्यामि रसानामत उत्तरम्|
षट् पञ्चभूतप्रभवाः सङ्ख्याताश्च यथा रसाः||३८||
Next, I would explain the six tastes which have been formed by various permutations and combinations of pancamahabhutas (basic elements of nature).

**Genesis of Rasa from five basic elements:**
सौम्याः खल्वापोऽन्तरिक्षप्रभवाः प्रकृतिशीता लघ्व्यश्चाव्यक्तरसाश्च, तास्त्वन्तरिक्षादभ्रश्यमाना भ्रष्टाश्च पञ्चमहाभूतगुणसमन्विता जङ्गमस्थावराणां भूतानां मूर्तीरभिप्रीणयन्ति, तासु मूर्तिषु षड्भिमूर्च्छन्ति रसाः||३९||

The moon is the presiding Deity of water. The water in the atmosphere (before it falls on the ground) is by nature cold and light, and its Rasa is not manifested at this stage. The moment it starts falling from atmosphere and after it falls on the ground, it gets impregnated with the qualities of the five Mahabhutas and it nourishes the individuals belonging to the vegetable and animal kingdom. At this stage the six tastes manifest themselves in these individuals. [39]

तेषां षण्णां रसानां सोमगुणातिरेकान्मधुरो रसः, पृथिव्यग्निभूयिष्ठत्वादम्लः, सलिलाग्निभूयिष्ठत्वाल्लवणः, वाय्वग्निभूयिष्ठत्वात्
कटुकः, वाय्वाकाशातिरिक्तत्वातिक्तः, पवनपृथिवीव्यतिरेकात् कषाय इति|
एवमेषां रसानां षट्त्वमुपपन्नं न्यूनातिरेकविशेषान्महाभूतानां भूतानामिव स्थावरजङ्गमानां नानावर्णाकृतिविशेषाः; षड्तुतुक्त्वाच्च
कालस्योपपन्नो महाभूतानां न्यूनातिरेकविशेषः||४०||

**Predominance of basic elements in individual Rasa:**
All the tastes have Jala Mahabhuta (water element) dominance.
Sweet taste – Madhura rasa = Prithvi + Ap (earth + water)
Sour taste – Amla rasa = Prathvi + Agni (earth + fire)
Salt taste – Lavana Rasa = Jala and Agni (water + fire)
Pungent taste – Katu Rasa = Vayu + Agni (air and fire)
Bitter taste – Tikta Rasa = Vayu + Akasha (air and ether)
Astringent taste – Kashaya Rasa = Vayu and Prithvi (air and earth).

Vegetables and animals are of diverse type, depending upon their color and shape (owing to the predominance
or otherwise of the various Mahabhutas (5 basic elements). Similarly, tastes are also six in number due to the
predominance or otherwise of the five Mahabhutas. The predominance or otherwise of five Mahabhutas in turn
depends on the six seasonal variations. [40]

**Flow of Rasas (taste):**
तत्राग्निमारुतात्मका रसाः प्रायेणोर्ध्वभाजः, लाघवादुत्प्लवनत्वाच्च वायोरूर्ध्वज्वलनत्वाच्च वह्नेः; सलिलपृथिव्यात्मकास्तु
प्रायेणाधोभाजः, पृथिव्या गुरुत्वान्निम्नगत्वाच्चोदकस्य; व्यामिश्रात्मकाः पुनरुभयतोभाजः||४१||

Rasas with qualities of fire (Agni) and air (Vayu) have a tendency of upward movement. This is because of the
lightness and upward mobility of Vayu and upward flames of Agni. The Rasas with the qualities of Jala and Prithvi on
the other hand have a tendency for downward movement because of the heaviness of Prithvi and downward flow of
Jala. The Rasas within both the categories of substances mentioned above share both the qualities. [41]

तेषां षण्णां रसानामेकैकस्य यथाद्रव्यं गुणकर्माण्यनुव्याख्यास्यामः||४२||
We shall now explain the properties and actions of each one of the six Rasa as they are found in various drugs and
diets. [42]

**Action of Sweet Taste:**
तत्र, मधुरो रसः शरीरसात्म्याद्रसरुधिरमांसमेदोस्थिमज्जौजःशुक्राभिवर्धन आयुष्यः षडिन्द्रियप्रसादनो बलवर्णकरः
पित्तविषमारुतघ्नस्तृष्णादाहप्रशमनस्त्वच्यः केश्यः कण्ठ्यो बल्यः प्रीणनो जीवनस्तर्पणो बृंहणः स्थैर्यकरः क्षीणक्षतसन्धानकरो
घ्राणमुखकण्ठौष्ठजिह्वाप्रह्लादनो दाहमूर्च्छाप्रशमनः षट्पदपिपीलिकानामिष्टतमः स्निग्धः शीतो गुरुश्च|

**Action of Sweet Taste:**
Shareera Satmya – congenial to the body, wholesome
Rasa, Rudhira, Mamsa Medo Asthi Majja Oja Shukra Abhivardhana – improves – Rasa (body fluid), blood, muscle,
fat, bone, marrow, ojas, semen and longevity and also Ojas
Ayushyaha – improves life expectancy.
Shadindriya Prasadana – They are soothing to the six sense organs (5 sense organs + mind)
Bala Varnakara – improves strength and skin complexion
Pitta Visha Marutaghna – balances Pitta, toxicity and Vata.
Trishna Daha Prashamana – relieves thirst and burning sensation

Tvachya – improves skin quality

Keshya – improves hair

Kanthya – improves voice quality

Balya – improves strength and immunity

Preenana – soothing

Jeevana – enlivening,

Tarpana – invigorating

Bruhmana – nourishing

Sthairyakara – improves body stamina and stability

Ksheena Kshata Sandhanakara – useful in relieving chest injury and bone fracture healing

Ghrana Mukha Kantha Oshta Jihva Prahladana – soothing to the nose, mouth, throat, lips and tongue

Daha Murcha Prashamana – relieves burning sensation and unconsciousness

Shat Pada Pipeelikaanaam ishtatamaha – attracts bees and ants

Snigdha sheeto guruscha – unctuous, coolant and heavy to digestion


**When sweet is used in excess**, it causes Kapha vitiation, leading to

स एवङ्गुणोऽप्येक एवात्यर्थमुपयुज्यमानः स्थौल्यं मार्दवमालस्यमतिस्वप्नं गौरवमनन्नाभिलाषमग्नेर्दौर्बल्यमास्यकण्ठयोर्मांसाभिवृद्धिं श्वासकासप्रतिश्यायालसकशीतज्वरानाहास्यमाधुर्यवमथुसञ्ज्ञास्वरप्रणाशगलगण्डगण्डमालाश्लीपद-गलशोफबस्तिधमनीगलोपलेपाक्ष्यामयाभिष्यन्दानित्येवम्प्रभृतीन् कफजान् विकारानुपजनयति )|४३|)


**When sweet is used in excess**, it causes Kapha vitiation, leading to

Sthoulya – obesity

Mardava – increased softness of the body

Alasyam Atisvapnam – increases laziness, and excess sleep,

Gauravam – increased feeling of heaviness

Ananna Abhilasha – lack of interest in food

Agner Daurbalya – low digestion strength

Aasya Kanthayor maamsaabhivruddhi – increased muscle growth in mouth and throat

Shwasa, Kasa – cough, cold, asthma

Pratisyaya, Alasaka - running nose, indigestion (intestinal torpor)

Sheeta jwara – fever of Kapha imbalance, with cold feeling

Anaha – bloating

Asya Madhurya - feeling of sweetness in mouth

Vamathu – vomiting

Sanjna svara pranasha - loss of sensation, loss of voice

Galaganda, Gandamala, Shleepada – Scrofula, cervical lymphadenitis, elephantiasis,

Gala Shopha – Pharayngitis

Bati Dhamani Galopalepa – Adhesion in the bladder, vessels (as in atherosclerosis – cholesterol deposition in blood vessels), throat

Akshi Amaya, Abhishyanda – eye disorders, conjunctivitis [43-i]


### Action of Sour Taste – Amla Rasa

अम्लो रसो भक्तं रोचयति, अग्निं दीपयति, देहं बृंहयति ऊर्जयति, मनो बोधयति, इन्द्रियाणि दृढीकरोति, बलं वर्धयति, वातमनुलोमयति, हृदयं तर्पयति, आस्यमास्रावयति, भुक्तमपकर्षयति क्लेदयति जरयति, प्रीणयति, लघुरुष्णः स्निग्धश्च|


### Action of Sour Taste – Amla Rasa

Bhaktam rochayati – improves taste of food

Agnim deepayati – improves digestion strength

Deham brimhayati, Urjayati – nourishes the body, improves enthusiasm

Mano Bodhayati – pleases the mind

Indriyani Drudhikaroti – strengthens sense organs

Balam Vardhayati – improves strength and immunity

Vatam Anulomayati – ensures movement of Vata in its natural direction

Hrudayam tarpayati – nourish the heart

Asyam Asravayati – causes salivation

Bhuktam Apakarshayati – help in swallowing

Kledayati, jarayati – moistens and digests food

Preenayati – refreshing

Laghu, Ushna, Snigdhascha – light, hot and unctuous

**When sour is used in excess,it leads to**

स एवङ्गुणोऽप्येक एवात्यर्थमुपयुज्यमानो दन्तान् हर्षयति, तर्षयति, सम्मीलयत्यक्षिणी, संवेजयति लोमानि, कफं विलापयति, पित्तमभिवर्धयति, रक्तं दूषयति,मांसं विदहति, कायं शिथिलीकरोति, क्षीणक्षतकृशदुर्बलानां श्वयथुमापादयति, अपि च क्षताभिहतदष्टदग्धभग्नशूनप्रच्युतावमूत्रितपरिसर्पितमर्दितच्छिन्नभिन्नविश्लिष्टोद्विद्धोत्पिष्टादीनि   पाचयत्याग्नेयस्वभावात्, परिदहति कण्ठमुरो हृदयं च |४३|

**When sour is used in excess,it leads to**

Dantan harshayati – causes tingling sensation in teeth

Tarshayati – causes excessive thirst

Sammeelayati akshini – causes drowsiness in eyes

Samvejayati lomani – horripulation

Kapham vilapayati – Liquefies and vitiates Kapha

Pittam Abivardhayati – increases Pitta

Raktam dushayati – vitiates blood

Mamsam vidahati – causes burning sensation in muscle tissue

Kayam shithilikaroti – makes the body brittle

Ksheenakshata krusha durbalaanaam shvayathum aapadayati – in lean, injured and weak persons, it causes swelling and inflammation

Due to heating property they cause suppuration of wounds caused by ulceration, trauma, contagious bites, burn, fracture, animals, (viz snakes like Karanda), bruise, excision, incision, separation, perforation and crushing.

Paridahati kantamuro hrudayam ca – Causes burning sensation in throat and heart region [43-ii]

**Action of Salt taste – Lavana Rasa Karma :**

लवणो रसः पाचनः क्लेदनो दीपनश्च्यावनश्छेदनो भेदनस्तीक्ष्णः सरो विकास्यधःस्रंस्यवकाशकरो वातहरः स्तम्भबन्धसङ्घातविधमनः सर्वरसप्रत्यनीकभूतः, आस्यमास्रावयति, कफं विष्यन्दयति, मार्गान् विशोधयति, सर्वशरीरावयवान् मृदूकरोति, रोचयत्याहारम्, आहारयोगी, नात्यर्थं गुरुः स्निग्ध उष्णश्च|

स एवङ्गुणोऽप्येक एवात्यर्थमुपयुज्यमानः पित्तं कोपयति, रक्तं वर्धयति, तर्षयति, मूर्च्छयति, तापयति, दारयति, कृष्णाति मांसानि, प्रगालयति कुष्ठानि, विषं वर्धयति, शोफान् स्फोटयति, दन्तांश्च्यावयति, पुंस्त्वमुपहन्ति, इन्द्रियाण्युपरुणद्धि, वलिपलितखालित्यमापादयति, अपि च लोहितपित्ताम्लपित्तविसर्पवातरक्तविचर्चिकेन्द्रलुप्तप्रभृतीन्विकारानुपजनयति |४३|

**Action of Salt taste – Lavana Rasa Karma :**

Pachanaha – help in digestion

Kledanaha – causes moistening effect

Deepanaha chyavana chedano -improves digestion, scraping effect, excision effect

Bhedana, teekshna – breaks down, piercing, sharp
Saro – causes / initiates movement
Vikaarasya adhaha sramsyavakaashakara – causes movement of Doshas in downward direction
Vatahara – Balances Vata
Stambhana bandha samghata vidhamana – breaks down stiffness, tightening effect and obstructions
Sarvarasa pratyaneekabhutaha – can dominate all other tastes
Aasyam aasraavayati – causes salivation
Kapham vishyandayati – liquifies Kapha
Maargaan vishodhayati – cleanses and clears body channels
Sarvashareera avayavaan mrudukaroti – softens and brings about tenderness in all body parts
Rochayati aahaaram – improves taste of food
Aahaarayogi naatyartham guru snigdha ushnascha – essential ingredient in foods. It is not too heavy, not too hot and not oily.

**When salt is used in excess :**
Pittam kopayati – causes vitiation of Pitta
Rakatm vardhayati – aggravates blood
Tarshayati – causes excessive thirst
Murchayati – causes fainting
Tapayati – causing heating sensation
Darayati – causes erosion
Krushnati mamsani – depletion of muscle tissue
Pragalayati kushtani – sloughing of skin diseases
Visham vardhayati – aggravates poison effects and symptoms
Shophan sphotayati – opens up swellings
Dantan chyavayati – causes teeth dislodgement
Pumstvam upahanti – causes impotency
Indriyani uparunaddhi – obstruction of the function of senses
Vali palita khalityam apadayati – premature wrinkling, graying and baldness
Lohitapitta amlapitta – bleeding disorders, gastritis
Visarpa – herpes
Vatarakta – gout
Vicharchika indralupta – eczema and alopecia [43-iii]

**Action of Pungent Taste – Katu Rasa**
कटुको रसो वक्त्रं शोधयति, अग्निं दीपयति, भुक्तं शोषयति, घ्राणमास्रावयति, चक्षुर्विरेचयति, स्फुटीकरोतीन्द्रियाणि, अलसकश्वयथूपचयोदर्दाभिष्यन्दस्नेहस्वेदक्लेदमलानुपहन्ति, रोचयत्यशनं, कण्डूर्विनाशयति , व्रणानवसादयति, क्रिमीन् हिनस्ति, मांसं विलिखति, शोणितसङ्घातं भिनत्ति, बन्धांश्छिनत्ति, मार्गान् विवृणोति, श्लेष्माणं शमयति, लघुरुष्णो रूक्षश्च|
स एवङ्गुणोऽप्येक एवात्यर्थमुपयुज्यमानो विपाकप्रभावात् पुंस्त्वमुपहन्ति, रसवीर्यप्रभावान्मोहयन्ति, ग्लापयति, सादयति, कर्शयति, मूर्च्छयति, नमयति, तमयति, भ्रमयति, कण्ठं परिदहति, शरीरतापमुपजनयति, बलं क्षिणोति, तृष्णां जनयति; अपि च वात्यग्निगुणबाहुल्याद्भ्रमदवथुकम्पतोदभेदैश्चरणभुजपार्श्वपृष्ठप्रभृतिषु मारुतजान् विकारानुपजनयति (४);

**Action of Pungent Taste – Katu Rasa**
Vaktram Shodhayati – cleanses mouth
Agnim deepayati – improves digestion strength
Bhuktam shoshayati – dries up food
Ghranam asravayati – causes watering of nose

Chakshur virechayati – causes lacrimation
Sphutikaroti indriyani – sharpens sense organs
cure diseases like Alasaka (intestinal toper), Shvayathu (inflammation), Upachaya (obesity), Udarda (urticaria), Abhishyanda (chronic conjunctivitis),
Sneha Sveda Kleda malan upahanti – helps in oleation, sweating, helps in elimination of sticky waste products
Rochyayati Ashanam – improves food taste
Kandur vinashayati – relieves itching
Vranan avasadayati – allay excessive growth of ulcers
Krimeen Hinasti – kills germs and worms
Mamsam vilikhati – scrapes down muscle tissue
Shonita Sanghatam bhinatti – breaks down blood clots
Bandhan chinatti – breaks down bonding,
Margan Vivrunoti – clears body channels
Shleshmanam shamayati – balances down Kapha
Laghu, Ushna, Rooksha – light, hot and dry in nature.

**Effect of excess of pungent taste -**
Pumstvam Apahanti – causes impotence
Glapayati, Sadayati, Karshayati – cause unconsciousness, weariness, leanness
Murchayati – causes unconsciousness
Namayati – causes body to bend forward
Tamayati – causes feeling of darkness
Bhramayati – causes dizziness
Kantam Paridahati – burning sensation in throat
Shareera tapam upajanayati – burning sensation in body
Balam kshinoti – depletes strength and immunity
Trushnam janayati – causes thirst

Because of the dominance of Vayu and Agnimahabhutas they also cause giddiness (bhrama), burning sensation (Davatu), tremor (kampa) piercing (toda) and stabbing pain (bheda) in legs, hands, back etc. [43-iv]

## Action of Bitter Taste – Tikta Rasa

तिक्तो रसः स्वयमरोचिष्णुरप्यरोचकघ्नो विषघ्नः क्रिमिघ्नो मूर्च्छादाहकण्डूकुष्ठतृष्णाप्रशमनस्त्वङ्मांसयोः स्थिरीकरणो ज्वरघ्नो दीपनः पाचनः स्तन्यशोधनो लेखनः क्लेदमेदोवसामज्जलसीकापूयस्वेदमूत्रपुरीषपित्तश्लेष्मोपशोषणो रूक्षः शीतो लघुश्च|
स एवङ्गुणोऽप्येक एवात्यर्थमुपयुज्यमानो रौक्ष्यात्खरविषदस्वभावाच्च रसरुधिरमांसमेदोस्थिमज्जशुक्राण्युच्छोषयति, स्रोतसां खरत्वमुपपादयति, बलमादत्ते, कर्शयति, ग्लपयति, मोहयति, भ्रमयति, वदनमुपशोषयति, अपरांश्च वातविकारानुपजनयति (५)

## Action of Bitter Taste – Tikta Rasa

Though not so good to taste, when taken, it improves taste in the person.
Vishaghna - detoxifies
Krimighna – kills germs and worms
Murcha daha kandu kushta – relieves unconsciousness, burning sensation, itching and skin disorders
Relieves thirst, strengthens and stabilizes body
Jvaraghna, Deepana, pachana – useful in fever, digestive and carminative
Stanya shodhana – cleanses, purifies breast milk
Lekhana – scraping
Dries up excess moisture, fat, marrow, lymph, pus, sweat, urine, Pitta and Shleshma.
Rooksha, Sheeta Laghu – dry, cold and light

## Excess of Bitter taste causes :

Due to dryness, roughness, non sliminess, bitter taste depletes Rasa dhatu (essence part of digestion), blood (rudhira), Mamsa (muscle tissue), Meda (fat tissue), Asthi (bone), Majja (marrow), Shukra (semen, female reproductive system)

Srotasam kharatvam upapadayati – brings about roughness to the body channels

Balamadatte - depletes strength and immunity

Karshayati – depletes body weight

Glapayati - weariness

Mohayati – unconsciousness

Bhramayati – giddiness

Vadanam upashoshayati -dryness of mouth

Vata Vikara anupajanayati - causes diseases of Vata imbalance [43-v]

### Action of Astringent Taste – Kashaya rasa :

कषायो रसः संशमनः सङ्ग्राही सन्धानकरः पीडनो रोपणः शोषणः स्तम्भनः श्लेष्मरक्तपित्तप्रशमनः शरीरक्लेदस्योपयोक्ता रूक्षः शीतोऽलघुश्च।

स एवङ्गुणोऽप्येक एवात्यर्थमुपयुज्यमान आस्यं शोषयति, हृदयं पीडयति, उदरमाध्मापयति, वाचं निगृह्णाति, स्रोतांस्यवबध्नाति, श्यावत्वमापादयति, पुंस्त्वमुपहन्ति, विष्टभ्य जरां गच्छति, वातमूत्रपुरीषरेतांस्यवगृह्णाति, कर्शयति, ग्लपयति, तर्षयति, स्तम्भयति, खरविशदरूक्षत्वात् पक्षवधग्रहापतानकार्दितप्रभृतींश्च वातविकारानुपजनयति॥४३॥

## Action of Astringent Taste – Kashaya rasa :

Samshamana – calming, healing

Sangrahi – absorbing, constipative

Sandhanakara – wound healing, bone healing

Peedana – causes pressure on body parts

Ropana – healing

Shoshana – dries up moisture

Stambhana – blocking

Shleshma raktapitta prashamana – balances down Kapha and Pitta, useful in bleeding disorders,

Shareera Kleda Upayokta -uses up body moisture

Rooksha, Sheeta, Laghu – dry, cold and light

## Excess of astringent taste causes :

Asyam shoshayati – dries up mouth

Hrudayam Peedayati – causes pressure pain in chest, heart

Udaram adhmapayati – distention of abdomen

Vacham nigruhnati – obstruction of speech

Srotamsi avabadhnati – constriction of channels

Shyavatvam apadayati – imparts black complexion

Pumstvam upahanti – causes impotency

Vishtabhya jaram gacchati – they get stuck in the gut and undergo digestion slowly

Causes obstruction to the passage of flatus, urine, stool and semen

Karshayati – causes emaciation

Glapayti – weariness

Tarshayati – excess thirst

Stambhayati – causes stiffness

Due to roughness, dryness and non-sliminess - astringent taste produces diseases like hemiplegia (pakshavadha), spasm (graha), convulsion (Apatanaka), facial paralysis (Ardita) etc, due to the vitiation of Vata.[43]

**All tastes bring about health and happiness**

इत्येवमेते षड्रसाः पृथक्त्वेनैकत्वेन वा मात्रशः सम्यगुपयुज्यमाना उपकाराय भवन्त्यध्यात्मलोकस्य, अपकारकराः पुनरतोऽन्यथा भवन्त्युपयुज्यमानाः; तान् विद्वानुपकारार्थमेव मात्रशः सम्यगुपयोजयेदिति||४४||

**All tastes bring about health and happiness**

All the six Rasas, if properly used jointly or individually, in proper dose, bring about happiness to all living beings. Otherwise they are equally harmful to all. So a wise person should use them properly in proper dose in order to have good result. [44]

**Determination of potency (Veerya) of a substance based on Rasa (taste):**

भवन्ति चात्र-

शीतं वीर्येण यद्द्रव्यं मधुरं रसपाकयोः|

तयोरम्लं यदुष्णं च यद्द्रव्यं कटुकं तयोः||४५||

The medicines and diet which are sweet in rasa and Vipaka (taste after digestion) are of Sheeta Veerya (cold potency). The medicines and diet which are sour or pungent in rasa and virya are of ushna veerya (hot potency). [45]

तेषां रसोपदेशेन निर्देश्यो गुणसङ्ग्रहः|

वीर्यतोऽविपरीतानां पाकतश्चोपदेक्ष्यते||४६||

यथा पयो यथा सर्पिर्यथा वा चव्यचित्रकौ|

एवमादीनि चान्यानि निर्दिशेद्रसतो भिषक्||४७||

For example, milk and ghee, with sweet taste and sweet Vipaka, have sheeta Veerya (cold potency) Chavya (Piper chaba Hunter) and chitraka (lead wort) are pungent in taste, pungent Vipaka, and have ushna veerya (hot potency) [46-47]

**Substances whose Veeryas (potency) are contradictory to Rasa (taste):**

मधुरं किञ्चिदुष्णं स्यात् कषायं तिक्तमेव च|

यथा महत्पञ्चमूलं यथाऽब्जानूपमामिषम्||४८||

लवणं सैन्धवं नोष्णमम्लमामलकं तथा|

अर्कागुरुगुडूचीनां तिक्तानामुष्णमुच्यते||४९||

**Substances whose Veeryas (potency) are contradictory to Rasa (taste):**

Some substances having sweet taste are of Ushna Veerya (hot) e.g. the meat of aquatic and marshy animals – Anupa and Abja mamsa. Some substances having astringent and bitter tastes are also of Ushnavirya (hot) e.g belonging to Mahat Panchamula (bilva, Agnimantha, Shynoaka, Gambhari and Patala), Arka – Calotropis gigantea R.Br), Aguru ( Aquilaria agallocha Roxb.) and Guduchi – all these have bitter taste. Similarly rock salt having saline taste has Ushna Veerya (hot) Amalaka (Emblica officinalis Gaertn) having sour taste has Anushna Virya (not hot).[48-49]

**Variation in the action of substances of similar tastes:**

किञ्चिदम्लं हि सङ्ग्राहि किञ्चिदम्लं भिनत्ति च|

यथा कपित्थं सङ्ग्राहि भेदि चामलकं तथा||५०||

पिप्पली नागरं वृष्यं कटु चावृष्यमुच्यते|

कषायः स्तम्भनः शीतः सोऽभयायामतोऽन्यथा||५१||

तस्माद्रसोपदेशेन न सर्वं द्रव्यमादिशेत्|

दृष्टं तुल्यरसेऽप्येवं द्रव्ये द्रव्ये गुणान्तरम्||५२||

**Variation in the action of substances of similar tastes:**

Some herbs having sour taste are absorbant – e.g. Kapittha (Feronia limonia Swingle); Some sour herbs are laxative, e.g Amalaka (Emblica officinalis Gaertn). Even though herbs having pungent taste are generally non-aphrodisiac, still Pippali (Piper longum Linn) and Shunti (Zingiber officinale Rosc) having such taste are aphrodisiac. Astringent herbs are usually Sheeta Veerya and absorbant, but Haritaki (Terminalia chebula Linn) is an exception to it – it is

Ushnavirya and laxative. Thus is to not possible to explain the properties of all the drugs and diets simply in term of Rasa because individual drugs having identical tastes vary in relation to their properties. [50-52]

## Relative superiority of Tastes based on certain qualities:

रौक्ष्यात् कषायो रूक्षाणामुत्तमो मध्यमः कटुः।
तिक्तोऽवरस्तथोष्णानामुष्णत्वाल्लवणः परः॥५३॥
मध्योऽम्लः कटुकश्चान्त्यः स्निग्धानां मधुरः परः।
मध्योऽम्लो लवणश्चान्त्यो रसः स्नेहान्निरुच्यते॥५४॥
मध्योत्कृष्टावराः शैत्यात् कषायस्वादुतिक्तकाः।
स्वादुर्गुरुत्वादधिकः कषायाल्लवणोऽवरः॥५५॥
अम्लात् कटुस्ततस्तिक्तो लघुत्वादुत्तमोत्तमः।
केचिल्लघूनामवरमिच्छन्ति लवणं रसम्॥५६॥
गौरवे लाघवे चैव सोऽवरस्तूभयोरपि।

## Relative superiority of Tastes based on certain qualities:

For Dryness quality (Rooksha), Kashaya (astringent) is best, Katu (pungent) is medium and Tikta (bitter) is inferior. For hotness quality (Ushna) – lavana (salt) is superior, sour is medium and Katu (pungent) is inferior. For Unctuousness, oiliness (Snigdha) quality, Sweet is superior, Pungent is medium and Bitter is inferior.

For Cooling quality (sheeta), Sweet – Astringent – Bitter

For Heaviness (guru) – Sweet- Astringent – salt

For lightness (laghu) – bitter – Pungent – Sour

Some authors are of the view that among light drugs and diets, those having saline taste are inferior. Thus drugs and diets having saline taste are inferior both in heaviness and lightness. [53-56]

### The Vipaka of Substances:

परं चातो विपाकानां लक्षणं सम्प्रवक्ष्यते॥५७॥
कटुतिक्तकषायाणां विपाकः प्रायशः कटुः।
अम्लोऽम्लं पच्यते स्वादुर्मधुरं लवणस्तथा॥५८॥

## The Vipaka of Substances:

Vipaka (taste after digestion) of susbstances having pungent, bitter and Astringent tastes is pungent (Katu Vipaka); Sour taste has Sour Vipaka (Amla Vipaka)

Sweet and salt tastes have Sweet (Madhura Vipaka) . [57-58]

## Role of tastes in evacuation of feces:

मधुरो लवणाम्लौ च स्निग्धभावात्त्रयो रसाः।
वातमूत्रपुरीषाणां प्रायो मोक्षे सुखा मताः॥५९॥
कटुतिक्तकषायास्तु रूक्षभावात्त्रयो रसाः।
दुःखाय मोक्षे दृश्यन्ते वातविण्मूत्ररेतसाम्॥६०॥

### Role of tastes in evacuation of feces:

Owing to their unctuousness (oiliness), sweet, sour and saline tastes are useful for the elimination of flatus, urine and stool. On the other hand, pungent, bitter and astringent tastes create difficulty in the elimination of flatus, stool, urine and semen in view of their drying property. [59-60]

## Action of Vipaka on Dosha and Evacuation:

शुक्रहा बद्धविण्मूत्रो विपाको वातलः कटुः।
मधुरः सृष्टविण्मूत्रो विपाकः कफशुक्रलः॥६१॥

पित्तकृत् सृष्टविण्मूत्रः पाकोऽम्लः शुक्रनाशनः|
तेषां गुरुः स्यान्मधुरः कटुकाम्लावतोऽन्यथा||६२||

**Action of Vipaka on Dosha and Evacuation:**
Katu Vipaka (pungent) aggravates Vata, reduces semen and obstructs the passage of stool and urine.
Madhura (Sweet) Vipaka aggravates Kapha, promotes semen and helps in the proper elimination of stool and urine.
Similarly (sour) Amla Vipaka aggravates Pitta, reduces semen and helps in the proper elimination of stool and urine.
Sweet Vipaka is heavy: pungent and sour ones are light. [61-62]

विपाकलक्षणस्याल्पमध्यभूयिष्ठतां प्रति|
द्रव्याणां गुणवैशेष्यात्रत तत्रोपलक्षयेत्||६३||

The relative superiority or inferiority of various types of Vipaka can be determined on the basis of the relative superiority and inferiority of the various properties of different drugs and diets. [63]

**The eight and the Two types of Veerya:**
मृदुतीक्ष्णगुरुलघुस्निग्धरूक्षोष्णशीतलम्|
वीर्यमष्टविधं केचित्, केचिद्द्विविधमास्थिताः||६४||
शीतोष्णमिति, वीर्यं तु क्रियते येन या क्रिया|
नावीर्यं कुरुते किञ्चित् सर्वा वीर्यकृता क्रिया||६५||

**The eight and the Two types of Veerya:**
Some opine there are eight types of Veerya –
Mridu (mild) X Teekshna (sharp),
Guru (heavy) X Laghu (light)
Snigdha (unctuous) X Rooksha (dry)
Ushna (hot) X Sheeta (cold).
Some others hold the view that it is only of two types viz, Sheeta Veerya – Cold potency and Ushna Veerya (hot). The term potency (Veerya) represents that aspect of drugs and diets by virtue of which they manifest their therapeutic action. There cannot be any action without potency; all actions are caused by potency (Veerya). [64-65]

**Determination of Rasa, Vipaka and Virya:**
रसो निपाते द्रव्याणां, विपाकः कर्मनिष्ठया|
वीर्यं यावदधीवासान्निपाताच्चोपलभ्यते||६६||

Rasa or taste can be ascertained immediately after their contact with the tongue; Vipaka is determined by the action (in the form of aggravation of Kapha etc). Virya can be determined in between the stages of Rasa and Vipaka, while in association with the body and or even immediately after coming into contact with the body. [66]

**Definition of Prabhava:**
रसवीर्यविपाकानां सामान्यं यत्र लक्ष्यते|
विशेषः कर्मणां चैव प्रभावस्तस्य स स्मृतः||६७||

Where there is similarity in two drugs in relation to their Rasa (taste), Vipaka and Virya (Potency) but in spite of this similarity these two drugs differ with regard to their action, the distinctive feature responsible for their distinctive effects not supported by their taste, Vipaka and potency is regarded as 'Prabhava' or Specific action.[67]

**Examples of Prabhava and the supremacy of Prabhava:**
कटुकः कटुकः पाके वीर्योष्णश्चित्रको मतः|

तद्वद्दन्ती प्रभावात् विरेचयति मानवम् ||६८||
विषं विषघ्नमुक्तं यत् प्रभावस्तत्र कारणम्|
ऊर्ध्वानुलोमिकं यच्च तत् प्रभावप्रभावितम्||६९||
मणीनां धारणीयानां कर्म यद्विविधात्मकम्|
तत् प्रभावकृतं तेषां प्रभावोऽचिन्त्य उच्यते ७०||

Both Chitraka – Leadword – Plumbago zeylanica and Danti (Baliospermum montanum) are pungent in taste, Pungent Vipaka and Ushna veerya (hot potency). But Danti acts as a purgative while chitraka does not. The purgative effect of Danti, therefore, can be explained only by taking recourse to its Prabhava or specific action.

The anti-toxic property of toxins, actions leading to the upward and or downward elimination of Doshas (Vamana, Virechana) and various effects of precious noble stones (Mani) when worn over the body all these are due to their specific action which are beyond all plausible explanations. Hence, they are said to act because of their Prabhava – special action.

**Ayurvedic Pharmacology – How a medicine acts?**

सम्यग्विपाकवीर्याणि प्रभावश्चाप्युदाहृतः|
किञ्चिद्रसेन कुरुते कर्म वीर्येण चापरम्||७१||
द्रव्यं गुणेन पाकेन प्रभावेण च किञ्चन|
रसं विपाकस्तौ वीर्यं प्रभावस्तानपोहति||७२||
बलसाम्ये रसादीनामिति नैसर्गिकं बलम्||७३|

**Ayurvedic Pharmacology – How a medicine acts?**

Certain drugs manifest their action by virtue of their taste:

Some by virtue of their potency (Veerya)

Some act by the virtue of Guna (quality) or Vipaka (taste conversion after digestion).

Some act by Prabhava (specific action).

In case the taste (Rasa), Vipaka, Veerya and Prabhava are all of equal strength, by nature,

taste is superseded by Vipaka,

both of them in turn are superseded by potency and

all the above are dominated by Prabhava – special action. [68-72]

**Characteristics of the Six Tastes:**

**Characteristc features of sweet taste:**

षण्णां रसानां विज्ञानमुपदेक्ष्याम्यतः परम्||७३||
स्नेहनप्रीणनाह्लादमार्दवैरुपलभ्यते|
मुखस्थो मधुरश्चास्यं व्याप्नुवँल्लिम्पतीव च||७४||

**Characteristc features of sweet taste :**

Sweetness is ascertained from

Snehana – oiliness, unctuousness,

Preenana – deliciousness,

Ahlada – delightfuness

Mardava – softness.

When taken in, it pervades all over the mouth as it is adhering to mouth.

**Characteristc features of Sour taste :**

दन्तहर्षान्मुखास्रावात् स्वेदनान्मुखबोधनात्|
विदाहाच्चास्यकण्ठस्य प्राश्यैवाम्लं रसं वदेत्||७५||

**Characteristc features of Sour taste :**

Sourness is ascertained from

Dantaharsha – tingling sensation in teeth

Mukha srava – Salivation,

Svedana – Sweating,

Mukha Bodhana – Clarity of mouth

Vidaha – burning sensation in the mouth and throat.

**Characteristc features of salt taste :**

प्रलीयन् क्लेदविष्यन्दमार्दवं कुरुते मुखे|

यः शीघ्रं लवणो ज्ञेयः स विदाहान्मुखस्य च||७६||

**Characteristc features of salt taste :**

Salt gets quickly dissolved in the mouth resulting in stickiness (kleda),

Vishyanda – moistness

Mardava – softness

Mukhasya Vidaha – produce burning sensation in the mouth.

**Characteristc features of pungent taste :**

संवेजयेद्यो रसानां निपाते तुदतीव च|

विदहन्मुखनासाक्षि संस्रावी स कटुः स्मृतः||७७||

Pungent taste is ascertained by

irritation and pain in tongue, burning and watering in the mouth, nose and eyes.

**Characteristc features of bitter taste :**

प्रतिहन्ति निपाते यो रसनं स्वदते न च|

स तिक्तो मुखवैशद्यशोषप्रह्लादकारकः ||७८||

Bitter taste is ascertained by –

weakening of taste perception of the tongue.

Such substances by themselves are not tasteful;

Causes non-sliminess, clarity (Vaishadya)

Shosha – dryness of tongue and

Prahlada – delightness.

**Characteristc features of astringent taste :**

वैशद्य स्तम्भजाड्यैर्यो रसनं योजयेद्रसः|

बध्नातीव च यः कण्ठं कषायः स विकास्यपि||७९||

Astringent taste is characterized by

Vaishadya – non-sliminess,

Stambha – stiffness,

Jadya – inaction in the tongue and

Badhnateeva Kantham – obstruct the throat as it were; they are not good for heart. [73-79]

**Agnivesha's question on unwholesome medicine and diets:**

एवमुक्तवन्तं भगवन्तमात्रेयमग्निवेश उवाच- भगवन्! श्रुतमेतदवितथमर्थसम्पद्युक्तं भगवतो यथावद्द्रव्यगुणकर्माधिकारे वचः, परं त्वाहारविकाराणां वैरोधिकानां लक्षणमनतिसङ्क्षेपेणोपदिश्यमानं शुश्रूषामह इति||८०||

After Lord Atreya explained the above theory, Agnivesha inquired, "Oh! Lord, we have listened to what you have stated about the medicines and diets- their properties and actions together with all relevant details. We would like to know in detail about the unwholesome properties of certain diets (that is alone which cause vitiation of the Dhatus (body tissues)" [80]

**Lord Atreya's reply – Incompatible combinations :**

देहधातुप्रत्यनीकभूतानि द्रव्याणि देहधातुभिर्विरोधमापद्यन्ते; परस्परगुणविरुद्धानि कानिचित्, कानिचित् संयोगात्, संस्कारादपराणि, देशकालमात्रादिभिश्चापराणि, तथा स्वभावादपराणि||८१||

The substances that are unwholesome to the body tissues and Doshas, oppose the body tissues.

1. Kanichit Paraspara guna viruddhani – Some act against the health, due to their mutually contradictory qualities;

2. Kanichit Samyogat – Some act against to health, by the combination of two (though, as individual substances, they may not be opposite to each other in qualities.)

3. Samskarat – Some by the method of preparation;

4. Desha Kala Matradibhihi – Some by virtue of the place (land and body), time and dose and

5. Svabhavat – Some others by their inherent) nature. [81]

**Examples:**

न मत्स्यान् पयसा सहाभ्यवहरेत्, उभयं ह्येतन्मधुरं मधुरविपाकं महाभिष्यन्दि शीतोष्णत्वादिविरुद्धवीर्यं विरुद्धवीर्यत्वाच्छोणितप्रदूषणाय महाभिष्यन्दित्वान्मार्गोपरोधाय च||८२||

तन्निशम्यात्रेयवचनमनु भद्रकाप्योऽग्निवेशमुवाच- सर्वानेव मत्स्यान् पयसा सहाभ्यवहरेदन्यत्रैकस्माच्चिलिचिमात्, स पुनः शकली लोहितनयनः सर्वतो लोहितराजी रोहिताकारः प्रायो भूमौ चरति, तं चेत् पयसा सहाभ्यवहरेन्निःसंशयं शोणितजानां विबन्धजानां च व्याधीनामन्यतममथवा मरणं प्राप्नुयादिति||८३||नेति भगवानात्रेयः- सर्वानेव मत्स्यान्न पयसा सहाभ्यवहरेद्विशेषतस्तु चिलिचिमं, स हि महाभिष्यन्दित्वात् स्थूललक्षणतरानेतान् व्याधीनुपजनयत्यामविषमुदीरयति च|

ग्राम्यानूपौदकपिशितानि च मधुतिलगुडपयोमाषमूलकबिसैर्विरूढधान्यैर्वा नैकध्यमद्यात्, तन्मूलं हि बाधिर्यान्ध्यवेपथुजाड्यकलमूकतामैण्मिण्यमथवा मरणमाप्नोति|

न पौष्करं रोहिणीकं शाकं कपोतान् वा सर्षपतैलभ्रष्टान्मधुपयोभ्यां सहाभ्यवहरेत्, तन्मूलं हि शोणिताभिष्यन्दधमनीप्रवि(ति)चयापस्मारशङ्खकगलगण्डरोहिणीनामन्यतमं प्राप्नोत्यथवा मरणमिति|

न मूलकलशुनकृष्णगन्धार्जकसुमुखसुरसादीनि भक्षयित्वा पयः सेव्यं, कुष्ठाबाधभयात्|

न जातुकशाकं न निकुचं पक्वं मधुपयोभ्यां सहोपयोज्यम्, एतद्दिध मरणायाथवा बलवर्णतेजोवीर्योपरोधायालघुव्याधये षाण्ढ्याय चेति|

तदेव निकुचं पक्वं न माषसूपगुडसर्पिर्भिः सहोपयोज्यं वैरोधिकत्वात्|

तथाऽऽम्राम्रातकमातुलुङ्गनिकुचकरमर्दमोचदन्तशठबदरकोशाम्रभव्यजाम्बवकपित्थतिन्तिडीक-पारावताक्षोडपनसनालिकेरदाडिमामलकान्येवम्प्रकाराणि चान्यानि द्रव्याणि सर्वं चाम्लं द्रवमद्रवं च पयसा सह विरुद्धम्|

तथा कङ्गुवनकमकुष्ठककुलत्थमाषनिष्पावाः पयसा सह विरुद्धाः|

पद्मोत्तरिकाशाकं शार्करो मैरेयो मधु च सहोपयुक्तं विरुद्धं वातं चातिकोपयति|

हारिद्रकः सर्षपतैलभृष्टो विरुद्धः पित्तं चातिकोपयति|

पायसो मन्थानुपानो विरुद्धः श्लेष्माणं चातिकोपयति|

उपोदिका तिलकल्कसिद्धा हेतुरतीसारस्य|

बलाका वारुण्या सह कुल्माषैरपि विरुद्धा, सैव शूकरवसापरिभृष्टा सद्यो व्यापादयति|

मयूरमांसमेरण्डसीसकावसक्तमेरण्डाग्निप्लुष्टमेरण्डतैलयुक्तं सद्यो व्यापादयति|

हारिद्रकमांसं हारिद्रसीसकावसक्तं हारिद्राग्निप्लुष्टं सद्यो व्यापादयति; तदेव भस्मपांशुपरिध्वस्तं सक्षौद्रं सद्यो मरणाय|

मत्स्यनिस्तालनसिद्धाः पिप्पल्यस्तथा काकमाची मधु च मरणाय|

मधु चोष्णमुष्णार्तस्य च मधु मरणाय|

मधुसर्पिषी समघृते, मधु वारि चान्तरिक्षं समघृतं, मधु पुष्करबीजं, मधु पीत्वोष्णोदकं, भल्लातकोष्णोदकं, तक्रसिद्धः कम्पिल्लकः, पर्युषिता काकमाची, अङ्गारशूल्यो भासश्चेति विरुद्धानि|

इत्येतद्यथाप्रश्नमभिनिर्दिष्टं भवतीति||८४||


**Milk with fish -**

Fish should not be taken together with milk, both of them have sweet taste, but due to the contradiction in their potency (fish is hot and milk is cold) they vitiate the blood and obstruct the channels of circulation. Having listened to Lord Atreya, Bharadvaja said to Agnivesha, "One can take all kinds of fish except Chilichima together with milk. The Chilichima fish has scales; its eyes are red and it has red spot all over the body; it is like the Rohita (red carp fish) fish and moves on the ground. If this fish is taken with milk, it is bound to cause constipation and diseases relating to blood and it may even cause death. [82-83]

Lord Atreya while disagreeing with the above view said, "One must not take milk along with fish specially with Cilicima type of fish. Cilicima fish considerably obstructs the channels of circulation and causes the above mentioned diseases whose symptoms are very clear; it also produces Amavisa (toxin due to improper digestion as well as metabolism).

**Meat combinations** - Meat of domestic, marshy and aquatic animals (Gramya, Anupa Audaka Pishita) should not be taken together with honey, sesame seeds, sugar candy, milk, black gram (Masha), radish, lotus stalk or germinated grains (Viruda dhanya). By doing so, one gets afflicted with deafness, blindness, trembling, loss of intelligence loss of voice and nasal voice, it may even cause death.

One should not take vegetable of Pushkara (Nelumbo nucifera Gaertn) and Katukarohini – Picrorhiza kurroa or meat of Kapota (dove) fried in mustard oil together with honey and milk, for this obstructs channels of circulation and causes dilatation of blood vessels, epilepsy, Shankhaka (a disease of the head characterized by acute pain in temporal region), Galaganda (Scrofula) or even death.

**Milk combinations** - Milk should not be taken after the intake of radish, garlic, Keshnagandha (Moringa oleifera Lam.) Arjaka (Ocimum gratissimum Linn), Sumukha Surasa (Tulsi – Holy basil), etc. this may cause skin diseases.

Leaves of Jatuka (Ferula narthex) or ripe fruit of Nikucha (Artocarpus lakoocha Roxb) should not be taken with honey and milk; it may cause loss of strength complexion, and semen, sterility and other serious types of diseases which may lead to death.

Ripe fruit of Nikucha (Artocarpus lakoocha Roxb) should not be taken with the soup of Masha (black gram), sugar candy and ghee because they are mutually contradictory.

**Milk with sour fruits** - Amra – mango, Amrataka – Spondias pinnata Kurz, Matulunga – Lemon variety – (Citrus decumana / Citrus limon Linn), Nikucha (Artocarpus lakoocha Roxb), Karamarda (Carissa carandas Linn), Mocha (Salmalia malabarica Schott & Endl), Dantashatha (Citrus medica Linn), Badara – Zizyphus jujuba, Koshamra Bhavya (Dillenia indica Linn), Jambava (Syzygium cumini Skeels), Kapittha (Feronia limonia), Tintidi (Tamarindus indica Linn), meat of Paravata (Pigeon), Akshoda ( Juglans regia Linn), Panasa (Jack fruit), Narikela (Coconut), Dadima – Pomegranate, Amalaka (Emblica officinalis Gaerth) and such other solid and liquid materials which are sour in taste become mutually contradictory when taken with milk. Similarly Kangu (Setaria italica Beauv), Vanaka Makustha (Phaseolus aconitifolius Jacq), Kulattha (Horse gram), Masha (black gram) Nishpava (pea), when taken with milk are mutually contradictory.

Padma (Nelumbo nucifera Gaertn); Leaves of Uttarika, Sharkara type of wine, Maireya type of wine and honey, if taken together are unwholesome and they aggravate, Doshas specially Vata.

Meat of Haritala bird fried with mustard oil is unwholesome and they aggravate Dohsas, especially Pitta. Payasa (milk prepration) when taken with Mantha (thin gruel) is unwholesome and they aggravate Doshas, especially Kapha.
Upodika (Basella rubra Linn) prepared with the paste of Tila (Sesame seed) causes diarrhorea.
Meat of a crane either with Varuni type of wine or Kulmasha (Paste of Barley mixed up with hot water and slightly boiled so as to form a cake) is unwholesome; again if fired with lard, it will cause instantaneous death.

**Meat of peacock** roasted on a castor spit, if burnt with castor wood fuel and mixed with castor oil causes instantaneous death. Similarly the meat of Haaridraka roasted on a turmeric spit and burnt with the fuel of turmeric wood and (or) when mixed with ashes, dust and honey, causes instantaneous death.

**Pippali – Long pepper** fruit, prepared with fish fat and Kakamachi (Black nightshade – Solanum nigrum), mixed with honey causes death. Hot honey or intake of honey by a person afflicted with heat causes death.

**Honey and ghee, Honey – hot water:**
Honey and ghee or honey and rain water, both in water both in equal quantity,
honey together with the seeds of Pushkara (Nelumbo nucifera Gaertn)
intake of hot water with honey,
Bhallataka (Semecarpus anacardium Linn.) together with hot water;
Kampilllaka (Mallotus philippinensis Muell Arg) boiled with meat of Bhasa (beared Vulture), roasted with the spit or fire-brand are unwholesome. So everything in accordance with the questions has been explained. [84]

**Definition of unwholesome diet – Ahita:**
यत् किञ्चिद्दोषमासाव्य न निर्हरति कायतः।
आहारजातं तत् सर्वमहितायोपपद्यते॥८५॥

All drugs and diets which dislodge the various Doshas from their proper place, but do not expel them out of the body are to be regarded as unwholesome. [85]

**18 Types of Viruddha :**

यच्चापि देशकालाग्निमात्रासात्म्यानिलादिभिः|
संस्कारतो वीर्यतश्च कोष्ठावस्थाक्रमैरपि||८६||
परिहारोपचाराभ्यां पाकात् संयोगतोऽपि च|
विरुद्धं तच्च न हितं हृत्सम्पद्विधिभिश्च यत्||८७||

**1. Desha Viruddha :**

विरुद्धं देशतस्तावद्रूक्षतीक्ष्णादि धन्वनि|
आनूपे स्निग्धशीतादि भेषजं यन्निषेव्यते||८८||

**Place** – Intake of dry and sharp substance in deserts; oily and cold substance in marshy land is place contradictory diet habit.

**2. Kala Viruddha :**

कालतोऽपि विरुद्धं यच्छीतरूक्षादिसेवनम्|
शीते काले, तथोष्णे च कटुकोष्णादिसेवनम्||८९||

**Time contradictory diet habit** – Intake of cold and dry substances in winter; pungent and hot substance in the summer.

**3. Agni Viruddha :**

विरुद्धमनले तद्वदन्नपानं चतुर्विधे|

**Power of Digestion contradictory diet** – Intake of heavy food when the power of digestion is mild (mandagni) and intake of light food when the power of digestion is sharp (Teekshnagni) are examples of this contradictory diet. Similarly, intake of food at various time with irregular and normal power of digestion fall under this category.

**4. Matra Viruddha :**

विरुद्धमनले तद्वदन्नपानं चतुर्विधे|
मधुसर्पिः समधृतं मात्रया तद्विरुध्यते||९०||

**Dose specific diet contradiction** – Intake of honey and ghee in equal quantity

**5. Satmya Viruddha :**

कटुकोष्णादिसात्म्यस्य स्वादुशीतादिसेवनम्|
यत्तत् सात्म्यविरुद्धं तु विरुद्धं त्वनिलादिभिः||९१||

**Habit specific diet contradiction** - Intake of sweet and cold substance by persons accustomed to pungent and hot substances

**6. Dosha Viruddha :**

**Dosha specific diet contradiction** - Utilization of drugs, diets and regimen having similar qualities with Dosas but at variance with the habit of the individual.

**7. Samskara Viruddha :**

या समानगुणाभ्यासविरुद्धान्नौषधक्रिया|
संस्कारतो विरुद्धं तद्यद्भोज्यं विषवद्भवेत्||९२||

Method of preparation specific diet contradiction:- Drugs and diets which when prepared in a particular way produce poisonous effects, for example, meat of peacock (Shikhi mamsa) roasted on a castor spit.

**8. Veerya Viruddha :**

एरण्डसीसकासक्तं शिखिमांसं यथैव हि|
विरुद्धं वीर्यतो ज्ञेयं वीर्यतः शीतलात्मकम्||९३||

**Potency specific diet contradiction**- Substances having cold potency in combination with those of hot potency.

**9. Koshta Viruddha :**

तत् संयोज्योष्णवीर्येण द्रव्येण सह सेव्यते|
क्रूरकोष्ठस्य चात्यल्पं मन्दवीर्यमभेदनम्||९४||

**Bowel specific diet contradiction –**
Administration of a mild purgative in a small dose for a person with hard bowel (Krura Koshta) and administration of strong purgatives food for a person with soft bowel (Mrudu Koshta)

**10. Avastha Viruddha :**

मृदकोष्ठस्य गुरु च भेदनीयं तथा बहु|
एतत् कोष्ठविरुद्धं तु, विरुद्धं स्यादवस्थया||९५||
श्रमव्यवायव्यायामसक्तस्यानिलकोपनम्|
निद्रालसस्यालसस्य भोजनं श्लेष्मकोपनम्||९६||

**Stage specific contradiction:**
Indulgence in Vata aggravating diet after physical stress, sexual intercourse, exercise.
Indulgence in Kapha aggravating diet by a lethargic, sleepy person.

**11. Krama Viruddha:**

यच्चानुत्सृज्य विण्मूत्रं भुङ्क्ते यश्चाबुभुक्षितः|
तच्च क्रमविरुद्धं स्याद्यच्चातिक्षुद्वशानुगः||९७||

**Order specific contradiction –** If a person takes food before his bowel and urinary bladder are clear (empty) or when he does not have appetite or after his hunger has been highly aggravated.

**12. Parihara Viruddha :**

परिहारविरुद्धं तु वराहादीन्निषेव्य यत्|

**Prescription specific contradiction -** Intake of hot things after taking pork

**13. Upachara Viruddha :**

सेवेतोष्णं घृतादींश्च पीत्वा शीतं निषेवते||९८||

**Treatment specific contradiction –** Taking cold things after taking ghee.

**14. Paka Viruddha :**

परिहारविरुद्धं तु वराहादीन्निषेव्य यत्|
सेवेतोष्णं घृतादींश्च पीत्वा शीतं निषेवते||९८||

**Cooking contradiction –** Preparation of food with bad or rotten fuel, under-cooking, over-cooking or burning during the process of preparation.

**15. Samyoga Viruddha :**

अपक्वतण्डुलात्यर्थपक्वदग्धं च यद्भवेत्|
संयोगतो विरुद्धं तद्यथाऽम्लं पयसा सह||९९||

**Combination –** Intake of sour substance with milk.

### 16. Hrudaya Viruddha :

अमनोरुचितं यच्च हृदिवरुद्धं तदुच्यते|

**Palatability:** - Any substance which is not pleasant in taste.


### 17.Sampat Viruddha -

सम्पद्विरुद्धं तद्विवद्यादसञ्जातरसं तु यत्||१००||

**Richness of quality:** - Intake of substance that are not mature, over mature or purified.


### 18. Vidhi Viruddha:

अतिक्रान्तरसं वाऽपि विपन्नरसमेव वा|

ज्ञेयं विधिविरुद्धं तु भुज्यते निभृते न यत्|

**Rules of eating :-** Taking meals in public [86-101]


### Effect of taking incompatible foods :

षाण्ढ्यान्ध्यवीसर्पदकोदराणां विस्फोटकोन्मादभगन्दराणाम्|

मूर्च्छामदाध्मानगलग्रहाणां पाण्डुवामयस्यामविषस्य चैव||१०२||

किलासकुष्ठग्रहणीगदानां शोथाम्लपित्तज्वरपीनसानाम् |

सन्तानदोषस्य तथैव मृत्योर्विरुद्धमन्नं प्रवदन्ति हेतुम्||१०३||


### Effect of taking incompatible foods :

Intake of unwholesome food is responsible for the

Shandya – causation of sterility ,

Andhya – blindness,

visarpa (herpes, spreading type of skin disease),

Dakodara – ascitis,

Visphota – eruptions,

Unmada – insanity,

Bhagandara – fistula,

Murcha – fainting,

Mada – intoxication,

Adhmana – bloating

Galagraha – spasmodic obstruction in throat,

Pandu – anemia, initial stage of liver disorder

Amavisha- poisoning due to Ama (indigestion and altered metabolism),

Kilasa type of skin disease,

Kushta – skin disorders

Grahani – sprue, IBS,

Shotha – oedema,

Amlapitta – acid dyspepsia,

Jvara – fever,

Peenasa – rhinitis,

Santana Dosha – foetal diseases and

Mrutyu – death. [102-103]


### Treatment for disorders of incompatible food and diet habits :

एषां खल्वपरेषां च वैरोधिकनिमित्तानां व्याधीनामिमे भावाः प्रतिकारा भवन्ति|

तद्यथा- वमनं विरेचनं च, तद्विरोधिनां च द्रव्याणां संशमनार्थमुपयोगः, तथाविधैश्च द्रव्यैः पूर्वमभिसंस्कारः शरीरस्येति||१०४||

**Treatment for disorders of incompatible food and diet habits –**
Diseases caused by the intake of unwholesome diets and drugs can be cured by Vamana – emesis, Virechana – purgation or administration of antidotes and by taking prophylactic measures. [104]
Virechana – Purgation,
Vamana – emesis,
antidotes and prophylaxis- these four cure the diseases caused/ to be caused by the intake of unwholesome drugs and diets.

**Changing from unwholesome habits to wholesome habits:**
भवतश्चात्र-
विरुद्धाशनजान् रोगान् प्रतिहन्ति विवेचनम्|
वमनं शमनं चैव पूर्वं वा हितसेवनम्||१०५||
सात्म्यतोऽल्पतया वाऽपि दीप्ताग्नेस्तरुणस्य च|
स्निग्धव्यायामबलिनां विरुद्धं वितथं भवेत्||१०६||

**Changing from unwholesome habits to wholesome habits:**
The diseases caused by consumption of unwholesome foods are destroyed (cured) by purgation, emesis and palliative (shamana) treatments. In those who are habituated to intake of wholesome foods and medicines from the beginning the diseases caused by consumption of unwholesome foods will not be manifested. If an individual is habituated to the intake of unwholesome medicines and diets or if they are taken in small quantity or intake by a person having strong digestive power or by a young person or by the one who has undergone oleation therapy (Snehakarma) or who is strong physique due to physical exercise, the wholesomeness of the various drugs diets does not have any effect. [105-106]

**Summary:**
तत्र श्लोकाः-
मतिरासीन्महर्षीणां या या रसविनिश्चये|
द्रव्याणि गुणकर्मभ्यां द्रव्यसङ्ख्या रसाश्रया||१०७||
कारणं रससङ्ख्याया रसानुरसलक्षणम्|
परादीनां गुणानां च लक्षणानि पृथक्पृथक्||१०८||
पञ्चात्मकानां षट्त्वं च रसानां येन हेतुना|
ऊर्ध्वानुलोमभाजश्च यद्गुणातिशयाद्रसाः||१०९||
षण्णां रसानां षट्त्वे च सविभक्ता विभक्तयः|
उद्देशश्चापवादश्च द्रव्याणां गुणकर्मणि||११०||
प्रवरावरमध्यत्वं रसानां गौरवादिषु|
पाकप्रभावयोर्लिङ्गं वीर्यसङ्ख्याविनिश्चयः||१११||
षण्णामास्वाद्यमानानां रसानां यत् स्वलक्षणम्|
यद्यद्विरुध्यते यस्माद्येन यत्कारि चैव यत्||११२||
वैरोधिकनिमित्तानां व्याधीनामौषधं च यत्|
आत्रेयभद्रकाप्यीये तत् सर्वमवदन्मुनिः||११३||

Discussion among the sages about the tastes, properties and actions of drugs of various categories, number of drugs depending upon their tastes, factors determining the number of tastes; definitions of taste (rasa) and Anurasa (after or subsidiary taste); definition of attributes like Para (superiority) etc; factors leading to the formation of six tastes out of the five Mahabhutas; qualities responsible for the upward and downward physical action of tastes; various permutations and combinations of six tastes; attributes and actions of various types along with their exceptions.

Superiority, mediocrity and inferiority of tastes for producing heaviness etc. definitions of Vipaka and Prabhava (specific action); determination of the number of Virya (potency); specific manifestations of the drugs having six tastes when administered; mutually contradictory drugs and diets; cause of contradiction and their specific manifestations; treatment of diseases produced by the intake of drugs and diets having mutually contradtictory properties- all these have ben discussed in this chapter entitled "Atreya bhadrakapyiya Adhyaya".[107-113]

इत्यग्निवेशकृते तन्त्रे चरकप्रतिसंस्कृते श्लोकस्थाने आत्रेयभद्रकाप्यीयो नाम षड्विंशोऽध्यायः||२६||

Thus ends the twenty sixth chapter on of Sutrasthana of Charaka Sahmita, Agnivesha's work as redacted by Charaka.[26]

# 27

# Sutrasthana Chapter 27 Annapana Vidhim

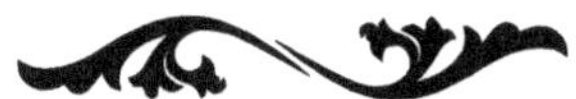

**Annapana Vidhi Adhyaya**

**Classification Of Foods and Drinks :**

अथातोऽन्नपानविधिमध्यायं व्याख्यास्यामः||१||

इति ह स्माह भगवानात्रेयः||२||

The 27th chapter of Charaka Samhita Sutrasthana is called Annapana Vidhi Adhyaya. It explains in detail about fruits, milk and dairy products, various types, qualities and benefits of vegetables, oils, grains, pulses, wines, meat, waters, sugarcane preparations, honey and its types, importance of after-drinks, and more.

## Importance of wholesome food:

इष्टवर्णगन्धरसस्पर्श विधिविहितमन्नपानं प्राणिनां प्राणिसञ्ज्ञकानां प्राणमाचक्षते कुशलाः, प्रत्यक्षफलदर्शनात्; तदिन्धना ह्यन्तरग्नेः स्थितिः; तत् सत्त्वमूर्जयति, तच्छरीरधातुव्यूहबलवर्णेन्द्रियप्रसादकरं यथोक्तमुपसेव्यमानं, विपरीतमहिताय सम्पद्यते||३||

## Importance of wholesome food:

Such diets and drinks whose colour, smell, taste and touch are pleasing (ishta) to the senses and conducive to the health are considered as equivalent to prana – life for the living beings by some experts due to the below mentioned reasons :

Vidhi vihitam anna paanam – If taken in accordance with the rules, it is responsible for the very life of living beings. In fact, such food itself is Prana (life, being).

Pratyaksha phala darshanaat – The results (life supporting) of ideal diets and drinks can be seen/perceived directly.

Tat indhanaa hyantaragnehe stitihi – The ideal diets and drinks form the fuel for the digestive fire.

Tat sattvam oorjayati – They promote satva – positive mental health and oorja – enthusiasm, positive energy.

Such diets and drinks, taken in ideal ways, nourish dhatu – body tissues, improve strength and immunity, and skin complexion and soothe sense organs. If the food is taken improperly, it can be harmful. [3]

## Types of food and their actions:

तत् स्वभावादुदक्तं क्लेदयति, लवणं विष्यन्दयति, क्षारः पाचयति, मधु सन्दधाति, सर्पिः स्नेहयति, क्षीरं जीवयति, मांसं बृंहयति, रसः प्रीणयति, सुरा जर्जरीकरोति, शीधुरवधमति, द्राक्षासवो दीपयति, फाणितमाचिनोति, दधि शोफं जनयति, पिण्याकशाकं ग्लपयति, प्रभूतान्तर्मलो माषसूपः, दृष्टिशुक्रघ्नः क्षारः, प्रायः पित्तलमम्लमन्यत्र दाडिमामलकात्, प्रायः श्लेष्मलं मधुरमन्यत्र मधुनः पुराणाच्च शालिषष्टिकयवगोधूमात्, प्रायस्तिक्तं वातलमवृष्यं चान्यत्र वेगाग्रामृतापटोलपत्रात्, प्रायः कटुकं वातलमवृष्यं चान्यत्र पिप्पलीविश्वभेषजात्||४||

## Types of food and their actions:

So, we shall now explain the properties of various diets and drinks in order to bring to light their useful effects on the body, Oh! Agnivesha.

Svabhaavaat udakam kledayati – By nature water moistens,

Lavanam vishyandayati – salt causes liquification, moistness, makes the things less viscous

Ksharam pachayati – Kshara (water insoluble ash part of certain herbs) – digest, cause conversion in wounds

Madhu Sandhadati – honey brings together the ruptured tissue elements, it joins (sandhaana)

Sarpim snehayati – ghee produces unctuousness, oiliness,

Ksheeram jeevayati – milk invigorates, enlivens, improves life, saves life.

Mamsam brumhayati – meat brings about corpulence, it nourishes

Rasaha preenayati – meat soup nourishes

Sura Jarjaree karoti – wine causes flabbiness, fragile

Sheeduravadhamati – Seedhu type of wine causes emaciation,

Drakshasavo deepyati – grape wine stimulates appetite,

Phanitam aachinoti – Phanita (penidium, a product of molasses) helps to accumulate Doshas,

Dadhi shopham janayati – curd causes oedema,

Pinyaka shaakam glapayati – vegetable of Pinyaka (Harita Shigru) causes depression;

prabhuta antarmalo maasha soopaha – Black gram soup increases bulk of faeces;

Drushti Shukraghnaha kshaaraha – alkalies impair the power of vision and reduce semen.

Except for pomegranate and Amla (Indian gooseberry), all sour tasting substances probably increase Pitta.

Except for honey, old rice and shastika types of rice, barley and wheat, all diets of sweet tasting substances generally aggravate Kapha.

Except the sprouts of Vetra (Salix caprea Linn), Guduchi (Tinospora cordifolia Miers) and leaves of Patola – pointed gourd, all bitter substances generally aggravate Vata and are un-aphrodisiac (Avrushya).

Similarly except Pippali – Long pepper fruit and Ardraka – Ginger Rhizome, all diets with pungent taste aggravate Vata and are un-aphrodisiac (Avrushya). [4]


**Classification of food articles:**

परमतो वर्गसङ्ग्रहेणाहारद्रव्याण्यनुव्याख्यास्यामः ||५||

शूकधान्यशमीधान्यमांसशाकफलाश्रयान्|

वर्गान् हरितमद्याम्बुगोरसेक्षुविकारिकान्||६||

दश द्वौ चापरौ वर्गौ कृतान्नाहारयोगिनाम्|

रसवीर्यविपाकैश्च प्रभावैश्च प्रचक्ष्महे||७||


**Classification of food articles:**

We shall now explain the tastes (rasa), potency (Veerya), Vipaka (taste conversion after digestion) and specific action (Karma) of the various diets and drinks classified according to the following 12 groups: -

1. Shooka dhanya (corns with bristles)
2. Shami Dhanya (Pulses)
3. Mamsa (Meat)
4. Shaaka (vegetables)
5. Phala (fruits)
6. Harita (greens, Salads)
7. Madya (Wine)
8. Ambu (Water)
9. Gorasa (Milk and milk products)
10. Ikshu Vikara (Products of sugarcane)
11. Kritanna (Food preparations, recipes)
12. Ahara Upayogi (Accessory food articles) [5-7]

**Shuka Dhanyas (Corns with Bristles)**

अथ शूकधान्यवर्गः-

रक्तशालिर्महाशालिः कलमः शकुनाहृतः |

तूर्णको दीर्घशूकश्च गौरः पाण्डुकलाङ्गुलौ||८||

सुगन्धको लोहवालः सारिवाख्यः प्रमोदकः|

पतङ्गस्तपनीयश्च ये चान्ये शालयः शुभाः||९||

शीता रसे विपाके च मधुराश्चाल्पमारुताः|

बद्धाल्पवर्चसः स्निग्धा बृंहणाः शुक्रमूत्रलाः||१०||

रक्तशालिर्वरस्तेषां तृष्णाघ्नस्त्रिमलापहः |

महांस्तस्यानु कलमस्तस्याप्यनु ततः परे||११||

यवका हायनाः पांसुवाप्यनैषधकादयः |

शालीनां शालयः कुर्वन्त्यनुकारं गुणागुणैः||१२||

**Shali (rice) class of corns are of the following varieties:-**

1. Rakta shaali – red variety of rice
2. Maha shaali – big sized rice
3. Kalama type of rice
4. Shakunahruta
5. Turnaka
6. Dirgha shooka
7. Gaura – white rice
8. Panduka – pale colored rice
9. Langula
10. Sugandhaka – rice with good smell
11. Lohavala
12. Sariva
13. Pramodaka
14. Patanga
15. Tapaniya

These rice types of corn are cold in potency (Sheeta Veerya) and sweet in taste as well as Vipaka (Madhura Rasa, Madhura Vipaka) – taste conversion after digestion;

Baddha Alpa varchasaha – they do not form much faeces, they may cause constipation,

Snigdha – impart oiliness to the body

Bruhmana – improve weight,

Shukrala – increase sperm production

Mootrala – diuretic, increases urine volume

Of them, the red variety of rice (Rakta shali) is the best.

Trushnaghna – It relieves thirst

Trimalaapaha – Balances all the three Doshas.

The next best is Maha shali (big sized rice); next to it is Kalama and others follow in the order of their description.

Besides, there are some other varieties of Shali viz, 1. Yavaka, 2. Hayana, 3. Pamshu, 4. Vapya, 5. Naishadhaka etc; which imitate good and bad qualities of the varieties of rice mentioned here. [8-12]

**Varieties of rice and their qualities:**

**Shashtika shali – rice that is harvested in 60 days –**

शीतः स्निग्धोऽगुरुः स्वादुस्त्रिदोषघ्नः स्थिरात्मकः|

षष्टिकः प्रवरो गौरः कृष्णगौरस्ततोऽनु च॥१३॥
वरकोद्दालकौ चीनशारदोज्ज्वलदर्दुराः।
गन्धनाः कुरुविन्दाश्च षष्टिकल्पान्तरा गुणैः॥१४॥

Shashtika rice is cold in potency, oily, light, sweet, balances all the three Doshas and stabilises. White variety of Shastika shali is good, black-white mixed variety is slightly inferior.

**The minor varieties of Shashtika shali:-**
1. Varaka
2. Uddalaka
3. Cheena
4. Shaarada
5. Ujwala
6. Dardura
7. Gandhana
8. Kuruvinda – These are slightly inferior in quality, compared to Shashtika

**Vreehi Shali – Rice harvested in autumn:**
मधुरश्चाम्लपाकश्च व्रीहिः पित्तकरो गुरुः।
बहुमूत्रपुरीषोष्मा त्रिदोषस्त्वेव पाटलः॥१५॥
Vreehi is sweet in taste, undergoes sour taste conversion after digestion (Amla Vipaka), heavy to digestion and increases Pitta.

बहुमूत्रपुरीषोष्मा त्रिदोषस्त्वेव पाटलः॥१५॥
Patala variety of rice produces urine and feces in large quantity and increases all the three Doshas. [13-15]

**Some inferior varieties:**
सकोरदूषः श्यामाकः कषायमधुरो लघुः।
वातलः कफपित्तघ्नः शीतः सङ्ग्राहिशोषणः॥१६॥
हस्तिश्यामाकनीवारतोयपर्णीगवेधुकाः।
प्रशान्तिकाम्भःश्यामाकलौहित्याणुप्रियङ्गवः॥१७॥
मुकुन्दो झिण्टिगर्मूटी वरुका वरकास्तथा।
शिबिरोत्कटजूर्णाह्वाः श्यामाकसदृशा गुणैः॥१८॥

**Some inferior varieties:**
Shyamaka (Setaria italica Beauv) and Koradusha (Paspalum scrobiculatum Linn) are

- astringent and sweet in taste (Kashaya, Madhura),
- cold in potency (sheeta veerya),
- increases Vata, balances Kapha and Pitta.
- drying, absorbent and light to digest

Corns similar to Shyamaka in property are:
1. Hastishyamaka (bigger variety of Syamaka)
2. Neevara (Udika, wild variety of rice)
3. Toyaparni
4. Gavedhuka (Ghuluncha – it is of two types viz, wild and cultivated)

5. Prashantika
6. Ambhaha shyamaka
7. Lauhitya
8. Anu
9. Priyangu (Kangani)
10. Mukunda (Vakastrna)
11. Jhintigarmuti
12. Varuka (Shana)
13. Varaka (Shyamabija)
14. Shibira(siddhaka)
15. Utkata
16. Jurnahva (Millet) [16-18]

## Barley benefits – Yava Dhanya :

रूक्षः शीतोऽगुरुः स्वादुर्बहुवातशकृद्यवः|
स्थैर्यकृत् सकषायश्च बल्यः श्लेष्मविकारनुत्||१९||

Barley is
Yava (barley) is
Rooksha – dry
Sheeta – cold, coolant
Aguru – not very heavy to digest
Svadu – sweet
Sakashaya – slightly astringent
Bahuvata Shakrut – produces wind and stool in large quantities.
Sthairyakrut – stabilises the body,
Balya – improves strength
Shleshma Vikaranut – Balances Kapha.
It is stabilising and strengthening. It alleviates the vitiated Kapha.

## Venu Yava – Bamboo Seed benefits:

रूक्षः कषायानुरसो मधुरः कफपित्तहा|
मेदःक्रिमिविषघ्नश्च बल्यो वेणुयवो मतः||२०||

Venuyava (bamboo seed) is
Dry,
sweet and slightly astringent in taste,
Meda Krimi Vishaghna – reduces fat, useful in worm infestation and poisoning.
Balya – improves strength and immunity [19-20]

## Wheat benefits – Godhuma:

सन्धानकृद्वातहरो गोधूमः स्वादुशीतलः|
जीवनो बृंहणो वृष्यः स्निग्धः स्थैर्यकरो गुरुः||२१||
नान्दीमुखी मधूली च मधुरस्निग्धशीतले|
इत्ययं शूकधान्यानां पूर्वो वर्गः समाप्यते||२२||
इति शूकधान्यवर्गः प्रथमः|

## Wheat :

Sandhanakrut – joins the ends (as in wound healing, fracture healing)

Vatahara – balances Vata,

Svadhu sheetala – Sweet, cold in potency,

Jeevana – invigorating,

Brumhana – nourishing

Vrushya – aphrodisiac,

Snigdha – unctuous, oily

Sthairyakrut – stabilising

Guru – heavy to digest.

Nandimukhi (Yavika) and Madhuli (a variety of wheat) are sweet, unctuous and cold in potency.

Thus completes explanation of Shooka Dhanya Varga – the first group consisting of corns with bristles. [21-22]

**Shami Dhanya Varga – Varieties of pulses and their qualities :**
**Green gram benefits – Mudga**

कषायमधुरो रूक्षः शीतः पाके कटुर्लघुः|
विशदः श्लेष्मपित्तघ्नो मुद्गः सूप्योत्तमो मतः||२३||

Of all the pulses, green gram is the best.

Kashaya, Madhura – astringent, sweet

Rooksha – dry

Sheeta – cold, coolant

Katu Vipaka – undergoes pungent taste conversion after digestion

Laghu – light to digest

Vishad – brings clarity to channels

Shleshma Pittaghna – balances Kapha and Pitta.

**Black gram benefits – Masha**

वृष्यः परं वातहरः स्निग्धोष्णो मधुरो गुरुः|
बल्यो बहुमलः पुंस्त्वं माषः शीघ्रं ददाति च||२४||

Vrushya – aphrodisiac

Param Vatahara – balances Vata to a great extent

Snigdha – oily, unctuous

Ushna – hot potency

Madhura – sweet

Guru – heavy to digest

Balya – improves digestion and strength

Bahumala – increases bulk of faeces

Pumstvam sheeghram dadaati- improves fertility quickly.

**Cow-pea benefits – Raja Masha:**

राजमाषः सरो रुच्यः कफशुक्राम्लपित्तनुत्|
तत्स्वादुर्वातलो रूक्षः कषायो विशदो गुरुः||२५||

Rajamasha – Cow pea is (Vigna unguiculata) is

Sara – eases movement, laxative

Rucha – palatable, useful in anorexia

Shukranut – decreases semen

Balances Kapha and Amla Pitta (acid dyspepsia).

It aggravates Vata.

Rooksha – dry

Kashaya – astringent,

Vishada – non-slimy and

Guru – heavy

## Horse gram benefits – Kulattha:

उष्णाः कषायाः पाकेऽम्लाः कफशुक्रानिलापहाः।

कुलत्था ग्राहिणः कासहिक्काश्वासार्शसां हिताः||२६||

Kulattha (Dolichos Biflorus Linn) – Horse gram is

Ushna – hot in potency,

Kashaya – astringent in taste and

Amla Vipaka – undergoes sour taste conversion after digestion.

Kapha Anlilapaha – Balances the vitiated Kapha and Vata.

Shukrapaha – decreases semen

Grahi – absorbent, may cause constipation,

useful for patients suffering from coughing (Kasa), hiccup (Hikka), dyspnoea, asthma (shwasa) and piles (Arsha).

## Moth bean benefits – Makushta

मधुरा मधुराः पाके ग्राहिणो रूक्षशीतलाः।

मकुष्ठकाः प्रशस्यन्ते रक्तपित्तज्वरादिषु||२७||

Moth bean – Makustha (Phaseolus aconitifolius/Vigna aconitifolia) is

Madura – sweet in taste and Vipaka,

Grahi – absorbent, causes mild constipation,

Rooksha – dry

Sheetala – coolant

Useful in Raktapiita – bleeding disorders such as nasal bleeding, heavy periods.

Jwara – useful in fever

## Bengal gram (Chickpea), Lentil, Grass pea

चणकाश्च मसूराश्च खण्डिकाः सहरेणवः।

लघवः शीतमधुराः सकषाया विरूक्षणाः||२८||

पित्तश्लेष्मणि शस्यन्ते सूपेष्वालेपनेषु च।

तेषां मसूरः सङ्ग्राही कलायो वातलः परम||२९||

Chickpea/Bengal gram – Chanaka (Cicer arietinum Linn), Lentil – Masura (Lens culinaris Medic) and Khandika (Grass pea – Lathyrus sativus Linn) and Harenu (a type of pea) are –

Laghu – light,

Sheeta – cold in potency,

Madhura – sweet with

Kashaya – astringent taste and

Rookshana – dry

In the form of soup and ointment, they are useful in patients suffering from diseases due to the vitiation of Pitta and Kapha. Of them, Lentil – Masura (Lens culinaris Medic) is absorbent, constipative.

Kalaya (Peanut) considerably aggravates Vata.

## Sesame seed – Tila:

स्निग्धोष्णो मधुरस्तिक्तः कषायः कटुकस्तिलः।

त्वच्यः केश्यश्च बल्यश्च वातघ्नः कफपित्तकृत्||३०||

**Tila – sesame is**

Snigdha – unctuous, oily

Ushna – hot in potency,

Madhura – sweet,

Tikta – bitter

Kashaya – astringent

Katu – pungent in taste.

Tvachya – good for skin

Keshya – promotes hair growth.

It is strength promoting.

It alleviates the vitiation of Vata and

Kapha Pittakrut – aggravates Kapha and Pitta.

**Indian bean/Lablab bean – Shimbi :**

मधुराः शीतला गुर्व्यो बलघ्न्यो रूक्षणात्मिकाः।

सस्नेहा बलिभिर्भोज्या विविधाः शिम्बिजातयः॥३१॥

शिम्बी रूक्षा कषाया च कोष्ठे वातप्रकोपिनी।

न च वृष्या न चक्षुष्या विष्टभ्य च विपच्यते॥३२॥

**Indian bean/Lablab bean – Shimbi –**

The various types of Shimbi (Dolichos lablab – Indian Bean/Lablab bean) are all

Madhura – sweet,

Sheetala – cold in potency and

Guru – heavy

Balaghna – They demote strength;

Rooksha – dry

They are to be taken together with some oily substance by sturdy persons

Kashaya – astringent

It aggravates Vata in the gastrointestinal tract.

   It is neither aphrodisiac nor couducive to eyes.

It produces wind during the process of digestion, hence causing bloating.

**Pigeon pea benefits – Adhaki –**

आढकी कफपित्तघ्नी वातला, कफवातनुत् ।

Adhaki – Pigeon pea/Toor dal (Cajanus cajan) balances Kapha and Pitta but aggravates Vata.

Avalguja (Psoralea corylifolia Linn) and Edagaja (Cassia tora) balance Kapha and Vata.

Nishpava (a type of cowpea) aggravates Vata and Pitta.

Properties of Kakandoma (a type of shimbi), Atmagupta (Mucuna prurita Hook.) and Uma (Linseed – Linum usitatissimum Linn) are the same as Black gram – Masha.

Thus the second group consisting of pulses – Shami Dhanya has been described. [23-34]

**Food derived from animal kingdom:**

**अथमांसवर्गः:- – group of meats**

अथ मांसवर्गः:-

गोखराश्वतरोष्ट्राश्वद्वीपिसिंहर्क्षवानराः।

वृको व्याघ्रस्तरक्षुश्च बभ्रुमार्जारमूषिकाः॥३५॥

लोपाको जम्बुकः श्येनो वान्तादश्चाषवायसौ।

शशघ्नी मधुहा भासो गृध्रोलूककुलिङ्गकाः॥३६॥

धूमिका कुररश्चेति प्रसहा मृगपक्षिणः

श्वेतः श्यामश्चित्रपृष्ठः कालकः काकुलीमृगः||३७||
कूर्चिका चिल्लटो भेको गोधा शल्लकगण्डकौ|
कदली नकुलः श्वाविदिति भूमिशयाः स्मृताः||३८||
सृमरश्चमरः खड्गो महिषो गवयो गजः|
न्यङ्कुर्वराहश्चानूपा मृगाः सर्वे रुरुस्तथा||३९||
कूर्मः कर्कटको मत्स्यः शिशुमारस्तिमिङ्गिलः|
शुक्तिशङ्खोद्रकुम्मीरचुलुकीमकरादयः||४०||
इति वारिशयाः प्रोक्ता...|४१|
..वक्ष्यन्ते वारिचारिणः|
हंसः क्रौञ्चो बलाका च बकः कारण्डवः प्लवः||४१||
शरारिः पुष्कराह्वश्च केशरी मणितुण्डकः |
मृणालकण्ठो मद्गुश्च कादम्बः काकतुण्डकः||४२||
उत्क्रोशः पुण्डरीकाक्षो मेघरावोऽम्बकुक्कुटी|
आरा नन्दीमुखी वाटी सुमुखाः सहचारिणः||४३||
रोहिणी कामकाली च सारसो रक्तशीर्षकः|
चक्रवाकस्तथाऽन्ये च खगाः सन्त्यम्बुचारिणः||४४||
पृषतः शरभो रामः श्वदंष्ट्रो मृगमातृका|
शशोरणौ कुरङ्गश्च गोकर्णः कोट्टकारकः||४५||
चारुष्को हरिणैणौ च शम्बरः कालपुच्छकः|
ऋष्यश्च वरपोतश्च विज्ञेया जाङ्गला मृगाः||४६||
लावो वर्तीरकश्चैव वार्तीकः सकपिञ्जलः|
चकोरश्चोपचक्रश्च कुक्कुभो रक्तवर्त्मकः||४७||
लावाद्या विष्किरास्त्वेते वक्ष्यन्ते वर्तकादयः|
वर्तको वर्तिका चैव बर्ही तित्तिरिकुक्कुटौ||४८||
कङ्कशारपदेन्द्राभगोनर्दगिरिवर्तकाः|
क्रकरोऽवकरश्चैव वारडश्चेति विष्किराः||४९||
शतपत्रो भृङ्गराजः कोयष्टिर्जीवजीवकः|
कैरातः कोकिलोऽत्यूहो गोपापुत्रः प्रियात्मजः||५०||
लट्टा लट्ट(टू)षको बभ्रुर्वटहा डिण्डिमानकः|
जटी दुन्दुभिपाक्कारलोहपृष्ठकुलिङ्गकाः ||५१||
कपोतशुकशारङ्गाश्चिरटीकङ्कुयष्टिकाः|
सारिका कलविङ्कश्च चटकोऽङ्गारचूडकः||५२||
पारावतः पाण्ड(न)विक इत्युक्ताः प्रतुदा द्विजाः|५३|
शतपत्रो भृङ्गराजः कोयष्टिर्जीवजीवकः|
कैरातः कोकिलोऽत्यूहो गोपापुत्रः प्रियात्मजः||५०||
लट्टा लट्ट(टू)षको बभ्रुर्वटहा डिण्डिमानकः|
जटी दुन्दुभिपाक्कारलोहपृष्ठकुलिङ्गकाः ||५१||
कपोतशुकशारङ्गाश्चिरटीकङ्कुयष्टिकाः|
सारिका कलविङ्कश्च चटकोऽङ्गारचूडकः||५२||
पारावतः पाण्ड(न)विक इत्युक्ताः प्रतुदा द्विजाः|५३|

The group of animals whose meat is commonly used as food are enumerated under the following eight categories.

1.  Prasaha – animals and birds which eat by snatching the food.

2.   Bhumishaya – Animals which live in burrows in earth

3.   Anupa – Animals living in marshy place

4.   Vaarishaya – aquatic animals

5.   Varichara – birds moving in water

6.   Jangala – Animals living in dry land forests

7.   Vishkira – Gallinaceous birds

8.   Pratuda – Packer birds

**A. Prasaha (animals and birds who eat by snatching)**

1. Go (cow)

2. Ashvatara (mule)

3. Khara (ass)

4. Ushtra (camel)

5. Ashva (horse)

6. Dveepi (panther)

7. Simha (Lion)

8. Ruksa (bear)

9. Vanara (monkey)

10. Vruka (wolf)

11. Vyaghra (tiger)

12. Tarakshu (hyena)

13. Babhru (large brown mangoose)

14. Marjara (cat)

15. Mooshika (mouse)

16. Lopaaka (fox)

17. Jambuka (jackal)

18. Shyena (hawk)

19. Vantada (dog)

20. Chaasha (blue jay)

21. Vaayasa (crow)

22. Shashaghni (golden eagle)

23. Madhuha (honey buzzard)

24. Bhasa (bearded vulture)

25. Grudhra (vulture)

26. Ulooka (owl)

27. Kulingaka (sparrow hawk)

28. Dhoomika (owlet)

29. Kurara (fish eagle)

**B. Bhumisaya (animals who live in burrows in earth)**

1. Shveta Kakuli Mriga (white python)

2. Shyama Kakuli Mriga (Greenish black python)

3. Chitraprushta Kakuli Mriga (spotted python)

4. Kaalaka Kakulimrga (black python)

5. Kurchika (hedgehog)

6. Chillata (musk shrew)

7. Bheka (frog)

8. Godha (inguana)

9. Shallaka (angolin)

10. Gandaka (gecko)

11. Kadali (marmet)

12. Nakula (mongoose)

13. Shvavit (prorcupiue)

### C. Anupa (animals inhabitingmarshy land)

1. Srumara (wild boar)

2. Chamara (yak)

3. Khadga (rhinoceros)

4. Mahisha (buffalo)

5. Gavaya (gayal cow)

6. Gaja (elephant)

7. Nyanku (antelope)

8. Varaha (hog)

9. Ruru (deer)

### D. Vaarisaya (aquatic animals)

1. Koorma (tortoise)

2. Karkataka (crab)

3. Matsya (fish)

4. Shishumaara (Estuarine crocodile)

5. Timingila (whale)

6. Shukti (pearl oyster)

7. Shankha (conch snail)

8. Udra (cat-fish)

9. Kumbheera (crocodile)

10. Chuluki (gangetic dolphin)

11. Makara (great Indian crocodile) etc

### E. Varichara (birds moving in water)

1. Hamsa (swan)

2. Krauncha (demoiselle crane)

3. Balaaka (sow wreath crane)

4. Baka (common crane)

5. Kaarandava (goose)

6. Plava (pelican)

7. Sharaari (skimmer)

8. Pushkaraahva (lilly trother)

9. Keshari (comb dock)

10. Manitundaka (red wattled lap-wing)

11. Mrunalakanta (snake bird)

12. Madgu (little cormorant)

13. Kaadamba (whistling teal)

14. Kaakatundaka (common river bird)

15. Utkrosha (trumpeter)

16. Pundareekaksha (white eyed pochard)

17. Megharaava (screamer)

18. Ambu Kukkuti (water hen)

19. Ara (cobbler's owl bird)

20. Nandimukhi (flamingo)

21. Vaati (grede)

22. Sumukha (laughing gull)

23. Sahacharina (petrel)

24. Rohini (tropic bird)

25. Kamakali (frigate bird)

26. Saarasa (sarus crane)

27. Rakta Sheershaka (sarada crane with a red head)

28. Chakravaaka (Ruddy sheldrake)

**F. Jangala (animals of dry land forests)**

1. Prushata (spotted deer)

2. Sarabha (wapiti)

3. Rama (Kashmir deer)

4. Shvadamshtra (mouse deer)

5. Mrugamatruka (hog deer)

6. Shasha (hare)

7. Urana (wild sheep)

8. Kuranga (roe deer)

9. Gokarna (mule deer)

10.Kottakaaraka (barking deer)

11.Arushka(gazelle)

12.Harina (red deer)

13.Ena (krsna) (black buck)

14. Sambara (Indian sambar)

15. Kaalapucchaka (black tailed deer)

16. Rushya (musk deer)

17. varapota (deerlet)

**G. Viskira (gallinaceous birds)**

**Group 1.**

1. Lava (common quail)

2. Varteeraka (rain quail)

3. Vartika (grey partridge)

4. Kapinjala (jungle bush quail)

5. Chakora (chukor)

6. Upacakra (sushi chukor)

7. Kukkubha (crow pheasant)

8. Raktavartma (red jungle fowl)

**Group II**

9. Vartaka (male bustard)

10. Vartika (female bustard)

11. Barhi (peacock)

12. Tittiri (partridge)

13. Kukkuta (cook)

14. Kanka (heron)

15. Shaarapada (stork)

16. Indrabha (adjutant)

17. Gonarda (Hill partridge)

18. Girivartaka (mountain quail)

19. Krakara (snipe)

20. Avakara (pea-fowl)

21. Vaarada (spoonbill)

   **H. Pratuda (packer birds)**

1. Shatapatra (woodpecker)

2. Bhringaraja (king bird of paradise)

3. Koyasti (coucal)

4. Jeevajeevaka (common myna)

5. Kairata (butcherbird)

6. Kokila (koel)

7. Atyuha (bulbul)

8. Gopapulra (cow-bird)

9. Priyatmaja (babbler)

10. Latta (scarlet minivet)

11. Lattasaka (minivet)

12.Babhru(Bengal-tree pie)

13.Vataha(tree pie)

14.Dindimanaka(toucan)

15.Jati (hoopoe)

16. Dundnbhi (horn bill)

17. Pakkara (green barbet)

18.Lohaprstha (kingfisher)

19.Kulingaka (baya or weaver bird)

20.Kapota (dove)

21.Suka (green parakeet)

22.Saranga (large Indian parakeet)

23.Cirati(window bird)

24.Kanku (blossom headed parakeet)

25. Yastika (sun bird)

26.Sarika (shama thrush)

27. Kalavinka (house sparrow)

28.Cataka (tree sparrow)

29.Angaracudaka (free crested wren)

30. Paravata (pigeon)

31. Pandavika (white pigeon) [35-52]


**Eight varieties of animals:**

प्रसह्य भक्षयन्तीति प्रसहास्तेन सञ्ज्ञिताः||५३||

भूशया बिलवासित्वादानूपानूपसंश्रयात् |

जले निवासाज्जलजा जलेचर्याज्जलेचराः||५४||

स्थलजा जाङ्गलाः प्रोक्ता मृगा जाङ्गलचारिणः|

विकीर्य विष्किराश्चेति प्रतुद्य प्रतुदाः स्मृताः||५५||

योनिरष्टविधा त्वेषा मांसानां परिकीर्तिता|५६|

Animals and birds which take their food by snatching are known as Prasaha;

Those residing in borrows are known as Bhushaya;

Those residing in marshy land are Anupa;

Those residing in water are known as Jalaja (aquatic);

Those birds which move on water are known as Jangala;

Those which disperse food before taking are known Vishkira (gallinaceous) and

Those which strike at the food articles before taking it are Pratuda (peckers) [53-55]

**Qualities of the food obtained from them:**

प्रसहा भूशयानूपवारिजा वारिचारिणः||५६||

गुरूष्णस्निग्धमधुरा बलोपचयवर्धनाः|

वृष्याः परं वातहराः कफपित्तविवर्धनाः||५७||

हिता व्यायामनित्येभ्यो नरा दीप्ताग्नयश्च ये|

प्रसहानां विशेषेण मांसं मांसाशिनां भिषक्||५८||

जीर्णार्शोग्रहणीदोषशोषार्तानां प्रयोजयेत्|

लावाद्यो वैष्किरो वर्गः प्रतुदा जाङ्गला मृगाः||५९||

लघवः शीतमधुराः सकषाया हिता नृणाम्|

पित्तोतरे वातमध्ये सन्निपाते कफानुगे||६०||

विष्किरा वर्तकाद्यास्तु प्रसहाल्पान्तरा गुणैः|६१|

Meat of the those which eat by snatching (Prasaha), marshy (Anupa) and aquatic animals (Varija), those which move in water (Varichara) and burrow- dwelling (Bhushaya) are –

Guru – heavy,

Ushna – hot in potency,

Snigdha – unctuous, oily

Madhura – sweet,

Balavardhana – improves strength and immunity

Upachaya vardhana – improves body nourishment, plumpness

Vrushya – aphrodisiac

Vatahara – Balances Vata and increases Kapha and Pitta.

It is useful for people who do daily exercise and for those having good digestion strength.

The meat of meat- eating Praasaha type of animals (those which eat by snatching) is especially useful for patients suffering from chronic piles (Arsha – Haemorrhoids), Grahani – Malabsorption syndrome, Irritable Bowel Syndrome and Shosha – emaciation.

The meat of the first group of the gallinaceous birds (Vishkira) beginning with quail, the packers (Pratuda) and animals of Jangala type (living in dry land forests) is

Laghu – light to digest

Sheeta – cold in potency and

Madhura – sweet

Sa Kashaya – slightly astringent.

It is useful for patients suffering from diseases due to the vitiation of all the three Doshas (highly vitiated Pitta, moderately vitiated Vata and slightly vitiated Kapha).

The meat of the second group of gallinaceous birds (Vishkira) beginning with male bustard is inferior to that of Prasahas in qualities. [56-60]


**Goat meat benefits – Ajamamsa :**

नातिशीतगुरुस्निग्धं मांसमाजमदोषलम्||६१||

शरीरधातुसामान्यादनभिष्यन्दि बृंहणम्|

**Goat meat is :**

Naati sheeta – not too cold

Guru – heavy

Snigdha – unctuous, oily

Adoshala – does not cause Dosha imbalance

It is homologous with the muscle of the human body. It does not obstruct/cause coating the channels of circulation and is nourishing (Bruhmana).

**Mutton benefits- (Sheep meat) – Avimamsa:**

मांसं मधुरशीतत्वाद्गुरु बृंहणमाविकम्||६२||

योनावजाविके मिश्रगोचरत्वादनिश्चिते|६३|

**Mutton (Sheep meat) is**

Madhura – sweet

Sheeta – cold,

Hence, it is Guru – heavy to digest.

Bruhmana – nourishing.

It is not possible to include goat and sheep in any of the eight categories mentioned above. They inhabit marshy land, at times deserts and sometimes both. [61-62]

**Qualities of specific variety of animal food:**

General properties of meat of various animals have been discussed above; some of them have specific properties and those are discussed below.

**Peacock meat – Barhi:**

दर्शनश्रोत्रमेधाग्निवयोवर्णस्वरायुषाम्||६४||

बर्ही हिततमो बल्यो वातघ्नो मांसशुक्रलः|

**Meat of peacock** is useful as a promoter of eye sight, power of hearing, intelligence, power of digestion, youth, complexion, voice, longevity, strength, Mamasadhatu (muscle) and semen. It alleviates Vata.

**Swan meat benefits:**

गुरूष्णस्निग्धमधुराः स्वरवर्णबलप्रदाः||६५||

बृंहणाः शुक्रलाश्चोक्ता हंसा मारुतनाशनाः|

Meat of swan is

Guru – heavy,

Ushna – hot

Snigdha – unctuous, oily

Madhura – sweet

Swaraprada – heavy,

Varnaprada – improves skin complexion

Balaprada – improves strength and immunity

Brumhana – improves nourishment

Shukrala – improves male and female reproductive system, improves semena and sperm quality and quantity

Maruta Nashana – Balances Vata

**Cock meat benefits – Charana:**

स्निग्धाश्चोष्णाश्च वृष्याश्च बृंहणाः स्वरबोधनाः||६६||

बल्याः परं वातहराः स्वेदनाश्चरणायुधाः|

Cock meat is

Snigdha – unctuous, oily

Ushna – hot

Vrushya – aphrodisiac

Brumhana – improves nourishment

Svarabodhana – improves voice

Swedana – induces sweating

Param Vatahara – Balances Vata, immensely

**Meat of partridge benefits – Tittira:**
गुरूष्णो मधुरो नातिधन्वानूपनिषेवणात्||६७||
तित्तिरिः सञ्जयेच्छीघ्रं त्रीन् दोषाननिलोल्बणान्|

Meat of partridge is neither heavy, nor hot, nor sweet, since it inhabits both the desert and the marshy land. It balances all the three Doshas, especially Vata.

**Meat of grey partridge benefits – Kapinjala:**
पित्तश्लेष्मविकारेषु सरक्तेषु कपिञ्जलाः||६८||
मन्दवातेषु शस्यन्ते शैत्यमाधुर्यलाघवात्|

The meat of grey partridge is

Sheeta – cold

Madhura – sweet

Laghu – light to digest

Because of these qualities, it is useful in Pitta and Kapha imbalance disorders, blood vitiation disorders. It is also useful in dull Vata conditions (leading to inactivity, slow movement etc).

**Meat of common quail benefits – Lava:**
लावाः कषायमधुरा लघवोऽग्निविवर्धनाः||६९||
सन्निपातप्रशमनाः कटुकाश्च विपाकतः|

Meat of common quail is

Kashaya – astringent,

Madhura – sweet

Laghu – light to digest

Agnivardhana – improves digestion strength

It balances all three Doshas.

**Iguana meat benefits:**
गोधा विपाके मधुरा कषायकटुका रसे||७०||
वातपित्तप्रशमनी बृंहणी बलवर्धनी|

**Iguana meat** is

Madhura Vipaka – sweet taste conversion after digestion

Kashaya – astringent

Katu – pungent taste

Vatapitta prashamana – balances Vata and Pitta

Brumhana – improves nourishment

Balavardhana – improves strength and immunity

**Pangolin meat benefits – Shallaka:**
शल्लको मधुराम्लश्च विपाके कटुकः स्मृतः||७१||
वातपित्तकफघ्नश्च कासश्वासहरस्तथा|

Pangolin meat is

Madhura – sweet

Amla – sour

Katu Vipaka – Pungent

balances all the three Doshas.

Kasahara – relieves cough, cold
Shwasahara – useful in asthma, COPD and other respiratory diseases

**Meat of domestic pigeon – Kapota**
कषायविशदाः शीता रक्तपितनिबर्हणाः||७२||
विपाके मधुराश्चैव कपोता गृहवासिनः|
The meat of the domesticated variety of pigeon is
Kashaya – astringent,
Vishada – non-slimy, clear
Sheeta – cold
Raktapitta – useful in bleeding disorders
Madhura Vipaka – sweet
The meat of wild pigeons is slightly lighter than the domesticated variety. It is cold in potency and astringent in taste.
It causes oliguria (Swalpa Mootrakara).

**Meat of green parakeet – Shuka Mamsa:**
शुकमांसं कषायाम्लं विपाके रूक्षशीतलम्||७४||
शोषकासक्षयहितं सङ्ग्राहि लघु दीपनम्|
The meat of green parakeet is
kashaya – astringent
Amla – sour in taste,
Rooksha – dry
Sheetala – cold in potency,
Useful in
Shosha – emaciation
Kasa – cough, cold
Kshaya – tuberculosis, chronic respiratory diseases
Sangrahi – absorbent
Laghu – light to digest
Deepana – improves digestion strength

**Sparrow meat benefits – Chataka**
चटका मधुराः स्निग्धा बलशुक्रविवर्धनाः||७५||
सन्निपातप्रशमनाः शमना मारुतस्य च|
The meat of sparrow is
Madhura – sweet
Snigdha – unctuous, oily
Balavardhana – improves strength and immunity
Shukravardhana – improves male and female reproductive system, improves semen and sperm quality and quantity
Useful in disorders of Tridosha imbalance, especially balances Vata.

**Hare meat benefits:**
कषायो विशदो रूक्षः शीतः पाके कटुलघुः||७६||
शशः स्वादुः प्रशस्तश्च सन्निपातेऽनिलावरे|
The meat of hare is
Kashaya – astringent,
Vishada – non-slimy, clear

Rooksha – Dry
Sheeta – cold in potency,
Katu Vipaka pungent in Vipaka,
Swadu – sweet in taste.
It is useful in sannipata (a condition caused by the vitiation of all the three Doshas) where the vitiated state of Vata is relatively mild.

**The meat of black buck benefits- Ena:**
मधुरा मधुराः पाके त्रिदोषशमनाः शिवाः||७७||
लघवो बद्धविण्मूत्राः शीताश्चैनाः प्रकीर्तिताः|
The meat of black buck is
Madhura – sweet in taste as well as Vipaka,
balances all the three Doshas
Shiva – wholesome
Laghu – light to digest
Sheeta – coolant
Baddha Vinmutra – obstructs the passage of stool and urine.

**Pork benefits – Varaha:**
स्नेहनं बृंहणं वृष्यं श्रमघ्नमनिलापहम्||७८||
वराहपिशितं बल्यं रोचनं स्वेदनं गुरु|
Pork is
Snigdha – oily, unctuous
Brumhana – improves nourishment
Vrushya – aphrodisiac
Shramaghna – relieves tiredness
Anilapaha – Balances Vata
Balya – improves strength and immunity
Rochana – improves taste
Svedaha – causes sweating
Guru – heavy to digest

**Beef benefits:**
गव्यं केवलवातेषु पीनसे विषमज्वरे||७९||
शुष्ककासश्रमात्यग्निमांसक्षयहितं च तत्|
Beef is useful in the
Kevala Vata roga – exclusive imbalance of Vata,
Peenasa – rhinitis,
Vishama Jwara – chronic recurrent fever
Shushka Kasa – dry cough
Shrama – tiredness
Atyagni – excessive digestion strength
Kshaya – tuberculosis, chronic respiratory diseases wasting of muscles.

**Buffalo meat benefits- Mahisha:**
स्निग्धोष्णं मधुरं वृष्यं माहिषं गुरु तर्पणम्||८०||
दाढर्यं बृहत्वमुत्साहं स्वप्नं च जनयत्यपि|

Buffalo meat is
Snigdha – oily, unctuous
Ushna – hot
Madhura – sweet
Vrushya – aphrodisiac
Guru – heavy to digest
Tarpana – refreshing
Dardhya – causes weight gain
Utsaha – increases enthusiasm
Svapna – induces sleep.

**Fish benefits:**

गुरूष्णा मधुरा बल्या बृंहणाः पवनापहाः||८१||
मत्स्याः स्निग्धाश्च वृष्याश्च बहुदोषाः प्रकीर्तिताः|

*Fish in general is*
Guru – heavy
Ushna – hot
Madhura – sweet
Balya – improves strength and immunity
Brumhana – improves nourishment
Pavanapaha – Balances Vata
Snigdha – unctuous, oily
Vrushya – aphrodisiac
Bahudosha – causes Dosha vitiation, hence can be injurious to health

**Rohita fish benefits:**

शैवालशष्पभोजित्वात्स्वप्नस्य च विवर्जनात्||८२||
रोहितो दीपनीयश्च लघुपाको महाबलः|

Rohita fish lives on moss and grass and does not sleep. Therefore, it promotes the power of digestion. It is light for digestion and it promotes strength considerably.

**Tortoise meat benefits:**

वर्ण्यो वातहरो वृष्यश्चक्षुष्यो बलवर्धनः||८३||
मेधास्मृतिकरः पथ्यः शोषघ्नः कूर्म उच्यते|

Tortoise meat
Varnya – promotes skin complexion,
Vatahara – Balances Vata
Vrushya – aphrodisiac
Chakshushya – useful in improving eye sight
Balavardhana – improves strength and immunity
Medhakara – improves intelligence
Smrutikara – improves memory
Pathya – wholesome
Shoshaghna – useful in emaciation

**The meat of rhinoceros benefits – Khanga Mamsa:**

खड्गमांसमभिष्यन्दि बलकृन्मधुरं स्मृतम्||८४||

स्नेहनं बृंहणं वर्ण्य श्रमघ्नमनिलापहम्|

The meat of rhinoceros is

Abhishyandi – causes obstruction to the channel of circulation, causes coating inside the channels

Balakrut – improves strength and immunity

Madhura – sweet

Snehana – oily

Brumhana – improves nourishment

Varnya – promotes skin complexion

Shramaghna – relieves tiredness

Anilapaha – Balances Vata

**Eggs benefits:**

धार्तराष्ट्रचकोराणां दक्षाणां शिखिनामपि||८५||

चटकानां च यानि स्युरण्डानि च हितानि च|

क्षीणरेतःसु कासेषु हृद्रोगेषु क्षतेषु च||८६||

मधुराण्यविदाहीनि सद्योबलकराणि च|

शरीरबृंहणे नान्यत् खाद्यं मांसादि विशिष्यते||८७||

इति वर्गस्तृतीयोऽयं मांसानां परिकीर्तितः|

इति मांसवर्गस्तृतीयः|

**Eggs benefits:**

Eggs of swan, choker, hen, peacock and sparrow promote strength instantaneously (Sadya balakara). They are sweet and do not cause burning sensation. They are useful in diseases like

Ksheenareta – oligospermia,

Kasa – cough, cold

Hrudroga – heart diseases

Kshata – injury

No other food excels meat in producing a nourishing effect. Thus ends the third group describing the meat of various animals. [63-87]

**Vegetables (leaves, tubers and fruits) – Shaka Varga – शाकवर्ग -**

अथ शाकवर्गः-

पाठाशुषाशटीशाकं वास्तुकं सुनिषण्णाकम्||८८||

विद्याद्ग्राहि त्रिदोषघ्नं भिन्नवर्चस्तु वास्तुकम्|

Now begins the description of the vegetable group.

Patha – Cissampelos pareira Linn,

Shusha – Cassia occidentalis Linn,

Shati – Zadoary (root) – Hedychium spicatum/Curcuma zedoaria,

Vastuka – Chenopodium album Linn and

Sunishannaka – Marsilea minuta var. Indica

These balance all the three Doshas.

All of them except Vastuka (Chenopodium album Linn) are Grahi – absorbent, bowel binding. Vastuka is, however, Laxative.

**Kakamachi**

त्रिदोषशमनी वृष्या काकमाची रसायनी||८९||

नात्युष्णशीतवीर्या च भेदिनी कुष्ठनाशिनी|

Kakamachi (Solanum nigrum Linn) balances all the three Doshas,

Vrushya – Aphrodisiac

Rasayani – anti ageing

Bhedini – purgative

Kushtanashini – useful in skin diseases

## Rajakshavaka

राजक्षवकशाकं तु त्रिदोषशमनं लघु||९०||

ग्राहि शस्तं विशेषेण ग्रहण्यर्शोविकारिणाम्|

Rajakshavaka (Euphorbia microphylla Heyne) balances all the three vitiated Doshas,

Laghu – light to digest

Grahi – absorbent,

Useful in

Grahani – Malabsorption syndrome, irritable bowel syndrome

Arsha – Haemorrhoids

**Kaala Shaaka** (Corchorus capsularis Linn) is pungent and promoter of digestion. It cures toxic conditions (Gara Visha) and oedema – Shopha.

**Kalaya** (Lathyrus sativus Linn) is light, hot in potency, dry and aggravation of Vata.

## Changeri :

दीपनी चोष्णवीर्या च ग्राहिणी कफमारुते||९२||

प्रशस्यतेऽम्लचाङ्गेरी ग्रहण्यर्शोहिता च सा|

Changeri (Rumex dentatus/Oxalis corniculata) is hot in potency

Ushna – hot

Grahi – absorbent

Useful in disorders of Kapha and Vata imbalance

Grahani – Malabsorption syndrome, irritable bowel syndrome

Arsha – Hemorrhoids

## Upodika – Malabar Spinach:

मधुरा मधुरा पाके भेदिनी श्लेष्मवर्धनी||९३||

वृष्या स्निग्धा च शीता च मदघ्नी चाप्युपोदिका|

**Upodika (Basella rubra Linn) is**

Madhura – sweet in taste as well as Vipaka,

Bhedini – purgative,

Shleshmavardhini – aggravator of Kapha,

Vrushya – aphrodisiac

Snigdha – unctuous, oily

Sheeta – cold in potency

Madaghni – causes intoxication.

## Tanduliyaka (Amaranthus tricolor Linn)

रूक्षो मदविषघ्नश्च प्रशस्तो रक्तपितिनाम्||९४||

मधुरो मधुरः पाके शीतलस्तण्डुलीयकः|

**Tanduliyaka (Amaranthus tricolor Linn) is**

Rooksha – dry

Mada Vishaghna – anti-poisonous, anti-toxic

Useful in Raktapitta – bleeding disorders
Madhura – sweet in taste and Vipaka
Sheeta – cold in potency.

**Gotu Kola and others :**

मण्डूकपर्णी वेत्राग्रं कुचेला वनतिक्तकम्||९५||
कर्कोटकावल्गुजकौ पटोलं शकुलादनी|
वृषपुष्पाणि शाङ्र्गेष्टा केम्बूकं सकठिल्लकम्||९६||
नाडी कलायं गोजिह्वा वार्ताकं तिलपर्णिका|
कौलकं कार्कशं नैम्बं शाकं पार्पटकं च यत्||९७||
कफपित्तहरं तिक्तं शीतं कटु विपच्यते|९८|

**Gotu Kola and others :**

Gotu kola, tender shoots of Vetra (Salix caprea), Kuchela (Cissampelos pareira Linn),Vanatiktaka (Cyclea peltata), Karkotaka (Momordica dioica Roxb), Avaluguja (Psoralea corylifolia Linn), Patola (Trichosanthes cucumerina Linn),Shakuladani – Picrorhiza kurroa, flowers of Vasa (Adhatoda vasica Nees), Sharngestha, Kembuka, Katillaka (Boerhaavia diffusa Linn), Nadi, round variety of Kalaya (Lathyrus aphaca Linn), Gojihva (Onosma bracteatum Wall), Vartaka (Solanum melongena Linn), Tilaparni (Gynandropsis gynandra Briquet), Karavelaka (Bitter gourd), Karkasha, Nimba – Neem, Prapataka (Fumaria parviflora Lam),- all these are alleviators of Kapha and Pitta, bitter in taste, cold in potency and pungent in Vipaka. [88-97]

**Qualities of different vegetables:**

सर्वाणि सूप्यशाकानि फञ्जी चिल्ली कुतुम्बकः||९८||
आलुकानि च सर्वाणि सपत्राणि कुटिञ्जरम्|
शणशाल्मलिपुष्पाणि कर्बुदारः सुवर्चला||९९||
निष्पावः कोविदारश्च पत्तुरश्चुच्चुपर्णिका|
कुमारजीवो लोट्टाकः पालङ्क्या मारिषस्तथा||१००||
कलम्बनालिकासूर्यः कुसुम्भवृकधूमकौ|
लक्ष्मणा च प्रपुन्नाडो नलिनीका कुठेरकः||१०१||
लोणिका यवशाकं च कूष्माण्डकमवल्गुजम्|
यातुकः शालकल्याणी त्रिपर्णी पीलुपर्णिका||१०२||

All types of Supyasaka viz,
Mashaparni – Teramnus labialis Spreng
Phanji (Rivea ornata Choisy),
Chilli (Chenopodium album Linn),
Kutumbaka (Leucas linifolia Spreng ),
all types of Aluka (potato and tubers) along with their leaves,
Kutinjara shana (Crotalaria juncea Linn).
Flower of Salmali (Salmalia malabarica Schott & Endl),
Karbudara (Bauhinia variegata Linn- White variety),
Suvarchala (Helianthus annuus Linn).
Nishpava (a variety of pea),
Kovidara (Bauhinia variegata Linn- red variety),
Pattura (Celosia argentea Linn),
Chucchuparni (Corchorus olitorius Linn),
Kumarajeeva (Putranjiva roxburghii Wall),
Lottaka (Eriobotrya japonica Lindl),
Palankya -Spinach (Spinacia oleracea Linn),

Maarisha (Amaranthus tricolor Linn),
Kalamba (Ipomoea reptans Poir),
Nalika (Onosma echioides Linn),
Lonika (Portulaca oleracea Linn),
Yavasaka (Alhagi pseudalhagi Desv),
Kushmanda – Ash gourd
Avalguja (Psoralea corylifolia Linn),
Yatuka, Salakalyani,
Triparni (Adiantum lunulatumBurm),
Peeluparni

**Properties of all these vegetables are -**
शाकं गुरु च रूक्षं च प्रायो विष्टभ्य जीर्यति|
मधुरं शीतवीर्यं च पुरीषस्य च भेदनम्||१०३||
**All these vegetables are -**
Vegetables of all these types are
Guru – heavy
Rooksha – dry
Madhura – sweet
Sheeta veerya – cold potency
Bhedana – purgative.
They produce wind during the process of digestion.
They become wholesome for intake when boiled and drained of the juice, and added with fatty substances in plenty.

**Flowers:**
पुष्पं ग्राहि प्रशस्तं च रक्तपित्ते विशेषतः|
न्यग्रोधोदुम्बराश्वत्थप्लक्षपद्मादिपल्लवाः||१०५||
Flowers of the below mentioned are Grahi – absorbent, bowel binding, useful for Raktapitta (a diseases characterised by bleeding from different parts of the body).
Shana (Crotalaria juncea Linn),
Kovidara (Bauhinia variegata Linn- red variety),
Karbudara (white variety of Kovidara) and
Shalmali (Salmalia malabarica Schott and Endl)

**Tender leaves**
न्यग्रोधोदुम्बराश्वत्थप्लक्षपद्मादिपल्लवाः||१०५||
कषायाः स्तम्भनाः शीता हिताः पित्तातिसारिणाम्|
Tender leaves of the below mentioned are Kashaya – astringent, Stambhana – causes constipation, stops bleeding, Sheeta – coolant, Useful in Diarrhoea of Pitta origin (Pitta Atisara).
Nyagrodha (Ficus bengalensis Linn),
Udumbara (Ficus racemosa Linn),
Ashvattha (Ficus religiosa Linn),
Plaksha (Ficus lacor Buch-Ham),
Kamala – Lotus etc.

वायुं वत्सादनी हन्यात् कफं गण्डीरचित्रकौ||१०६||
श्रेयसी बिल्वपर्णी च बिल्वपत्रं तु वातनुत्|

भण्डी शतावरीशाकं बला जीवन्तिकं च यत्||१०७||

पर्वण्याः पर्वपुष्प्याश्च वातपित्तहरं स्मृतम्|

लघु भिन्नशकृत्तिक्तं लाङ्गलक्युरुबूकयोः||१०८||

तिलवेतसशाकं च शाकं पञ्चाङ्गुलस्य च|

वातलं कटुतिक्ताम्लमधोमार्गप्रवर्तनम्||१०९||

रूक्षाम्लमुष्णं कौसुम्भं कफघ्नं पित्तवर्धनम्|

त्रपुसैर्वारुकं स्वादु गुरु विष्टम्भि शीतलम्||११०||

मुखप्रियं च रूक्षं च मूत्रलं त्रपुसं त्वति|

एर्वारुकं च सम्पक्वं दाहतृष्णाक्लमार्तिनुत्||१११||

वर्चोभेदीन्यलाबूनि रूक्षशीतगुरूणि च|

चिर्भटैर्वारुके तद्वद्वर्चोभेदहिते तु ते||११२||

Vatasadani (Tinospora cordifolia Miers), Alleviates Vata,

Gandira (Euphorbia antiquorum Linn) and Chitraka – Leadwort – Plumbago zeylanica Linn, alleviate Kapha.

Shreyasi (Scindapsus officinalis) Alleviate Vata.

Bhandi, Shatavari (Asparagus racemosusWild), Bala – Country mallow (root) – Sida cordifolia Linn, Jivanti – Leptadenia reticulata, Parvani and Parvapushpa, alleviate Vata and Pitta.

Langalika (Gloriosa superba Linn) and Urubuka (a variety of Ricinus communis Linn) are light, Laxative and bitter.

Tila (Sesamum indicum Linn) sesame leaves, Vetasa (Salix caprea Linn), and the small variety of Eranda castor aggravate Vata.

They are pungent, bitter and sour in taste and purgative.

Kusumbha (Carthamus tinctorius Linn) is unctuous, sour, hot in potency, balances Kapha and aggravator of Pitta.

Both Trapusa (Cucumis sativus Linn) and Ervaruka (Cucumis melo var utilissmus) are sweet, heavy, producers of wind in the intestine and cold in potency.

Trapusha, however, is palatable, unctuous and exceedingly diuretic.

Ripe fruit of Ervaruka cures burning sensation, thirst and exhaustion.

Alabu (Lagenaria siceraria Standl), is Purgative, unctuous, cold in potency and heavy.

Chirbhata (Cucumis melo Linn) and Ervaruka share the properties of Alabu (Lagenaria sicerariaStandl) but the former two are useful in Diarrhoea.

**Ripe ash gourd benefits – Kushmanda :**

सक्षारं पक्वकूष्माण्डं मधुराम्लं तथा लघु|

सृष्टमूत्रपुरीषं च सर्वदोषनिबर्हणम्||११३||

Ash gourd is sweet and sour in taste, slightly alkaline and light. It helps elimination of urine and faces and alleviates all the three vitiated Dosas. [113]

**Water plants and others:**

केलूटं च कदम्बं च नदीमाषकमैन्दुकम्|

विशदं गुरु शीतं च समभिष्यन्दि चोच्यते||११४||

**Water plants and others:**

Keluta, Kadamba (Anthocaphius indicus A. Rich),

Nadi mashaka and Enduka are –

Vishada – non-slimy, clear

Guru – heavy

Sheeta – cold

Abhishyandi – causes obstruction to the channel of circulation, causes coating inside the channels.

**Various types of blue lotus Utpala (Nymphaea alba) are**

उत्पलानि कषायाणि रक्तपित्तहराणि च|
तालप्रलम्बं स्यादुरःक्षतरुजापहम्||११५||

astringent and cure Raktapitta (a disease characterised by bleeding from different parts of the body).

खर्जूरं तालशस्यं च रक्तपित्तक्षयापहम्|
तरूटबिसशालूक्क्रौञ्चादनकशेरुकम्||११६||
शृङ्गाटकाङ्कलोड्यं च गुरु विष्टम्भि शीतलम्|
कुमुदोत्पलनालास्तु सपुष्पाः सफलाः स्मृताः||११७||
शीताः स्वादुकषायास्तु कफमारुतकोपनाः|
कषायमीषद्विष्टम्भि रक्तपित्तहरं स्मृतम्||११८||
पौष्करं तु भवेद्बीजं मधुरं रसपाकयोः|
बल्यः शीतो गुरुः स्निग्धस्तर्पणो बृंहणात्मकः||११९||
वातपित्तहरः स्वादुर्वृष्यो मुञ्जातकः परम्|
जीवनो बृंहणो वृष्यः कण्ठ्यः शस्तो रसायने||१२०||
विदारिकन्दो बल्यश्च मूत्रलः स्वादुशीतलः|
अम्लिकायाः स्मृतः कन्दो ग्रहण्यर्शोहितो लघुः||१२१||
नात्युष्णः कफवातघ्नो ग्राही शस्तो मदात्यये|
त्रिदोषं बद्धविण्मूत्रं सार्षपं शाकमुच्यते||१२२||
(तद्वत् स्याद्रक्तनालस्य रूक्षमम्लं विशेषतः|) तद्वत् पिण्डालुकं विद्यात् कन्दत्वाच्च मुखप्रियम्|
सर्पच्छत्रकवर्ज्यास्तु बह्व्योऽन्याश्छत्रजातयः||१२३||
शीताः पीनसकर्त्र्यश्च मधुरा गुर्व्य एव च|
चतुर्थः शाकवर्गोऽयं पत्रकन्दफलाश्रयः||१२४||
इति शाकवर्गश्चतुर्थः

**Sprout of Palm** - Tala (Borassus flabellifer Linn) cures pain due to chest injury (Urakshata ruja)

**Dates – Khajura (**Phoenix sylvestris Roxb) and the kernel of Tala – Palm (Borassus flabellifer Linn) are curative of Raktapitta ( a disease characterised by bleeding from various parts of the body) and Kshataruja – pain due to injury. Taruta, Bisa (Nelumbo nucifera Gaertn), Shaaluka (Nymphaea alba Linn), Kraunchaadana, Kasheruka (Scirpus grossus Linn), Shringataka (Trapa bispinosa Roxb), Ankalodya (small variety of Nymphaea alba Linn) are –

Guru – heavy

Vishtambhi – productive of wind in the abdomen, causes bloating

Sheeta – cold in potency.

Rhizome, flower and fruit of Kumuda (a variety of lotus) and utpala (Nymphaea alba Roxb.) are cold in potency, sweet and astringent in taste. They aggravate Kapha and vata.

**Seeds of Pushkara** (Nelumbo nucifera Gaertn) are slightly astringent, productive of wind in the abdomen, creative of wind in the abdomen, curative of Raktapitta (a disease characterised by bleeding from different of the body) and sweet both in taste and in Vipaka.

**Munijaataka** (Eulophia campestris wall) is strength promoting, cold in potency, heavy, unctuous, refreshing, and nourishing, sweet and exceeding aphrodisiac. It alleviates Vata and Pitta.

Vidari (Ipomoea paniculata R. Br) is invigorating, nourishing, aphrodisiac, tonic, diuretic, sweet in taste and cold in potency. It promotes strength and voice.

**The root of tamarind** Amlika (Tamarindus indica Linn) is beneficial for malabsorptionsyndrome (IBS), piles and alcoholism. It is light, bowel- binding and not very hot in potency. It alleviates both Vata and Kapha.

**Leaves of Sarshapa** – Mustard leaf (Brassica nigra Koch) vitiate all the three Dosas and obstruct the elimination of urine and stool.

**Raktanala** (Hibiscus sabdariffa Linn) shares all the properties of Sarshapa (Brassica nigra Koch) but it is especially unctuousand sour in taste.

**Pindalu** (Dioscorea alata Linn) shares all the qualities of Sarapa (Brassica nigra Koch) and being an edider root, it is palatable.

In addition to Sarpachatraka (a type of Chatra), there are many other types of Chatra (Psalliota campestris) which are cold in potency, heavy and sweet in taste. They aggravate Vata.

Thus ends the group of vegetables which include leaves, roots including rhizomes, fruits, flowers etc. [114-124]

**Fruits and their qualities – Phala Vargha**

**Raisin benefits:**

तृष्णादाह ज्वरश्वास रक्तपित्त क्षतक्षयान्|
वातपित्तमुदावर्तं स्वरभेदं मदात्ययम्||१२५||
तिक्तास्यतामास्यशोषं कासं चाशु व्यपोहति|
मृद्वीका बृंहणी वृष्या मधुरा स्निग्धशीतला||१२६||

Raisin provides immediate cure for

Trishna – excessive thirst,

Daha – Burning sensation

Jwara – fever

Shwasa – asthma, respiratory disorders involving difficulty in breathing

Raktapitta – bleeding disorders like nasal bleeding and menorrhagia

Kshata – chest injury

Kshaya – tuberculosis, chronic respiratory diseases wasting of muscles

Vata Pitta disorders

Udavarta – bloating

Swarabheda – hoarse voice

Madatyaya – alcoholism

Tiktasyata – bitter taste in tongue

Asya Shosha – mouth dryness

Kasa – cold, cough

Raisins are

Bruhmani – improves nourishment

Vrushya – aphrodisiac

Madhura – sweet

Snigdha – unctuous, oily

Sheetala – coolant

**Dates benefits:**

मधुरं बृंहणं वृष्यं खर्जूरं गुरु शीतलम्|
क्षयेऽभिघाते दाहे च वातपित्ते च तद्धितम्||१२७||

Dates (Phoenix sylvestris Roxb) are –

Madhura – sweet

Brumhana – improves nourishment

Vrushya – aphrodisiac

Guru – heavy

Sheetala – coolant

Useful in

Kshaya – tuberculosis, chronic respiratory diseases wasting of muscles

Abhighata – injury

Daha – Burning sensation
Balances Vata and Pitta.

**Different fruits:**

तर्पणं बृंहणं फल्गु गुरु विष्टम्भि शीतलम्।
परूषकं मधूकं च वातपित्ते च शस्यते||१२८||
मधुरं बृंहणं बल्यमामातं तर्पणं गुरु|
सस्नेहं श्लेष्मलं शीतं वृष्यं विष्टभ्य जीर्यति||१२९||
तालशस्यानि सिद्धानि नारिकेलफलानि च|
बृंहणस्निग्धशीतानि बल्यानि मधुराणि च||१३०||
मधुराम्लकषायं च विष्टम्भि गुरु शीतलम्|
पित्तश्लेष्मकरं भव्यं ग्राहि वक्रविशोधनम्||१३१||
अम्लं परूषकं द्राक्षा बदराण्यारुकाणि च|
पित्तश्लेष्मप्रकोपीणि कर्कन्धुनिकुचान्यपि||१३२||
नात्युष्णं गुरु सम्पक्वं स्वादुप्रायं मुखप्रियम्|
बृंहणं जीर्यति क्षिप्रं नातिदोषलमारुकम्||१३३||
द्विविधं शीतमुष्णं च मधुरं चाम्लमेव च|
गुरु पारावतं ज्ञेयमरुच्यत्यग्निनाशनम्||१३४||
भव्यादल्पान्तरगुणं काश्मर्यफलमुच्यते|
तथैवाल्पान्तरगुणं तूदमम्लं परूषकात्||१३५||
कषायमधुरं टङ्कं वातलं गुरु शीतलम्|

**Different fruits:**

**Phalgu (Ficus hispida Linn)** Is refreshing, nourishing, heavy and cold in potency. It produces wind in the stomach. Parushaka (Grewia asiatica Linn) and Madhuka (Madhuca indica J.F. Gmel) are useful in alleviating vitiated Vata as well as Pitta. Sweet variety of Amrataka (Spondias pinnata Kurz) is sweet in taste, nourishing, strength promoting, refreshing, heavy, unctuous, aggravator of Kapha, cold in potency and aphrodisiac. During digestion, it produces wind in the abdomen.

Ripe fruits of palmyra and coconut, Palm and coconut fruit are

Brumhana – improves nourishment

Snigdha – unctuous, oily

Sheeta – cold

Balya – improves strength and immunity

Madhura – sweet

**Bhavya (Dillenia indica Linn)** is sweet, sour and astringent in taste, productive of wind in the abdomen, heavy, cold in potency, aggravator of Pitta as well as Kapha and bowel- binding. It clears the mouth. Sour variety of Parushaka (Grewia asiatica Linn), Draksha (sour grapes), Badara (Ziziphus jujuba Lam), Aruka (Prunus persica Linn), Karkandhu (Ziziphus nummularia W. and A) and Nikucha (Artocarpus lakoocha Roxb) aggravate Pitta and Kapha.

**Ripe aruka** (Prunus persica Linn) is not very hot in potency. It is very heavy, sweetish, palatable, nourishing and easily digestible. It does not aggravate much of Dosas. There are two types of Paravata (Psidium guajava Linn). Fruits-one is sweet in taste and cold in potency and the other is sour in taste and hot in potency. Both of them are heavy to digest and curative of anorexia as well as excessive digestion and metabolism.

**Fruit of Kasmarya** (Gmelina arborea Linn) is only slightly different from Bhavya (Dillenia indica Linn) in quality. Sour variety of Tuda (Morus acidosa Griff) is also slightly different from Parusaka (Grewia asiatica Linn) in quality.

**Tanka** (Pyrus communis Linn) is astringent, sweet in taste and cold in potency. It aggravates Vata.

### Curd fruit/Elephant apple/Wood apple benefits – Kapittha

कपित्थमामं कण्ठघ्नं विषघ्नं ग्राहि वातलम् ||१३६||
मधुराम्लकषायत्वात् सौगन्ध्याच्च रुचिप्रदम्|
परिपक्वं च दोषघ्नं विषघ्नं ग्राहि गुर्वपि||१३७ |

### Unripe curd fruit (Feronia limonia Swingle) is

Kantaghna – harmful for voice.
Vishaghna – anti-poisonous, anti-toxic
Grahi – absorbent, bowel binding
Vatala – causes Vata increase
Madhura – sweet, Amla – sour, Kashaya – astringent
Sugandha –has a good smell.
Ruchiprada – improves taste
Ripe fruit balances all the three Doshas,
Vishaghna – anti-poisonous, anti-toxic
Grahi – absorbent, bowel binding
Guru – heavy.

### Bael fruit benefits:

बिल्वं तु दुर्जरं पक्वं दोषलं पूतिमारुतम्|
स्निग्धोष्णतीक्ष्णं तद्बालं दीपनं कफवातजित्||१३८||

**Ripe fruit of bael** (Aegle marmelos Corr) is
Durjara – difficult for digestion,
Doshala – aggravates all the Doshas
Pooti Maruta – producer of foul-smelling flatus.
The young unipe bael fruits
Snigdha – unctuous, oily
Ushna – hot
Teekshna -Piercing
Pittavardhana – increases Pitta.
Deepana – improves digestion strength
Kapha Vatajit – Balances Kapha and Vata.

### Ripe mango benefits:

रक्तपित्तकरं बालमापूर्ण पित्तवर्धनम्|
पक्वमाम्रं जयेद्वायुं मांसशुक्रबलप्रदम्||१३९||

Unripe mango worsens bleeding disorders, and Pitta.
Ripe mango balances Vata, increases muscle, semen, strength and immunity.

### Jamun fruit benefits-

कषायमधुरप्रायं गुरु विष्टम्भि शीतलम्|
जाम्बवं कफपित्तघ्नं ग्राहि वातकरं परम्||१४०||

Jambu (Syzygium cumini Skeels) is

Madhura – sweet

Kashaya – slightly astringent,

Guru – heavy

Vishtambhi – producer of wind in abdomen, causes bloating

Sheetala – coolant

balances Kapha and Pitta,

Grahi – absorbent, bowel binding

Vatakara – aggravation of Vata.


**Jujube – Badara (Ziziphus jujuba Lam)**

बदरं मधुरं स्निग्धं भेदनं वातपित्तजित्|

तच्छुष्कं कफवातघ्नं पित्ते न च विरुध्यते||१४१||

**Jujube fruit** is sweet, unctuous, laxative, and balances Vata as well as Pitta. Its dried fruits alleviate Vata and Kapha but do not go against Pitta.


कषायमधुरं शीतं ग्राहि सिम्बि(न्चि)तिकाफलम्|

गाङ्गेरुकी करीरं च बिम्बी तोदनधन्वनम्||१४२||

मधुरं सकषायं च शीतं पित्तकफापहम्|

सम्पक्वं पनसं मोचं राजादनफलानि च||१४३||

स्वादूनि सकषायाणि स्निग्धशीतगुरूणि च|

कषायविशदत्वाच्च सौगन्ध्याच्च रुचिप्रदम्||१४४||

अवदंशक्षमं हृद्यं वातलं लवलीफलम्|

नीपं शताह्वकं पीलु तृणशून्यं विकङ्कतम्||१४५||

प्राचीनामलकं चैव दोषघ्नं गरहारि च|

ऐङ्गुदं तिक्तमधुरं स्निग्धोष्णं कफवातजित्||१४६||

तिन्दुकं कफपित्तघ्नं कषायं मधुरं लघु|

Simbitika Phala is astringent and sweet in taste, cold in potency and constipating in nature.

Gangeruki (Grewia papulitalia Vahl), Karira (Capparis decidua Edgew), Bimbi (Coccinia indica W and A) Todana a variety of (Grewia tiliaefolia Vahl) and Dhanvana (Grewia tiliaefolia Vahl) are sweet accompanied with astringent in taste, cold in potency and balances Pitta as well as Kapha.

**Jackfruit benefits:** Ripe fruits of Panasa (jackfruit – Artocarpus heterophyllus Lam), Mocha (Musa paradisiaca Linn) and Rajadana (Mimusops hexandra Roxb) are sweet accompanied with astringent in taste, cold in potency, unctuous and heavy to digest.

Fruits of Lavali (Cicca acida Merrill) are palatable because of astringent taste, non-sliminess and fragrance. When taken in, they produce palatability in other food articles. It is good for the heart but aggravates Vata.

Nipa (Anthocephalns indicus A. Rich), Shatahvaka (AsparagusracemousWilld), Pilu (Salvadora persica Linn), Trunasunya (Pandanus tectorius Soland), Vikankata (Gymnosporia spinosa Fiori) and Pracinamalaka (Flacourtia jangomas Raeusch) alleviate vitiated Doshas and toxic conditions.

Ingudi (Balanites aegyptiaca Delile) is bitter and sweet in tast, unctuous, hot in potency and balances Kapha as well as Vata.

Tindnka (Diospyros peregrina Gurke) is astringent , sweet, light and balances Kapha as well as Pitta.

**Amla benefits – Amalaki**

विद्यादामलके सर्वान् रसाँल्लवणवर्जितान्||१४७||

रूक्षं स्वादु कषायाम्लं कफपितहरं परम्|

Amla (Emblica officinalis Gaertn.) contains all tastes except salt

Rooksha – dry

Swadu – sweet

Kashaya – astringent

Balances Kapha and Pitta.

### Bibhitaka (Terminalia Belerica Roxb)

रसासृङ्मांस मेदोजान्दोषान् हन्ति बिभीतकम्||१४८||

स्वरभेद कफोत्क्लेद पित्तरोग विनाशनम्|

Vibheetaki cures the diseases relating to Rasa (Plasma), Rakta (blood), Mamsa (flesh) and Mrdas (fat).

Useful in

Swarabheda – hoarse voice

Kapha Utkleda – kapha is increased

Pitta roga

### Pomegranate benefits:

रसासृङ्मांसमेदोजान्दोषान् हन्ति बिभीतकम्||१४८||

स्वरभेदकफोत्क्लेदपित्तरोगविनाशनम्|

अम्लं कषायमधुरं वातघ्नं ग्राहि दीपनम्||१४९||

स्निग्धोष्णं दाडिमं हृद्यं कफपित्ताविरोधि च|

रूक्षाम्लं दाडिमं यत्तु तत् पित्तानिलकोपनम्||१५०||

मधुरं पित्तनुत्तेषां पूर्वं दाडिममुत्तमम्|

There are three types of Dadima – Pomegranate.

The first variety which is the best of all is sour, astringent and sweet in taste, balances Vata, bowel – binding, promoter of digestion, unctuous, hot in potency and cardiac tonic. It does not provoke Kapha and Pitta. It cures hoarseness of voice and disease due to the vitiation of Kapha as well as Pitta. The second variety is unctuousand sour in taste. It aggravates Pitta and Vata. The third variety is sweet and it alleviates Pitta.

### Vrikshamla – Garcinia morella

वृक्षाम्लं ग्राहि रूक्षोष्णं वातश्लेष्मणि शस्यते||१५१||

**Vrikshamla – Garcinia morella** is bowel- binding, unctuous, hot in potency and useful in vitiated Vata and Kapha.

### Tamarind, Amlavetasa -

अम्लिकायाः फलं पक्वं तस्मादल्पान्तरं गुणैः|

गुणैस्तैरेव संयुक्तं भेदनं त्वम्लवेतसम्||१५२||

**Ripe fruit of Amlika (tamarind)** is slightly different in quality.

Amlavetasa (Rheum emodi Wall) shares all the qualities of Vrikshamla – Garcinia morella. In addition, it is laxative.

### Matulunga – Lemon variety :

शूलेऽरुचौ विबन्धे च मन्देऽग्नौ मद्यविप्लवे |

हिक्काश्वासे च कासे च वम्यां वर्चोगदेषु च||१५३||

वातश्लेष्मसमुत्थेषु सर्वेष्वेवोपदिश्यते|

केसरं मातुलुङ्गस्य लघु शेषमतोऽन्यथा||१५४||

The filaments of Matulunga – Lemon variety – Citrus decumana/Citrus limon are useful in colic pain, anorexia, constipation, impairment of digestion, alcoholisms, hiccough, dyspnoea, cough, vomiting, disorders relating to faces and such other diseases as arise from the vitiated Vata as well as Kapha. Filaments, unlike other parts of this plant, are light.

रोचनो दीपनो हृद्यः सुगन्धिस्त्वग्निववर्जितः|

कर्चूरः कफवातघ्नः श्वासहिक्काशसां हितः||१५५||
मधुरं किञ्चिदम्लं च हृद्यं भक्तप्ररोचनम्|
दुर्जरं वातशमनं नागरङ्गफलं गुरु ||१५६||
वातामाभिषुकाक्षोटमुकूलकनिकोचकाः|
गुरूष्णस्निग्धमधुराः सोरुमाणा बलप्रदाः||१५७||
वातघ्ना बृंहणा वृष्याः कफपित्ताभिवर्धनाः|
प्रियालमेषां सदृशं विद्यादौष्ण्यं विना गुणैः||१५८||
श्लेष्मलं मधुरं शीतं श्लेष्मातकफलं गुरु|
श्लेष्मलं गुरु विष्टम्भि चाङ्कोटफलमग्निजित्||१५९||
गुरूष्णं मधुरं रूक्षं केशघ्नं च शमीफलम्|
विष्टम्भयति कारञ्जं वातश्लेष्माविरोधि च||१६०||
आम्रातकं दन्तशठमम्लं सकरमर्दकम्|
रक्तपितकरं विद्यादैरावतकमेव च||१६१||
वातघ्नं दीपनं चैव वार्ताकं कटु तिक्तकम्|
वातलं कफपितघ्नं विद्यात् पर्पटकीफलम्||१६२||
पित्तश्लेष्मघ्नमम्लं च वातलं चाक्षिकीफलम्|
मधुराण्यम्लपाकीनि पित्तश्लेष्महराणि च||१६३||
अश्वत्थोदुम्बरप्लक्षन्यग्रोधानां फलानि च|
कषायमधुराम्लानि वातलानि गुरूणि च||१६४||
भल्लातकास्थ्यग्निसमं तन्मांसं स्वादु शीतलम्|
पञ्चमः फलवर्गोऽयमुक्तः प्रायोपयोगिकः||१६५||
इति फलवर्गः

    **Karcura** (Hedychium spicatum Ham ex Smith) without skin is palatable, digestive stimulant, cordial, fragrant, and balances Kapha as well as Vata. It is useful for suffering from dyspnea, hiccough and piles.

Fruit Nagaranga (Citrus reticulata Blanco) is slightly sour, cordial, difficult to digest and heavy. It makes other foods palatable.

**Vatama** (Prunus amygdalus Batsch), Abhisuka Aksota (Juglans regia Linn) Mukula (Pistacia vera Linn), nikuca (Artocarpus lakoocha Roxb) and Urumana (Prunus armeniaca Linn) are heavy, hot in potency, unctuous, sweet, strength promoting, balances Vata, nourishing, aphrodisiac and aggravator of Kaphas as well as Pitta. Priyala (Buchanania lazan Spreng) shares all the qualities except their potency in which it is cold.

**Fruit of Sleshmataka** (Cordia dichotoma) is sweet in taste, cold in potency, heavy and aggravator of Kapha.

**Fruit of Ankota** (Alangium salvifolium Wang) is heavy and aggravator of Kapha. It produces wind in the abdomen and alleviates heat of the body.

**Fruit of Sami** (Prosopis spicigera Linn) is heavy, hot sweet in taste, unctuous and depilatory of hair.

**Fruit of Karanja** (Pongamia pinnata) produces wind in the abdomen and does not provoke Vata or Kapha.

Sour variety of Amrataka – Spondias pinnata Kurz, Dantasatha Airavataka are sour in taste and they cause Raktapitta (a condition charactised by bleeding from different parts of the body.

Vartaka (Solanum melongena Linn) alleviates Vata. It is pungent and bitter in taste. It stimulates digestion.

Fruit of parpataki aggravates Vata and alleviates Kapha as well as Pitta.

Fruits of Aksiki are sour. It aggravates Vata but alleviates Pitta as well as Kapha.

Fruits of Asvattha, (Ficus religiosa Linn), Udumbara (Ficus racemosa Linn), Plaksa (Ficus lacor Buch Ham) and Nyagrodha (Ficus Bengalaensis Linn0 are astringent sweet, sour and heavy. They aggravate Vata.

Marking nut – Nut of Bhallataka (Semecarpus Anacardium Linn) is caustic like fire but it is sweet and cold in potency.

Thus ends the fifth group dealing with fruits that are commonly used. [125-165]


**Vegetables Used uncooked – Harita Varga**

**Fresh ginger benefits – Ardraka - Vishva Bheshaja:**

रोचनं दीपनं वृष्यमार्द्रकं विश्वभेषजम्|

वातश्लेष्मविबन्धेषु रसस्तस्योपदिश्यते||१६६||

Green ginger is

Rochaka – appetiser,

Deepana – improves digestion strength

Vrushya – aphrodisiac

Its juice is useful in Vata and Kapha disorders

Vibandha – constipation.

**Lemon juice benefits: – Jambira**

रोचनो दीपनस्तीक्ष्णः सुगन्धिर्मुखशोधनः|

जम्बीरः कफवातघ्नः क्रिमिघ्नो भक्तपाचनः||१६७||

Jambira (Citrus medica Linn) is

Rochana – appetizer,

Deepana – improves digestion strength

Teekshna -Piercing

Sugandhi – good smelling

Mukha Shodhana – mouth- cleanser,

balances Kapha as well as Vata and

Krimighna – anti- infective.

Pachana – It helps digestion of food.

**Radish benefits:**

बालं दोषहरं, वृद्धं त्रिदोषं, मारुतापहम्|

स्निग्धसिद्धं, विशुष्कं तु मूलकं कफवातजित्||१६८||

Tender radish alleviates Doshas. When overgrown, it provokes these doshas. When cooked with unctuous substance, it alleviates Vata. When dried, it alleviates Kapha and Vata.

**Tulsi benefits:**

हिक्काकासविषश्वासपार्श्वशूलविनाशनः|

पित्तकृत् कफवातघ्नः सुरसः पूतिगन्धहा||१६९||

Surasa (Ocimum Sanctum Linn) cures

Hikka – hiccough,

Kasa – cold, cough

Visha – toxic conditions

Shwasa – asthma, respiratory disorders involving difficulty in breathing

Parshva Shoola – pain in the flanks, side of chest and abdomen

Pittakrut – increases Pitta

Balances Kapha and Vata

relieves bad odor.

यवानी चार्जकश्चैव शिग्रुशालेयमृष्टकम्|

हृद्यान्यास्वादनीयानि पित्तमुत्क्लेशयन्ति च||१७०||

**Yavani** (Trachyspermum ammi Sprague), Arjaka (Ocimum gratissimum Linn), Shigru (Moringa oleifera Lam), Shaleya (Trigonella foenum- graecum Linn) and Mrustaka (Brassica nigra Koch) are Hrudya – cardiac tonic, good for heart and palatable. They provoke Pitta.

गण्डीरो जलपिप्पल्यस्तुम्बरुः शृङ्गवेरिका|

तीक्ष्णोष्णकटुरूक्षाणि कफवातहराणि च||१७१||

पुंस्त्वघ्नः कटुरूक्षोष्णो भूस्तृणो वक्त्रशोधनः|

**Gandira** (Euphorbia antiquorum Linn), Jalapippali (Commelina salicifolia Roxb), Tumburu (Zanthoxylum alatum

Roxb) and sprouts of Shringavera – Ginger – Zingiber officinale Rosc. are Teekshna – Piercing, sharp, hot in potency, pungent in taste and unctuous. They alleviate Kapha and Vata.

**Bhustrna** (Cymbopogon citratus Stapf) is Pumstvaghna – unaphodisiac, pungent, unctuous, hot in potency, and cleanser of mouth.

खराह्वा कफवातघ्नी बस्तिरोगरुजापहा||१७१||

धान्यकं चाजगन्धा च सुमुखश्चेति रोचनाः|

सुगन्धा नातिकटुका दोषानुत्क्लेशयन्ति च||१७३||

ग्राही गृञ्जनकस्तीक्ष्णो वातश्लेष्मार्शसां हितः|

स्वेदनेऽभ्यवहारे च योजयेतमपितिनाम्||१७४||

**Kharahva** (Trachyspermum roxburghianum) alleviates Kapha, Vata and the disorders of the urinary bladder.

### Coriander benefits:

Dhanyaka (Coriandrum sativum Linn), Ajagandha (Gynandropsis gynandra Briquet) and Sumukha are appetisers and fragrant. They are not very pungent. They also do not provoke Dosas.

Grunjanaka is bowel- binding and sharp. It is useful for piles and diseases due to the vitiation of Vata and Kapha. It is used for fomentation and as a food for such people who do not have Pitta in excess.

### Onion benefits:

श्लेष्मलो मारुतघ्नश्च पलाण्डुर्न च पितनुत्|

आहारयोगी बल्यश्च गुरुवृष्योऽथ रोचनः||१७५||

**Palandu** –Onion (Allium cepa Linn) aggravates Kapha and alleviates Vata, but it does not alleviate Pitta. It is useful as a food.

It is heavy and aphrodisiac. It promotes strength and appetite.

### Garlic benefits:

क्रिमिकुष्ठकिलासघ्नो वातघ्नो गुल्मनाशनः|

स्निग्धश्चोष्णश्च वृष्यश्च लशुनः कटुको गुरुः||१७६||

Garlic – Lasuna (Allium sativum Linn) cures infectious, obstinate skin disease, disease due to the vitiation of Vata and abdominal tumour. It is unctuous, hot in potency, aphrodisiac pungent and heavy.

शुष्काणि कफवातघ्नान्येतान्येषां फलानि च|

हरितानामयं चैष षष्ठो वर्गः समाप्यते||१७७||

इति हरितवर्गः

In dried form as also the fruits of these plants that are used in salad form, alleviate Kapha and Vata.

Thus ends the sixth group consisting of such plants that are used in salad form. [176-177]

### Qualities of wines – Madya (intoxicants liquors) – Madya Varga

प्रकृत्या मद्यमम्लोष्णमम्लं चोक्तं विपाकतः|

सर्वं सामान्यतस्तस्य विशेष उपदेक्ष्यते||१७८||

Now begins the group of wines. By nature, wines in general are

Amla – sour in taste as well as Vipaka and Ushna – hot in potency. The properties of specific types of wine will now be described. [178]

### Different varieties of liquors and their qualities: -

कृशानां सक्तमूत्राणां ग्रहण्यर्शोविकारिणाम्|

सुरा प्रशस्ता वातघ्नी स्तन्यरक्तक्षयेषु च||१७९||

Sura type of wine is useful for patients from emaciation, suppression of urine, malabsorption syndrome (IBS) and piles. It alleviates Vata and is useful in deficient lactation as well as anaemia.

हिक्काश्वासप्रतिश्यायकासवर्चोग्रहारुचौ|

वम्यानाहविबन्धेषु वातघ्नी मदिरा हिता||१८०||

**Madira type of wine** is useful in hiccups, dyspnoea, coryza, cough, constipation, anaemia, emesis and obstruction of faces and urine. It also alleviates Vata.

शूलप्रवाहिकाटोपकफवातार्शसां हितः|
जगलो ग्राहिरूक्षोष्णः शोफघ्नो भक्तपाचनः||१८१||

**Jagala type** of wine is useful in colic pain, dysentery, meteorism, piles and oedema. It alleviates Kapha and Vata. It is constipative, unctuous, hot and carminative.

शोषार्शोग्रहणीदोषपाण्डुरोगारुचिज्वरान्|
हन्त्यरिष्टः कफकृतान् रोगान्रोचनदीपनः ||१८२||

Arishta type of wine is useful in Kshaya – emaciation, piles, malabsoprtion syndrome (IBS), anemia, anorexia, fever and diseases caused by the vitiation of Kapha. It is both digestive and carminative.

**Shaarkara type of wine**

मुखप्रियः सुखमदः सुगन्धिर्बस्तिरोगनुत् |
जरणीयः परिणतो हृद्यो वर्ण्यश्च शार्करः||१८३||

**Sharkara** wine is palatable, of light intoxicating effect ragrant, and curative of bladder diseases. It is digestive stimulant, cordial and conducive to good complexion after it is well digested.

रोचनो दीपनो हृद्यः शोषशोफार्शसां हितः|
स्नेहश्लेष्मविकारघ्नो वर्ण्यः पक्वरसो मतः||१८४||

**Pakvarasa** type of wine is palatable, digestive, cordial and useful in Kshaya – emaciation, oedema and piles. It cures diseases caused by the improper administration of unctuous substances and vitiation of Kapha. It promotes complexions.

जरणीयो विबन्धघ्नः स्वरवर्णविशोधनः|
लेखनः शीतरसिको हितः शोफोदरार्शसाम्||१८५||

**Sitarasika type** of wine helps digestion. Alleviates constipation, promotes voice as well as complexion and is useful in oedema, abdominal diseases and piles.

सृष्टभिन्नशकृद्वातो गौडस्तर्पणदीपनः|
पाण्डुरोगव्रणहिता दीपनी चाक्षिकी मता ||१८६||

**Gauda** type of wine produces more faeces and flatus. It caused diarrhoea and excessive elimination of flatus. It is nourishing and digestive.The Aksiki type of wine is useful for anaemia and ulcers. It is a digestive stimulant.


सुरासवस्तीव्रमदो वातघ्नो वदनप्रियः|

**Sursava** type of wine is a very strong intoxicant. It alleviates Vata and is palatable.

छेदी मध्वासवस्तीक्ष्णो मैरेयो मधुरो गुरुः||१८७||
धातक्याऽभिषुतो हृद्यो रूक्षो रोचनदीपनः|

**Madhvasava** type of wine is depletive and sharp.

Maireya type of wine is sweet and heavy.

Dhatakyasava (Asava prepared with the fruits - actually flowers are used in practice - of Dhataki – Woodfordia fruticosa) type of wine is cordial, unctuous, palatable and digestive.

माध्वीकवन्न चात्युष्णो मृद्वीकेक्षुरसासवः||१८८||
रोचनं दीपनं हृद्यं बल्यं पित्ताविरोधि च|
विबन्धघ्नं कफघ्नं च मधु लघ्वल्पमारुतम्||१८९||
सुरा समण्डा रूक्षोष्णा यवानां वातपित्तला|
गुर्वी जीर्यति विष्टभ्य श्लेष्मला तु मधूलिका||१९०||
दीपनं जरणीयं च हृत्पाण्डुक्रिमिरोगनुत्|
ग्रहण्यर्शोहित भेदि सौवीरकतुषोदकम्||१९१||
दाहज्वरापहं स्पर्शात् पानाद्वातकफापहम्|
विबन्धघ्नमवस्रंसि दीपनं चाम्लकाञ्जिकम्||१९२||

Asava prepared with grape and sugarcane juice shares all the Madhvika but it is not too hot in potency.

Wine prepared with honey is palatable, digestives; cordial and strength promoting. It doesn't aggravate Pitta and

Vata to a great extent. It alleviates Kapha and cures constipation. Wine prepared with barley together with its Manda (scum) is unctuous and hot. It aggravates Vata and Pitta.

Wine prepared with Madhulika (Ragi – Finger millet - Eleusine coracana), a type of Godhuma – wheat – Triticum sativum) is heavy. It produces wind during digestion. It aggravates Kapha. Sauviraka and Tushodaka are digestive and carminative. They are useful in heart diseases, anemia, parasitic infections, malabsorprtion syndrome (IBS) and piles. They are also laxative. Sour congee alleviates burning sensation and fever by external application. When taken in, it alleviates Vata, Kapha and constipation. It is laxative and digestive.

**Qualities and benefits of wine – fresh and old -**

प्रायशोऽभिनवं मद्यं गुरुदोषसमीरणम्|

स्रोतसां शोधनं जीर्णं दीपनं लघु रोचनम्||१९३||

हर्षणं प्रीणनं मद्यं भयशोकश्रमापहम्|

प्रागल्भ्यवीर्यप्रतिभातुष्टिपुष्टिबलप्रदम्||१९४||

सात्त्विकैर्विधिवद्युक्त्या पीतं स्यादमृतं यथा|

Generally speaking, fresh wine is heavy and it aggravates all Doshas.

Old wine clarifies the channels of circulation. It is digestive, light and palatable.

Wine in general is exhilarating, and nourishing. It eliminates fear, grief and exhaustion. It promotes confidence, energy, intelligence, contentment, nourishment and strength. If taken by good people observing all the rules, it works as an elixir.

Thus the seventh group pertaining to wine is described. [179-195]

**Water:**

अथजलवर्गः:-

जलमेकविधं सर्वं पतत्यैन्द्रं नभस्तलात्|१९६|

Now begins the description of the group consisting of various types of water.

The entire water is ultimately of only one type viz, the one which falls from sky as directed by Indra.

**Rain water:**

तत् पतत् पतितं चैव देशकालावपेक्षते||१९६||

खात् पतत् सोमवाय्वर्कैः स्पृष्टं कालानुवर्तिभिः|

शीतोष्णस्निग्धरूक्षाद्यैर्यथासन्नं महीगुणैः||१९७||

While falling and also after fall from the sky, the properties of water vary depending upon the time and space.[196]

**Contamination:**

Water falling from the sky comes in contact with the moon, the air and the sun-all ordained by the time. Similarly, after its fall on the earth, it gets in touch with the proximal properties of the earth; like cold, heat, unctuousness, un-unctuousness etc. [197]

**Qualities of Rain water:**

शीतं शुचि शिवं मृष्टं विमलं लघु षड्गुणम्|

प्रकृत्या दिव्यमुदकं,...|१९८|

By nature rain water has six qualities viz, coldness, purity, benevolence, pleasantness and clearness.

**Effects of Receptable and season on rain water:**

श्वेते कषायं भवति पाण्डरे स्यातु तिक्तकम्|

कपिले क्षारसंसृष्टमूषरे लवणान्वितम्||१९९||

कटु पर्वतविस्तारे मधुरं कृष्णमृत्तिके|

एतत् षाड्गुण्यमाख्यातं महीस्थस्य जलस्य हि|

तथाऽव्यक्तरसं विद्यादैन्द्रं कारं हिमं च यत्||२००||

यदन्तरिक्षात् पततीन्द्रसृष्टं चोक्तैश्च पात्रैः परिगृह्यतेऽम्भः|

तदैन्द्रमित्येव वदन्ति धीरा नरेन्द्रपेयं सलिलं प्रधानम्||२०१||

ईषत्कषायमधुरं सुसूक्ष्मं विशदं लघु|

अरूक्षमनभिष्यन्दि सर्वं पानीयमुत्तमम्||२०२||
गुर्वभिष्यन्दि पानीयं वार्षिकं मधुरं नवम्|
तनु लघ्वनभिष्यन्दि प्रायः शरदि वर्षति||२०३||
तत्तु ये सुकुमाराः स्युः स्निग्धभूयिष्ठभोजनाः|
तेषां भोज्ये च भक्ष्ये च लेह्ये पेये च शस्यते||२०४||
हेमन्ते सलिलं स्निग्धं वृष्यं बलहितं गुरु|
किञ्चित्ततो लघुतरं शिशिरे कफवातजित्||२०५||
कषायमधुरं रूक्षं विद्याद्वासन्तिकं जलम्|
ग्रैष्मिकं त्वनभिष्यन्दि जलमित्येव निश्चयः|
ऋतावृताविहाख्याताः सर्व एवाम्भसो गुणाः||२०६||
विश्रान्तेषु तु कालेषु यत् प्रयच्छन्ति तोयदाः|
सलिलं तत्तु दोषाय युज्यते नात्र संशयः||२०७||
राजभी राजमात्रैश्च सुकुमारैश्च मानवैः|
सुगृहीताः शरद्यापः प्रयोक्तव्या विशेषतः||२०८||

**Effects of Receptable and season on rain water:**

After it has fallen down on the earth, its properties are determined by the place where it falls.

If it falls on the earth of white colour, it becomes astringent in taste;

on yellowish white earth it is bitter;

on brown earth it is alkaline,

on salt soil it is of salt taste; on the mountain valley it is pungent in taste and on the black soil it is sweet in taste. These are the six properties of rainwater that has fallen on the ground. Tastes are not manifested in the rain- water, hailstone or snow water.

The rain water falling from the sky as ordained by Indra and collected in the suitable receptacle is known as Aindra. This is the water par excellence fit to be taken by kings. The water which is slightly astringent and sweet in taste, exceedingly thin, non-slime, light, soft and non-greasy is best to be taken.

Rainwater available in the rainy season is heavy and greasy. The one available during the autumn is thin, light and non-greasy. Persons with tender bodily constitution and those who are accustomed to taking predominantly unctuous food are advised to use this water in the preparation of mistakable and eatable food, linctuses and drinks.

Water available during the Hemanta (winter) season is unctuous, aphrodisiac, strength promoting and heavy; Water of the Shishira (later part of winter) is slightly lighter and balances Kapha and Vata. Water available during spring is astringent as well as sweet in taste and unctuous. Summer water is not greasy.

Thus the properties of various types of water in different seasons have been described. Water collected from untimely rains is undoubtedly unwholesome.Water of autumn season collected in suitable receptacles should specially be used by kings, those enjoying royal authority and persons having tender heaths. [198-208]

**River water:**

नद्यः पाषाणविच्छिन्नविक्षुब्धाभिहतोदकाः |
हिमवत्प्रभवाः पथ्याः पुण्या देवर्षिसेविताः||२०९||
नद्यः पाषाणसिकतावाहिन्यो विमलोदकाः|
मलयप्रभवा याश्च जलं तास्वमृतोपमम्||२१०||
पश्चिमाभिमुखा याश्च पथ्यास्ता निर्मलोदकाः|
प्रायो मृदुवहा गुर्व्यो याश्च पूर्वसमुद्रगाः||२११||
पारियात्रभवा याश्च विन्ध्यसह्यभवाश्च याः|
शिरोहृद्रोगकुष्ठानां ता हेतुः श्लीपदस्य च||२१२||

The (water) of rivers originating from the Himalayas and with their water dispersed, disturbed and hit by stones are sacred and wholesome. The divine sages use this water. The rivers originating from the Malayas and those carryingstones and sand possess clear water. The water of such rivers is just like nectar.

The rivers flowing towards the west possess wholesome and clear water. Those flowing towards the eastern sea generally possess soft and heavy water. Rivers originating from the Pariyatra (Western Vindhya Range), Vindhya and Sahya ranges are responsible for diseases of head, heart, obstinate skin diseases including leprosy and filarial. [209-212]

**Water reservoirs and rivers of rainy season:**

वसुधाकीटसर्पाखुमलसन्दूषितोदकाः।

वर्षाजलवहा नद्यः सर्वदोषसमीरणाः॥२१३॥

वापीकूपतडागोत्ससरःप्रस्रवणादिषु।

आनूपशैलधन्वानां गुणदोषैर्विभावयेत्॥२१४॥

पिच्छिलं क्रिमिलं क्लिन्नं पर्णशैवालकर्दमैः।

विवर्णं विरसं सान्द्रं दुर्गन्धं न हितं जलम्॥२१५॥

विस्रं त्रिदोषं लवणमम्बु यद्वरुणालयम्।

इत्यम्बुवर्गः प्रोक्तोऽयमष्टमः सुविनिश्चितः॥२१६॥

इति जलवर्गोऽष्टमः

**Water reservoirs and rivers of rainy season:**

The rivers carrying rainwater which are vitiated by the mud, insects, snakes, mice and dirt are responsible for all kinds of diseases. The water of the pond, well, lake, spring, tank and cascade shares the merits and demerits of the places in which they are situated, e.g marshy land, hilly area, desert etc. The water which is slimy, full of parasites and vitiated with leaves, moss and mud, of ugly color, high density, having bad taste, and smell is not wholesome. Water of the sea possesses a fishy smell and is salty. It is responsible for the aggravation of the three doshas. Thus the eighth group of water consisting of various types of water are described. [213-216]

**Milk and dairy products -Gorasa Varga**

**10 qualities of cow milk:**

स्वादु शीतं मृदु स्निग्धं बहलं श्लक्ष्णपिच्छिलम्।

गुरु मन्दं प्रसन्नं च गव्यं दशगुणं पयः॥२१७॥

तदेवङ्गुणमेवौजः सामान्यादभिवर्धयेत्।

प्रवरं जीवनीयानां क्षीरमुक्तं रसायनम्॥२१८॥

Cow milk has ten properties viz,

Swadu – Sweetness,

Sheeta – cold

Mrudu – soft

Snigdha – unctuous, oily

Bahala – density, thick

Shlakshna – smoothness,

Picchila – slimeness, stickiness

Guru – heavy

Manda – slowness

Prasanna – calming, clarity.

These are also the properties of Ojas. So, milk having identical properties is conducive to the promotion of Ojas. Thus, milk is an elixir per excellence (Rasyana).

**Buffalo milk benefits:**

महिषीणां गुरुतरं गव्याच्छीततरं पयः।

स्नेहान्यूनमनिद्राय हितमत्यग्नये च तत्॥२१९॥

Milk of buffalo is Guru – heavier than cow milk, cold in comparison with the cow's milk. It has more of an unctuousness, oiliness and it is useful for persons suffering from insomnia and too rapid digestion.

**Camel milk:**

रूक्षोष्णं क्षीरमुष्ट्रीणामीषत्सलवणं लघु।

शस्तं वातकफानाहक्रिमिशोफोदरार्शसाम्||२२०||

Milk of the camel is

Rooksha – dry

Ushna – hot

slightly salt,

Laghu – light to digest

Useful in Anaha (bloating, constipation), parasitic infection, odema, ascites, piles and other diseases due to the vitiation of Vata and Kapha.

**Ekashapha**

बल्यं स्थैर्यकरं सर्वमुष्णं चैकशफं पयः।

साम्लं सलवणं रूक्षं शाखावातहरं लघु||२२१||

**Ekashapha** - The milk of Animals having one hoof (that is, mare, ass etc) is all

Balya – improves strength and immunity

Stairyakara – stabilising,

Ushna – hot

sour, salt, unctuous, cures Vata diseases of extremities and light.

**Goat milk, sheep milk, Elephant milk**

साम्लं सलवणं रूक्षं शाखावातहरं लघु||२२१||

छागं कषायमधुरं शीतं ग्राहि पयो लघु।

रक्तपित्तातिसारघ्नं क्षयकासज्वरापहम्||२२२||

हिक्काश्वासकरं तूष्णं पित्तश्लेष्मलमाविकम्।

हस्तिनीनां पयो बल्यं गुरु स्थैर्यकरं परम्||२२३||

Goat milk – Ajaksheera

Milk of the goat is astringent as well as sweet in taste,

cold,

Grahi – absorbent, bowel binding

Laghu – light to digest

and it is useful for persons suffering from Raktapitta (a disease characterized by bleeding from various parts of the body), diarrhoea, Kshaya – emaciation, coughing and fever.

Milk of sheep is hot. It aggravates hiccups and dyspnoea. It also alleviates Pitta and Kapha.

Milk of elephants is strength- giving, heavy and stabilising.

**Human milk benefits:**

जीवनं बृंहणं सात्म्यं स्नेहनं मानुषं पयः।

नावनं रक्तपित्ते च तर्पणं चाक्षिशूलिनाम्||२२४||

Human breast milk is invigorating, nourishing, wholesome and oleating. As an inhalation, it is useful for Rakta Pitta (haemothemia). It is also soothing for persons having pain in their eyes. [217-224]

**Curds qualities and benefits:**

रोचनं दीपनं वृष्यं स्नेहनं बलवर्धनम्।

पाकेऽम्लमुष्णं वातघ्नं मङ्गल्यं बृंहणं दधि||२२५||

पीनसे चातिसारे च शीतके विषमज्वरे।

अरुचौ मूत्रकृच्छ्रे च कार्श्ये च दधि शस्यते||२२६||

शरद्ग्रीष्मवसन्तेषु प्रायशो दधि गर्हितम्।

रक्तपित्तकफोत्थेषु विकारेष्वहितं च तत्||२२७||

**Curd is**

Rochana – improves taste, appetiser

Deepana – improves digestion strength

Vrushya – aphrodisiac

Snehana – imparts oiliness

Balavardhana – improves strength and immunity

Amla Vipaka – Sour taste conversion after digestion

Ushna – hot

Vataghna – Balances Vata

Mangalya – auspicious

Brumhana – improves nourishment

Useful in

Pinasa (rhinitis),

Atisara – diarrhoea,

Sheetaka (fever with cold),

Vishamajwara – irregular fever,

Aruchi – Anorexia, lack of interest in food

Mutrakrichra – dysuria, difficulty to pass urine

Karshya – emaciation

It is generally harmful during autumn, summer and spring seasons. It is invariably harmful in diseases caused by the vitiation of blood, Pitta and Kapha. [225-227]

**Creams:**

त्रिदोषं मन्दकं, जातं वातघ्नं दधि, शुक्रलः।

सरः, श्लेष्मानिलघ्नस्तु मण्डः स्रोतोविशोधनः॥२२८॥

Immature curd aggravates all the three Dosas. Curd in its primary stage alleviates Vata.

Cream of curd is Shukrala – improves male and female reproductive system, improves semen and sperm quality and quantity. Whey alleviates Kapha as well as Vata and also clears the channels of circulation. [228]

**Buttermilk:**

शोफार्शोग्रहणीदोषमूत्रग्रहोदरारुचौ।

स्नेहव्यापदि पाण्डुत्वे तक्रं दद्याद्गरेषु च॥२२९॥

**Buttermilk is useful in**

Shopha – oedema,

Arsha – Haemorrhoids

Grahani – Malabsorption syndrome, irritable bowel syndrome

Mutragraha – urine retention

Udara – Ascites

Aruchi – Anorexia, lack of interest in food

Snehavyapat – in case of ghee and fat indigestion

affliction with Gara type of poison.

Pandu – Anaemia, initial stages of liver disorders

It is also used for alleviating the complications of oleation therapy.[229]

**Butter benefits:**

सङ्ग्राहि दीपनं हृद्यं नवनीतं नवोद्धृतम्।

ग्रहण्यर्शो विकारघ्नमर्दितारुचि नाशनम्॥२३०॥

Fresh butter is digestive, stimulant and cardiotonic. It is useful in malabsorption syndrome (IBS), Piles, facial paralysis and anorexia. [230]

**Ghee:**

स्मृतिबुद्ध्यग्निशुक्रौजःकफमेदोविवर्धनम्।

वातपित्तविषोन्मादशोषालक्ष्मीज्वरापहम् ||२३१||

सर्वस्नेहोत्तमं शीतं मधुरं रसपाकयोः|

सहस्रवीर्यं विधिभिर्घृतं कर्मसहस्रकृत्||२३२||

मदापस्मारमूर्च्छायशोषोन्मादगरज्वरान्|

योनिकर्णशिरःशूलं घृतं जीर्णमपोहति||२३३||

सर्पीष्यजावि महिषीक्षीरवत् स्वानि निर्दिशेत्|२३४|

**Cow ghee** promotes memory, intellect, power of digestion, semen, Ojas,

Kapha and fat.

It alleviates Vata, Pitta

Visha – toxic conditions

Unmada – insanity,

Shosha – emaciation

Alakshmihara – it is auspicious.

It is the best of all the unctuous substances, cold in potency and sweet both in taste as well as Vipaka.

When administered according to the prescribed procedure, it increases, thousand times in potency and develops manifold utilities.

**Purana Ghrita – Old cow ghee is useful in**

Mada – intoxication,

Apasmara – epilepsy,

Moorcha – fainting,

Shosha – emaciation

Unmada – schizophrenia, insanity

Gara – remnant poisons

Jwara – fever

Pain in the ear, head as well as female genital tract.

Properties of ghee of other animals viz, goat, sheep and buffalo are the same as those of their milk. [231-233]

**Other milk products:**

पीयूषो मोरटं चैव किलाटा विविधाश्च ये||२३४||

दीप्ताग्नीनामनिद्राणां सर्व एव सुखप्रदाः|

गुरवस्तर्पणा वृष्या बृंहणाः पवनापहाः||२३५||

विशदा गुरवो रूक्षा ग्राहिणस्तक्रपिण्डकाः|

गोरसानामयं वर्गो नवमः परिकीर्तितः||२३६||

इति गोरसवर्गो नवमः|

Colostrums, Morata (Milk of a cow seven days after calving MW) and various types of Kilata (inspissated milk) are useful for patients having strong digestion and insomnia. They are heavy, refreshing, aphrodisiac and alleviators of Vata. Takrapinda (cheese) is non-slimy, heavy, unctuous and bowel- binding.

Thus ends the ninth group consisting of milk and milk products of cows and other animals. [234-236]

**Varieties of sugarcane – Ikshu Varga:**

वृष्यः शीतः सरः स्निग्धो बृंहणो मधुरो रसः|

श्लेष्मलो भक्षितस्येक्षोर्यान्त्रिकस्तु विदह्यते||२३७||

शैत्यात् प्रसादान्माधुर्यात् पौण्ड्रकाद्वंशको वरः|२३८|

When taken by chewing, sugarcane juice is

Vrushya – aphrodisiac

Sheeta – cold

Sara – laxative, promotes movement of liquids in channels

Snigdha – unctuous, oily

Brumhana – improves nourishment

Madhura – sweet

Shleshmala – increases Kapha

But the machine pressed juice causes burning sensation (indigestion).

Paundraka type of sugarcane (near to white colour) is superior to Vamshaka and is also good. [236]

**Products of Sugarcane:**

**Jaggery -**

प्रभूतक्रिमिमज्जासृङ्मेदोमांसकरो गुडः||२३८||

क्षुद्रो गुडश्चतुर्भागत्रिभागार्धावशेषितः|

रसो गुरुर्यथापूर्वं धौतः स्वल्पमलो गुडः||२३९||

ततो मत्स्यण्डिकाखण्डशर्करा विमलाः परम्|

यथा यथैषां वैमल्यं भवेच्छैत्यं तथा तथा||२४०||

वृष्या क्षीणक्षतहिता सस्नेहा गुडशर्करा|

कषायमधुरा शीता सतिक्ता यासशर्करा||२४१||

रूक्षा वम्यतिसारघ्नी च्छेदनी मधुशर्करा|

तृष्णासृक्पित्तदाहेषु प्रशस्ताः सर्वशर्कराः||२४२||

Treacle/jaggery (Guda) causes increased parasitic infection.

Majjakara – It increases the quantity of marrow,

Asruk kara – improves blood,

medo Mamsakara – increases fat and muscles.

Before its formation as treacle (guda) the sugar cane juice undergoes four stages viz.

Ardhavasheshita ( when only ½ of the juice remains in the process of boiling),

Tribhaga avaseshishita (when 1/3 rd remains),

Chaturbhag Avasheshita (when ¼th remains) and

Kshudra Guda or Phanita (Inspissated juice black in color).

The juice undergoing transformation through all these four stages is progressively heaviest.

That is to say, the Phanita (inspissated juice) is the heaviest.

**Dhauta** is that variety of treacle which is cleaned and which contains increase in parasites etc. Matsyandika (crude sugar when the juice is inspissated so as to take the shape of eggs of fish), Khanda (sugar candy) and Sarkara (sugar) are all progressively better refined and cooler in relation to Dhauta Guda.

That is to say, sugar represents the best refined stage of juice. It is also the coldest of all varieties.

**Sugar prepared of sugar cane juice is**

Vrushya – aphrodisiac

useful in emaciation and unctuous.

The sugar prepared by boiling the decoction or Duralabha (Fagonia cretica Linn) is known to be bitter in taste and cold in potency.

Sugar deposited in the vessel containing honey is unctuous and useful in vomiting as well as diarrhea. It is depleting.

Sugar in general is useful in thirst, Raktapitta (a disease characterized by bleeding from different parts of the body) and burning sensation. [238-242]

**Types of honey and benefits:**

माक्षिकं भ्रामरं क्षौद्रं पौतिकं मधुजातयः|

माक्षिकं प्रवरं तेषां विशेषाद्भ्रामरं गुरु||२४३||

माक्षिकं तैलवर्णं स्याद्घृतवर्णं तु पौतिकम्|

क्षौद्रं कपिलवर्णं स्याच्छ्वेतं भ्रामरमुच्यते||२४४||

वातलं गुरु शीतं च रक्तपित्तकफापहम्|

सन्धातृ च्छेदनं रूक्षं कषायं मधुरं मधु ||२४५||

हन्यान्मधूष्णमुष्णार्तमथवा सविषान्वयात्|

गुरूरूक्षकषायत्वाच्छैत्याच्चाल्पं हितं मधु||२४६||

**Honey has four types viz.**

1. Makshika (honey collected by the red variety of honey bee)

2. Bhramara (honey collected by Bhrunara type of bee)

3. Kshaudra (honey collected by small type of honey bee)

4. Paittaka (honey collected Puttika type of bee- they are of big size.)

Of them, Makshika is the best; Bhramara is especially heavy.

Makshika type of honey is of the color of til oil.

Paittika is the color of ghee.

Kshaudra is brown in color and

Bhramara is of white color.

Honey in general is the aggravation of Vata, heavy, cold in potency and detoxifies blood, Pitta as well as Kapha. It promotes healing and depletion. Warm honey or honey taken by an individual suffering from heat is fatal because during the process of collection it is contaminated with poisonous material from the bees themselves or from the various poisonous plants. Honey should be taken in small quantities because it is heavy, unctuous, astringent in taste and cold in potency. [243-246]

**Precaution for honey consumption: - Madhu ama/Madhvama**

नातः कष्टतमं किञ्चिन्मध्वामात्तिद्धि मानवम्|

उपक्रमविरोधित्वात् सद्यो हन्याद्यथा विषम्||२४७||

आमे सोष्णा क्रिया कार्या सा मध्वामे विरुध्यते|

मध्वामं दारुणं तस्मात् सद्यो हन्याद्यथा विषम्||२४८||

Nothing is so troublesome as Ama caused by the improper intake of honey.

Heat is considered to be wholesome in the case of Ama, but it is not conducive to honey. So by virtue of these therapeutic contradictions, Ama produced by the improper intake of honey causes instantaneous death like poison. [247-248]

**Importance of honey:**

नानाद्रव्यात्मकत्वाच्च योगवाहि परं मधु|

Since it originates from flowers having different tastes, potencies etc. honey is the best Yogavahi – catalyst substance. That is to say, it carries the properties of the drugs added to it.

Thus, ends the 10th group dealing mostly with sugarcane and its products. [249]

**Cooked food preparations – Kritanna Varga**

Now begins the group consisting of food preparations.

**Thin gruel – Peya**

क्षुत्तृष्णाग्लानि दौर्बल्य कुक्षिरोगज्वरापहा|

स्वेदाग्निजननी पेया वातवर्चोनुलोमनी||२५०||

**Thin gruel (Peya) is useful in**

Kshut –excess hunger

Trushna –excess thirst

Glani – tiredness

Daurbalya – weakness

Kukshiroga – abdominal disorders

Jwara – fever

It promotes sweating. It is digestive and is conducive to downward movement of the flatus as well as faeces.

Thick gruel (Vilepi) is refreshing, bowel binding, light and cardiac tonic.

**Gruel water (Manda)**

तर्पणी ग्राहिणी लघ्वी हृद्या चापि विलेपिका।

मण्डस्तु दीपयत्यग्निं वातं चाप्यनुलोमयेत्।।२५१।।

मृदूकरोति स्रोतांसि स्वेदं सञ्जनयत्यपि।

लङ्घितानां विरिक्तानां जीर्णे स्नेहे च तृष्यताम्।।२५२।।

दीपनत्वाल्लघुत्वाच्च मण्डः स्यात् प्राणधारणः।

**Water part of the gruel – Manda** stimulates the power of digestion and

Vata Anulomana – facilitates the downward movement of flatus.

It softens the channels of circulation, and produces sweating.

By virtue of its lightness and the capacity to promote digestion, gruel water is the sustainer of life for those who have
undergone fasting and Vamana – vomiting therapies and those who are suffering from excessive thirst caused after
consuming oil/ fat, Peya –gruel water is best.

**Thick gruel of paddy– Laja Peya -**

लाजपेया श्रमघ्नी तु क्षामकण्ठस्य देहिनः।।२५३।।

तृष्णातीसारशमनो धातुसाम्यकरः शिवः।

Shramaghni – relieves fatigue

restores voice

Useful in

Trushna – excessive thirst

Atisara – diarrhoea

It maintains the normalcy of tissue elements and is a wholesome diet.

**Lajamanda – Thin gruel of paddy -**

लाजमण्डोऽग्निजननो दाहमूर्च्छानिवारणः ।।२५४।।

मन्दाग्निविषमाग्नीनां बालस्थविरयोषिताम्।

देयश्च सुकुमाराणां लाजमण्डः सुसंस्कृतः।।२५५।।

क्षुत्पिपासापहः पथ्यः शुद्धानां च मलापहः।

शृतः पिप्पलिशुण्ठीभ्यां युक्तो लाजाम्लदाडिमैः।।२५६।।

कषायमधुराः शीता लघवो लाजसक्तवः।२५७।

**Thick gruel of** paddy promotes digestion and cures burning sensation as well as fainting. It is auspicious. These types
of gruel water when properly prepared with Dhanyaka (Coriander), Pippali – Long pepper fruit – Piper longum Linn,
is prescribed for persons of tender- health, children, and women and those persons suffering from indigestion and
irregularity in digestion. The gruel water of fried paddy when prepared with sour pomegranate, boiled with Pippal
(Piper longum Linn) and Sunthi (Ginger) allays hunger and thirst. It is wholesome and it helps eliminate of waste
products from the body of those who have undergone the purificatory therapies. Roasted flour of the fried paddy is
astringent as well as sweet in taste, cold in potency and light. [250-256]

**Different rice preparations:**

सुधौतः प्रसुतः स्विन्नः सन्तप्तश्चौदनो लघुः।।२५७।।

भृष्टतण्डुलमिच्छन्ति गरश्लेष्मामयेष्वपि।

अधौतोऽप्रसुतोऽस्विन्नः शीतश्चाप्योदनो गुरुः।।२५८।।

मांसशाकवसातैलघृतमज्जफलौदनाः।

बल्याः सन्तर्पणा हृद्या गुरवो बृंहयन्ति च।।२५९।।

तद्वन्माषतिलक्षीरमुद्गसंयोगसाधिताः।२६०।

Rice prepared on the boiled (dehusked) paddy, well cleaned and filtered is light when taken hot. Fried rice is useful
even in toxic conditions as well as diseases due to Kapha. The rice prepared of unboiled paddy, not cleaned as well
as filtered, is heavy, especially when taken after it has become cold. Rice prepared with meat, vegetable, muscle fat,
oil, ghee, marrow and fruit is strength promoting, refreshing, cardiac tonic, heavy and nourishing. Similar are the

properties of the rice prepared of Masha (black gram), Tila – Sesame (Sesamum indicum), Mudga (green gram) and milk. [257-259]

### Preparation of yava and others:

कुल्माषा गुरवो रूक्षा वातला भिन्नवर्चसः||२६०||

स्विन्नभक्ष्यास्तु ये किंचित् सौप्यगौधूमयाविकाः|

भिषक् तेषां यथाद्रव्यमादिशेद्गुरुलाघवम्||२६१||

**Kulmasha** is heavy, unctuous, aggravator of Vata and laxative. Edibles are also prepared with pulses, wheat, and barley by steam boiling. The physician should determine their heaviness or lightness in accordance with the properties of the material used in their preparation. [260-261]

### Juices and soups:

अकृतं कृतयूषं च तनुं सांस्कारिकं रसम्|

सूपमम्लमनम्लं च गुरुं विद्याद्यथोत्तरम्||२६२||

Juice is of two types - the one without fat, salt and pepper, and the other prepared with fat, salt and pepper- wide Susruta: Sutra 46: 379. The former is thin owing to the presence of meat in a small quantity. The latte is thick owing to its preparation with plenty of fat, meat etc. Similarly, soup is of two types viz, one which is sour and the other which is not sour. The latter is heavier than the former. [262]

### Flours – Saktu

सक्तवो वातला रूक्षा बहुवर्चोनुलोमिनः|

तर्पयन्ति नरं सद्यः पीताः सद्योबलाश्च ते||२६३||

मधुरा लघवः शीताः सक्तवः शालिसम्भवाः|

ग्राहिणो रक्तपित्तघ्नास्तृष्णाच्छर्दिज्वरापहाः||२६४||

### Saktu - Flour

The roasted corn-flour aggravates Vata. It is unctuous. It produces faeces in large quantities and is laxative. It provides instantaneous refreshment and strengths when taken in. Roasted flour of rice is sweet, light, cool, bowel- binding, useful in Rakthapitta (a diseases characterised by bleeding from various parts of the body), thirst, vomiting and fever.293-264]

### Indications for Yava – Barley (Hordeum vulgare) preparation:

हन्याद्व्याधीन् यवापूपो यावको वाट्य एव च|

उदावर्तप्रतिश्यायकासमेहगलग्रहान्||२६५||

धानासञ्ज्ञास्तु ये भक्ष्याः प्रायस्ते लेखनात्मकाः|

शुष्कत्वात्तर्पणाश्चैव विष्टम्भित्वाच्च दुर्जराः||२६६||

विरूढधाना शष्कुल्यो मधुक्रोडाः सपिण्डकाः|

पूपाः पूपलिकाद्याश्च गुरवः पैष्टिकाः परम्||२६७||


**Yava - Barley**

Vatya preparation of barley or pastry made of barley alleviates diseases like Udavarta (a type of abdominal disease characterised by the retention of faeces), Pratisyaya (Coryza), cough urinary diseases and obstruction in throat. Fried barely is generally depletive. Owing to its dryness, it is refreshing and due to its heaviness, it is difficult to digest. Geminated barley, Shashkuli, Madhukroda, Pindaka, Pupa, Pupalika etc are difficult for digestion. [256-267]


**Mixed preparations of Vegetables and meat:**

फलमांसवसाशाकपललक्षौद्रसंस्कृताः|

भक्ष्या वृष्याश्च बल्याश्च गुरवो बृंहणात्मकाः||२६८||

वेशवारो गुरुः स्निग्धो बलोपचयवर्धनः|

गुरवस्तर्पणा वृष्याः क्षीरेक्षुरसपूपकाः ||२६९||

सगुडाः सतिलाश्चैव सक्षीरक्षौद्रशर्कराः|

भक्ष्या वृष्याश्च बल्याश्च परं तु गुरवः स्मृताः||२७०||

**Eatables prepared with** fruit, meat, muscle fat, vegetables, powder of sesamum and honey are aphrodisiac, strength promoting, heavy, unctuous, promoter of strength and plumpness. Pesties made predominantly of milk and sugarcane juice are heavy, refreshing and aphrodisiac. Eatables prepared with sugar candy, sesamum, milk, honey and sugar are aphrodisiac and strength promoting but they are heavy. [268-270]

**Wheat preparations:**

सस्नेहाः स्नेहसिद्धाश्च भक्ष्या विविधलक्षणाः|
गुरवस्तर्पणा वृष्या हृद्या गौधूमिका मताः||२७१||
संस्काराल्लघवः सन्ति भक्ष्या गौधूमपैष्टिकाः|
धानापर्पटपूपाद्यास्तान् बुद्ध्वा निर्दिशेत्तथा||२७२||

**Various types of eatables of wheat** prepared by adding fat or fried with fat are heavy, refreshing, aphrodisiac and cardio tonic. Pastry preparations of wheat like fried wheat, Chapati cake are light by virtue of the method involved in their preparation. Their properties can be explained accordingly. [271-272]

**Pressed Paddy preparation:**

पृथुका गुरवो भृष्टान् भक्षयेदल्पशस्तु तान्|
यावा विष्टभ्य जीर्यन्ति सरसा भिन्नवर्चसः||२७३||

**Pruthuka (pressed paddy)** is heavy and strength promoting. It should be taken only in a small quantity. Yavacipita (pressed barley) produces wind during the process of digestion. Prthuka, if prepared without frying is laxative. [273]

**Supya (pulses) preparation:**

सूप्यान्नविकृता भक्ष्या वातला रूक्षशीतलाः|
सकटुस्नेहलवणानल्पशो भक्षयेत्तु तान्||२७४||

Eatables prepared of pulses like Mudga (Green gram) and Masa (Phaseolus radiates Linn) aggravates Vata. They are unctuous and cold. They should be taken in small quantities together with pungent things, fat and salt. [274]

**Food that gives nourishment and strength:**

मृदुपाकाश्च ये भक्ष्याः स्थूलाश्च कठिनाश्च ये|
गुरवस्ते व्यतिक्रान्तपाकाः पुष्टिबलप्रदाः||२७५||

Eatables which are cooked fully, coarse and hard, are heavy, and they take a long time to get digested. They promote nourishment as well as strength. [275]

**Assessment of diet:**

द्रव्यसंयोगसंस्कारं द्रव्यमानं पृथक् तथा|
भक्ष्याणामादिशेद्बुद्ध्वा यथास्वं गुरुलाघवम्||२७६||

Lightness or heaviness of eatables is determined by the types of combination, methods of preparation and properties in which ingredients are added to them. [276]

**Vimardaka:**

नानाद्रव्यैः समायुक्तः पक्वामक्लिन्नभर्जितैः|
विमर्दको गुरुर्हृद्यो वृष्यो बलवतां हितः) ||२७७||

**Vimardaka** is prepared by the combination of several ingredients- ripe, unripe, soft and fried. It is heavy, cardio-tonic, and aphrodisiac. It is useful only for persons who are physically strong. [277]

**Rasala and Lassi:**

रसाला बृंहणी वृष्या स्निग्धा बल्या रुचिप्रदा|
स्नेहनं तर्पणं हृद्यं वातघ्नं सगुडं दधि||२७८||
द्राक्षाखर्जूरकोलानां गुरु विष्टम्भि पानकम्|
परुषकाणां क्षौद्रस्य यच्चेक्षुविकृतिं प्रति||२७९||

**Rasala** is nourishing, aphrodisiac, unctuous, strength promoting and palatable
Curd mixed with sugar candy is unctuous, refreshing, cardio- tonic and balances Vata.[278]

**Juice – Panaka (Linctus) preparations:**

Beverages prepared of Darksha – Raisin – Vitis vinifera Linn, Kharjura (Phoenix sylvestris roxb), Kola (Ziziphus jujuba Lam), Parusaka (Grewia asiatica Linn), honey and products of sugarcane are heavy and they produce wind during the process of digestion. However, their properties can be determined by taking into account the ingredients and the proportion in which they are added.

### Raga and Shadava

तेषां कट्वम्लसंयोगान् पानकानां पृथक् पृथक्|
द्रव्यं मानं च विज्ञाय गुणकर्माणि चादिशेत्||२८०||

कट्वम्लस्वादुलवणा लघवो रागषाडवाः|
मुखप्रियाश्च हृद्याश्च दीपना भक्तरोचनाः||२८१||

आम्रामलकलेहाश्च बृंहणा बलवर्धनाः|
रोचनास्तर्पणाश्चोक्ताः स्नेहमाधुर्यगौरवात्||२८२||

बुद्ध्वा संयोगसंस्कारं द्रव्यमानं च तच्छ्रितम्|
गुणकर्माणि लेहानां तेषां तेषां तथा वदेत्||२८३||

Various types of Ragasadava (Raga and Sadava) are pungent, sour, sweet and salty in taste and they are light, palatable, cardio-tonic and carminative. They cause palatability in other food when added to it.

Linctuses prepared of Amra – mango – (Mangifera indica Linn) and Amalaka (Emblica officinalis Gaertn) are nourishing and strength promoting. Because of their unctuousnessand sweetness, they are palatable and refreshing. Properties and actions of various types of linctuses which are not described here are to be determined by the type of combination, method of preparation and the proportion in which ingredients are added to it. [279-283]

### Fermented preparation of rice and other vegetables:

रक्तपित्तकफोत्क्लेदि शुक्तं वातानुलोमनम्|
कन्दमूलफलाद्यं च तद्वदि्वद्यात्तदासुतम्||२८४||

शिण्डाकी चासुतं चान्यत् कालाम्लं रोचनं लघु|
विद्याद्वर्गं कृतान्नानामेकादशतमं भिषक्||२८५||

Shukta aggravates bleeding disorders, as well as Kapha and alleviates Vata. Even the rhizomes, roots and fruits carry the same property when fermented in it. Sindaki and other beverages which have become sour in taste due to prolonged storage after fermentation are palatable and light. Thus ends the eleventh group consisting of food preparation. [284-285]

### Adjuvant of food & oils:

कषायानुरसं स्वादु सूक्ष्ममुष्णं व्यवायि च|
पित्तलं बद्धविण्मूत्रं न च श्लेष्माभिवर्धनम्||२८६||

वातघ्नेषूत्तमं बल्यं त्वच्यं मेधाग्निवर्धनम्|
तैलं संयोगसंस्कारात् सर्वरोगापहं मतम्||२८७||

तैलप्रयोगादजरा निर्विकारा जितश्रमाः|
आसन्नतिबलाः सङ्ख्ये दैत्याधिपतयः पुरा||२८८||

ऐरण्डतैलं मधुरं गुरु श्लेष्माभिवर्धनम्|
वातासृग्गुल्महृद्रोगजीर्णज्वरहरं परम्||२८९||

कटूष्णं सार्षपं तैलं रक्तपित्तप्रदूषणम्|
कफशुक्रानिलहरं कण्डूकोठविनाशनम् [२] ||२९०||

प्रियालतैलं मधुरं गुरु श्लेष्माभिवर्धनम्|
हितमिच्छन्ति नात्यौष्ण्यात्संयोगे वातपित्तयोः||२९१||

आतस्यं मधुराम्लं तु विपाके कटुकं तथा|
उष्णवीर्यं हितं वाते रक्तपित्तप्रकोपणम्||२९२||

कुसुम्भतैलमुष्णं च विपाके कटुकं गुरु।
विदाहि च विशेषेण सर्वदोषप्रकोपणम्॥२९३॥
फलानां यानि चान्यानि तैलान्याहारसंविधौ।
युज्यन्ते गुणकर्मभ्यां तानि ब्रूयाद्यथाफलम्॥२९४॥

**Now begins the group consisting of the adjuvants of food:**
**Sesame oil** is sweet with accompanying astringent taste, suitable (can penetrate through the suitable channels of the body), hot in potency and Vyavayi (which undergoes Paka or chemical change after it is pervaded all over the body). It aggravates Pitta, binds bowel and reduces the quantity of urine but it does not aggravate kapha. It is the best among those which balance Vata. It promotes strength, skin health, intelligence and power of digestion. In combination with various drugs (Samyoga), sesamum oil is said to cure all diseases. In the ancient time, kings of demons, by virtue of the use of oil overcame aging, got rid of diseases as well as fatigue-less, acquired great strength instantaneously and fought battles (successfully).

**Castor oil** is sweet in taste, heavy, increases Kapha and balances Vata, Raktagulma (a type of abdominal tumour especially in females), heart disease, indigestion and fever.

Mustard oil is pungent in taste and hot in potency. It aggravates Rakta as well as Pitta and reduces Kapha, semen as well as Vata. It cures itching and urticaria.

**Oil of Priyala** (Buchanania lanzan Spreng) is sweet in taste, heavy and aggravator of Kapha. Since it is not very hot, it is useful when Vata and Pitta are jointly aggravated.

**Oil of Atasi** (Linum usitatissimumLinn) is sweet as well as sour in taste, pungent in Vipaka and hot in potency. It alleviates Vata but aggravates Rakta and Pitta.

**Oil of Kusumbha** (Carthamus tinctorius Linn) is hot in potency, pungent in Vipaka and heavy. It produces a burning sensation and aggravates all the Dosas.

Several other oils are also used for the preparation of food. Their properties and actions are similar to those of the fruits from which these oils are extracted. [286-294]

**Animal fat:**
मधुरो बृंहणो वृष्यो बल्यो मज्जा तथा वसा।
यथासत्वं तु शैत्योष्णे वसामज्ज्योर्विनिर्दिशेत्॥२९५॥
Muscle fat and marrow are sweet in taste, nourishing, aphrodisiac and strength promoting. Their potencies, viz hot and coldness, are to be determined according to the nature of the animal from which they are collected. [295]

**Condiments, spices and salts:**
सस्नेहं दीपनं वृष्यमुष्णं वातकफापहम्।
विपाके मधुरं हृद्यं रोचनं विश्वभेषजम्॥२९६॥
श्लेष्मला मधुरा चार्द्रा गुर्वी स्निग्धा च पिप्पली।
सा शुष्का कफवातघ्नी कटूष्णा वृष्यसम्मता॥२९७॥
नात्यर्थमुष्णं मरिचमवृष्यं लघु रोचनम्।
छेदित्वाच्छोषणत्वाच्च दीपनं कफवातजित्॥२९८॥
वातश्लेष्मविबन्धघ्नं कटूष्णं दीपनं लघु।
हिङ्गु शूलप्रशमनं विद्यात् पाचनरोचनम्॥२९९॥
रोचनं दीपनं वृष्यं चक्षुष्यमविदाहि च।
त्रिदोषघ्नं समधुरं सैन्धवं लवणोत्तमम्॥३००॥
सौक्ष्म्यादौष्ण्याल्लघुत्वाच्च सौगन्ध्याच्च रुचिप्रदम्।
सौवर्चलं विबन्धघ्नं हृद्यमुद्गारशोधि च॥३०१॥
तैक्ष्ण्यादौष्ण्याद्व्यवायित्वाद्दीपनं शूलनाशनम्।
ऊर्ध्वं चाधश्च वातानामानुलोम्यकरं बिडम्॥३०२॥
सतिक्तकटु सक्षारं तीक्ष्णमुत्क्लेदि चौदि्भदम्।

न काललवणे गन्धः सौवर्चलगुणाश्च ते॥३०३॥
सामुद्रकं समधुरं, सतिक्तं कटु पांशुजम्।
रोचनं लवणं सर्वं पाकि संस्यनिलापहम्॥३०४॥

**Dry ginger** is unctuous, promoter of digestion, aphrodisiac, hot in potency, balances vata as well as Kapha, sweet in Vipaka, cardio- tonic and palatable.

**Green but ripe** Pippali – Long pepper fruit is aggravator of Kapha, Sweet in taste, heavy and unctuous. Dried Pippali – Long pepper fruit – Piper longum however balances Kapha as well as Vata, pungent in taste, hot in potency, and aphrodisiac.

**Maricha – Black pepper fruit** - piper nigrum is not very hot in potency, non-aphrodisiac, light and palatable. Due to its depleting and absorbing properties, it promotes digestion and alleviates Kapha as well as Vata.

The gum resin of Hingu – Asafetida (Ferula narthex Boiss) balances colic pain, is carminative and palatable.

**Saindhava (rock salt)** is the best among salts. It is palatable, promoter of digestion, aphrodisiac, conducive for eye sight, balances all the three Dosas and slightly sweet in taste. It does not cause burning sensation.

Sauvarcala (Sonchal salt) is suitable (capable of permeating though the subtle channels of body), hot, light and fragrant. By virtue of these properties, it is palatable, laxative and cardiotonic and it purifies eructations.

**Bida** type of salt is sharp, hot and Vyavayi (which undergoes Paka or chemical change after it is pervaded all over the body). By virtue of these qualities, it promotes digestion, cures colic pain and helps eliminating of gas from abdomen both through the upper as well as lower tract (mouth and anus)

**Aubdhida type of salt** which is also known as Utkarika is pungent and slightly bitter in taste. It is alkaline, sharp and softening.

**Kala type** of salt is only a variety of sonchal salt having all the attributes of the latter except that in the former there is no fragrance.

**Samudra** (salt collected from the southern coast- also known as Karakaca) is slightly sweet in taste whereas Pamsuja (salt collected from the eastern coast) is pungent with a bitter taste.

Salts in general are palatable, promotes digestion, is laxative and balances Vata [296-304]

**Kshara (Alkalies):-**

हृत्पाण्डुग्रहणीरोगप्लीहानाहगलग्रहान्।
कासं कफजमर्शांसि यावशूको व्यपोहति॥३०५॥
तीक्ष्णोष्णो लघुरूक्षश्च क्लेदी पक्ता विदारणः।
दाहनो दीपनश्छेता सर्वः क्षारोऽग्निसन्निभः ॥३०६॥

**Yava Kshara** (an alkali preparation from the plant barley) is useful in

Hrudroga – heart diseases,

Pandu – anaemia,

Grahani – malabsorptionsyndrome (IBS)

Pleeha – enlargement of spleen,

Anaha – bloating, constipation,

Galagraha – obstruction in throat,

Kasa – coughing and

Kaphaja Ashmari – piles of Slaismika variety.

Alkali preparations (Ksharas) in general are sharp, hot, light, unctuous, softening, carminative, corrosive, and caustic, digestive stimulant and depletive. They cause burns and thereby work like life. [305-306]

**Others:**

कारवी कुञ्चिकाऽजाजी यवानी धान्यतुम्बुरु।
रोचनं दीपनं वातकफदौर्गन्ध्यनाशनम्॥३०७॥

**Karavi** (Carum carvi Linn), Kuncika (Nigella sativa Linn), Ajaji( Cuminum cyminum Linn), Yavani (Trachyspermum ammi Sprague ), Dhanya (Corindarum sativum Linn) and Tumburu (Zanthoxylum alatum Roxb) are palatable, digestive stimulant, alleviator Vata as well as Kapha and remover of foul odor.[307]

आहारयोगिनां भक्तिनिश्चयो न तु विद्यते।
समाप्तो द्वादशश्चायं वर्ग आहारयोगिनाम्॥३०८॥
इत्याहारयोगिवर्गो द्वादशः।

Adjutants of food are ultimately in number. Thus, ends the twelfth group consisting of adjustments of food. [308]

**Choice of grains:**

शूकधान्यं शमीधान्यं समातीतं प्रशस्यते।
पुराणं प्रायशो रूक्षं प्रायेणाभिनवं गुरु ॥३०९॥
यद्यदागच्छति क्षिप्रं ततत्ल्लघुतरं स्मृतम्।
निस्तुषं युक्तिभृष्टं च सूप्यं लघु विपच्यते॥३१०॥

**Corns and grains**, one year after their harvesting, are whole some. Old corn and grains are mostly unctuous and fresh ones are heavy. Corns and grains which take a shorter time for cultivation as well as harvesting are lighter than those taking longer time. Dehusked pulse when slightly fried becomes light for digestion. [309-310]

**Choice of animals:**

मृतं कृशं चातिमेद्यं वृद्धं बालं विषैर्हतम्।
अगोचरभृतं व्यालसूदितं मांसमुत्सृजेत्॥३११॥
अतोऽन्यथा हितं मांसं बृंहणं बलवर्धनम्॥३१२।

Meat of animals who have died a natural death, who are emaciated (or dried up after death), who are fatty in excess, who are old, who are too young, who are killed by poisonous arrows, who graze in a land not commensurate with their natural habitat and who are bitten by snakes and tigers etc. are unwholesome. Otherwise, meat is wholesome, nourishing and strength promoting. [311]

**Meat soup and its qualities:**

प्रीणनः सर्वभूतानां हृद्यो मांसरसः परम्॥३१२॥
शुष्यतां व्याधिमुक्तानां कृशानां क्षीणरेतसाम्।
बलवर्णार्थिनां चैव रसं विद्याद्यथामृतम्॥३१३॥
सर्वरोगप्रशमनं यथास्वं विहितं रसम्।
विद्यात् स्वर्यं बलकरं वयोबुद्धीन्द्रियायुषाम्॥३१४॥
व्यायामनित्याः स्त्रीनित्या मद्यनित्याश्च ये नराः।
नित्यं मांसरसाहारा नातुराः स्युर्न दुर्बलाः॥३१५॥

Meat soup is refreshing for all animals. For those who are dehydrated or emaciated, who are in the convalescence stage, those having semen, in small quantities and those who aspire better strength and complexion, meat soup is like ambrosia. When taken according to the prescribed method, it promotes voice, youth, intelligence, power of sensory organs and longevity. If those who habitually indulge in exercise, sex and wine, take meat soup regularly, thy neither succumb to decreases nor less their strength. [312-315]

**Unwholesome vegetable preparations:**

क्रिमिवातातपहतं शुष्कं जीर्णमनार्तवम्।
शाकं निःस्नेहसिद्धं च वर्ज्यं यच्चापरिसूतम्॥३१६॥
पुराणमामं सङ्क्लिष्टं क्रिमिव्यालहिमातपैः।
अदेशकालजं क्लिन्नं यत्स्यात्फलमसाधु तत्॥३१७॥
हरितानां यथाशाकं निर्देशः साधनादृते।
मद्याम्बुगोरसादीनां स्वे स्वे वर्गे विनिश्चयः॥३१८॥

**Vegetables infested with insects**, exposed to wind, the sun, long, dried up, old and unseasonal are unwholesome. When they are cooked without adding fat and residual water after boiling is not filtered out, vegetables become unwholesome for use.

Fruits which are old, unripe, afflicted by insects and serpents, exposed to snow or sun for long, growing in the land and season other than the normal habitat and time and putrefied are unwholesome.

Rules regarding salads are the same as vegetables except that the rules regarding the latter are not applicable to the former. Rules regarding the unwholesomeness of wines, water and milk products are described in the respective groups. [316-318]

**Anupana – Varieties of drinks used after food :**

यदाहारगुणैः पानं विपरीतं तदिष्यते।
अन्नानुपानं धातूनां दृष्टं यन्न विरोधि च॥३१९॥
आसवानां समुद्दिष्टामशीतिं चतुरुत्तराम्।
जलं पेयमपेयं च परीक्ष्यानुपिबेद्दिधतम्॥३२०॥
स्निग्धोष्णं मारुते शस्तं पित्ते मधुरशीतलम्।
कफेऽनुपानं रूक्षोष्णं क्षये मांसरसः परम्॥३२१॥
उपवासाध्वभाष्यस्त्रीमारुतातपकर्मभिः।
क्लान्तानामनुपानार्थं पयः पथ्यं यथाऽमृतम्॥३२२॥
सुरा कृशानां पुष्ट्यर्थमनुपानं विधीयते।
काश्र्यार्थं स्थूलदेहानामनु शस्तं मधूदकम्॥३२३॥
अल्पाग्नीनामनिद्राणां तन्द्राशोकभयक्लमैः।
मद्यमांसोचितानां च मद्यमेवानुशस्यते॥३२४॥

**Anupana- Post prandial drink:**

Generally post-prandial drinks should have the properties opposite to those of the food taken. But at the same time, such drinks should not be harmful to the tissue elements of the body. Water as well as the eighty-four varieties of alcoholic preparations (described in the 25th chapter of this section) are to be examined and with a view to ascertain their wholesomeness or otherwise and only useful drinks are to be taken.

In conditions caused by the aggravation of vata, Oily and hot after drinks are useful.

Similarly in Pitta sweet and cold, and

Kapha – oily and hot post drinks are useful.

For Kshaya – emaciation meat soup is the useful post-prandial drink. Milk is the post-prandial drink like ambrosia for those fatigued due to indulgence in fasting, long walk, long speeches, sex and exposure to wind and sun. For nourishing emaciated individuals, wine is the best post-prandial drink. For causing emaciation of over corpulent individuals honey water is the useful post-prandial drink. Alcohol serves as useful post-prandial drink for those accustomed to alcoholic drinks as well as meat, and suffering from loss of digestion, insomnia, accompanied with drowsiness, grief, fear and exhaustion. [319-324]

**Effects of after-food drinks on the individual and the food :**

अथानुपानकर्मगुणान् प्रवक्ष्यामः- अनुपानं तर्पयति, प्रीणयति, ऊर्जयति, बृंहयति, पर्याप्तिमभिनिर्वर्तयति, भुक्तमवसादयति, अन्नसङ्घातं भिनत्ति, मार्दवमापादयति, क्लेदयति, जरयति, सुखपरिणामितामाशुव्यवायितां चाहारस्योपजनयतीति॥३२५॥

**Effects of after-food drinks (Anupana) on the individual and the food:**

Now we shall explain the actions and properties of post-prandial drinks. Post- prandial drinks in general, bring about refreshment, pleasure, energy, nourishment, satisfaction and steadiness in the food eaten. It helps in breaking down, softening, digesting, proper assimilation and instant diffusion of the food taken. [325]

**Summing up:-**

अनुपानं हितं युक्तं तर्पयत्याशु मानवम्।
सुखं पचति चाहारमायुषे च बलाय च॥३२६॥

Thus, it is said:

Administration of wholesome post-prandial drinks refreshes instantaneously and helps an individual in easy digestion resulting in the promotion of longevity and strength. [326]

**Contra inditations of Anupana (after-drinks)**

नोध्र्वाङ्गमारुताविष्टा न हिक्काश्वासकासिनः।

न गीतभाष्याध्ययनप्रसक्ता नोरसि क्षताः||३२७||
पिबेयुरुदकं भुक्त्वा तद्धि कण्ठोरसि स्थितम्|
स्नेहमाहारजं हत्वा भूयो दोषाय कल्पते||३२८||

Water should not be taken after food by those suffering from diseases of the head due to the vitiation of Vata, Hiccup, dyspnea, cough as well as tuberculosis. It is also prohibited for those who indulge in singing, speech and study with loud sound because it remains in the throat and chest, and removes from there the unctuous substances taken along with food resulting in the further aggravation of the condition. [327-328]

**Purpose of brief description:**

अन्नपानैकदेशोऽयमुक्तः प्रायोपयोगिकः|
द्रव्याणि न हि निर्देष्टुं शक्यं कात्स्न्र्येन नामभिः||३२९||
यथा नानौषधं किञ्चिद्देशजानां वचो यथा|
द्रव्यं तत्तथा वाच्यमनुक्तमिह यद्भवेत्||३३०||

Only such diets and drinks as are mostly used by people, are described here. In terms of description, it is even impossible to enumerate by names all the drugs as it is said, in the previous chapter, "There is no substance which is not useful as a drug". (Vide Sutra 26:12) Properties of such drugs which are not mentioned here may be determined by taking into account attributes made from them by the people of that locality. [329-330]

**Factors determining the qualities of dietetic articles:**

चरः शरीरावयवाः स्वभावो धातवः क्रिया|
लिङ्गं प्रमाणं संस्कारो मात्रा चास्मिन् परीक्ष्यते||३३१||

Animals, habitat and food, organs (parts) of the body, nature, tissues, activity, sex, size/quantity as well as mode of preparation and quantity are (also) to be examined to determine the properties of foods that are not described in this text.[331]

**Effect of Desha (Place):**

चरोऽनूपजलाकाशधन्वाद्यो भक्ष्यसंविधिः|
जलजानूपजाश्चैव जलानूपचराश्च ये||३३२||
गुरुभक्ष्याश्च ये सत्त्वाः सर्वे ते गुरवः स्मृताः|
लघुभक्ष्यास्तु लघवो धन्वजा धन्वचारिणः||३३३||

**Effect of Desha (Place):**

Chara (habitat and food) consists of habitats like marshy land, water, sky and desert as well as food intake of the animal. Meat of those animals which are born or who move in water and marshy land, and who take heavy food is heavy (for digestion). Similarly, the meat of those animals which take light food and are born or move in the desert are light. [332-333]

**Parts of animals:**

शरीरावयवाः सक्थिशिरःस्कन्धादयस्तथा|
सक्थिमांसाद्गुरुः स्कन्धस्ततः क्रोडस्ततः शिरः||३३४||
वृषणौ चर्म मेढ्रं च श्रोणी वृक्कौ यकृद्गुदम्|
मांसाद्गुरुतरं विद्याद्यथास्वं मध्यमस्थि च||३३५||

**Parts of animals:**

Different parts of the body are thigh, head, shoulder etc. Flesh of the shoulder is heavier than the thigh. Similarly, the chest is heavier than the shoulder and head is heavier than the chest. In comparison to all the above, flesh of testicles, skin, phallus, hips, kidneys, liver and rectum, middle parts of the body, and muscles attached with bones is heavier. This comparison of lightness and heaviness is in respect of the same animal. [334-335]

**Guru – heavy and Laghu – light to digest:**

स्वभावाल्लघवो मुद्गास्तथा लावकपिञ्जलाः|
स्वभावाद्गुरवो माषा वराहमहिषास्तथा||३३६||
धातूनां शोणितादीनां गुरुं विद्याद्यथोत्तरम्|

अलसेभ्यो विशिष्यन्ते प्राणिनो ये बहुक्रियाः||३३७||

**Mudga (Green gram)**, Lava (common quail) and Kapinjala (jungle bush quail) are light by nature. Similarly, Masha (black gram), Varaha (pork) and buffalo are heavy by nature.

Tissue elements, viz, Rakta (blood), Mamsa (muscle, Medas (fat), Asti(bone), Majja (marrow) and Sukrs (semen) are progressively heavier. Animals that are more active are lighter than the lazy ones. [336-337]

### Sex and stature:

गौरवं लिङ्गसामान्ये पुंसां स्त्रीणां तु लाघवम्|

महाप्रमाणा गुरवः स्वजातौ लघवोऽन्यथा||३३८||

Of the species of quadruped animals, males are heavy and females are light. Similarly, among them, those of larger size are heavy and smaller ones are light. [338]

### Processing:

गुरूणां लाघवं विद्यात् संस्कारात् सविपर्ययम्|

व्रीहेर्लाजा यथा च स्युः सक्तूनां सिद्धपिण्डिकाः||३३९||

Heaviness of food articles can be converted into lightness and vice versa by the process of preparation. For example, the Vrihi is heavy in nature but when processed and converted into Laja/sattu it becomes light. But when boiled on fire so as to form a cake of bolus, the laja once again becomes heavy in nature. [339]

### Dose:

अल्पादाने गुरूणां च लघूनां चातिसेवने|

मात्रा कारणमुद्दिष्टं द्रव्याणां गुरुलाघवे||३४०||

गुरूणामल्पमादेयं लघूनां तृप्तिरिष्यते|

मात्रां द्रव्याण्यपेक्षन्ते मात्रा चाग्निमपेक्षते||३४१||

The quantity of intake is also responsible for the heaviness or lightness of food articles. Even a heavy food article if taken in small quantities is light in effect and so a light one taken in large quantities results in heaviness. Thus, heavy things should be taken in small quantities and light things until one is satisfied. Action of food articles (as well as drugs) is conditioned by the quantity of intake and the proper quantity in which food articles are to be taken is dependent on the power of digestion including metabolism of individual. [3340-341]

### Diet and Agni (digestive power):

बलमारोग्यमायुश्च प्राणाश्चाग्नौ प्रतिष्ठिताः|

अन्नपानेन्धनैश्चाग्निर्ज्वलति व्येति चान्यथा ||३४२||

Strength, health, longevity and vital breath are dependent upon the power of digestion including metabolism. When supplied with fuel in the form of food and drinks, this power of digestion is sustained; it dwindles when deprived of it. [342]

### Dietetic consideration – heavy and light:

गुरुलाघवचिन्तेयं प्रायेणाल्पबलान् प्रति|

मन्दक्रियाननारोग्यान् सुकुमारान्सुखोचितान्||३४३||

Heaviness and lightness of food articles is to be considered mostly for the individuals who are weak, indolent, unhealthy, of tender health and who are given to luxury.[343]

### Dialectic consideration- essential:

दीप्ताग्नयः खराहाराः कर्मनित्या महोदराः|

ये नराः प्रति तांश्चिन्त्यं नावश्यं गुरुलाघवम्||३४४||

For those who have strong power of digestion, who are accustomed to the intake of heavy (hard) food articles, who are pot-belly (obese) and accustomed to hard labor, heaviness or lightness of food articles does not matter much [344]

### Food – intake is a sacrifice (yaga)

हिताभिर्जुहुयान्नित्यमन्तरग्निं समाहितः|

अन्नपानसमिद्भिर्ना मात्राकालौ विचारयन्||३४५||

आहिताग्निः सदा पथ्यान्यन्तरग्नौ जुहोति यः|

दिवसे दिवसे ब्रह्म जपत्यथ ददाति च||३४६||

नरं निःश्रेयसे युक्तं सात्म्यज्ञं पानभोजने|

भजन्ते नामयाः केचिद्भाविनोऽप्यन्तरादृते||३४७||

### Food – intake is a sacrifice(yaga)

Paying due consideration to the quantity and time, a self- controlled man should regularly and carefully take useful, beneficial and wholesome foods and drinks and offer them to the digestive fire as in a fire sacrifice. This process should be methodical and should take place daily in a consistent and monitored way. Like an Aahitagni (a man who always puts efforts to keep the fire kindled and balanced regularly) who takes diet conducive to the power of digestion, being aware of the wholesomeness of food and drinks, who is on the pathway of righteousness (which would provide him salvation) and who resorts to meditation of "Brahman' and Charity enjoys blissful life without any disease during the present as well as future lives. Since such persons would keep away from unwholesome foods which are root causes of diseases and also from non-righteousness things, they will never suffer from any disease in the present as well as in future. [345-347]

### To live for one hundred years:

षड्त्रिंशतं सहस्राणि रात्रीणां हितभोजनः|

जीवत्यनातुरो जन्तुर्जितात्मा सम्मतः सताम्||३४८||

A self controlled man, blessed by noble-men lives for hundred years free from diseases by the intake of wholesome food.{348}

### Utility of the consideration of foods and drinks:

प्राणाः प्राणभृतामन्नमन्नं लोकोऽभिधावति|

वर्णः प्रसादः सौस्वर्यं जीवितं प्रतिभा सुखम्||३४९||

तुष्टिः पुष्टिर्बलं मेधा सर्वमन्ने प्रतिष्ठितम्|

लौकिकं कर्म यद्वृत्तौ स्वर्गतौ यच्च वैदिकम्||३५०||

कर्मापवर्गे यच्चोक्तं तच्चाप्यन्ने प्रतिष्ठितम्|३५१|

Food sustains the life of living beings. All living beings in the universe requires food. Complexion, clarity, good voice, longevity, geniuses, happiness, satisfaction, nourishment, strength and intellect are all conditioned by food. Professional activities leading to happiness in this world, Vedic rituals leading to abode in heaven and observance of truth, Brahmacarya leading to salvation are all based on food. [349-350]

### Summary:

प्राणाः प्राणभृतामन्नमन्नं लोकोऽभिधावति|

वर्णः प्रसादः सौस्वर्यं जीवितं प्रतिभा सुखम्||३४९||

तुष्टिः पुष्टिर्बलं मेधा सर्वमन्ने प्रतिष्ठितम्|

लौकिकं कर्म यद्वृत्तौ स्वर्गतौ यच्च वैदिकम्||३५०||

कर्मापवर्गे यच्चोक्तं तच्चाप्यन्ने प्रतिष्ठितम्|३५१|

### Summary:

Properties of food and drinks in general, ingredients having fore most qualities, twelve groups, post- prandial drinks along with their properties, brief statements on heaviness and lightness of food ingredients- all these necessitating special studies are mentioned in this chapter on "The Properties of Diets and Drinks. [351-352]

इत्यग्निवेशकृते तन्त्रे चरकप्रतिसंस्कृते श्लोकस्थानेऽन्नपानविधिर्नाम सप्तविंशोऽध्यायः||२७||

Thus ends the twenty seventh chapter on the "Properties of the Diets and Drinks" of the Sutra section of Agnivesas work as redacted by Charaka.

# 28

# Sutrasthana Chapter 28 Vividha Ashita Peeteeyam

**Vividha Ashita Peeteeya Adhyaya**

**Process of Digestion, How Food Causes Disease –**

अथातो विविधाशितपीतीयमध्यायं व्याख्यास्यामः||१||

इति ह स्माह भगवानात्रेयः||२||

The 28th chapter of Charaka explains how different types of foods undergo digestion, how they nourish different body tissues, how wholesome diet and regimen causes health and unwholesomeness causes disease and so on. The chapter name is Vividha Ashita Peeteeya Adhyaya

**Digestion of food and nourishment of body tissues:**

विविधमशितं पीतं लीढं खादितं जन्तोर्हितमन्तरग्निसन्धुक्षितबलेन यथास्वेनोष्मणा सम्यग्विपच्यमानं कालवदनवस्थितसर्वधातुपाकमनुपहतसर्वधात्वूष्ममारुतस्रोतः केवलं शरीरमुपचयबलवर्णसुखायुषा योजयति शरीरधातूनूर्जयति च|

धातवो हि धात्वाहाराः प्रकृतिमनुवर्तन्ते||३||

**Digestion of food and nourishment of body tissues:**

Antaragni (internal fire) empowers digestive fire to digest various types of food –

Ashita – eatables

Peeta – liquid foods

Leeda – linctus, jams,

Khadita – foods which can be masticated

Then the foods are taken to Dhatu level (level of body tissues – blood, muscle, bone tissue etc). Here, the food is subjected to Dhatu agni – a digestive process that converts a particular part of food into the native Dhatu. There are seven Dhatus. So, obviously there are seven dhatu agnis i.e. tissue fires. These agnis convert respective parts of food into body tissue.

The food which is thus digested causes:

Upachaya – body nourishment, plumpness

Bala – strength and immunity

Varna – skin tone and complexion

Sukha – comfort, good mental health

Ayusha – improves life expectancy.

Thus all the body tissues get well nourished. [3]

**How waste products of the body get support:**

तत्राहारप्रसादाख्यो रसः किट्टं च मलाख्यमभिनिर्वर्तते|

किट्टात् स्वेदमूत्रपुरीषवातपित्तश्लेष्माणः कर्णाक्षिनासिकास्यलोमकूपप्रजननमलाः केशश्मश्रुलोमनखादयश्चावयवाः पुष्यन्ति|

**How waste products of the body get support:**
Food, after digestion takes two forms viz,

- Prasada – the essence part, which is formed in the first stage. This is also called as 'Rasa'
- Kitta – the waste part

The waste part further nourishes
Sweda – sweat,
Mootra – urine
Pureesha – faeces
Tridosha – Vata, Pitta and Kapha
Excreta of the ear, eye, nose, mouth, hair follicles, as well as genitals organs and also to
Kesha – hair of the head,
Shmashru – beard,
Loma – small hair of the body,
Nakha – nails etc.,

**How the body tissues – Dhatu gets nourishment?**
पुष्यन्ति त्वाहाररसाद्रसरुधिरमांसमेदोस्थिमज्जशुक्रौजांसि पञ्चेन्द्रियद्रव्याणि धातुप्रसादसञ्ज्ञकानि शरीरसन्धिबन्धपिच्छादयश्चावयवाः।
ते सर्व एव धातवो मलाख्याः प्रसादाख्याश्च रसमलाभ्यां पुष्यन्तः स्वं मानमनुवर्तन्ते यथावयःशरीरम्।
एवं रसमलौ स्वप्रमाणावस्थितावाश्रयस्य समधातोर्धातुसाम्यमनुवर्तयतः।
निमित्ततस्तु क्षीणवृद्धानां प्रसादाख्यानां धातूनां वृद्धिक्षयाभ्यामाहारमूलाभ्यां रसः साम्यमुत्पादयत्यारोग्याय, किट्टं च मलानामेवमेव।
स्वमानातिरिक्ताः पुनरुत्सर्गिणः शीतोष्णपर्यायगुणैश्चोपचर्यमाणा मलाः शरीर धातुसाम्यकराः समुपलभ्यन्ते॥४॥

**How the body tissues – Dhatu gets nourishment:**
From the Rasa – essence part of food digestion, the successive dhatus –
Rudhira – blood
Mamsa – muscle
Meda – fat tissue
Asthi – bone tissue
Majja – contents inside bone, bone marrow
Shukra – reproductive system get nourished successively
Then all the sense organs and body joints get nourished.
Thus the essence part (Rasa (taste) and waste part (Kitta or Mala) of food nourishes the body tissues and body waste products respectively and thus the proper portions of tissues and waste products are maintained in balance, according to the size and shape of the body. Due to certain causes, the tissue elements may get Kshaya (depletion) or Vruddhi (excessive increase). Similarly, even the waste products can undergo Kshaya or Vruddhi. The right amount of food, with correct opposing qualities of hot and cold, causes re-balancing of this increase / decrease. [4]

**Relation of foods with body and Diseases:**
तेषां तु मलप्रसादाख्यानां धातूनां स्रोतांस्ययनमुखानि।
तानि यथाविभागेन यथास्वं धातूनापूरयन्ति।
एवमिदं शरीरमशितपीतलीढखादितप्रभवम्।
अशितपीतलीढखादितप्रभवाश्चास्मिन् शरीरे व्याधयो भवन्ति।
हिताहितोपयोगविशेषास्त्वत्र शुभाशुभविशेषकरा भवन्तीति॥५॥

**Relation of foods with body and Diseases:**
The pure as well as waste products (of digestion and metabolism) enter into the various channels of circulation (Srotas) and circulate through them. Each tissue (Dhatu) has its own channel (Srotas). These channels (Srotas) carrying specific nutrient material provide nourishment in required quantity to various Dhatus. Thus the body is

the result of nourishment drawn (in fourfold manner) from eatables, beverages, linctuses, and masticates. Diseases are also manifested in the body by the four types of foods (viz, eating, drinking, licking and masticating). Intake of wholesome and unwholesome food is the cause for health and disease respectively. [5]

**Agnivesha inquired:**

एवंवादिनं भगवन्तमात्रेयमग्निवेश उवाच- दृश्यन्ते हि भगवन्! हितसमाख्यातमप्याहारमुपयुञ्जाना व्याधिमन्तश्चागदाश्च, तथैवाहितसमाख्यातम्; एवं दुष्टे कथं हिताहितोपयोगविशेषात्मकं शुभाशुभविशेषमुपलभामह इति||६||

**Agnivesha inquired**

"Oh! Lord, people taking so called wholesome foods are found to suffer from diseases even though some of them are healthy. And a few people taking unwholesome food are found to be healthy. In view of this, how to draw the conclusion that health and diseases are conditioned by wholesome and unwholesome food respectively. [6]

**Cause for disease:**

तमुवाच भगवानात्रेयः- न हिताहारोपयोगिनामग्निवेश! तन्निमित्ता व्याधयो जायन्ते, न च केवलं हिताहारोपयोगादेव सर्वव्याधिभयमतिक्रान्तं भवति, सन्ति ह्यृतेऽप्यहिताहारोपयोगादन्या रोगप्रकृतयः, तद्यथा- कालविपर्ययः, प्रज्ञापराधः, शब्दस्पर्शरूपरसगन्धाश्चासात्म्या इति|

ताश्च रोगप्रकृतयो रसान् सम्यगुपयुञ्जानमपि पुरुषमशुभेनोपपादयन्ति; तस्माद्धिताहारोपयोगिनोऽपि दृश्यन्ते व्याधिमन्तः|

अहिताहारोपयोगिनां पुनः कारणतो न सद्यो दोषवान् भवत्यपचारः|

न हि सर्वाण्यपथ्यानि तुल्यदोषाणि, न च सर्वे दोषास्तुल्यबलाः, न च सर्वाणि शरीराणि व्याधिक्षमत्वे समर्थानि भवन्ति|

तदेव ह्यपथ्यं देशकालसंयोगवीर्यप्रमाणातियोगाद्भूयस्तरमपथ्यं सम्पद्यते|

स एव दोषः संसृष्ट्योनिर्विरुद्धोपक्रमो गम्भीरानुगतश्चिरस्थितः प्राणायतनसमुत्थो मर्मोपघाती कष्टतमः क्षिप्रकारितमश्च सम्पद्यते|

शरीराणि चातिस्थूलान्यतिकृशान्यनिविष्टमांसशोणितास्थीनि दुर्बलान्यसात्म्याहारोपचितान्यल्पाहाराण्यल्पसत्त्वानि च भवन्त्यव्याधिसहानि, विपरीतानि पुनर्व्याधिसहानि|

एभ्यश्चैवापथ्याहारदोषशरीरविशेषेभ्यो व्याधयो मृदवो दारुणाः क्षिप्रसमुत्थाश्चिरकारिणश्च भवन्ति|

त एव वातपित्तश्लेष्माणः स्थानविशेषे प्रकुपिता व्याधिविशेषानभिनिर्वर्तयन्त्यग्निवेश!||७||

**Cause for disease:**

Lord Atreya replied, "It is not that individuals accustomed to wholesome food suffer from diseases, due to the food that they are taking.

न च केवलं हिताहारोपयोगादेव सर्व व्याधिभयमतिक्रान्तं भवति

It is not only by taking wholesome food one can overcome all diseases.

Apart from an unwholesome diet, there are other factors for the causation of diseases. They are –

Kaala Viparyaya – seasonal abnormality,

Prajnaparadha – intellectual blasphemy – knowingly committing mistakes

Shabda Sparsha Rupa Rasa (taste) Gandha Asatmya – unwholesome contents of sense faculties with their objects like sound, touch, vision, taste and smell. These factors may produce diseases even in individuals accustomed to wholesome food.

नहि सर्वाण्यपथ्यानि तुल्यदोषाणि, न च सर्वेदोषास्तुल्यबलाः, नचसर्वाणिशरीराणिव्याधिक्षमत्वेसमर्थानिभवन्ति|

Due to certain factors, even unwholesome food does not produce diseases immediately. All unwholesome foods are not equally bad: all Doshas are neither of equal strength, nor all bodies capable of resisting diseases equally.

तदेवह्यपथ्यं देश काल संयोग वीर्य प्रमाणातियोगाद्भूयस्तरमपथ्यंसम्पद्यते|

An unwholesome food article – Apathya is harmful (or not) depending upon the

Desha – nature of the locality,

Kala – season / time

Samyoga – combination

Veerya (potency) and

Pramana – quantity.

So, an unwholesome diet becomes more unwholesome, if taken in the wrong season, in the wrong place, with bad food combination, in improper quantity.

The Doshas become more acute and difficult-to-cure if they are combined with each other, if they require mutually contradictory therapies (for example, Kapha needs hot treatment but if it is associated with Pitta, then, Pitta needs cold treatment) if they are deep seated, if chronic, if vitiated in body parts where life is situated and if they afflict the vital organs.

People with obese or emaciated body, or having loose muscle, blood and bone tissues or weak or nourished with unwholesome food or accustomed to the intake of less food or having feeble mind, are unable to resist diseases. On the other hand, individuals having opposite types of physical constitution are capable of resisting diseases.

The intake of unwholesome food, as well as the Doshas and physical constitution of above description gives rise to diseases of many types, viz mild or severe and acute or chronic. The Doshas, viz, Vata, Pitta and Kapha give rise to various types of diseases depending upon the site of Dosha vitiation. [7]

तत्र रसादिषु स्थानेषु प्रकुपितानां दोषाणां यस्मिन् स्थाने ये ये व्याधयः सम्भवन्ति तांस्तान् यथावदनुव्याख्यास्यामः॥८॥

We shall now describe the various diseases which occurs in different sites (Dhatus) like Rasa due to the aggravation of the Doshas.[8]

**Rasa Pradoshaja Roga – Diseases due to vitiated Rasa Dhatu (the first essence part got after digestion process):**

अश्रद्धा चारुचिश्चास्यवैरस्यमरसज्ञता।

हल्लासो गौरवं तन्द्रा साङ्गमर्दो ज्वरस्तमः॥९॥

पाण्डुत्वं स्रोतसां रोधः क्लैब्यं सादः कृशाङ्गता।

नाशोऽग्नेरयथाकालं वलयः पलितानि च॥१०॥

रसप्रदोषजा रोगा,...।११।

Following diseases are caused by the vitiation of Rasadhatu.

Ashraddha – Disinclination for food,

Aruchi – anorexia

Asya Vairasya – foul taste in mouth

Arasanjnata – lack of taste sensing capacity

Hrullasa – nausea,

Gaurava – heaviness

Tandra – drowsiness, fatigue

Angamarda – Malaise, body ache

Jwara – fever

Tama – darkness in front of eyes

Pandutva – anaemia, pale discolouration of skin

Srotasam rodha – obstruction of body channels

Klaibya – impotency

Saada – heaviness of body, as if the body is struck and cannot function.

Krushangata – emaciation, shrunken body parts

Nasho Agnehe – loss of digestion strength

Ayatha Kala Vali Palita – premature wrinkling of skin and greying of hairs. [9-10]

**Rakta Pradoshaja Vyadhis – Diseases due to vitiated Blood tissue:**

...वक्ष्यन्ते रक्तदोषजाः।

कुष्ठवीसर्पपिडका रक्तपित्तमसृग्दरः॥११॥

गुदमेढ्रास्यपाकश्च प्लीहा गुल्मोऽथ विद्रधिः।

नीलिका कामला व्यङ्गः पिप्पलवस्तिलकालकाः॥१२॥

ददुश्चर्मदलं श्वित्रं पामा कोठासमण्डलम्|
रक्तप्रदोषाज्जायन्ते,...|१४|

Kushta – Skin diseases

Visarpa ( acute spreading diseases of the skin)

Pidaka – carbuncle, Pimples,

Raktapitta (a diseases characterized by bleeding from different parts of the body),

Asrugdhara – menorrhagia, heavy periods

Guda Medhra Paka – inflammation and suppuration in rectum and penis

Asya Paka – mouth ulcers,

Pleeha – Disease of the spleen, Splenomegaly

Gulma - Tumors of the abdomen

Vidradhi – Abscess

Neelika – blue moles,

Kaamala – Jaundice,

Vyanga (freckles),

Piplava (portwine mark),

Tilakaalaka (black mole),

Dadru – ringworm ,

Charmadala- dermatitis, skin tags

Shvitra – leukoderma,

Pama – papules,

Kotha (urticaria) and

Asra Mandala – red circular patches. [11-12]

**Mamsa Pradoshaja Vikara – Diseases causes by vitiated Muscle tissue:**

...शृणु मांसप्रदोषजान्||१३||
अधिमांसार्बुदं कीलं गलशालूकशुण्डिके|
पूतिमांसालजीगण्डगण्डमालोपजिह्विकाः||१४||
विद्यान्मांसाश्रयान्,...|१५|

Adhimamsa – Granuloma,

Arbuda – Myoma

Keela – Piles,

Gala Shalooka – Uvulitis,

Gala shundika – tonsillitis,

Pootimamsa – Sloughing of flesh,

Alaji – boils,

Ganda – goiter,

Gandamala – cervical adenitis

Upajihvika – inflammation of epiglottis. [13-14]

**Meda Pradoshaja Vikara – Diseases due to vitiation of fat tissue**

... मेदःसंश्रयांस्तु प्रचक्ष्महे|
निन्दितानि प्रमेहाणां पूर्वरूपाणि यानि च||१५||

Premonitory signs and symptoms of Prameha (Urinary tract disorders, diabetes mellitus). [15]

**Asthi Pradoshaja Vikara – Diseases caused by vitiated bone tissue:**

अध्यस्थिदन्तौ दन्तास्थिभेदशूलं विवर्णता|
केशलोमनखश्मश्रुदोषाश्चास्थिप्रदोषजाः||१६||

Adhyasthi – Hypertrophy of the bones

Adhi danta – excess teeth,

Dantabheda – cracking sensation in the teeth

Asthibheda, Shoola – crackling sensation and pain in bone,

Vivarnata – discoloration of hair

Deformity of hair of head, body hairs, nail as well as beard.[16]

**Majja Pradoshaja Vikara – Diseases due to vitiated bone marrow tissue:**

रुक् पर्वणां भ्रमो मूर्च्छा दर्शनं तमसस्तथा।

अरुषां स्थूलमूलानां पर्वजानां च दर्शनम्॥१७॥

मज्जप्रदोषात्, ...।१८।

Parva Ruk – Pain in small joints

Bhrama – Delusion, Dizziness

Murcha – fainting, loss of consciousness

Tamo Darshana – seeing darkness in front of eyes

Manifestation of deep-seated abscesses in joints [17]

**Shukra Pradoshaja Vikara – Diseases due to vitiated Semen / reproductive system:**

...शुक्रस्य दोषात् क्लैब्यमहर्षणम्।

रोगि वा क्लीबमल्पायुर्विरूपं वा प्रजायते॥१८॥

न चास्य जायते गर्भः पतति प्रसवत्यपि।

शुक्रं हि दुष्टं सापत्यं सदारं बाधते नरम्॥१९॥

Due to the vitiation of Shukra or semen the individual suffers from

Klaibya – impotent

Aharshana – lack of erection and enjoyment in sex

His progeny, if any, will be sick, sterile, short lived and disfigured.

Either there is no conception or there will be abortion or miscarriage. Thus the vitiation of Shukra (semen) brings misery to the couple and progeny. [18-19]

**Affection of Sense organs:**

इन्द्रियाणि समाश्रित्य प्रकुप्यन्ति यदा मलाः।

उपघातोपतापाभ्यां योजयन्तीन्द्रियाणि ते॥२०॥

**Affection of Sense organs:**

Sense organs are either totally or partially destroyed when Doshas get vitiated and lodge in them. [20]

**Affection of tendons and ligaments:**

स्नायौ सिराकण्डराभ्यो दुष्टाः क्लिश्नन्ति मानवम्।

स्तम्भसङ्कोचखल्लीभिर्ग्रन्थिस्फुरणसुप्तिभिः॥२१॥

**Affection of tendons and ligaments:**

Doshas when vitiated in tendons (Snayu), vessels (Sira) and ligaments (Kandara), they cause

Stambha – stiffness

Samkocha – contraction,

Khalli – neuralgia of the upper and lower extremities,

Granthi – tumour, fibroid

Sphurana – throbbing sensation and

Supti – numbness.[21]

**Vitiation of waste products:**

मलानाश्रित्य कुपिता भेदशोषप्रदूषणम्|

दोषा मलानां कुर्वन्ति सङ्गोत्सर्गावतीव च||२२||

When Doshas get vitiated in waste products, they cause

Bheda – dislodgement of stool,

Shoshana – drying up,

Pradushana – impairment

Sanga – absolute retention or

Utsarga – excessive elimination of these waste products [22]

**Treatment principle for management of diseases caused by Errors in Food:**

विविधादशितात् पीतादहिताल्लीढखादितात्|

भवन्त्येते मनुष्याणां विकारा य उदाहृताः||२३||

तेषामिच्छन्ननुत्पत्तिं सेवेत मतिमान् सदा|

हितान्येवाशितादीनि न स्युस्तज्जास्तथाऽऽमयाः||२४||

**Treatment principle for management of diseases caused by Errors in Food:**

Diseases enumerated for Dhatu (tissues), waste products (mala), ligaments, tendons etc are caused by the improper intake of food comprising eatables, beverages, lickable and foods which are masticated. One should always take wholesome food with a view to preventing the occurrence of such diseases.

**Rasa Dhatu treatment:**

ररसजानां विकाराणां सर्वं लङ्घनमौषधम्|

For diseases caused by bad foods, affecting Rasa Dhatu, Langhana treatment should be adopted (such as fasting, exercise etc. which brings about lightness to the body).

**Rakta Dhatu treatment:**

विधिशोणितिकेऽध्याये रक्तजानां भिषग्जितम्||२५||

Treatment of diseases caused by the vitiation of Rakta is described in the 24th chapter of Sutrasthana - Vidhi Shniteeya Adhyaya

**Mamsa Dhatu (muscle tissue) treatment:**

मांसजानां तु संशुद्धिः शस्त्रक्षाराग्निकर्म च|

For muscle tissue disorders,

Samshuddhi – Panchakarma purification treatment

Shastrakarma – surgery

Ksharakarma – application of Kshara (water insoluble ash of herbs)

Agnikarma – cautery treatment

**Medo Dhatu (fat tissue) treatment:**

अष्टौनिन्दितिकेऽध्याये मेदोजानां चिकित्सितम्||२६||

The fat tissue disorder treatment is explained 21st chapter of Sutrasthana - Asthau Ninditeeya Adhyaya.

**Asthi Dhatu (bone tissue) treatment:**

अस्थ्याश्रयाणां व्याधीनां पञ्चकर्माणि भेषजम्|

बस्त्यः क्षीरसर्पींषि तिक्तकोपहितानि च||२७||

For diseases of bone tissue, Panchakarma treatment especially Basti (enema) with milk, ghee and bitter herbs is useful.

**Majja (marrow) and Shukra Dhatu (reproductive system) treatment:**

मज्जशुक्रसमुत्थानामौषधं स्वादुतिक्तकम्|

अन्नं व्यवायव्यायामौ शुद्धिः काले च मात्रया||२८||

Majja and Shukra Dhatu diseases are treated with diets of sweet and bitter tastes, sexual intercourse, exercise and timely elimination of Doshas (Panchakarma) in proper quantity.

**For diseases of sensory organs**

शान्तिरिन्द्रियजानां तु त्रिमर्मीये प्रवक्ष्यते।
स्नाय्वादिजानां प्रशमो वक्ष्यते वातरोगिके||२९||
नवेगान्धारणेऽध्याये चिकित्सासङ्ग्रहः कृतः।
मलजानां विकाराणां सिद्धिश्चोक्ता क्वचित्क्वचित्||३०||

The treatment will be explained in detail in 26th chapter of Chikithsasthana (the sensation on the treatment of diseases). Treatment of diseases of ligaments etc. will be described in the chapter 28th of Chikithsasthana – Trimarmeeya Chikithsa Adhyaya.

Treatment of diseases of waste products, the line of treatment is already explained in 7th chapter of Sutrasthana - Na Vegan Dharaneeya Adhyaya [29-30]

**How do Doshas move from gastrointestinal tract to limbs?**

व्यायामादूष्मणस्तैक्ष्ण्यादिधतस्यानवचारणात्।
कोष्ठाच्छाखा मला यान्ति द्रुतत्वान्मारुतस्य च||३१||
तत्रस्थाश्च विलम्बन्ते कदाचिन्न समीरिताः।
नादेशकाले कुप्यन्ति भूयो हेतुप्रतीक्षिणः||३२||

**How do Doshas move from gastrointestinal tract to limbs?**

Due to Vyayama – exercise
Ushmana – excess heat, acuteness of the digestion, intake of excessive hot and spicy food,
Teekshna – intake of foods having piercing and strong nature
non-observation of wholesome regimen and
By the force and pressure of Vata,
The vitiated Doshas from the alimentary tract spread to the periphery – limbs, muscles, bones etc.
In the absence of any exciting cause, the vitiated Doshas at times remain in dormant stage till they meet with the causative factors at appropriate time, place for the manifestation of their effects. [31-32]

**Traction of Doshas from periphery to the alimentary tract:**

वृद्ध्या विष्यन्दनात् पाकात् स्रोतोमुखविशोधनात्।
शाखा मुक्त्वा मलाः कोष्ठं यान्ति वायोश्च निग्रहात्||३३||

Due to
Vruddhi – further aggravation,
Vishyandana – due to liquefication / increase in fluidity,
Paaka – due to suppuration,
removal of the obstructions in the channel of circulation (Srotas)
the vitiated Doshas leave the periphery and come to the alimentary tract. [33]

**Ideal approach:**

अजातानामनुत्पत्तौ जातानां विनिवृत्तये।
रोगाणां यो विधिर्दृष्टः सुखार्थी तं समाचरेत्||३४||

In order to prevent the unmanifested diseases and to cure the manifested ones, an individual desirous of happiness, should follow the regimen prescribed in this text.

सुखार्थाः सर्वभूतानां मताः सर्वाः प्रवृत्तयः।
ज्ञानाज्ञानविशेषात् मार्गामार्गप्रवृत्तयः||३५||

All the mental and physical activities of all the living beings are to achieve Sukha – happiness. A wise man follows the proper path. An ignorant one takes the unwholesome path. [34-35]

**Importance of following wholesome regimen:**

हितमेवानुरुध्यन्ते प्रपरीक्ष्य परीक्षकाः।

रजोमोहावृतात्मानः प्रियमेव तु लौकिकाः॥३६॥

**Importance of following wholesome regimen:**

The wise person observes wholesome regimen, after proper examination. The ignorant person, with his mind covered with Rajas (attraction) and Tamas (illusion) runs after an apparently pleasing regimen.

**How can a person avoid disease?**

श्रुतबुद्धिः स्मृतिर्दाक्ष्यं धृतिर्हित निषेवणम् |
वाग्विशुद्धिः शमो धैर्यमाश्रयन्ति परीक्षकम्॥३७॥
लौकिकं नाश्रयन्त्येते गुणामोहरजःश्रितम् |
तन्मूलाबहवोयन्तिरोगाःशारीरमानसाः॥३८॥

**How can a person avoid disease?**

The wise man is endowed with

Shruta – sound knowledge

Buddhi – intellect

Smruti – memory,

Daksha – skill, discipline

Dhruti – good retention power

Hita Nishevana – ability to stick to wholesome regimen,

Vak Vishuddhi – clarity in speech

Shama – tranquillity and

Dhairya – courage

Ignorant individuals being shrouded with illusion (Tamas) and Rajas (attraction) are deprived of those virtues and therefore, succumb to various disorders of body and mind. [37-38]


**Consequence of ignorance:**

प्रज्ञापराधाद्ध्यहितानर्थान् पञ्च निषेवते|
सन्धारयति वेगांश्च सेवते साहसानि च॥३९॥
तदात्वसुखसङ्गेषु भावेष्वज्ञोऽनुरज्यते|
रज्यते न तु विज्ञाता विज्ञाने ह्यमलीकृते॥४०॥


**Consequence of ignorance:**

Due to

Prajnaparadha – intellectual blasphemy, knowingly doing the wrong things,

Ahita Indriyartha Sannikarsha – the ignorant indulges in unwholesome gratification of five senses,

Vega Dharana – suppression of natural urges,

Saahasa – straining beyond one's capacity and

adoption of such regimes yields only temporary pleasure. But the wise do not indulge in them because of their clarity of vision. [39-40]

**Selection of food:**

न रागान्नाप्यविज्ञानादाहारानुपयोजयेत्|
परीक्ष्य हितमश्नीयाद्देहो ह्याहारसम्भवः॥४१॥

**Selection of food:**

The body is constituted of food hence one should take wholesome food only, after careful examination and should not indulge in unwholesome ones out of greed or ignorance.[41]

**Observation of eight factors:**

आहारस्य विधावष्टौ विशेषा हेतुसञ्ज्ञकाः|
शुभाशुभसमुत्पत्तौ तान् परीक्ष्य प्रयोजयेत्॥४२॥

There are eight factors (described in Vimana Sthana 1ˢᵗ chapter, in future) to be considered in dietetics. They are responsible for causing happiness or misery. These factors are to be examined before taking any food.[42]

**Need to observe wholesome rules:**

परिहार्याण्यपथ्यानि सदा परिहरन्नरः|
भवत्यनृणतां प्राप्तः साधूनामिह पण्डितः||४३||
यत्तु रोगसमुत्थानमशक्यमिह केनचित्|
परिहर्तुं न तत् प्राप्य शोचितव्यं मनीषिभिः||४४||

**Need to observe wholesome rules:**

The wise who always avoid the intake of unwholesome food are held in high esteem by saints. However, there are certain diseases which no one can avoid and in such events the wise need not worry. [43-44]

**Summing up the contents:**

तत्र श्लोकाः:-
आहारसम्भवं वस्तु रोगाश्चाहारसम्भवाः|
हिताहितविशेषाच्च विशेषः सुखदुःखयोः||४५||
सहत्वे चासहत्वे च दुःखानां देहसत्त्वयोः |
विशेषो रोगसङ्घाश्च धातुजा ये पृथक्पृथक्||४६||
तेषां चैव प्रशमनं कोष्ठाच्छाखा उपेत्य च|
दोषा यथा प्रकुप्यन्ति शाखाभ्यः कोष्ठमेत्य च||४७||
प्राज्ञाज्ञयोर्विशेषश्च स्वस्थातुरहितं च यत्|
विविधाशितपीतीये तत् सर्वं सम्प्रकाशितम्||४८||


**Summing up the contents:-**

How food causes health and disease, wholesome and unwholesome foods, being responsible for happiness and misery respectively, individuals who have immunity from and susceptibility to the various psychosomatic diseases, various diseases specific to each of the Dhatus (tissue elements), therapies for their cure, the method by which Doshas get vitiated and come to the periphery from the alimentary tract and vice versa, specific characteristics of wise and ignorant individuals, regime useful for healthy individuals as well as patients all these are described in this chapter – Vividha Ashita Peeteeya Adhyaya

इत्यग्निवेशकृते तन्त्रे चरकप्रतिसंस्कृते सूत्रस्थाने विविधाशितपीतीयो नामाष्टाविंशोऽध्यायः||२८|| इत्यन्नपानचतुष्कः||७||

Thus ends the 28ᵗʰ of Charaka Samhita Sutrasthana of Agnivesha's work as redacted by Charaka.[45]

This ends Annapana Chatushka.

# 29

# Sutrasthana Chapter 29 Dasha Prana Ayataneeyam

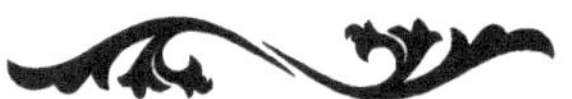

**Dasha Prana Ayataneeya Adhyaya**

**10 Abodes of Life**

अथातो दशप्राणायतनीयमध्यायं व्याख्यास्यामः||१||

इति ह स्माह भगवानात्रेयः||२||

The 29th chapter of Charaka Samhita Sutrasthana is called Dasha Praana Aayataneeya Adhyaya – 10 abodes of life. It explains about 10 vital places where life is situated in the body, qualities of good and bad physicians.

**Dasha Prana Aayatana – places where Prana (vital life energy) resides:**

दशैवायतनान्याहुः प्राणा येषु प्रतिष्ठिताः [१] |

शङ्खौ मर्मत्रयं कण्ठो रक्तं शुक्रौजसी गुदम्||३||

तानीन्द्रियाणि विज्ञानं चेतनाहेतुमामयान्|

जानीते यः स वै विद्वान् प्राणाभिसर उच्यते||४||

In the body, Prana – Vital life force resides in 10 places.

Shankhau – 2 Shankha places – temporal region

Marma Traya – Three Marmas - heart, urinary system and head

Kantha – Throat

Rakta – blood,

Shukra – reproductive system,

Ojas - immune system

Guda – rectum.

The wise physician who is well acquainted with these ten important abodes of life and knowledge about sense organs, intelligence, and soul, causes of diseases, treatment and signs and symptoms of diseases is known as the saviour of life – Praanaabhisara. [3-4]

**Two types of physicians – good and the bad:**

द्विविधास्तु खलु भिषजो भवन्त्यग्निवेश! प्राणानामेकेऽभिसरा हन्तारो रोगाणां, रोगाणामेकेऽभिसरा हन्तारः प्राणानामिति||५||

Oh! Agnivesha, there are two types of physicians.

Pranabhisara – who saves lives and kills diseases.

Rogabhisara – who worsen diseases and kill life. [5]

**Qualities of a good Ayurvedic physician:**

एवंवादिनं भगवन्तमात्रेयमग्निवेश उवाच- भगवंस्ते कथमस्माभिर्वेदितव्या भवेयुरिति||६||

भगवानुवाच- य इमे कुलीनाः पर्यवदातश्रुताः परिदृष्टकर्माणो दक्षाः शुचयो जितहस्ता जितात्मानः सर्वोपकरणवन्तः सर्वेन्द्रियोपपन्नाः प्रकृतिज्ञाः प्रतिपत्तिज्ञाश्च ते ज्ञेयाः प्राणानामभिसरा हन्तारो रोगाणां; तथाविधा हि केवले शरीरज्ञाने शरीराभिनिर्वृत्तिज्ञाने प्रकृतिविकारज्ञाने च निःसंशयाः, सुखसाध्यकृच्छ्रसाध्ययाप्यप्रत्याख्येयानां च रोगाणां समुत्थानपूर्वरूपलिङ्गवेदनोपशयविशेषज्ञाने व्यपगतसन्देहाः,

त्रिविधस्यायुर्वेदसूत्रस्य ससङ्ग्रहव्याकरणस्य सत्रिविधौषधग्रामस्य प्रवक्तारः, पञ्चत्रिंशतो मूलफलानां चतुर्णां च स्नेहानां पञ्चानां च लवणानामष्टानां च मूत्राणामष्टानां च क्षीराणां क्षीरत्वग्वृक्षाणां च षण्णां शिरोविरेचनादेश्च पञ्चकर्माश्रयस्यौषधगणस्याष्टाविंशतेश्च यवागूनां द्वात्रिंशतश्चूर्णप्रदेहानां षण्णं च विरेचनशतानां पञ्चानां च कषायशतानां प्रयोक्तारः, स्वस्थवृत्तविहितभोजनपाननियमस्थानचङ्क्रमणशयनासनमात्राद्रव्याञ्जनधूमनावनाभ्यञ्जन- परिमार्जनवेगाविधारणविधारणव्यायामसात्म्येन्द्रियपरीक्षोपक्रमणसद्वृत्तकुशलाः , चतुष्पादोपगृहीते च भेषजे षोडशकले सविनिश्चये सत्रिपर्येषणे सवातकलाकलज्ञाने व्यपगतसन्देहाः, चतुर्विधस्य च स्नेहस्य चतुर्विंशत्युपनयस्योपकल्पनीयस्य चतुःषष्टिपर्यन्तस्य च व्यवस्थापयितारः, बहुविधविधानयुक्तानां च स्नेह्यस्वेद्यवम्यविरेच्यविविधौषधोपचाराणां च कुशलाः, शिरोरोगादेर्दोषांश्विकल्पजस्य च व्याधिसङ्ग्रहस्य सक्षयपिडकाविद्रधेस्त्रयाणां च शोफानां बहुविधशोफानुबन्धानामष्टचत्वारिंशतश्च रोगाधिकरणानां चत्वारिंशदुत्तरस्य च नानात्मजस्य व्याधिशतस्य तथा विगर्हितातिस्थूलातिकृशानां सहेतुलक्षणोपक्रमाणां स्वप्नस्य च हिताहितस्यास्वप्नातिस्वप्नस्य च सहेतूपक्रमस्य षण्णां च लङ्घनादीनामुपक्रमाणां सन्तर्पणापतर्पणजानां च रोगाणां सरूपप्रशमनानां शोणितजानां च व्याधीनां मदमूर्च्छायासन्न्यासानां च सकारणरूपौषधोपचाराणां कुशलाः, कुशलाश्चाहारविधिविनिश्चयस्य प्रकृत्या हिताहितानामाहारविकाराणामग्र्यसङ्ग्रहस्यासवानां च चतुरशीतेर्द्रव्यगुणकर्मविनिश्चयस्य रसानुरससंश्रयस्य सविकल्पवैरोधिकस्य द्वादशवर्गाश्रयस्य चान्नपानस्य सगुणप्रभावस्य सानुपानगुणस्य नवविधस्यार्थसङ्ग्रहस्याहारगतेश्च हिताहितोपयोगविशेषात्मकस्य च शुभाशुभविशेषस्य धात्वाश्रयाणां च रोगाणां सौषधसङ्ग्रहाणां दशानां च प्राणायतनानां यं च वक्ष्याम्यर्थैर्दशमहामूलीये त्रिंशत्तमाध्याये तत्र च कृत्स्नस्य तन्त्रोद्देशलक्षणस्य तन्त्रस्य च ग्रहणधारणविज्ञानप्रयोगकर्मकार्यकालकर्तृकरणकुशलाः , कुशलाश्च स्मृतिमतिशास्त्रयुक्तिज्ञानस्यात्मनः शीलगुणैरविसंवादनेन च सम्पादनेन सर्वप्राणिषु चेतसो मैत्रस्य मातापितृभ्रातृबन्धुवत्, एवंयुक्ता भवन्त्यग्निवेश! प्राणानामभिसरा हन्तारो रोगाणामिति॥७॥

**Qualities of a good Ayurvedic physician:**

Agnivesha inquired from Lord Atreya, " How to recognize the two types of Physicians – the good and the bad.

Lord Atreya explained the qualities of a good physician.

Kuleena – Physicians who are born in Noble families,

Paryavadaata Shruta – who are well read,

Pari Drushta Karma – who have practical experience,

Daksha – disciplined, skilful,

Shuchi – clean, hygienic

Jitahasta – with expert hands

Jitaatmana – who have a very good self- control over mind

Sarva Upakaranavanta – having all the equipment

Sarvendriya Upapanna – have healthy sense organs,

Prakrutijna – who are acquainted with natural manifestations

Pratipattijna – who have presence of mind

The doctors with such qualities are Prana Abhisara Vaidya – saviours of life and destroyers of diseases.

Such physicians are well acquainted with the Anatomy and physiology of the entire body, manifestation and growth of the body and origin and aetiology, prodromal signs and symptoms, actual signs and symptoms as well as managements of diseases. They also can easily categorize patients as – easily curable, curable with difficulty palliable and incurable.

Such a physician will have sound knowledge of

1. Trisutra – Three principles of Ayurveda –

   1. Hetu – etiology,
   2. Linga – symptomatology and
   3. Prashamana – treatment

2. Sound knowledge of acronyms, formulae
3. Three sources of medicines: animal, mineral and plant

4.  35 types of roots and fruits: 4 types of fat; 5 types of salt, 8 types of wine, eight types of milk and six plants whose latest and bark are useful:

5.  Various types of drugs used in Panchakarma therapies

6.  28 types of gruel (Yavagu)

7.  32 types of powders and ointments

8.  600 types of purgatives

9.  500 types of decoction:

10. Knowledge of the factors responsible for the maintenance of positive health including diets, drug, regimen, residence, movement, sleep, rest, quantity, drugs, collieries, smoking, inhalation, unction, washing, non-suppression of body urges, suppression of mental urges. Physical exercise, wholesomeness for examining the sense organs;

11. Knowledge of the four aspects of therapeutics having sixteen factors:

12. Determination of nature of diseases

13. Three pursuits of life.

14. Various actions of Vata Dosha.

15. Four types of unctuous substances prepared according to twenty four methods with drugs of various tastes permutation and combination and which are of sixty four types

16. Various methods of preparation of drugs and therapies for oleation (Snehana), sweating (Svedana), emesis (Vamana) and purgation (Virechana)

17. Diseases of head etc

18. Summary of diseases caused by permutation and combination of various Doshas.

19. Ailments like Oja kshaya, carbuncle and abscess

20. These types of oedema and other diseases having swelling in one or the other part of the body

21. Forty eight types of diseases

22. One hundred forty types of diseases of Nanatmaja variety (diseases caused specifically by one Dosha)

23. Etiology , signs, symptoms and management of despicable individuals who are either very crapulent or emaciated

24. Useful and harmful nature of sleep, sleeplessness and excessive sleep along with their etiology and management

25. Six therapeutic measures like Langhana, Brumhana etc.,

26. Signs, symptoms and treatment of diseases due to over nourishment and

27. Under-nourishment diseases caused by vitiation of blood. Viz. intoxication, fainting and syncope along with their etiology, signs and symptoms and treatment by medicines and regimen

28. Rules of dietetics, food preparations which are wholesome and unwholesome by nature

29. The diets and regimen which are foremost in nature amongst their class

30. Forty types of alcoholic preparation

31. Determination of Dravya (matter) Guna (Quality), Karma (action) primary and secondary tastes,

32. Ingredients of food and drinks classified into twelve groups along with their properties

33. Properties of postprandial drink

34. Nine factors are required to be examined for determining the properties of food.

35. Digestive and metabolic processes

36. Various types of incompatible food ingredients

37. Good and till effects of wholesome and unwholesome food

38. Diseases caused by the vitiation of various tissue elements along with their treatment in brief

39. Ten resorts of life and other things which will be explained in the 30th chapter.

They understand the eight sections of Ayurveda (science of life) in their entirety along with the scope of the science. They have the power of grasping, retention and understanding of the text. They apply their knowledge so acquired for the treatment of diseases with a view to bringing the Dhatus to their normal state after determining the stage of the diseases, their own ability and the properties of the drugs employed. They are gifted with memory;

intelligence, theoretical and practical knowledge. They have cordial feelings towards other creatures. Doctors with such qualities give life to patients and cure their diseases. [6-7]

**A bad physician:**

अतो विपरीता रोगाणामभिसरा हन्तारः प्राणानां, भिषक्छद्मप्रतिच्छन्नाः कण्टकभूता लोकस्य प्रतिरूपकसधर्माणो राज्ञां प्रमादाच्चरन्ति राष्ट्राणि||८||

Opposite to this, are the pseudo- physicians who, instead of taking away the diseases, take away life itself like thorns, and move around the world due to the lack of vigilance on the part of the rulers. [8]

**Identification of a bad physician :**

तेषामिदं विशेषविज्ञानं भवति- अत्यर्थं वैद्यवेशेन श्लाघमाना विशिखान्तरमनुचरन्ति कर्मलोभात्, श्रुत्वा च कस्यचिदातुर्यमभितः परिपतन्ति, संश्रवणे चास्यात्मनो वैद्यगुणानुच्चैर्वदन्ति, यश्चास्य वैद्यः प्रतिकर्म करोति तस्य च दोषान्मुहुर्मुहुरुदाहरन्ति, आतुरमित्राणि च प्रहर्षणोपजापोपसेवादिभिरिच्छन्त्यात्मीकर्तुं, स्वल्पेच्छुतां चात्मनः ख्यापयन्ति, कर्म चासाद्य मुहुर्मुहुरवलोकयन्ति दाक्ष्येणाज्ञानमात्मनः प्रच्छादयितुकामाः, व्याधिं चापावर्तयितुमशक्नुवतो व्याधितमेवानुपकरणमपरिचारकमनात्मवन्तमुपदिशन्ति , अन्तगतं चैनमभिसमीक्ष्यान्यमाश्रयन्ति देशमपदेशमात्मनः कृत्वा, प्राकृतजनसन्निपाते चात्मनः कौशलमकुशलवद्वर्णयन्ति, अधीरवच्च धैर्यमपवदन्ति धीराणां, विद्वज्जनसन्निपातं (चाभिसमीक्ष्य) प्रतिभयमिव कान्तारमध्वगाः परिहरन्ति दूरात्, यश्चैषां कश्चित् सूत्रावयवो भवत्युपयुक्तस्तमप्रकृते प्रकृतान्तरे वा सततमुदाहरन्ति, न चानुयोगमिच्छन्त्यनुयोक्तुं वा, मृत्योरिव चानुयोगादुद्विजन्ते, न चैषामाचार्यः शिष्यः सब्रह्मचारी वैवादिको वा कश्चित् प्रज्ञायत इति||९||


**Identification of a bad physician :**

Too much self- praise.

They move about from one street to another in search of livelihood in the garb of physicians.

Once they hear about somebody's sickness, they would surround him and start listing their own qualities loudly so that the patient could listen to them.

In case a physician is already attending to him they try to find fault again and again with the attending physician.

They win over the friends of the patients by pleasing them, back- biting and flattering.

They propagate that they are interested in a nominal remuneration only.

After they succeed in winning over the patient, they look at him again and again skilfully trying to cover their ignorance.

If they are unable to alleviate the disease, they blame that the patient lacked proper equipment, attendance and self control.

As soon as the patient dies, they fly away to some other place in some other garb.

In the congregation of ordinary men they proclaim their ability in self- contradicting tones.

Like an impatient person they speak ill of the patience of courageous individuals.

In the event of their coming across a seminar of the wise, they immediately leave the place from the very distance as the travellers keep themselves away from the frightful forests.

In case they happen to have knowledge of some therapeutic formula, they will never hesitate in quoting them without caring for the relevance to the topic.

They do not relish any questions from others nor do they like to put any queries to others.

They get perturbed by the question as if attacked by death. Nobody would know anything about their preceptor, disciple, classmate or even their opponents [9]


भवन्ति चात्र-

भिषक्छद्म प्रविश्यैवं व्याधितांस्तर्कयन्ति ये|

वीतंसमिव संश्रित्य वने शाकुन्तिका द्विजान्||१०||

श्रुतदृष्टक्रियाकालमात्राज्ञानबहिष्कृताः|

वर्जनीया हि ते मृत्योश्चरन्त्यनुचरा भुवि||११||

वृत्तिहेतोर्भिषङ्मानपूर्णान् मूर्खविशारदान्|

वर्जयेदातुरो विद्वान् सर्पास्ते पीतमारुताः||१२||
ये तु शास्त्रविदो दक्षाः शुचयः कर्मकोविदाः|
जितहस्ता जितात्मानस्तेभ्यो नित्यं कृतं नमः||१३||

तत्र श्लोकः:-
दशप्राणायतनिके श्लोकस्थानार्थसङ्ग्रहः|
द्विविधा भिषजश्चोक्ताः प्राणस्यायतनानि च||१४||

Pseudo- physicians in the guise of doctors try to catch the patients as the bird- catchers catch their prey in the net. They are far away from the textual and practical experience, knowledge about the time of administering the therapy and its dosage. They are like the messengers of death on the earth; hence they should be boycotted.

A wise patient should avoid such egoistic dummy doctors, the worst among idiots who have taken to this profession only to earn livelihood. They are as dangerous as snakes satiated with the wind.
On the other hand, the real physicians well-versed in the science of medical knowledge and surgical operations and self- control deserve respect and honour. [10-13]

इत्यग्निवेशकृते तन्त्रे चरकप्रतिसंस्कृते श्लोकस्थाने दशप्राणायतनीयो नामोनत्रिंशोऽध्यायः||२९||
Thus, ends 29th chapter – Dasha Prana Ayataneeya Adhyaya, of Charaka Samhita Sutrasthana of Agnivesha's work as redacted by Charaka

# 30

# Sutrasthana Chapter 30 Arthe Dashamahamooleeyam

**Arthe Dasha Mahamuliya Adhyaya**
**Essence And Purpose of Ayurveda**

अथातोऽर्थेदशमहामूलीयमध्यायं व्याख्यास्यामः||१||

इति ह स्माह भगवानात्रेयः||२||

This chapter explains about the purpose of Ayurveda – the science of life, its eight branches, scope of Ayurveda, synonyms, how this science of life should be studied, and importance of heart, Ojas, Different sections and chapters of Charaka Samhita etc. This is the 30th Chapter of Charaka Samhita Sutrasthana, called Dasha Mahamooliya Adhyaya – the 10 vessels and their roots in heart.

**Heart, its synonyms and importance:**

अर्थे दश महामूलाः समासक्ता महाफलाः|

महच्चार्थश्च हृदयं पर्यायैरुच्यते बुधैः||३||

षडङ्गमङ्गं विज्ञानमिन्द्रियाण्यर्थपञ्चकम्|

आत्मा च सगुणश्चेतश्चिन्त्यं च हृदि संश्रितम्||४||

**Heart, its synonyms and importance:**

There are ten channels of great biological importance attached to the heart. The synonyms of heart are –
Mahat- big, of huge importance
Artha – means for life
Hrudaya
Shadanga – 6 parts of the body – 2 upper and lower limbs, trunk and head,
other viscera,
Vijnana – consciousness,
Indriya – 5 Sense organs (nose, tongue, eye, skin and ear)
Indriya Artha – objects of sense organs ( smell, taste, shape, touch, sound)
Atma – soul
Atma guna – qualities of soul – Iccha – desire, Dvesha – hatred, Sukha –happiness, Dukha – grief, Buddhi – intellect,
Prayatna – effort
Cheta and Chintya – mind and objects of the mind are all located in the heart. [3-4]

**Result of injury to heart:**

प्रतिष्ठार्थं हि भावानामेषां हृदयमिष्यते|

गोपानसीनामागार कर्णिकेवार्थचिन्तकैः||५||

"

तस्योपघातान्मूच्छयं भेदान्मरणमृच्छति|६|

As the central wooden grid supports the thatch, the heart supports all the factors explained above. Even a small injury to the heart result in

Murcha – fainting, loss of consciousness or

Marana – death. [5]


## Heart, the Seat of Ojas:

यद्धि तत् स्पर्शविज्ञानं धारि तत्त्र संश्रितम्||६||

तत् परस्यौजसः स्थानं तत्र चैतन्यसङ्ग्रहः|

हृदयं महदर्थश्च तस्मादुक्तं चिकित्सकैः ||७||


The heart is indispensable for all the normal mental and physical activities. In the heart, resides Para Ojas – the superior Ojas, which controls the mind. This is why; the physicians have designated the heart as 'Hridaya', 'Mahat' and 'Artha' [6-7]


## Vessels (channels) attached to the heart:

तेन मूलेन महता महामूला मता दश|

ओजोवहाः शरीरेऽस्मिन् विधम्यन्ते समन्ततः||८||

Attached to the heart are the ten vessels which carry Ojas and pulsate all over the body.[8]


## Ojas and its importance:

येनौजसावर्तयन्तिप्रीणिताःसर्वदेहिनः |

यद्तेसर्वभूतानांजीवितंनावतिष्ठते||९||

यत्सारमादौगर्भस्ययतद्गर्भरसाद्रसः |

संवर्तमानं हृदयंसमाविशतियत्पुरा ||१०||

यस्य नाशातुनाशोऽस्तिधारियद्धृदयाश्रितम् |

यच्छरीररसस्नेहःप्राणायत्रप्रतिष्ठिताः||११||

तत्फलाबहुधा वाताःफलन्तीव(ति) महाफलाः|१२|


## Ojas and its importance:

It is the Ojas which keeps all the living begins nourished and refreshed.

There can be no life without Ojas.

Ojas marks the beginning of the formation of embryos. It is the nourishing fluid from the embryo. It enters the heart right at the stage of the embryo's initial formation.

Loss of Ojas amounts to the loss of life itself.

It sustains life and is located in the heart.

It constitutes the essence of all the Dhatus (tissues).

The Elan Vital owes its existence to it. But all this action of Ojas manifests itself in different ways, by flowing through the 10 vessels (channels) attached to it. Hence, these 10 channels attached to the heart are also very important. [9-11]


## Definition of Dhamani (artery), Srotas (channels) and Sira (veins)

ध्मानाद्धमन्यः स्रवणात् स्रोतांसि सरणात्सिराः||१२||


Dhmyanaat Dhamanyaha – because of pulsation, some channels of the body are called as Dhamani – arteries

Sravaraat srotamsi – because of transudation, movement of fluids inside some channels, they are called Srotas.

Saranaat sira – due to sarana – simple movement, some channels are called as Sira. [12]

## Tips for preservation of Ojas:

*तन्महत्ता महामूलास्तच्चोजः परिरक्षता|*
*परिहार्या विशेषेण मनसो दुःखहेतवः||१३||*
*हृदयं यत् स्याद्यदौजस्यं स्रोतसां यत् प्रसादनम्|*
*तत्तत् सेव्यं प्रयत्नेन प्रशमो ज्ञानमेव च||१४||*

## Tips for preservation of Ojas:

Those who want to preserve / protect Ojas and maintain heart and the vessels in good condition, should avoid such factors that lead to unhappiness (worries, stress).
Diets and medicine which are conducive to the heart (Hrudya), ojas and body channels should be taken.
The herbs that maintain good health of Srotas (body channels) should be taken. [13-14]

## Desirable habits:

*अथ खल्वेकं प्राणवर्धनानामुत्कृष्टतममेकं बलवर्धनानामेकं बृंहणानामेकं नन्दनानामेकं हर्षणानामेकमयनानामिति |*
*तत्राहिंसा प्राणिनां प्राणवर्धनानामुत्कृष्टतमं, वीर्यं बलवर्धनानाम्, विद्या बृंहणानाम्, इन्द्रियजयो नन्दनानां, तत्त्वावबोधो हर्षणानां,*
*ब्रह्मचर्यमयनानामिति ; एवमायुर्वेदविदो मन्यन्ते||१५||*

## Desirable habits:

According to Ayurveda, the foremost factors to promote longevity, nourishment, delightfulness and happiness and lead to salvation are -
*तत्राहिंसा प्राणिनां प्राणवर्धनानामुत्कृष्टतमं,*
tatrāhiṃsā prāṇināṃ prāṇavardhanānāṃ utkṛṣṭatamaṃ, - Non-violence is the best tool to improve life quality and expectancy.
Veeryam balavardhananam – potency and courage are the best tools to improve strength and immunity
Vidya Brumahanaanam – knowledge is the best promoter of nourishment
Indriyajayo nandanaanaam – control over sense organs is the best tool for rejoicing.
Tatva Avabhodo harshanaanaam – self-realization / self-awareness is the best tool for happiness
Brahmacharyam ayanaanaan – Celibacy is the best tool for salvation. [15]

## Proper study of Ayurveda:

*तत्रायुर्वेदविदस्तन्त्रस्थानाध्यायप्रश्नानां पृथक्त्वेन वाक्यशो वाक्यार्थशोऽर्थावयवशश्च प्रवक्तारो मन्तव्याः|*
*तत्राह- कथं तन्त्रादीनि वाक्यशो वाक्यार्थशोऽर्थावयवशश्चोक्तानि भवन्तीति||१६||*
*अत्रोच्यते- तन्त्रमार्षं कात्स्न्र्येन यथाम्नायमुच्यमानं वाक्यशो भवत्युक्तम्||१७||*
*बुद्ध्या सम्यगनुप्रविश्यार्थतत्त्वं वाग्भिर्व्यासससमासप्रतिज्ञाहेतूदाहरणोपनयनिगमनयुक्ताभिस्त्रिविधशिष्यबुद्धिगम्याभिरुच्यमानं वाक्यार्थशो भवत्युक्तम्||१८||*
*तन्त्रनियतानामर्थदुर्गाणां पुनर्विभावनैरुक्तमर्थावयवशो भवत्युक्तम्||१९||*

## Proper study of Ayurveda:

Ayurvedic scholars should be in a position to explain clearly, the whole textbook, its different sections, chapters and specific topics in each chapter. They should be able to faithfully recite the contents of the text, interpret them and give their gist. How could this be done?
The entire text transmitted through the sages is to be recited in the appropriate order. After proper understanding, the meanings underlying the text are to be interpreted with due regard to the principles of elaboration, contraction, thesis, reasoning, exemplification, correlation and conclusion, understandable to all the three- superior, inferior and modest types of disciples. The concepts difficult to grasp from the text are to be clarified again and again so that a clear picture of the context is understood. [17-19]

**Ayurveda, source and scope:**

तत्र चेत् प्रष्टारः स्युः- चतुर्णामृक्सामयजुरथर्ववेदानां कं वेदमुपदिशन्त्यायुर्वेदविदः? किमायुः?, कस्मादायुर्वेदः?, किमर्थमायुर्वेदः?, शाश्वतोऽशाश्वतो वा?, कति कानि चास्याङ्गानि?, कैश्चायमध्येतव्यः?, किमर्थं च? इति||२०||

**Ayurveda, source and scope:**

Again the question arises – out of the four Vedas – Rigveda, Samaveda, Yajurveda and Atharvaveda – which Veda(s) should Ayurvedic scholars follow? What is Ayu – lifespan? Why is it called Ayurveda? What is the object of Ayurveda? Is it eternal or ephemeral? What are its branches and how many are they? Who is eligible to study it and what for? [20]

**Source of Ayurveda:**

तत्र भिषजा पृष्टेनैवं चतुर्णामृक्सामयजुरथर्ववेदानामात्मनोऽथर्ववेदे भक्तिरादेश्या, वेदो ह्याथर्वणो दान स्वस्त्ययन बलि मङ्गल होम नियम प्रायश्चित्तोपवासमन्त्रादिपरिग्रहाच्चिकित्सां प्राह; चिकित्सा चायुषो हितायोपदिश्यते||२१||

Of the four Vedas, Ayurvedic doctors owe their loyalty to the Atharva Veda, because this deals with the worship, auspicious observances, oblations, observance of spiritual rules, atonement, fast, incantations etc. they are prescribed for the sake of longevity. [21]

**Definition of Ayu:**

वेदं चोपदिश्यायुर्वाच्यं [१] ; तत्रायुश्चेतनानुवृत्तिर्जीवितमनुबन्धो धारि चेत्येकोऽर्थः||२२||

After instructions about the Veda, various aspects of the life span are to be described.

Ayu – Life span is nothing but the continuation of consciousness, the act of keeping alive, Anubandha (which keeps the soul bonded to the body) and Dhari (one that holds the body and life together).

So, Anubandha and Dhari are synonyms of Ayu. [22]

**Definition of Ayurveda:**

तदायुर्वेदयतीत्यायुर्वेदः; कथमितिचेत्? उच्यते- स्वलक्षणतः सुखासुखतो हिताहिततः प्रमाणाप्रमाणतश्च; यतश्चायुष्याण्यनायुष्याणि च द्रव्यगुण कर्माणि वेदयत्यतोऽप्यायुर्वेदः|

तत्रायुष्याण्यनायुष्याणि च द्रव्यगुण कर्माणि केवलेनोपदेक्ष्यन्ते तन्त्रेण||२३||

The science which imparts knowledge about life, with special reference to its definition, and the description of happy and unhappy life, useful and harmful life, long and short spans of life promote and demote longevity, which explains medicine, its qualities and functions is called Ayurveda. It will be described in the entire treatise.[23]

**Happy life and unhappy life- Hitayu and Ahitayu:**

तत्रायुरुक्तं स्वलक्षणतो यथावदिहैव पूर्वाध्याये च|

तत्र शारीरमानसाभ्यां रोगाभ्यामनभिद्रुतस्य विशेषेण यौवनवतः समर्थानुगतबलवीर्ययशःपौरुषपराक्रमस्य ज्ञानविज्ञानेन्द्रियेन्द्रियार्थबलसमुदये वर्तमानस्य परमर्द्धिरुचिरविविधोपभोगस्य समृद्धसर्वारम्भस्य यथेष्टविचारिणः सुखमायुरुच्यते; असुखमतो विपर्ययेण; हितैषिणः पुनर्भूतानां परस्वादुपरतस्य सत्यवादिनः शमपरस्य परीक्ष्यकारिणोऽप्रमत्तस्य त्रिवर्ग परस्परेणानुपहतमुपसेवमानस्य पूजार्हसम्पूजकस्य ज्ञानविज्ञानोपशमशीलस्य वृद्धोपसेविनः सुनियतरागरोषेष्यर्म्यादमानवेगस्य सततं विविधप्रदानपरस्य तपोज्ञानप्रशमनित्यस्याध्यात्मविदस्तत्परस्य लोकमिमं चामुं चावेक्षमाणस्य स्मृतिमतिमतो हितमायुरुच्यते; अहितमतो विपर्ययेण||२४||

**Happy life and unhappy life- Hitayu and Ahitayu:**

In this chapter as well as in the first chapter of this section life has been defined.

Those who are not afflicted with physical and mental ailments, who are endowed with youth, enthusiasm, strength, virility, success, manliness, boldness, special knowledge of arts and sciences, senses organs, their objects and ability, riches and various luxurious articles for enjoyment, who achieve what even they want and move as they like, lead a happy life. Others lead an unhappy life.

Those who are the well-wishers of all creatures, who do not aspire for the wealth of others, who are truthful, who love peace, who examine things before acting upon them, who are vigilant, who enjoy the three important desires of life viz, virtue, wealth and pleasure without the one affecting the other, who respect seniors, who are endowed with elders, who are endowed with the knowledge of arts, sciences and tranquillity, who serve the elders, who have full control over passion, anger, envy, pride and prestige, who are constantly given to various types of charity, meditation, acquisition of knowledge and solitude, who make efforts both for the existing as well as the next life and are endowed with memory and intelligence, lead a useful life. Others do not. [24]

## Determination of life span – Ayu Pramana:

प्रमाणमायुषस्त्वर्थेन्द्रियमनोबुद्धिचेष्टादीनां विकृतिलक्षणैरुपलभ्यतेऽनिमित्तैः, अयमस्मात् क्षणान्मुहूर्तादिदिवसात् त्रिपञ्चसप्तदशद्वादशाहात् पक्षान्मासात् षण्मासात् संवत्सराद्वा स्वभावमापत्स्यत इति; तत्र स्वभावः प्रवृत्तेरुपरमो मरणमनित्यता निरोध इत्येकोऽर्थः; इत्यायुषः प्रमाणम्; अतो विपरीतमप्रमाणमरिष्टाधिकारे; देहप्रकृतिलक्षणमधिकृत्य चोपदिष्टमायुषः प्रमाणमायुर्वेदे ||२५||

## Determination of life span – Ayu Pramana:

The limitation of the span of life is known from the sudden abnormal change in the sense organs and the reception of their objects in the mind, intellect and general movement. They help in the prediction of the death of an individual after a particular moment, time or day, after three, five, and seven or ten days and after a fortnight, a month, six months or a year.

Svabhava (reversion to the original state), Uparama of Pravritti (decrease in activities), Marana (death), Anityata (not-permanent state) Nirodha (obstruction in the continuity of living process) – all these are synonymous for death. This is about the limited span of life. In the absence of such signs and symptoms, the span of life is to be determined as unlimited from the point of view of prognosis.

In Ayurveda, the span of life is described to be determined by special signs.

## Purpose of Ayurveda :

प्रयोजनं चास्य स्वस्थस्य स्वास्थ्यरक्षणमातुरस्य विकार प्रशमनंच||२६||

The utility of this science is to help maintain the health of a healthy individual and cure the disease of the patient. [25-26]

## Eternity of Ayurveda:

सोऽयमायुर्वेदःशाश्वतोनिर्दिश्यते, अनादित्वात्, स्वभावसंसिद्धलक्षणत्वात्, भावस्वभावनित्यत्वाच्च|

Ayurveda or the science of life is eternal because of the following:

Anaditvaat – Ayurveda has no beginning

Svabhava Samsidda lakshanatvaat – It deals with things that are inherent in Nature; and

Bhava Svabhava nityatvaat – Such natural manifestations are eternal.

There is no discontinuity either in the living process or in the knowledge of things. Knowledge of various factors relating to the science of life is eternal.

सद्रव्यहेतुलक्षणमपरापरयोगात्|

एष चार्थसङ्ग्रहो विभाव्यते आयुर्वेदलक्षणमिति|

गुरुलघुशीतोष्णस्निग्धरूक्षादीनां द्रव्याणां सामान्यविशेषाभ्यां वृद्धिह्रासौ, यथोक्तं- गुरुभिरभ्यस्यमानैर्गुरूणामुपचयो भवत्यपचयो लघूनां, एवमेवेतरेषामिति, एष भावस्वभावो नित्यः, स्वलक्षणं च द्रव्याणां पृथिव्यादीनां; सन्ति तु द्रव्याणि गुणाश्च नित्यानित्याः|

न ह्यायुर्वेदस्याभूत्वोत्पत्तिरुपलभ्यते, अन्यत्रावबोधोपदेशाभ्याम्; एतद्वै द्वयमधिकृत्योत्पत्तिमुपदिशन्त्येके|

स्वाभाविकं चास्य लक्षणमकृतं, यदुक्तमिहाद्येऽध्याये च; यथा- अग्नेरौष्ण्यम्, अपां द्रवत्वम्|

भावस्वभावनित्यत्वमपि चास्य, यथोक्तं- गुरुभिरभ्यस्यमानैर्गुरूणामुपचयो भवत्यपचयो लघूनामिति||२७||

The knowledge of happiness (good health) and unhappiness (ill health) along with their etiology, symptomatology and therapeutics has a continuity and is without any beginning. This is exactly described in the Ayurveda. Substances having properties live heaviness, lightness, cold, heat, unctuousness etc. get increased when other substances having similar properties are added; Substances having dissimilar qualities, on the other hand decrease their quantity. E.g., habitual intake of heavy things increases the heavy factors and decreases the lightness in the body. Similar is the case with other qualities. This is the eternity of natural manifestations.

Origin of Ayurveda is not available. It is not known if ever Ayurveda was non-existent at any time after which it was propagated. Like the heat of the fire and liquidity of water, the Ayurveda or the science of life is innate and it does not involve any artificiality (effort of Mortals). This is what is described in this chapter as well as in the first chapter of Sutrasthana [27]

### The eight branches of Ayurveda:

तस्यायुर्वेदस्याङ्गान्यष्टौ; तद्यथा- कायचिकित्सा, शालाक्यं, शल्यापहर्तृकं, विषगरवैरोधिकप्रशमनं, भूतविद्या, कौमारभृत्यकं, रसायनं, वाजीकरणमिति||२८||

### Ayurveda has eight branches viz.

Kayachikitsa – Internal medicine

Shalakya – Science of diseases specific to supra- clavicle region, eye , ear nose, mouth, throat etc

Shalya – Surgery

Visha, Gara Chikitsa – Toxicology

Bhuta Chikitsa – science of demonic seizures(Psychology, psychiatry)

Kaumara Bhrutya – Paediatrics

Rasayana – Science of rejuvenation, anti-aging treatment

Vajikarana – Science of aphrodisiacs.[28]

### Role of Ayurveda: To whom is it beneficial?

स चाध्येतव्यो ब्राह्मणराजन्यवैश्यैः|

तत्रानुग्रहार्थं प्राणिनां ब्राह्मणैः, आरक्षार्थं राजन्यैः, वृत्त्यर्थं वैश्यैः; सामान्यतो वा धर्मार्थकामपरिग्रहार्थं सर्वैः|

तत्र यदध्यात्मविदां धर्मपथस्थानां धर्मप्रकाशकानां वा मातृपितृभ्रातृबन्धुगुरुजनस्य वा विकारप्रशमने प्रयत्नवान् भवति, यच्चायुर्वेदोक्तमध्यात्ममनुध्यायति वेदयत्यनुविधीयते वा, सोऽस्य परो धर्मः; या पुनरीश्वराणां वसुमतां वा सकाशात् सुखोपहारनिमित्ता भवत्यर्थावाप्तिरारक्षणं च, या च स्वपरिगृहीतानां प्राणिनामातुर्यादारक्षा, सोऽस्यार्थः; यत् पुनरस्य विद्वद्ग्रहणयशः शरण्यत्वं च, या च सम्मानशुश्रूषा, यच्चेष्टानां विषयाणामारोग्यमाधत्ते सोऽस्य कामः|

इति यथाप्रश्नमुक्तमशेषेण||२९||

### Role of Ayurveda: To whom is it beneficial?

Ayurveda is suitable for Brahmanas (priests) for providing benefits to all creatures.

It is suitable for Kshatriyas (warriors) for protection and for Vaishyas (business people) livelihood. In general, Ayurveda can be studied by all for the attainment of virtues, wealth and pleasure. Virtues are attained by treating individuals who have spiritual knowledge, who practise and propagate righteousness and others like mother; father, brother, friends, and superiors. These are also achieved by spiritual knowledge contained in the science of life. With a view to leading a comfortable life, one can earn wealth and protection by treating kings and other wealthy individuals. He can also protect his subordinates and servants by this science. He draws pleasure by the respect shown to him by learned people, by his ability to protect others, by the prestige and obligation and by keeping his beloved ones like wife. Free from diseases.

Thus all the queries are answered in their entirety.[29]

**Mutual scholarly discussion:**

अथ भिषगादित एव भिषजा प्रष्टव्योऽष्टविधं भवति- तन्त्रं, तन्त्रार्थान्, स्थानं, स्थानार्थान्, अध्यायम्, अध्यायार्थान्, प्रश्नं, प्रश्नार्थाश्चेति; पृष्टेन चैतद्वक्तव्यमशेषेण वाक्यशो वाक्यार्थशोऽर्थावयवशश्चेति ||३०||

**Mutual scholarly discussion:**

One physician can examine the knowledge of the other physician by asking questions related to the below mentioned eight aspects –

Tantra – treatise,

Tantra Artha – scope of treatise,

Sthana – sections of treatise

Sthana artha – scope / meaning of sections

Adhyaya – chapters

Adhyaya Artha – scope of chapters

Prashna – topics

Prashnartha – scope of topics.

Being put to such questions, a physician should recite the textual data, interpret them and give the gist in their entirety.[30]

**Synonymous of Ayurveda and its scope:**

तत्रायुर्वेदः शाखा विद्या सूत्रं ज्ञानं शास्त्रं लक्षणं तन्त्रमित्यनर्थान्तरम् ||३१||

Shakha – having branches,

Vidya -knowledge,

Sutra – things explained in the form of formula,

Jnana – knowledge,

Lakshana – explains the features of good and bad life and

Tantra – treatises is synonymous with the Ayurveda.

**The scope of this science**

स चार्थः प्रकरणैर्विभाव्यमानो भूय एव शरीरवृत्तिहेतुव्याधिकर्मकार्यकालकर्तृकरणविधिविनिश्चयाद्दशप्रकरणः, तानि च प्रकरणानि केवलेनोपदेक्ष्यन्ते तन्त्रेण||३२||

The scope of this science has already been explained in its definition. Various topics discussed in this science are

1. Anatomy
2. Physiology
3. Etiology
4. Pathology
5. Therapeutics
6. Achievement of good health
7. Climatology including the stage of the disease.
8. Physicians
9. Therapies including wholesome locality and
10. Procedure. Descriptions of these topics are spread over the entire treatise. [31-32]

**Divisions of the treatise:**

तन्त्रस्यास्याष्टौ स्थानानि; तद्यथा- श्लोकनिदानविमानशारीरेन्द्रियचिकित्सितकल्पसिद्धिस्थानानि|
तत्र त्रिंशदध्यायकं श्लोकस्थानम्, अष्टाष्टाध्यायकानि निदानविमानशारीरस्थानानि, द्वादशकमिन्द्रियाणां, त्रिंशकं चिकित्सितानां, द्वादशके कल्पसिद्धिस्थाने भवतः||३३||

**The following are the eight sections of sections of the treatise:**

1. Slokasthana / Sutrasthana the section on general principles having thirty chapters.
2. Nidanasthana or the section on diagnosis of diseases having eight chapters;
3. Vimanasthana or the section on specific determination of drugs etc, havig eight chapter
4. Sarirasthana or the section on anatomy including embroyology having eight chapters.
5. Cikitsthana or the section on therapeutics having thirty chapters
6. Indriyasthana or the section on prognostic signs having twelve chapters.
7. Kalpasthana or the section on pharmaceutics having twelve chapters
8. Siddhisthana or the section on the successful administration of Pancakarma (five elimination therapies) having twelve chapters. [33]

भवति चात्र-
द्वे त्रिंशके द्वादशकं त्रयं च त्रीण्यष्टकान्येषु समाप्तिरुक्ता|
श्लोकौषधारिष्टविकल्पसिद्धिनिदानमानाश्रयसङ्ग्रकेषु||३४||
स्वे स्वे स्थाने यथास्वं च स्थानार्थ उपदेक्ष्यते|
सविंशमध्यायशतं शृणु नामक्रमागतम्||३५||

In brief:
Thus it is said:
Sutra and Chikitsa sthana have thirty chapters each,
Indriya, Kapha and Siddhi sections have twelve chapters each, and
Nidana, Vimana and Sharira Sections have eight chapters each. This is about the entire treatise.[34]
The scope of each section is described in respective places (sections) in the order of their occurrence, the names of one hundred twenty chapters are given below: -[35]

**The chapter names of all the entire Charaka Samhita are enlisted.**
दीर्घञ्जीवोऽप्यपामार्गतण्डुलारग्वधादिकौ|
षड्विरेकाश्रयश्चेति चतुष्को भेषजाश्रयः||३६||
मात्रातस्याशितीयौ च नवेगान्धारणं तथा|
इन्द्रियोपक्रमश्चेति चत्वारः स्वास्थ्यवृत्तिकाः ||३७||
खुड्डाकश्च चतुष्पादो महांस्त्रिस्रैषणस्तथा|
सह वातकलाख्येन विद्यान्नैर्देशिकान् बुधः||३८||
स्नेहनस्वेदनाध्यायावुभौ यश्चोपकल्पनः|
चिकित्साप्राभृतश्चैव सर्व एव प्रकल्पनाः||३९||
कियन्तःशिरसीयश्च त्रिशोफाष्टोदरादिकौ|
रोगाध्यायो महांश्चैव रोगाध्यायचतुष्टयम्||४०||
अष्टौनिन्दितसङ्ख्यातस्तथा लङ्घनतर्पणे|
विधिशोणितिकश्चैव व्याख्यातास्तत्र योजनाः||४१||
यज्जःपुरुषसङ्ख्यातो भद्रकाप्यान्नपानिकौ|
विविधाशितपीतीयश्चत्वारोऽन्नविनिश्चयाः||४२||
दशप्राणायतनिकस्तथाऽर्धदशमूलिकः|
द्वावेतौ प्राणदेहार्थौ प्रोक्तौ वैद्यगुणाश्रयौ||४३||
औषधस्वस्थनिर्देशकल्पनारोगयोजनाः|
चतुष्काः षट् क्रमेणोक्ताः सप्तमश्चान्नपानिकः||४४||

द्वौ चान्त्यौ सङ्ग्रहाध्यायाविति त्रिंशकमर्थवत्|
श्लोकस्थानं समुद्दिष्टं तन्त्रस्यास्य शिरः शुभम्||४५||
चतुष्काणां महार्थानां स्थानेऽस्मिन् सङ्ग्रहः कृतः|
श्लोकार्थः सङ्ग्रहार्थश्च श्लोकस्थानमतः स्मृतम्||४६||
ज्वराणां रक्तपित्तस्य गुल्मानां मेहकुष्ठयोः|
शोषोन्मादनिदाने च स्यादपस्मारिणां च यत्||४७||
इत्यध्यायाष्टकमिदं निदानस्थानमुच्यते|
रसेषु त्रिविधे कुक्षौ ध्वंसे जनपदस्य च||४८||
त्रिविधे रोगविज्ञाने स्रोतःस्वपि च वर्तने|
रोगानीके व्याधिरूपे रोगाणां च भिषग्जिते||४९||
अष्टौ विमानान्युक्तानि मानार्थानि महर्षिणा|
कतिधापुरुषीयं च गोत्रेणातुल्यमेव च||५०||
खुड्डिका महती चैव गर्भावक्रान्तिरुच्यते|
पुरुषस्य शरीरस्य विचयौ द्वौ विनिश्चितौ||५१||
शरीरसङ्ख्या सूत्रं च जातेरष्टममुच्यते |
इत्युद्दिष्टानि मुनिना शारीराण्यत्रिसूनुना||५२||
वर्णस्वरीयः पुष्पाख्यस्तृतीयः परिमर्शनः|
चतुर्थ इन्द्रियानीकः पञ्चमः पूर्वरूपिकः||५३||
कतमानिशरीरीयः पन्नरूपोऽप्यवाक्शिराः|
यस्यश्यावनिमित्तश्च सद्योमरण एव च||५४||
अणुज्योतिरिति ख्यातस्तथा गोमयचूर्णवान्|
द्वादशाध्यायकं स्थानमिन्द्रियाणामिति स्मृतम्||५५||
अभयामलकीयं च प्राणकामीयमेव च|
करप्रचितकं वेदसमुत्थानं रसायनम्||५६||
संयोगशरमूलीयमासिक्तक्षीरकं तथा|
माषपर्णभृतीयं च पुमाञ्जातबलादिकम्||५७||
चतुष्कद्वयमप्येतदध्यायद्वयमुच्यते|
रसायनमिति ज्ञेयं वाजीकरणमेव च||५८||
ज्वराणां रक्तपित्तस्य गुल्मानां मेहकुष्ठयोः|
शोषोन्मादेऽप्यपस्मारे क्षतशोथोदरार्शसाम्||५९||
ग्रहणीपाण्डुरोगाणां श्वासकासातिसारिणाम्|
छर्दिवीसर्पतृष्णानां विषमद्यविकारयोः||६०||
द्विव्रणीयं त्रिमर्मीयमूरुस्तम्भिकमेव च|
वातरोगे वातरक्ते योनिव्यापत्सु चैव यत्||६१||
त्रिंशच्चिकित्सितान्युक्तान्यतः कल्पान् प्रचक्ष्महे|
फलजीमूतकेक्ष्वाकुकल्पो धामार्गवस्य च||६२||
पञ्चमो वत्सकस्योक्तः षष्ठश्च कृतवेधने|
श्यामात्रिवृतयोः कल्पस्तथैव चतुरङ्गुले||६३||
तिल्वकस्य सुधायाश्च सप्तलाशङ्खिनीषु च|
दन्तीद्रवन्त्योः कल्पश्च द्वादशोऽयं समाप्यते||६४||
कल्पना पञ्चकर्माख्या बस्तिसूत्री तथैव च|
स्नेहव्यापदिकी सिद्धिर्नेत्रव्यापदिकी तथा||६५||
सिद्धिः शोधनयोश्चैव बस्तिसिद्धिस्तथैव च|
प्रासृती मर्मसङ्ख्याता सिद्धिर्बस्त्याश्रया च या||६६||

फलमात्रा तथा सिद्धिः सिद्धिश्चोतरसञ्ज्ञिता|
सिद्धयो द्वादशैवैतास्तन्त्रं चासु समाप्यते||६७||
स्वे स्वे स्थाने तथाऽध्याये चाध्यायार्थः प्रवक्ष्यते|
तं ब्रूयात् सर्वतः सर्वं यथास्वं ह्यर्थसङ्ग्रहात्||६८||

**The names of all the chapters of the entire Charaka Samhita are enlisted –**
The first 28 chapters are grouped into four chapters each – called chatushka.
The first set four chapters are grouped as – Bheshaja chatushka – explaining about medicines
The second set of four chapters are grouped as – Swaasthya chatushka – explaining about health
The third set of four chapters are grouped as – Nirdesha chatushka – explaining about directions for good health
The fourth set of four chapters are grouped as – Kalpana chatushka – explaining about medicine making
The fifth set of four chapters are grouped as – Roga chatushka – explaining about diseases
The sixth set of four chapters are grouped as – Yojana chatushka – explaining about planning of treatment
The seventh set of four chapters are grouped as – Annapana chatushka – explaining about dietetics.
The last two chapters are grouped as – Sangraha dvaya deal with the resorts of life and qualities of physicians. [36-43]

**Sub classification of Sutrasthana:**
औषधस्वस्थनिर्देशकल्पनारोगयोजनाः|
चतुष्काः षट् क्रमेणोक्ताः सप्तमश्चान्नपानिकः||४४||
द्वौ चान्त्यौ सङ्ग्रहाध्यायाविति त्रिंशकमर्थवत्|
Thus, the first section of thirty chapters is very important. In fact, it serves as the brain of the whole treatise. In this section quadrates of great importance are collected. Because of the compilation of fundamental principles concerning various aspects of the Ayurveda, this is known as the "Shloka" section [44]

श्लोकस्थानं समुद्दिष्टं तन्त्रस्यास्य शिरः शुभम्||४५||
चतुष्काणां महार्थानां स्थानेऽस्मिन् सङ्ग्रहः कृतः|
श्लोकार्थः सङ्ग्रहार्थश्च श्लोकस्थानमतः स्मृतम्||४६||
ज्वराणां रक्तपित्तस्य गुल्मानां मेहकुष्ठयोः|
शोषोन्मादनिदाने च स्यादपस्मारिणां च यत्||४७||
इत्यध्यायाष्टकमिदं निदानस्थानमुच्यते|
रसेषु त्रिविधे कुक्षौ ध्वंसे जनपदस्य च||४८||
त्रिविधे रोगविज्ञाने स्रोतःस्वपि च वर्तने|
रोगानीके व्याधिरूपे रोगाणां च भिषग्जिते||४९||
अष्टौ विमानान्युक्तानि मानार्थानि महर्षिणा|
कतिधापुरुषीयं च गोत्रेणातुल्यमेव च||५०||
खुड्डिका महती चैव गर्भावक्रान्तिरुच्यते|
पुरुषस्य शरीरस्य विचयौ द्वौ विनिश्चितौ||५१||
शरीरसङ्ख्या सूत्रं च जातेरष्टममुच्यते [४]|
इत्युद्दिष्टानि मुनिना शारीराण्यत्रिसूनुना||५२||
वर्णस्वरीयः पुष्पाख्यस्तृतीयः परिमर्शनः|
चतुर्थ इन्द्रियानीकः पञ्चमः पूर्वरूपिकः||५३||
कतमानिशरीरीयः पन्नरूपोऽप्यवाक्शिराः|
यस्यश्यावनिमित्तश्च सद्योमरण एव च||५४||
अणुज्योतिरिति ख्यातस्तथा गोमयचूर्णवान्|

द्वादशाध्यायकं स्थानमिन्द्रियाणामिति स्मृतम् ||७५||
अभयामलकीयं च प्राणकामीयमेव च|
करप्रचितकं वेदसमुत्थानं रसायनम्||७६||
संयोगशरमूलीयमासिक्तक्षीरकं तथा|
माषपर्णभृतीयं च पुमाञ्जातबलादिकम्||७७||
चतुष्कद्वयमप्येतदध्यायद्वयमुच्यते|
रसायनमिति ज्ञेयं वाजीकरणमेव च||७८||
ज्वराणां रक्तपित्तस्य गुल्मानां मेहकुष्ठयोः|
शोषोन्मादेऽप्यपस्मारे क्षतशोथोदरार्शसाम्||७९||
ग्रहणीपाण्डुरोगाणां श्वासकासातिसारिणाम्|
छर्दिवीसर्पतृष्णानां विषमद्यविकारयोः||८०||
द्विव्रणीयं त्रिमर्मीयमूरुस्तम्भिकमेव च|
वातरोगे वातरक्ते योनिव्यापत्सु चैव यत्||८१||
त्रिंशच्चिकित्सितान्युक्तान्यतः कल्पान् प्रचक्ष्महे|
फलजीमूतकेक्ष्वाकुकल्पो धामार्गवस्य च||८२||
पञ्चमो वत्सकस्योक्तः षष्ठश्च कृतवेधने|
श्यामात्रिवृतयोः कल्पस्तथैव चतुरङ्गुले||८३||
तिल्वकस्य सुधायाश्च सप्तलाशङ्खिनीषु च|
दन्तीद्रवन्त्योः कल्पश्च द्वादशोऽयं समाप्यते||८४||
कल्पना पञ्चकर्माख्या बस्तिसूत्री तथैव च|
स्नेहव्यापदिकी सिद्धिर्नेत्रव्यापदिकी तथा||८५||
सिद्धिः शोधनयोश्चैव बस्तिसिद्धिस्तथैव च|
प्रासृती मर्मसङ्ख्याता सिद्धिर्बस्त्याश्रया च या||८६||
फलमात्रा तथा सिद्धिः सिद्धिश्चोत्तरसञ्ज्ञिता|
सिद्धयो द्वादशैवैतास्तन्त्रं चासु समाप्यते||८७||
स्वे स्वे स्थाने तथाऽध्याये चाध्यायार्थः प्रवक्ष्यते|
तं ब्रूयात् सर्वतः सर्वं ह्यर्थसङ्ग्रहात्||८८||

Madana Kalpa Adhyaya
Jimutaka Kalpa Adhyaya
Ikshvaku Kalpa Adhyaya
Dhamargava Kalpa Adhyaya
Vatsaka Kalpa Adhyaya
Kritavedhana Kalpa Adhyaya
Shyamatrivrita Kalpa Adhyaya
Chaturangula Kalpa Adhyaya
Tilvaka Kalpa Adhyaya
Sudha Kalpa Adhyaya
Saptalashankhini Kalpa Adhyaya
Dantidravanti Kalpa Adhyaya
    Kalpana Siddhi Adhyaya
Panchakarmiya Siddhi Adhyaya
Bastisutriyam Siddhi Adhyaya
Snehavyapat Siddhi Adhyaya
Netrabastivyapat Siddhi Adhyaya
Vamana Virechana Vyapat Siddhi Adhyaya
Bastivyapat Siddhi Adhyaya
Prasrita Yogiyam Siddhi Adhyaya
Trimarmiya Siddhi Adhyaya
Basti Siddhi Adhyaya
Phalamatra Siddhi Adhyaya
Uttar Basti Siddhi Adhyaya

Then further, chapters of Vimana sthana, Shareera Sthana, Indriya Sthana, Chikitsa Sthana, Kalpa Sthana, Siddhi Sthana, are enlisted. Contents of each chapter will be described in the respective chapters and sections. All these in brief will be described in all the respective chapters and sections. [45 - 68]

## Definitions of Technical terms:

पृच्छा तन्त्राद्यथाम्नायं विधिना प्रश्न उच्यते|
प्रश्नार्थो युक्तिमांस्तस्य तन्त्रेणैवार्थनिश्चयः ||६९||
निरुक्तं तन्त्रणातन्त्रं, स्थानमर्थप्रतिष्ठया|
अधिकृत्यार्थमध्यायनामसञ्ज्ञा प्रतिष्ठिता ||७०||
इति सर्वं यथाप्रश्नमष्टकं सम्प्रकाशितम्|
कात्स्न्र्येन चोक्तस्तन्त्रस्य सङ्ग्रहः सुविनिश्चितः||७१||

An inquiry from the treatise, in proper order and without contradicting the context, is called 'Prashna' or a question. Elucidating the question with reasoning and precise explanation with tactual implications is known as Prashnartha or the exposition of the question. Because it provides information about the measures to be followed for the maintenance of health, it is called 'Tantra' or treatise (tantrana means to sustain the body or to observe the rules of health). A sthana or section deals with a particular topic and the specific problems of these topics are discussed in the chapters concerned (Abhyayas)

Thus, replies to all the eight questions (raised in para 20 of this chapter) along with a well ascertained summary of the entire treatise are given. [69-71]

## Semi doctors :

सन्ति पाल्लविकोत्पाताः सङ्क्षोभं जनयन्ति ये|

वर्तकानामिवोत्पाताः सहसैवाविभाविताः||७२||
तस्मात्तान् पूर्वसञ्जल्पे सर्वत्राष्टकमादिशेत्|
परावरपरीक्षार्थं तत्र शास्त्रविदां बलम्||७३||
शब्दमात्रेण तन्त्रस्य केवलस्यैकदेशिकाः|
भ्रमन्त्यल्पबलास्तन्त्रे ज्याशब्देनेव वर्तकाः||७४||

**Semi doctors :**

Some individuals having only partial knowledge of the science, at times create difficulties for others like the sudden flights of the male bustards. Therefore, with a view to knowing their actual acquaintance with the science and assessing their superiority or otherwise, one should put these eight questions to them before a formal discussion. Only persons well versed in science can face such questions. Those who are not acquainted with the science as a whole and know it only partially get frightened by the very sound of the treatise in its entirety like the male bustards by the sound of the bowstring. [72-74]

**Similes for Pseudo physician and Genuine Physicians:**

पशुः पशूनां दौर्बल्यात् कश्चिन्मध्ये वृकायते|
स सत्यं वृकमासाद्य प्रकृतिं भजते पशुः||७५||
तद्वदज्ञोऽज्ञमध्यस्थः कश्चिन्मौखर्यसाधनः|
स्थापयत्याप्तमात्मानमाप्तं त्वासाद्य भिद्यते||७६||
बभ्रुर्गूढ इवोर्णाभिरबुद्धिरबहुश्रुतः|
किं वै वक्ष्यति सञ्जल्पे कुण्डभेदी जडो यथा||७७||
सद्वृत्तैर्न विगृह्णीयादि्भिषगल्पश्रुतैरपि|
हन्यात् प्रश्नाष्टकेनादावितरांस्त्वाप्तमानिनः||७८||
दम्भिनो मुखरा ह्यज्ञाः प्रभूताबद्धभाषिणः|
प्रायः, प्रायेण सुमुखाः सन्तो युक्ताल्पभाषिणः||७९||
तत्त्वज्ञानप्रकाशार्थं महङ्कारमनाश्रितः|
स्वल्पाधाराज्ञमुखरान्मर्षयेन्न विवादिनः||८०||
परो भूतेष्वनुक्रोशस्तत्त्वज्ञान(ने)परा दया|
येषां तेषामसद्वादनिग्रहे निरता मतिः||८१||

**Similes for Pseudo physician and Genuine Physicians:**

Taking advantage of the weakness of others, any animal may play the role of a wolf; but when it comes across a real wolf, its true nature is exposed. Similarly, an ignorant individual, because of his garrulous nature tries to bully the ignorant ones but he breaks down when a real scholar is met with.

A man deprived of wisdom and knowledge is not well acquainted with science. But one who poses to be an expert should not be spared; he must be challenged with the eight categories of questions.

Ignorant individuals who are egoistic usually speak in excess with much inconsistency. Saintly individuals who are well versed in science usually speak less but they speak only relevant to the topic of discussion.

It is not for the sake of ego but for the purpose of keeping the light of knowledge burning that one must challenge a garrulous individual of little learning.

Those who have great compassion towards creatures and are even prepared to impart knowledge for this, should be ever vigilant in putting down false arguments. [75-81]

**Characteristics of ignorant and learned physician:**

असत्पक्षाक्षणित्वार्तिदम्भपारुष्यसाधनाः|
भवन्त्यनाप्ताः स्वे तन्त्रे प्रायः परविकत्थकाः||८२||
तान् कालपाशसदृशान् वर्जयेच्छास्त्रदूषकान्|

प्रशमज्ञानविज्ञानपूर्णाः सेव्या भिषक्तमाः||८३||

## Characteristics of ignorant and learned physician:

Those who are not well versed in the science of their own profession resort to dogmatic views, make excuses for lack of time or sudden illness, try to show their ability by demonstrating books, equipment etc. use harsh and abusive language and speak ill of others during debates. They should therefore be shunned. On the other hand, one should serve good physicians who are full of tranquility and have the knowledge of arts and sciences of the profession. [82-83]

## Causes of unhappiness and happiness:

समग्रं दुःखमायतमविज्ञाने द्वयाश्रयम्|

सुखं समग्रं विज्ञाने विमले च प्रतिष्ठितम्||८४||

इदमेवमुदारार्थमज्ञानां न प्रकाशकम्|

शास्त्रं दृष्टिप्रणष्टानां यथैवादित्यमण्डलम्||८५||

All psycho- somatic ailments are caused by the ignorance of the individual whereas understanding of things leads to complete happiness to body and mind. Just as the Sun in spite of providing all its light and brightness cannot help a blind man to see the things around him, Ayurveda shastra (science) also which provides instructions for the benefit of mankind in the present and also next life doesn't help or guide someone who is in darkness about the shastra i.e. devoid of the power of understanding the science of health. **[84-85]**

तत्र श्लोकाः:-

अर्थे दशमहामूलाः सञ्ज्ञा चासां यथा कृता|

अयनान्ताः षड्द्व्याश्च रूपं वेदविदां च यत्||८६||

सप्तकश्चाष्टकश्चैव परिप्रश्नाः सनिर्णयाः|

यथा वाच्यं यदर्थं च षड्विधाश्चैकदेशिकाः||८७||

अर्थेदशमहामूले सर्वमेतत् प्रकाशितम्|

सङ्ग्रहश्चायमध्यायस्तन्त्रस्यास्यैव केवलः||८८||

यथा सुमनसां सूत्रं सङ्ग्रहार्थं विधीयते|

सङ्ग्रहार्थं तथाऽर्थानामृषिणा सङ्ग्रहः कृतः||८९||

इत्यग्निवेशकृते तन्त्रे चरकप्रतिसंस्कृते श्लोकस्थानेऽर्थदशमहामूलीयो नाम त्रिंशोऽध्यायः||३०||

## Summary:

The reason for designating the ten vessels attached to the hearts as Mahamula, the foremost ones among the six categories of regimen, the characteristic features of learned physicians, the eight types of questions along with their replies, methods of reply and elaboration and six types of entire replies, methods of reply and elaboration and six types of pseudo- physicians all these are described in this chapter on the "Arthe Dasha Maha Mooleeya Adhyaya "

इत्यग्निवेशकृते तन्त्रे चरकप्रतिसंस्कृते श्लोकस्थानेऽर्थदशमहामूलीयो नाम त्रिंशोऽध्यायः||३०|| अग्निवेशकृते तन्त्रे चरकप्रतिसंस्कृते|
इयताऽवधिना सर्वं सूत्रस्थानं समाप्यते|

A summary of the entire treatise is given in this chapter. As a garland is prepared of flowers by the help of thread (Sutra) so also the topics for the treatise are summarized. [86-89]

Thus ends the 30th chapter of Sutrasthana of Charaka Samhita, of the work by Agnivesa as redacted by Charaka.(31)

Here ends the Sutra Sthana – the first section of Charaka Samhita.

अग्निवेशकृते तन्त्रे चरकप्रतिसंस्कृतेइयताऽवधिना सर्वं सूत्रस्थानं समाप्यते |

# Other Publications Of Easy Ayurveda

All our book publications are available at
www.EasyAyurveda.com/Books

**English Books:**
Charaka Samhita Volume 1,2,3 and 4 - English Translation
Ashtanga Hrudayam Sutrasthanam - English Translation
Living Easy With Ayurveda
Easy Ayurveda Home Remedies
Tridosha Made Easy
Ayurveda Tarka

**Hindi Books:**
Ayurved Samadhan

**Kannada Books:**
Sugama Jivanakkagi Ayurveda
Ayurveda Santvana

**Malayalam Books**
Ayurveda Asvasam
Jeevitha Soukhyathinu Ayurvedam

All our book publications are available at
www.EasyAyurveda.com/Books